WATER AND COMMUNITY HEALTH

Dr. Chebli Akli Islam

ALLIED
HEALTH
PRESS

Water and Community Health

Author: **Dr. Chebli Akli Islam**

Allied Health Press
4164 Lakeshore Road
Burlington ON L7L 1A4
Canada
www.alliedhealthpress.com
Email: orders@arclereducation.com

ISBN: 978-1-77956-789-5

ABOUT THE AUTHOR

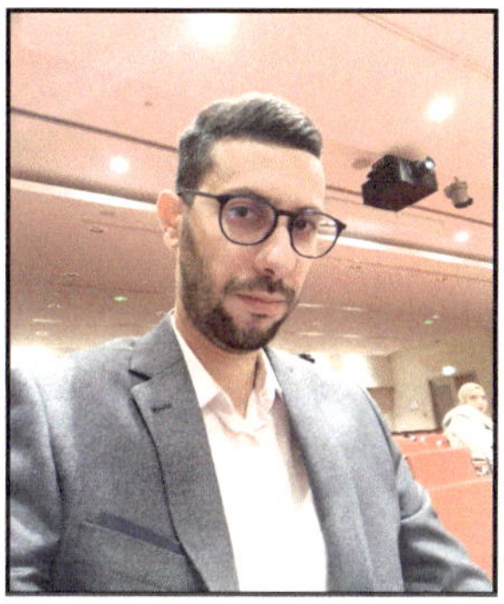

Dr. Chebli Akli Islam, PharmD, and holder of a PhD in Toxicology, epitomizes excellence in the field of hospital-university research. As a researcher at the University of Constantine, Faculty of Medicine, he passionately dedicates himself to studying various aspects of toxicology, including medicolegal, clinical, kinetic, food, and environmental toxicology. With over 10 years of experience, Dr. Chebli Akli Islam has cultivated expertise in a multitude of toxicological domains. His academic and professional career showcases an unwavering commitment to advancing knowledge in the field of toxicology. Dr. Chebli Akli Islam not only earned a pharmacy degree but also deepened his skills by pursuing a PhD in Toxicology, demonstrating his dedication to academic and scientific excellence. As a hospital-university researcher, Dr. Chebli Akli Islam tackles critical issues related to toxicology, such as toxic risk assessment in various contexts, identification of harmful substances in food and environmental products, and innovative solutions to mitigate the adverse effects of toxins on human health. His multidisciplinary expertise enables him to address the complex challenges of toxicology from different angles, ranging from clinical data analysis to the search for practical solutions to prevent poisonings and improve treatment protocols. Within the academic and scientific community, Dr. Chebli Akli Islam is recognized for his dedication to teaching and mentoring students, thereby inspiring future generations of researchers and healthcare professionals to pursue excellence in the field of toxicology. With his ambitious vision and unwavering commitment to scientific research, Dr. Chebli Akli Islam has become a prominent figure in the field of toxicology, making significant contributions to the safety and well-being of society.

Brief Table of Contents

Detailed Table of Contents

CHAPTER 7

The Role of Hygiene in Waterborne Disease Prevention 193

CHAPTER 8

The Link Between Water, Nutrition, and Health 223

CHAPTER 9

Climate Change and Water Health 255

CHAPTER 10

Water and Gender: Roles, Health Risks, Inequalities, and Community Solutions in Water Management 281

LIST OF FIGURES

PREFACE

Water is the essential foundation of all communities, facilitating the existence of human, animal, and plant life in a fragile balance that underpins public health. Where water supplies are plentiful and free of pollution, communities benefit from lower infectious disease rates, better nutritional status, and increased economic security. In contrast, restricted access to or poor-quality water leads to the outbreak of cholera, typhoid, dysentery, and other water-borne diseases and hence undermines social order and local development. Additionally, the absence of water creates hard choices between the needs of households, drinking, cooking, hygiene, and agriculture, tending to leave the most vulnerable groups at a disproportionately high risk.

In addition to acute health effects, water management influences larger determinants of health: sanitation infrastructure, waste management, and ecosystem health all depend on how communities access and protect their freshwater supplies. From microbial pathogens to chemical toxins, contaminants move through aquifers and distribution systems, accumulating in human tissues and interfering with physiological processes. Climate variability adds to these risks, as changing rainfall patterns manipulate water availability and concentrate contaminants. In the absence of timely interventions—point-of-use treatment, watershed protection, and behavior change—populations are faced with mounting burdens of diarrhea, malnutrition, and chronic disease.

Water and Community Health integrates the latest evidence, everyday practice, and case studies to assist practitioners, policymakers, and students in exerting a positive impact on water-related outcomes at the local level. This book provides an unambiguous overview of the scientific principles, technical options, and social factors guiding effective water supply, sanitation, and hygiene programs. It is utilized to bridge theory and practice and to determine scalable solutions for rural villages, urban neighborhoods, and humanitarian environments.

Chapter 1 sets the background with definitions of safe water, basic epidemiological principles, and an analysis of worldwide access deficits. Chapter 2 describes principal waterborne diseases—cholera, typhoid, cryptosporidiosis, giardiasis—taking into account their modes of transmission, clinical features, and control measures. Chapter 3 presents chemical, physical, and biological water quality parameters—pH, turbidity, heavy metals, microbial indicators—and routine sampling and laboratory analysis procedures. Chapter 4 discusses treatment technologies at the community and domestic levels, ranging from sedimentation tanks and rapid sand filtration to chlorination, solar water disinfection, and ceramic filtration. Chapter 5 discusses sanitation technologies, pit latrines, septic tanks, sewer systems, and sludge management, with a focus on pathogen reduction in wastewater streams.

Chapter 6 describes drinking water distribution network design and operation, from piped networks to reservoir siting, network hydraulics, leak detection, and fair apportionment. Chapter 7 describes individual and institutional hygiene practices—handwashing campaigns, menstrual hygiene management, handling and storing water—to interrupt disease transmission chains. Chapter 8 explores access to water, food preparation, and nutritional status interrelationships, explaining how water limitation and contamination result in undernutrition and foodborne illness. Chapter 9 addresses how rising temperature, altered precipitation, and extreme weather events affect water quantity and quality, driving shifts in disease patterns and resource conflict.

Chapter 10 addresses the gender dimensions of water management, detailing how women and girls disproportionately shouldered water collection, were exposed to special health hazards, and took leadership roles in water committees. Chapter 11 gives a general description of environmental pollutants—industrial effluent, agricultural runoff, and microplastics—and their pathways into drinking water supplies, and describes new monitoring technologies. Chapter 12 sets out national and international policy frameworks, including SDG 6 targets, WHO guidelines, and regulatory requirements, and assesses challenges to implementation. Chapter 13 gives a survey of diverse health interventions and programs, from large-scale vaccination campaigns with the provision of clean water to behavior change communication and capacity-building measures. Chapter 14 presents examples of community-managed water governance, collective governance arrangements, and participatory monitoring systems that promote long-term sustainability. Chapter 15 finally addresses the design of new technologies and approaches, such as real-time sensor networks, remote water quality monitoring, and decentralized treatment technologies, and speculates about directions for integrated research and practice.

This book will be of use to a variety of readers. Public health practitioners, water and sanitation engineers, environmental scientists, and urban planners will appreciate the technical advice required for project design and project evaluation. Community organizers, NGO field workers, and local government officials can draw on case examples and implementation advice to mobilize resources and build partnerships. Graduate students in public health, environmental studies, and development studies will appreciate the theoretical basis and liberal references. Most importantly, community leaders and activists seeking to enhance water access and health benefits will be inspired and given practical suggestions to put concepts into practice.

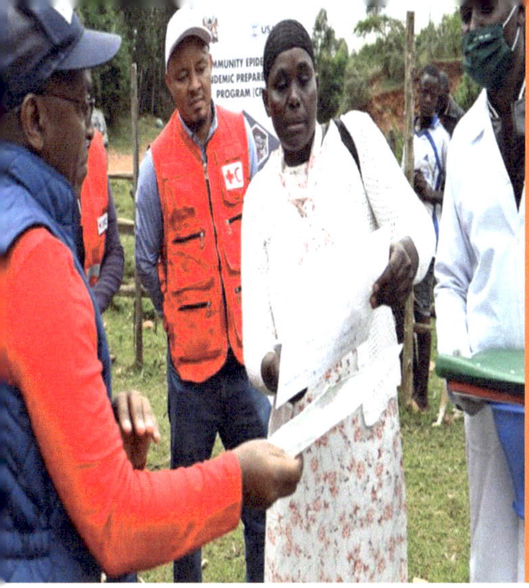

Chapter 1

INTRODUCTION TO WATER AND COMMUNITY HEALTH

Contents

Introduction

Clean water lies at the center of community life and daily living. Research goes on teaching us that when water is clean, it not only keeps disease away but maximizes overall wellbeing. Research has competing theories regarding how water, water use, and even general environmental concerns all intersect, and communities—so frequently burdened by pollution, old pipes, and changing climate patterns—find themselves needing safe water more than ever before. The effort to clean up water shows points of intersection among dollars and sense, grassroots organization, and long-term health (and yes, these can become a little unsavory). In most scenarios, knowing the way people think about and respond to water danger is determinative for creating solutions in the real world. Individuals are having more discussions about health issues related to water these days, and such discussion joins forces with advocacy efforts and research initiatives. For example, in Canada, concerns with the quality and accessibility of pediatric cancer care helped motivate the creation of the ACCESS consortium; a group dedicated to giving kids with cancer an even shot at good health. Such work illustrates a broader movement where communities are coming together in water and health to enhance well-being in the community. Everywhere across the board in Central America and beyond, projects put center stage the urgent need to clean up water and sanitation, leading public health work forward. Joining hands allows communities not only to decide what they need but also to establish trust within the systems supposed to serve. It's also worth looking into how people perceive and use water—psychology comes into play. In rural El Salvador, experience indicates that people's responses to water pollution are very advanced, and their awareness levels sometimes generate the risky type of denial of risk. At times, people minimize the dangers of polluted water, which in turn influences their daily life and general attitude toward health. All these have to be addressed by applying smart and focused education campaigns. In general, the integration of knowledge from environmental science, psychology, and community health appears to be the solution if we want to design interventions that improve water security and public health in general.

Definition of Community Health

Health outcomes and our surroundings mix together in ways that really matter—it's not just about individual well-being. Communities are shaped by things like clean water, proper sanitation, and education, which in most cases, all play their part in determining how people take care of themselves. When you take a closer look at water quality, you quickly see that contaminants can hit the community's health hard; a poor water system often opens the door to diseases, widens health gaps, and stresses local resources.

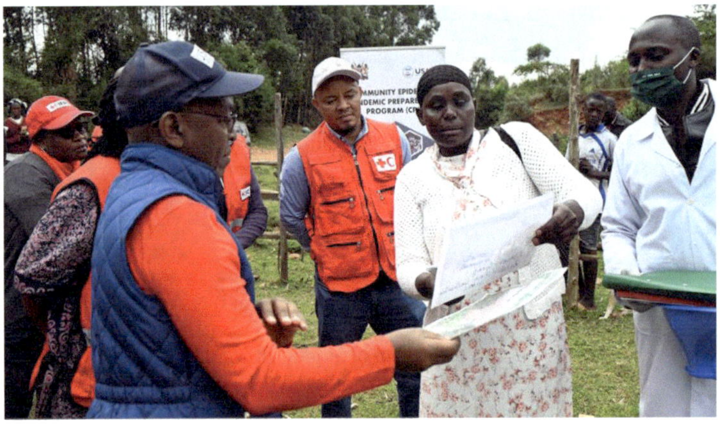

Source: International Federation of Red Cross and Red Crescent Societies. (2023). *DRR Day Story in Rural Kenya.*

Tackling these challenges calls for people to work together, as shared responsibilities among residents and service providers become key. Everyone involved in community health tends to get pulled into tackling these connected problems. A strong community often starts with combining resources—safe drinking water, public education, and even outreach efforts all working side by side. Public policies, like those that back vaccinations and health screenings, add extra resilience against crises. Communities that roll up their sleeves and get involved usually end up spotting local needs and practical fixes, which can be more lasting than those top-down solutions. For example, organizations like the IPCC remind us that climate change is shaking up natural resources, especially freshwater supplies, which means we need both immediate action and long-term plans (Intergovernmental Panel on Climate Change, 2023). Building a broad plan for community health can really set the stage for even the most vulnerable to thrive. It's not just local; water quality and community health mesh with bigger global challenges too, like antimicrobial resistance (AMR) and environmental sustainability. Recent studies point out that clean water is crucial for keeping infections in check and managing diseases effectively (Intergovernmental Panel on Climate Change, 2023). Without enough clean water, the risks of infections and complications from drug-resistant microbes jump noticeably. Facing these issues means mixing ideas from public health, environmental science, and community involvement in a practical way. Future policies, generally speaking, should lean more toward investing in water systems and health education; by doing so, communities can be empowered to take charge of their own well-being. In the end, nurturing strong systems that care about both water and community health not only eases current problems but also lays down a foundation for a healthier future.

Importance of Water in Public Health

Pure water is downright essential, it's the foundation of any successful society. Filthy water is full of all kinds of microbes that cause diseases such as cholera, dysentery, and typhoid fever. This problem strikes low-income communities particularly hard, where subpar sanitation only serves to exacerbate the danger. As a general rule, when people have consistent access to clean water, disease falls significantly and hospitals, which are already trying to manage an enormous number of issues, are relieved. In reality, investing in water infrastructure provides rapid health benefits and creates long-term system resilience, illustrating just how intricately water and public health are intertwined (Gatta, 2022). Water not only keeps sickness at bay; it intersects with everyday aspects of life like nutrition and mental health. Clean water is essential for cooking, watering crops, and even the simple hygiene that wards off infection. When there is a shortage of water, it's challenging for individuals to keep themselves clean, which of course increases the likelihood of getting sick. In addition, the stress and even slight stigma accompanying water shortages can add up to anxiety and fatigue. In most instances, public health programs expanding access to water not only decrease sickness—they also cultivate dignity and positive mental health among residents. Undoubtedly, water's value extends far beyond physical well-being, supporting a town's overall morale (Enayat et al., 2019). Dealing with water access issues isn't a task for one group; it requires a variety package of inputs from governments, NGOs, and communities. In many cases, that means spending money on improved pipes, clever technology, and even educational campaigns that get the word out about sustainable water behaviors. When the locals are engaged in decision-making, a little cultural flavor is introduced and the solutions are made more suitable to what works on the ground. Such an inclusive and sometimes lopsided process allows for strategies that provide equitable, dependable access to clean water. Typically, such interventions don't just check international target boxes, such as those under the UN's Sustainable Development Goals (SDGs)—but also bolster local systems of health, paving the way for harder, healthier communities in the future (Enayat et al., 2019).

Overview of the Relationship Between Water and Community Health

Clean water is important—a big deal. It's the type of essential need that swings the door wide open for community health, particularly in areas where resources are lean. In low- and middle-income communities, lacking adequate water, sanitation, and hygiene can seriously derail health opportunities, and too often lead families into a cycle of sickness and poverty. Tools such as Geographic Information Systems emerge as unlikely allies; they allow people to plot where water and sanitation are in short supply and verify how these variables relate to health. While this technology is not without its flaws, it tends to provide decision-makers with an edge when designing how to address water quality issues and protect against the threats that unclean water supplies pose (Pradhan et al., 2025). Examine more closely the interaction between water quality and health, and you soon find boundaries dissolving. When individuals have difficulty accessing safe water, malnutrition and stunting tend to make their appearance. For example, one study near the Sikabu Community Health Center found that a decline in good hygiene and proper sanitation accompanies lower water quality—resulting, in most instances, in increased stunting among children. The study, with its combination of hygiene practice observations and environmental surveys, just continues to make us believe that water access and daily habits must collaborate to eliminate these health inequalities (Yuniarti et al., 2024). It's not as straightforward as giving people clean water and then closing up shop. The overall picture is all about the way in which communities engage with water in their daily lives—everything from daily hygiene practices to a collective sense of responsibility for maintaining their environment in good health. Local knowledge does count, and with the addition of some contemporary technology monitoring water quality and usage, new avenues of addressing entrenched problems are opened. In the majority of instances, linking infrastructure development with grassroots education sets the stage for healthier communities that can recover from debacles a little bit better (Yuniarti et al., 2024).

1.1. The Role of Clean Water in Disease Prevention

Clean water is not merely a luxury, it's strictly necessary for maintaining healthy communities and reducing illness. In too many places, particularly those still underdeveloped, contaminated water allows infections such as cholera, dysentery, and typhoid fever to spread easily. When dangerous microbes insinuate themselves into water that consumers drink, at-risk groups are put in jeopardy. Ensuring water is safe to drink can significantly cut down on waterborne illnesses, increasing overall well-being within a community.

Health programs that blend a little sanitation instruction assist in establishing a culture where cleanliness and health remain top of mind, conveying the same vital message in various ways. If you dig deeper, the connection between clean water and disease prevention feeds into a broad spectrum of environmental and social variables. For example, climate change in general disrupts water availability and quality, which then alters health outcomes within communities. The IPCC, for instance, has identified that human health and climate impacts are enmeshed together, stating that access to clean water is a central element in ensuring that communities are better able to deal with these changes (Panel, 2023). In order to truly address disease, however, it would appear to be necessary to merge water quality management with strategies for adapting to our shifting climate. Public health policies need to balance environmental realities with advocating for water use practices that support community health—not only currently but also in the long term. Securing water systems against sudden changes, after all, yields rapid gains and invests in long-term community resilience. Clean water also enters into daily lifestyle habits that enhance wellbeing. As the WHO's new guidelines point out, when there is a reliable supply of safe water in communities, individuals will get out more, be active and not sit for long periods (Bull et al., 2020). Safe water not only aids in hydration but also good nutrition, which again helps to avoid disease. This combination—hydration, some exercise, and chronic disease management—truly illustrates why access to water deserves a place in public health strategies. Where water is consistently clean, public and individual health both benefit, opening up natural, sustainable paths to improved overall health (Figure 1.1).

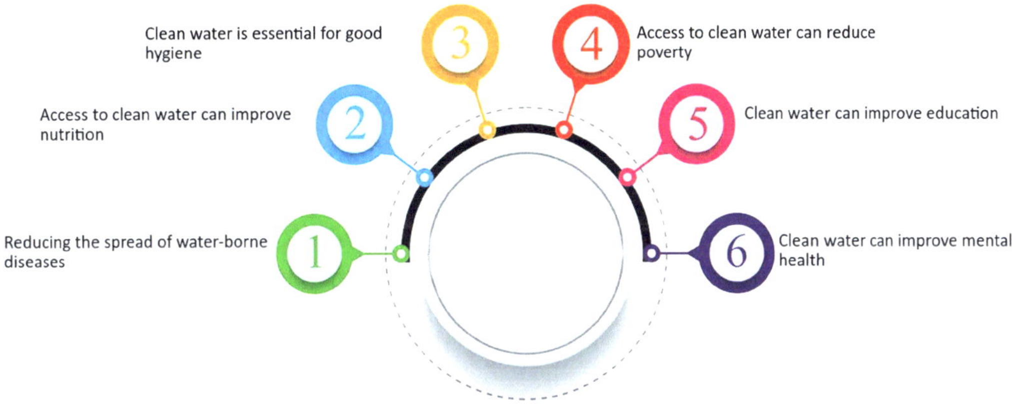

Figure 1.1. The impact of clean water on disease prevention.

Source: FasterCapital. (n.d.). *Water Provision – Quenching Thirst – The Essentiality of Water Provision – The Impact of Clean Water on Disease Prevention.*

1.1.1. Waterborne Diseases and Their Impact

Clean water is an absolute lifeline, yet millions still face waterborne diseases because of poor sanitation and polluted sources. It isn't just a matter of numbers—water quality really shapes how well a community can bounce back. With climate change making water scarcer and messier, managing our water becomes even more urgent, generally speaking. Consider, for example, the uptick in detection and treatment devices that are rising to combat perilous pathogens. The new developments keep water in check in real time while enhancing local security measures. When communities receive clean water, illness and mortality from the diseases decrease considerably. In effect, uniting research and tech opens the door to long-term solutions that alleviate the heavy burden on community health and well-being (Khant et al., 2025). Community responses to waterborne conditions tend to mix traditional practices with contemporary health measures. History attests that local measures sometimes prove surprisingly effective in controlling these diseases, particularly at difficult times. For instance, following the 2004 Aceh tsunami, health interventions were directly linked to community efforts, a definite indication of the strength of local know-how and collaboration in enforcing sanitation and tidiness. Neighbors relied on tried-and-tested methods such as boiling and filtering water to ensure it was safe to use, even when destroyed infrastructure and poor healthcare services made it more challenging. This combination of traditional practices and contemporary concepts truly emphasizes a people-centered strategy for combating waterborne diseases (Cipta et al., 2025).

The relationship between waterborne disease and public policy is becoming increasingly complicated as emerging global health threats arise. Policymakers, in general, must focus on ensuring water quality, updating sanitation infrastructure, and engaging communities at the forefront when addressing these concerns. The SDGs provide a rough outline that coordinates health efforts with environmental stewardship, hoping to deter waterborne disease with better water management.

And getting scientists, health professionals, and locals together tends to bring well-rounded solutions—cross-disciplinary collaboration is essential. Add machine learning and remote sensing to the mix, and our vision for how pathogens spread gets clearer, setting us up for more precise outbreak prevention. Overall, by addressing both the social and environmental determinants of health, leaders can build a strong system to safeguard communities from the far-reaching effects of these diseases (Khant et al., 2025) (Figure 1.2).

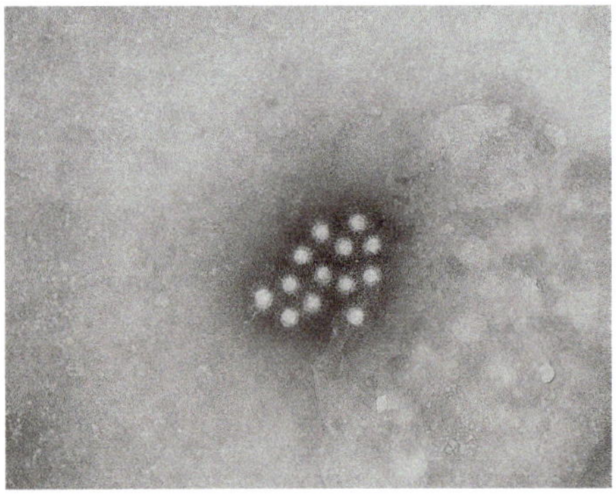

Figure 1.2. Waterborne diseases.

Source: By Photo Credit:Content Providers(s): CDC/Betty Partin - This media comes from the Centers for Disease Control and Prevention's Public Health Image Library (PHIL), with identification number #2739.Note: Public Domain, https://commons.wikimedia.org/w/index.php?curid=1097459

1.1.2. Importance of Sanitation and Hygiene

Seeing infectious diseases spread truly illustrates the close relationship between sanitation, hygiene, and overall public health. Wherever WASH conditions simply aren't good enough, outbreaks such as cholera can strike with force in much of the world, particularly where water, sanitation, and hygiene, , or WASH, conditions simply aren't adequate. In most cases, integrating WASH strategies into public health strategies reduces such outbreaks. For instance, improving water quality and sanitation infrastructure will reduce disease transmission a great deal. Local, community-based initiatives that encourage safe water access and simple, effective purification technologies are important, not just for short-term solutions but for creating longer-term practices that enhance health benefits (Izah et al., 2024).

Urban slums, however, appear to be especially challenging concerning good hygiene. A recent survey in Delhi slums, for example, identified some key gaps in practice and knowledge on drinking water and sanitation. As it happens, despite the fact that approximately 76.4% of households had toilets, many residents still engaged in unsafe hygiene practices, and poor water disposal simply compounded the issue (Chishti et al., 2023). More often than not, these results illustrate just how much targeted education is necessary, education that does not merely inform individuals what to do but empowers them to make safer decisions over the long term. At the end of it all, it isn't sufficient merely to give access to sanitation and hygiene facilities—there's a greater cultural and behavioral component at issue. There are also educational initiatives that must address not just the nuts and bolts of sanitation but also the social forces that determine our habits. For example, examining socio-economic variables can go some way to explain why some communities may continue to practice risky behavior, even where facilities exist. Once communities join in planning and executing WASH projects, there is an innate feeling of ownership and responsibility that comes in—something vital to sustained change. With the incorporation of these blended methods, we can raise public health levels and remind everyone that every community deserves a clean, safe place (Izah et al., 2024) (Figure 1.3).

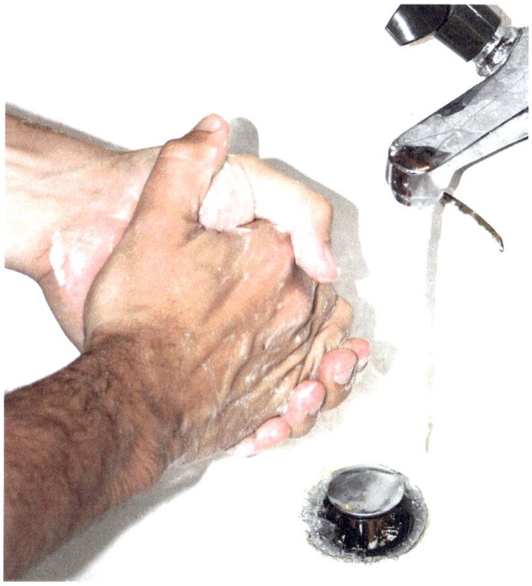

Figure 1.3. A person washing their hands is a personal hygiene practice.

Source: By Lars Klintwall Malmqvist (Larsklintwallmalmqvist) - Own work, Public Domain, https://commons.wikimedia.org/w/index.php?curid=4112060

1.2. Access to Safe Drinking Water

Water shortages disproportionately affect communities, particularly in impoverished locations. Consider Nigeria—about 66.3 million individuals lack water they can rely on for consumption, creating a huge void in local health services.

Water issues and complex sanitation go hand in hand with epidemics such as cholera and typhoid, adding to pressure on individuals already on the brink. It is not about pipe repair alone; the people must be informed about what's on, local activities must receive additional appropriations, and teat-up maintenance of ruptured systems is imperative. Across the board, if we fail to intervene with the proper programs, the pressure toward targets like SDG 6 is in actual jeopardy (Fatunmibi, 2024). Disparities in access to safe water reveal more than ecological slight—they enlarge health disparities in impacted communities. A lot of research highlights that if everybody just speaks about health effects, they pass up examining the work of figuring out how water really gets to people.

Environmental justice literature usually connects unjust distributions with bumbling procedures and missed acknowledgments, but most of the information we encounter is wedged in single-frame snapshots rather than going deep into what members of a community experience day in and day out. This limited approach leaves us still not fully understanding how individuals fight back against unequal access to water or the innovative means they resist. For the most part, making governments accountable for these fiascos continues to be a difficult problem for future research and policy solutions (Karasaki et al., 2023).

Drinking water is more than an amenity—it's the keystone of a healthy, prosperous community. Upgrading water systems not only reduces frustrating illnesses but also strengthens local economies when individuals aren't constantly sick. An open-minded solution to water issues must bring in community voices, ensuring those too-often-ignored help guide the decision. As projects are implemented, frequent check-ins and adjustments are necessary to combat continued water injustice. Ultimately, prioritizing safe water is essential to actual sustainable development and keeping everyone, particularly in the most vulnerable places, in line, even if at times the process does get a little complex (Fatunmibi, 2024) (Figure 1.4).

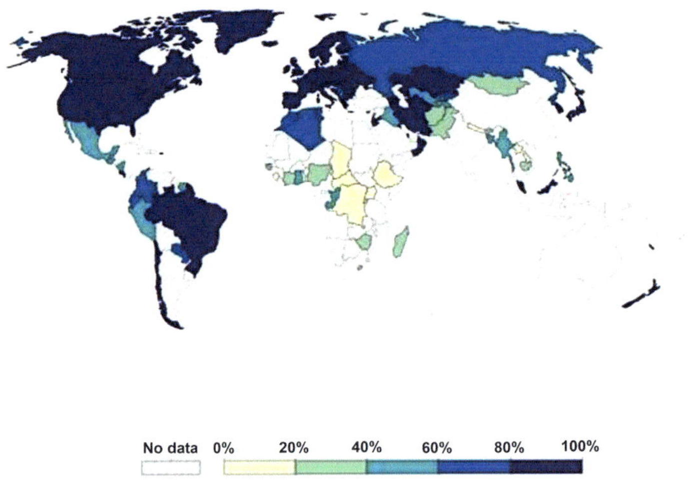

Figure 1.4. Distribution of the world population having access to safe drinking water in percentage in 2020.

Source: ResearchGate. (2024). *Distribution of the World Population Having Access to Safe Drinking Water in Percentage in 2020.*

1.2.1. Global Statistics on Water Access

Clean water is totally vital for community well-being, communities all over rely on it. Recently, international efforts to increase water, sanitation, and hygiene (WASH) have emerged in different corners. Consider the UK government for instance; they aimed to deliver clean water and sanitation to 60 million individuals from 2011–2015, and by the end, they had reached approximately 62.9 million people. It reveals that intense working can get things done, although it did question some issues about long-term sustainability. The impact review for the DFID WASH portfolio broadly highlighted the fact that improved immediate access apart, the overall longer-term is somewhat unstable—the security of water and more solid local institutions are yet to be seriously focused on (WSP, 2011). See the statistics, and you find yourself faced with a very stark portrayal of the disparity of global water accessibility. By 2020, almost 2 billion individuals globally continued to lack safely managed drinking water. This is a challenge that disproportionately affects marginalized communities, where unequal access combines with other social determinants to exacerbate health challenges. In most instances, closing these gaps requires creative financing strategies, particularly as new impact investment markets are on the rise. This new category of investment offers a number of opportunities that are specifically designed to increase infrastructure and access in WASH-related areas. Adjusting profit expectations with actual impact can ultimately provide both health and economic gains to under-served regions (Bugg-Levine & Brandenburg, 2010). To look toward the future, ensuring global water access becomes improved really hinges on cooperative efforts with local stakeholders with sustainability in mind. It is not sufficient to simply invest in good infrastructure without also constructing resilience at the community level and enhancing governance capacities—both must complement each other. For example, providing local institutions with the ability to manage and sustain these services is critical to ultimate success. Absent this, any advances may prove to be only temporary and could potentially perpetuate poverty and health disparities. Clearly, we require an integrated approach that does not leave any community behind, one that addresses urgent needs while also constructing enduring systems for the future (WSP, 2011) (Figure 1.5).

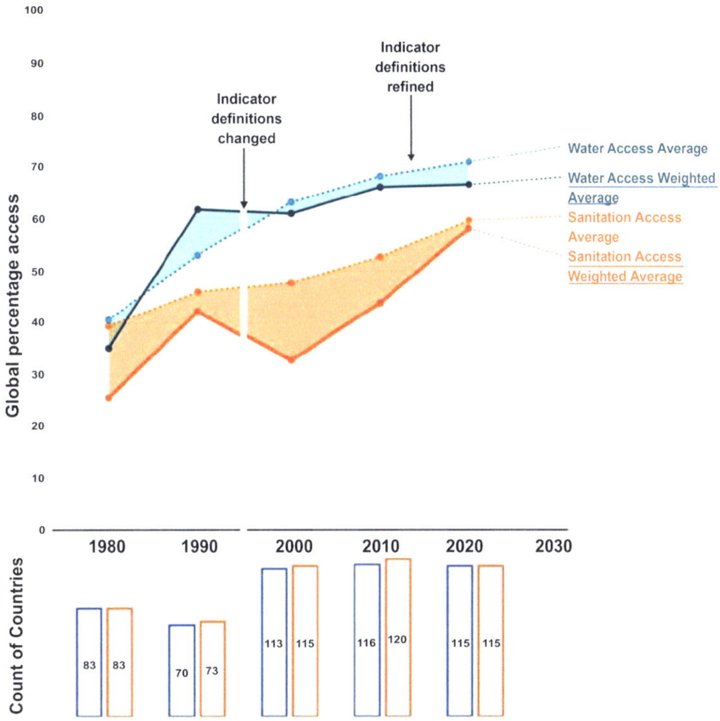

Figure 1.5. Worldwide progress towards access to safely managed drinking water and sanitation.

Source: Grafton, R. (2023). *Worldwide Progress Towards Access to Safely Managed Drinking Water and Sanitation*. ResearchGate.

1.2.2. Disparities in Water Access Among Different Communities

Safe, clean drinking water is supposed to be for all, but for many, they don't receive what they deserve, and that disparity manifests in large health disparities. In some places, particularly where incomes are low or communities are excluded, not having secure water tends to have a lot of negative consequences such as increased cases of waterborne diseases, malnutrition, and even reduced lifespans. Where you are, your status, and the surrounding arrangement all come together to determine who has clean water and who does not. Cities may have advanced systems while individuals in more dispersed regions sometimes rely on water that is not exactly safe. All of this effectively points towards directed investments and undertakings within water infrastructure, , a fact that prior research has also respectfully noted through an examination of relationships between finance, place, and access to water. Posing deeper questions, the human angle of water stress brings into relief the implications on day-to-day existence through the perceived scarcity of safe water. In areas such as coastal Peru, for instance, studies identify a direct correlation between where individuals place on the income spectrum and what sort of water they are able to attain. The poorer families have more difficult times—not only do they struggle with short-term health hazards but they suffer long-term consequences to child development and family nutrition overall. Lots of people have begun to view the inconvenience of water scarcity as merely another mundane issue, even though it conceals some fairly dangerous risks. So, repairing these problems requires us to marry pragmatic infrastructure improvement with an actual awareness of what the residents experience—something that a number of qualitative studies have noted in their own terms. Where the solution to such a mixed bag of water issues is concerned, there is no one method that succeeds. Rather, combining efforts with government agencies, local opinion, and health specialists appears to be the way to go. Consolidating sectors can implement sound, sustainable water management strategies that also enhance community expertise in water preservation—particularly since climate change continues to bring new issues our way. Policies that are intended to support the most vulnerable have already proved useful for reducing some of the health consequences associated with water shortages, with evidence of better water systems frequently being matched with higher overall health. With things moving as quickly as they are, it is possible that a responsive strategy that uses the community's energy and resources could be precisely what we require in order to finally get everyone access to safe drinking water.

1.2.3. Initiatives to Improve Access to Safe Drinking Water

Access to clean drinking water is usually addressed by combining several strategies. Mobilization of communities, local leaders, women's organizations, NGOs, everyone becomes engaged in the dissemination of information on water treatment methods. In a rural Ethiopian research, group discussions came up with the finding that individuals' habits are not only influenced by personal decisions but also by family routines, community atmosphere, and even the environment at large. The way people feel and perceive their water quality tends to determine if and how they treat it, and the open dialogue emphasizing local values for water serves to ignite a common sense of responsibility, ultimately improving public health results (Tamene, 2021). Education will be a big part of solidifying these gains. Health extension workers—science's everyday ambassadors to everyday life—have proven capable of transmitting effective safe water advice. Nevertheless, their training oftentimes requires a boost to prepare them with approaches for community members who are at varying levels of readiness (Tamene, 2021).

Providing these employees additional tools and resources sometimes truly reverses the game. When health education campaigns are tailored to address specific groups, the message has more punch, answering cultural idiosyncrasies and family routines as well as promoting a larger commitment to health and safety. The construction of strong infrastructure goes hand in hand with community initiatives to close water inequality gaps. Investment in items such as purifiers, boreholes, and piped water can, in the majority of instances, reduce health dangers associated with tainted sources. Governmental and global assistance programs tend to provide materials to communities that are in need, but these types of initiatives must accompany capacity-building efforts if they are to remain long-term. Implementing systems for tracking progress is also essential in keeping water safety standards on the right path. When concrete infrastructure projects combine with vibrant education campaigns, communities notice an overall increase in health corresponding to international patterns toward sustainable water management and good-being (Figure 1.6).

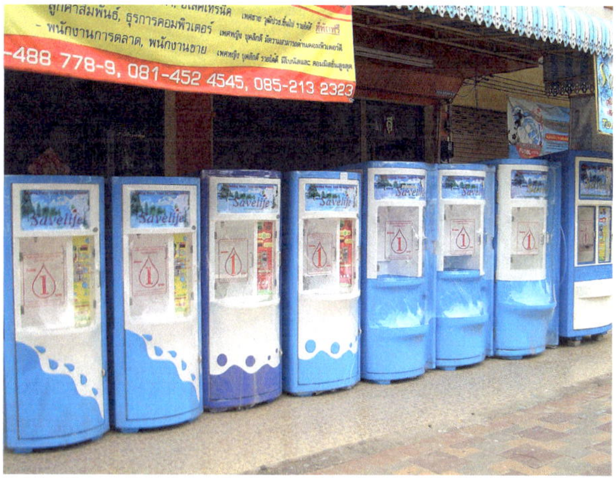

Figure 1.6. Implementing initiatives for improved access to safe clean water.

Source: By Vmenkov - Own work, CC BY-SA 4.0, https://commons.wikimedia.org/w/index.php?curid=3307263

1.3. Water Quality and Its Effects on Health

Clean drinking water counts, a great deal. It's the foundation of sound health for individuals worldwide, but severe weather these days, arriving harder and more frequently, disrupts water quality and exposes homes (HWI) to more risk. Fluctuating temperatures and shifting precipitation aren't abstract concepts; they determine how much water we receive and whether it's clean. One systematic review of seasonal weather and HWI highlighted that fluctuations in access to freshwater can lead to severe health issues, particularly for those on the margins. With climate change muddling our traditional weather patterns, gaining control over these seasonal changes becomes crucial for informing intelligent policies and practical engineering solutions that maintain water supplies stable and secure (Lauren et al., 2022). Waste management and water quality go hand in hand in maintaining a healthy community. If waste is not disposed of in the right manner, local water sources tend to become contaminated – raising the likelihood of waterborne diseases. Studies from such locations as Yamunanagar district in India indicate that insufficient knowledge about household waste management tends to accompany worse water quality.

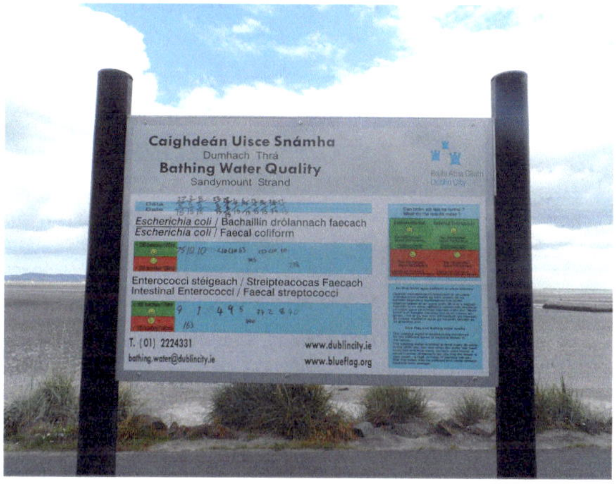

Figure 1.7. Water quality.

Source: By Sheila1988 - Own work, CC BY-SA 4.0, https://commons.wikimedia.org/w/index.php?curid=75791269

In reality, research shows that most homemakers tend to exhibit only a moderate understanding of proper wastage practices, thereby increasing the likelihood of diseases such as cholera and dysentery. Addressing this through education and outreach is rather critical in order to safeguard water for all (Arasi et al., 2022). Keeping water clean is not just an environmental concern; it is inextricably linked with social justice and public welfare. Vulnerable populations , such as low-income families – are frequently in more danger when water quality deteriorates and waste management breaks down.

With insufficient resources to obtain safe drinking water or properly deal with water-borne waste, these groups fall into the trap of health inequalities. In most cases, overcoming this is a matter of combining public health efforts, community education, and sound infrastructural investment. Increased knowledge regarding the importance of clean water and good waste management can enhance health benefits, with benefits today and ensuring resilience to withstand future challenges (Arasi et al., 2022; Lauren et al., 2022) (Figure 1.7).

1.3.1. Common Contaminants Found in Water Sources

Having access to safe drinking water simply means that we can't avoid the combination of threats that may be present in it. Small organisms such as bacteria and viruses breed quite rapidly when water is not properly treated or becomes contaminated in the first instance. Diseases like cholera or typhoid fever erupt when sanitation lags behind, and by and large, this is just how deadly such pathogens are. Current studies attribute millions of deaths to drug-resistant bacteria infections ; a cold, hard lesson that keeping an eye out for these unwelcome visitors is imperative for the health of the community. Chemical problems introduce an added level of danger (Intergovernmental Panel on Climate Change, 2023). Heavy metals , such as lead or mercury – tend to contaminate our water supply through such means as industrial runoff or deteriorating old pipes. Their existence is not a one-time concern; it can result in long-term neurological injury and developmental issues. It's strange that so many water analyses of the past targeted an individual pollutant at a time without considering how several toxins may act collectively to exacerbate health threats (Stoiber et al., 2019). This limited perspective indicates that we must obtain a new, full view of water quality to further safeguard public health.

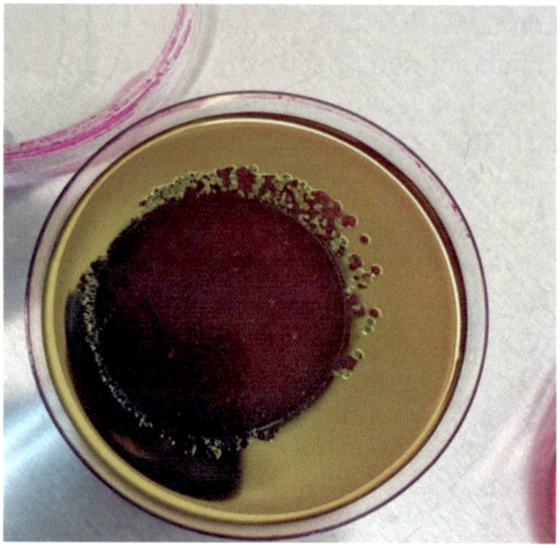

Figure 1.8. Aerobic mesophilic bacteria from a water sample that have formed colonies on a solid medium (left). Colonies of the Intestinal Bacterium *Escherichia coli* cultured on an agar plate with a selective nutrient medium, allowing differentiation between E. coli and related coliform bacteria (right).

Source: Abu-Sini MK, Maharmah RA, Abulebdah DH, Al-Sabi MNS. Isolation and Identification of Coliform Bacteria and Multidrug-Resistant *Escherichia coli* from Water Intended for Drug Compounding in Community Pharmacies in Jordan. *Healthcare*. 2023; 11(3):299. https://doi.org/10.3390/healthcare11030299 Escherichia coli

And then there's the newer class of pollutants such as pharmaceuticals and personal care products. These chemicals tend to pass through conventional water treatment facilities, lingering in our environment and imperceptibly changing human health. And small concentrations appear to be sufficient to disrupt endocrine systems—sometimes causing everything from reproductive problems to a greater risk of cancer. The chaotic interaction of these chemicals indicates a demand for a more mixed response in tracking water, especially by those depending on vulnerable sources. With growing awareness, it's increasingly apparent policymakers and health professionals need to pressure strong, comprehensive risk assessment and monitoring frameworks (Stoiber et al., 2019) (Figure 1.8).

1.3.2. Health Effects of Long-Term Exposure to Contaminated Water

Toxins in our drinking water have become a serious problem, with populations usually ending up with poor health. Regular exposure to contaminated water welcomes a range of waterborne diseases, a fact that rings especially true when you think about it because children, with their fragile systems, are more likely to suffer from both chemical toxins and pathogens. Mwale et al. (2025a) even indicate the way that compromised water quality typically coincides with increasing reports of gastrointestinal illness as well as other long-term problems. It's a little crazy when you consider it; inconsistent water means we need good, hands-on monitoring configurations to identify where contamination begins and then try to keep health threats contained. The effect extends beyond health, significantly disrupting the economic texture of communities. When water quality deteriorates, it's not merely a matter of getting ill; employment, particularly in industries such as fishing and farming where clean water is a requirement, suffers as well. Alvernia et al. (2021) remind us that events such as oil spills are not just environmental accidents—also destabilizing regional economies, quite frequently precipitating greater levels of unemployment and poverty. While families attempt to recover, their overall health, physical and mental, tends to decline, perpetuating a vicious cycle of economic and health-based struggles that linger long past resulting illnesses. Addressing these pervasive effects necessitates combination of solutions. First off, consolidating regulations on the way industries and farms dispose of waste is important; Mwale et al. (2025a) emphasize that more regulation can prevent runoff and other avenues for pollution. Meanwhile, public education among communities has a similar role to play, educating people on sustainable water use and empowering them to demand cleaner water. Mixing scientific study with shrewd public policy appears to be the direction to head. Finally, if local communities, policymakers, and public health agencies can naturally make sustained collaborations, there's a greater opportunity to adjust to and lessen the chronic hazard posed by polluted water, guiding all of us to a healthier, safer future (Figure 1.9).

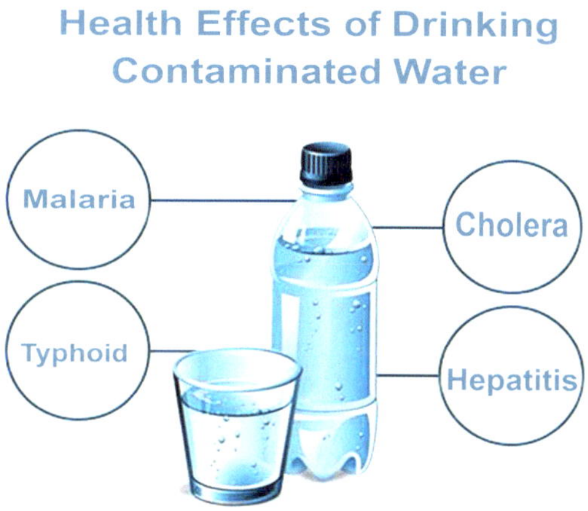

Figure 1.9. Health effects of drinking contaminated water.

Source: KENT RO Systems. (2017). *Health Effects of Drinking Contaminated Water.*

1.3.3. Methods for Testing and Improving Water Quality

Water safety is important to our people's well-being. There are plenty of means to test and improve water quality. Some individuals utilize a combination of chemical and biological analyses – consider testing for heavy metals and bacteria in water samples. One approach, spectrophotometry, provides very accurate measurements of contaminants, while microbiological tests can identify dangerous pathogens.

Regular surveillance like this provides both real-time updates and long-term information, so communities can better be ready when making water choices. Healthcare professionals, the majority of the time, do consider these results when making use of their professional judgment (Mancia et al., 2013). Another aspect is introducing treatment technology into the mix. Sophisticated filters , such as reverse osmosis (RO) and UV disinfection , come a long way in purifying water supplies of impurities and pathogens. These technologies tend to excel where the aging infrastructure is inadequate or has suffered, e.g., in rural or underserved communities.

Educating local residents about these systems can create a sense of local ownership and keep maintenance on schedule. Investing in sustainable solutions to water problems generally ends up benefitting public health as well, opening up safe drinking water to all, which is absolutely essential for public well-being (WSP, 2011). And then there is the community's role too. In addition to chemicals and technology, engaging people in water management creates a sense of responsibility and collective purpose. Some initiatives even allow residents to contribute to testing and monitoring – not only does this raise people's awareness of the value of clean water, but it encourages people to act when necessary. Citizen science can provide some fantastic additional data, supplementing what is already being monitored. Finally, when everyone works together to provide clean water, the combined effort enhances public health and keeps waterborne illness at bay, so that community health projects are that much more powerful.

1.4. The Economic Impact of Water on Community Health

Clean water has an enormous impact on keeping individuals and communities healthy, as well as local economies in significant ways. When water is not so good, the potential health risks have the tendency to send costs soaring high. For instance, a few studies indicate that in the Pusur River region, payments for illnesses brought about by contaminated water increase rapidly, particularly when people must run to healthcare centers. Illnesses such as typhoid and diarrhea impose significant expenditures that affect community clinics as well as larger hospitals. Increased healthcare costs then cause families to slash other essentials, locking them into a poverty-ill health cycle. In the majority of situations, maintaining water resources in order is not solely a matter of improved health—there is also reduced money tension in at-risk neighborhoods (Andesgur et al., 2025). Water problems are not all about quality; they become even more insidious in areas mired in geopolitical conflict. In Palestine, for example, constant wars run up against mundane concerns with accessing clean water, damaging people who are already marginalized. Usually, families suffering from water shortage end up passing the burden on women in charge of domestic water supplies, which tends to create additional stress and periodic family disputes, besides adverse effects on children's development and well-being. The economic cost is profound, when funds are scarce, households end up using what little they have to ensure that there is water, with less going to food, education, and other necessities. Overall, managing these multi-layered problems involves addressing both the social and financial dimensions simultaneously (Walther et al., 2025). Intelligent, strategic measures are required to mitigate the economic burden of water insecurity on public health.

Policymakers must advocate for initiatives that improve the quality of water as well as educate people about the danger posed by dirty water. These outreach efforts among communities can enable individuals to guard themselves, reducing waterborne diseases and consequently treatment expenses in the long run. Concurrently, directing funds towards improved water infrastructure can assist in alleviating the burden on marginalized communities. Overall, a balanced approach that considers both economic and health concerns is central to creating resilience and improved outcomes. It's very important that research with local realities informs policies so the solutions fit what people require (Andesgur et al., 2025; Walther et al., 2025).

1.4.1. Cost of Water-Related Health Issues

Lack of clean water hits communities severely—it not only raises the cost of medical care but also reduces the quality of life. Many low-income communities already struggling with shortages of resources see individuals suffering from water-borne illnesses hit hardest. Hospitals fill up and work or school days are lost, all of which ultimately hinder long-term community advancement and drain local coffers. It's obvious that understanding how water quality fits into health counts in making policy decisions, particularly where resources are constrained and the cost is high. Improved water, sanitation and hygiene (WASH) measures prove to be an important ingredient in mitigating such issues. Low-cost investments in these sectors reduce the incidence of ailments such as cholera or dysentery, which in turn reduces individuals' and societal health expenses in most instances. Frequently, spreading good information regarding safe water procedures empowerment communities beyond anticipated levels, improving general welfare in not always overtly apparent ways. There is ample documentation indicating strong WASH initiatives correlate with better health and more stable economies. Addressing these problems along with other ailments, such as HIV/AIDS, brings into focus why a mixed, integrated strategy makes so much sense (Tulenko, 2007). Overall, the economic burden of water-borne health problems weighs on government coffers and saps international aid efforts as well. Sickness spending that is preventable places tremendous strain on healthcare. Tackling these issues requires several strategies, switching to sustainable water infrastructure and intensifying community education on health and sanitation are among them. Studies typically find that long-term financial savings from the likes of eco-friendly housing tied in with improved access to water can be dramatic. Getting safe water to all isn't only a matter of health; it's economic, too (Beatley, 2011). The actual test is in allocating these investments the priority they deserve and fully understanding how water, health, and economic resilience come together.

1.4.2. Economic Benefits of Investing in Clean Water Infrastructure

Clean water is not merely about staying healthy, it tends to initiate local economic development. When clean water arrives, households spend less on medicine and more on school or work; local business activity increases, generating a cycle where improved health and greater prosperity continue to spur each other on. You can witness this come to life when quality water, through the reduction of waterborne disease, triggers a cascade: lower health expenditure, enhanced household purchasing power, and eventually, enhanced community living standards that perfectly align with main global standards such as the United Nations SDGs—most notably Goal 6: Clean Water and Sanitation (Onifade, 2024). In general, spending on clean water proves to be an actual building block for both short-term health benefits as well as long-term economic security. It doesn't end there. Investing in water infrastructure tends to unlock unsuspected opportunities for employment and skills building. Constructing, repairing, and even operating these facilities require a variety of hands-on skills, and that tends to trigger local workforce expansion. In communities like the Black Belt of Alabama, where socioeconomic conditions are fairly dire, focused water projects can close gaps in inequality. Neighbors coming together with their abilities to put these systems online foster not only a feeling of shared ownership but also attract businesses that had previously avoided communities with low-quality facilities. With increased companies moving into the area, communities gain improved tax collections and additional resources to invest in public services (Tillett, 2013)—an echo effect that stretches far beyond localized improvements in health. Simultaneously, resilient water systems have defenses in place against future shocks, such as droughts, floods, or unforeseen events of contamination. When communities invest in resilient infrastructure and sustainable water management, they typically position themselves to better manage climate fluctuations. These water conservation practices not only guard our existing assets, but they also rationalize water consumption and cut costs associated with treatment and distribution, sometimes in remarkably effective methods. In addition to that, a robust water system also protects surrounding agriculture, preserving food safety and boosting local economies. Therefore, clean water infrastructure performs a dual role—it's a solution for the health problems of today but also an insurance policy for tomorrow's environment and community health (Onifade, 2024) (Figure 1.10).

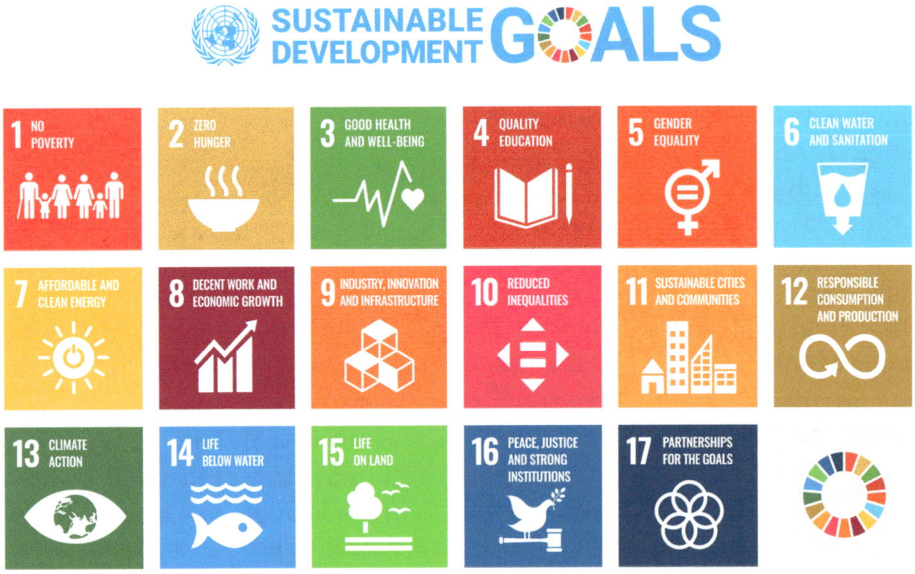

Figure 1.10. Sustainable development goal 6: Clean water and sanitation.

Source: By United Nations - un.org, Public Domain, https://commons.wikimedia.org/w/index.php?curid=80531292

1.4.3. Economic Improvements Through Water Access

Improvements in water access in poor neighborhoods are confronted with a whole mess of interconnected challenges. In urban locations, market-driven schemes and state initiatives both collide with issues; collective action problems tend to prevent locals from organizing effectively, and occasionally the state even resists allowing communities to take the lead, which complicates matters further. One can observe, for instance, that in India and Pakistan, once citizens become engaged with sanitation, solutions become viable. In many instances, overcoming obstacles, such as inadequate technical expertise and the absence of concerted actions—not only sanitizes the environment but also streamlines relations between citizens and government. These fluctuations suggest that with the proper type of push, strategic steps can ignite economic development and increase public health in a manner that has a ripple effect on all else. Access to water and economic development extend far beyond merely making individuals healthy immediately. Sanitation initiatives led by communities, for example, tend to introduce long-term economic dividends, such as improved work productivity and reduced healthcare costs. When groups of people invest in improved water and sanitation services, they create environments that enable all members to get on board economically; healthy individuals typically mean an active workforce, after all. Initiatives in India and Pakistan remind us of how critical it is to have intelligent partnerships and to rely on local capacity—both of which truly get the jobs done and translate into action. Addressing the money side of water access-related issues can alleviate the health burden as well as propel communities ahead in other socio-economic directions. Truly, cleaner, communal sanitary victories become central to enhancing local resilience and improving living standards. Another turn in the tale is the way that environmental issues bring additional layers to the entire water access and community health scenario. Affordable, sustainable housing projects these days often throw in water and sanitation upgrades, linking health, the environment, and economic well-being together in unexpected ways. Clean water and proper sanitation aren't just about avoiding sickness; they also touch on how good housing is and even how energy gets used. Consider green housing developments by way of example—they are forcing water access enhancements along with improving living standards and staying green all at the same time. This sort of integrated strategy is what results in communities not only addressing immediate health concerns; they are also laying the groundwork for long-term economic enhancements and overall higher living standards, as demonstrated in such research (Beatley, 2011; McGranahan, 2013).

1.5. Community Engagement and Education

Community participation in health initiatives has truly come into its own when addressing water issues. Locals participating isn't merely a sentimental notion; it translates to them having input on how water quality and sanitation levels get better where they are. On the whole, when people know what the problem is, they are more likely to adopt healthier habits, such as handwashing, more seriously. For instance, such efforts as promoting hygiene are more effective when members of the community participate in the development and operation of such campaigns; it creates not just awareness but a sense of ownership that has a tendency to result in greater overall health. Even a review by Mwaura (2024) highlights that in those areas where financial and cultural factors render clean water scarce, these community-centered efforts truly help make a difference. Getting local leaders, health workers, and residents together, then, is fairly instrumental in building a healthier setting. Much of the world, particularly in low- and middle-income nations—still has the very real danger of contaminated water hanging over its head. Educating people about the risks of unclean water can reduce waterborne illness by a substantial rate. Basic education workshops and campaigns regarding proper water treatment and sanitation practices set the stage for sustainable changes. Respected local leaders, when engaged, can influence public opinion and promote behavior change. Mwaura (2024) overall shows that consistent community involvement not only empowers people but also catalyzes broader changes in public health policy. In short, placing education at the center of water-health efforts can pay dividends in spades in terms of community resilience. Education isn't merely a matter of serving up facts, it's also about ensuring everyone has an equal shot at health resources. All too often, communities are struggling with uneven health because socio-economic conditions keep them from getting access to clean water and sanitation. When custom-designed educational interventions can identify and fill in the gaps, the entire community will gain. For example, fluoride treatment programs in Saudi Arabia show that a lot of children have dental caries because they do not have sufficient access to quality dental care. This case sort of highlights the necessity to create education suited to the particular cultural and pragmatic requirements of every community. Overall, implementing inclusive education policies is essential not just for improved water health but also for enhanced overall community wellness, and that linkage drives further increased health equity (Figure 1.11).

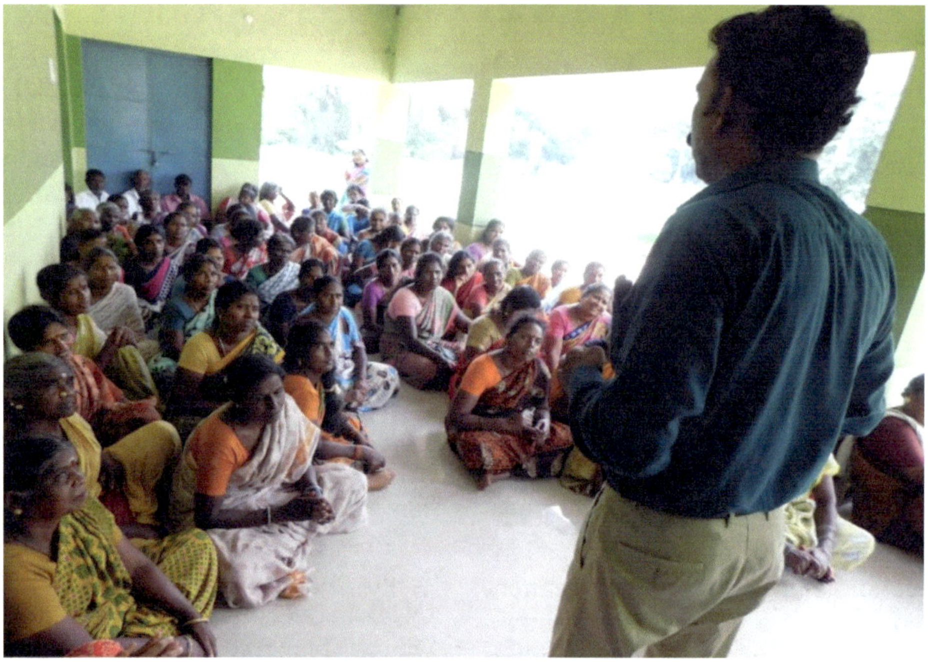

Figure 1.11. Community engagement in water management empowering individuals for collective impact.

Source: ADI International. (2023). *Community Engagement in Water Management Empowering Individuals for Collective Impact.*

1.5.1. Importance of Community Involvement in Water Management

Water management today truly relies on individuals getting engaged. Communities are the ones that devise and implement solutions that just suit the local culture and customs—this sort of grassroots assistance counts a great deal for safeguarding the environment as well as public health. When people get involved, projects can draw on local expertise and foster a shared sense of pride over water resources. Consider Zambia's strategy to curb cholera, for instance—the integrated community strategy for cholera control (ICSCC) indicates that a community-based approach can reduce disease transmission by encouraging improved hygiene and sanitation. Local participation generated faster discussions between different groups and even enabled tailor-made responses in cholera-endemic areas, evidently highlighting the way community contributions enhance overall public health (Mwale et al., 2025b). The connection between getting ordinary people on board and cleaner water just can't be disregarded. Doing things together for such activities as coordinating a watershed or operating an on-the-ground water treatment operation truly emphasizes just how crucial it is to involve regular people in the decision-making process. Better natural resource stewardship in nearly every instance has produced a discernible reduction of pollution, leading to improved water quality, and health outcomes. Research has shown that when residents assist in monitoring and maintaining local water sources, they are more likely to remain with environmentally friendly habits. This style of doing things not only enhances water quality but also provides individuals with the assurance and the voice to advocate for their own health requirements, connecting hands-on governance with healthier results (Elmadani et al., 2024). Ultimately, making water management initiatives sustainable depends on ongoing community engagement. Regular participation develops some sort of adaptive muscle required to address water issues that appear to shift on a whim. Through collaboration at the local level and listening to input from the locals, such water projects are better placed to cope with climatic and environmental fluctuations. Lessons from everywhere indicate that policies to improve public health must heed local economic and social conditions. Where local community involvement is the emphasis, decision-makers and planners can assist in building sustainable improvements in water quality and public health, which in turn consolidate the support system in the locality for the well-being of all (Elmadani et al., 2024; Mwale et al., 2025a) (Figure 1.12).

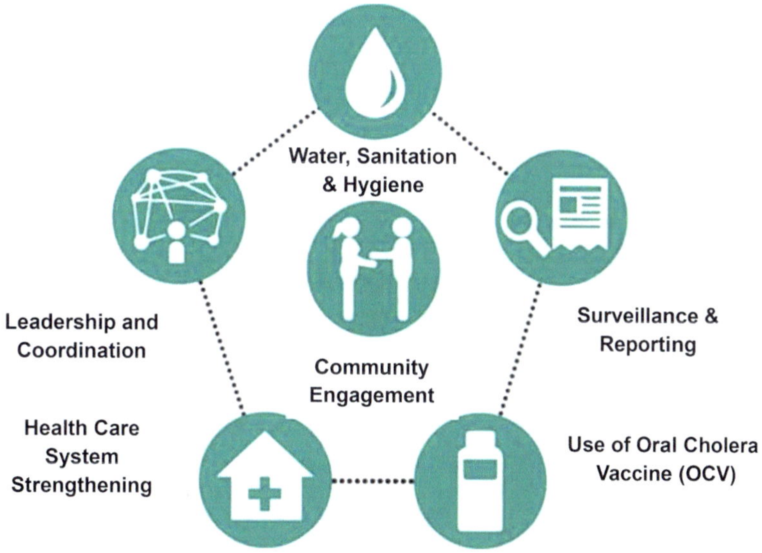

Figure 1.12. A multisectoral approach to cholera response.

Source: UNICEF. (2024). *Epidemiology, Preparedness, and Response to Cholera Epidemics – Training Package: Day 2, Module 2 – Multisectoral Response (Version 3.0).*

1.5.2. Educational Programs on Water Conservation and Health

Water conservation education is crucial for healthy communities. It's not simply a matter of teaching facts—people learn how water is directly connected to public health. Children, especially, come to see their own responsibility in defending nature when they develop eco-literacy through experiential learning. One study even indicates that Environment-Based Education tends to enhance children's eco-literacy and naturalistic intelligence, encouraging them toward greener behaviors (Setyaningsih et al., 2024). This type of knowledge not only enables people to start simple, sustainable practices but also allows communities to have water management and public health side by side. Local curriculum designs play a significant role here as well. Customizing lessons to what is important in a community allows individuals to relate what they learn in class to everyday challenges, often in surprising manners. It may sound like all conversation at the beginning, but discussing water-saving strategies creates ownership that, in the majority of instances, translates into more responsible behavior. Hands-on measures such as rainwater harvesting (RWH) or efficient irrigation can reduce the health consequences associated with contaminated water, and that is what connects conservation efforts to improved health outcomes (Vizzarri, 2024). The actual effectiveness of water conservation education is achieved through a combination of local governments, community organizations, and schools collaborating. Such collaborations introduce resources as well as expertise, making the programs even more valuable. Outdoor classes and hands-on workshops, for instance, can make the entire idea seem much more tangible. If individuals see the advantages firsthand, they are likely to remain committed to sustainable methods as well. Ultimately, by connecting clean water availability with better environmental situations, such education interventions solve greater health and nature issues (Setyaningsih et al., 2024) (Figure 1.13).

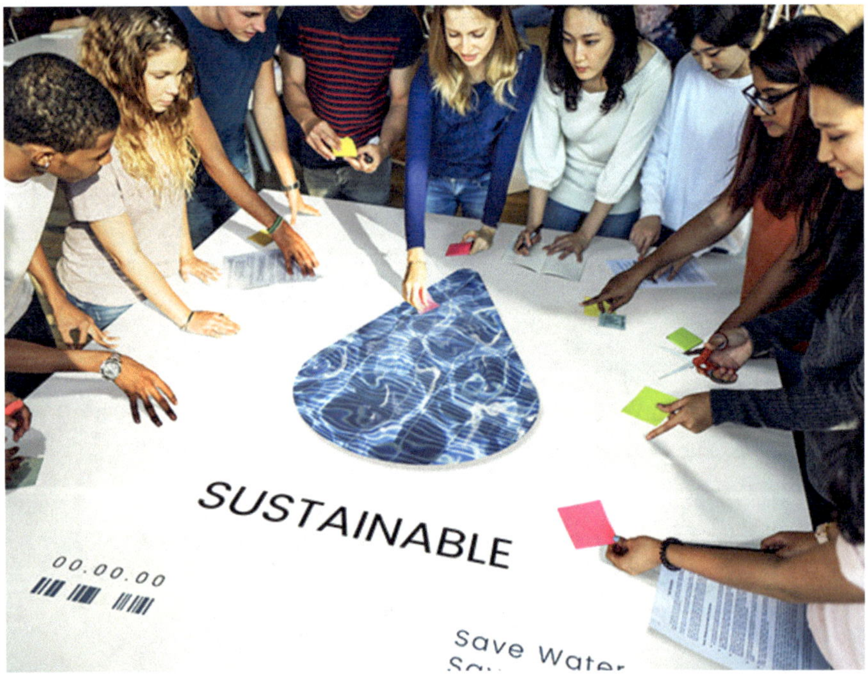

Figure 1.13. Water education program.

Source: Saving Water Partnership. (2021). *Water Education Program.*

1.5.3. Success Stories of Community-Led Water Initiatives

From all over the globe, day-to-day communities have risen up as a flesh-and-blood solution to deteriorating water crises – crises that, in most instances, only become more challenging due to climate change and less-than-optimal local governance. Folks are banding together in unexpected, quirky manners, not just repairing water deficits but creating their own resilience. Consider community-managed disaster risk reduction (CMDRR) as an example: it gives locals control over anticipating and managing water disasters in terms that combine age-old expertise with new, down-to-earth ideas. This action-ready strategy enhances security in the area and, plain and simple, is a nice model for other troubled areas to follow, suggesting that small, local solutions may trigger greater, system-wide reform (Broekhuijsen, 2009). In a different example, the tale of rainfed agricultural communities presents an equally fascinating picture. Indian farmers, in particular, have gotten together – sometimes in surprising configurations – to reimagine how they acquire and utilize water. They've altered their agricultural approaches to manage irregular weather that imperils their crops, and these adaptations have resulted in not just improved crop yields but also in smoother overall water management. Cooperation, mutual responsibility, and even some trial-and-error have prompted a few to design irrigation strategies that optimize each drop. In a number of respects, the initiative from these practical projects illuminates the path for subsequent concepts that might, hopefully, fan out to reinforce both agriculture and the general well-being of native communities (Appadurai et al., 2015). At its core, the boost from these local water projects shows how essential it is for people to get involved directly when it comes to handling water sustainably. Every one of these efforts emphasizes community ownership over just installing new pipes or infrastructure—they also teach folks about saving water and keeping things hygienic. In some sense, these efforts strengthen connections by continually demonstrating that taking care of water isn't simply a matter of a resource; it's about building a healthier, more connected style of life. As communities increasingly control their own water futures, despite a few bumps along the way, there is an unmistakable increase in health and overall well-being, toward a more resilient future in a volatile world (Broekhuijsen, 2009).

SUMMARY

Community health and water quality are connected in such a way that action needs to be taken sooner than later. Research appears to indicate that merely keeping water safe isn't sufficient – when locals take action, however, things get better. The research from Tehuledere, for example, indicates that even with good security measures, the question of how people deal with water collection and storage daily is what ends up being important. Approximately 64.1% of households practice hand washing during water collection, suggesting encouraging progress despite further learning being quite evident. Resident training and increasing hands-on hygiene knowledge allow people to take responsibility for making their water safe, which can raise overall health (Endale et al., 2016). Floods further obscure the issue of the safety of the water. In areas vulnerable to heavy rainfalls such as areas in Indonesia, flooding would aggravate health hazards by bringing down the quality of water in homes. If about 40% of the population experiences diarrhea episodes during flooding, it well indicates the cost to public health. In all instances, indigenous knowledge regarding sanitation proves to be an actual game-changer. Arming community members with the appropriate information regarding water management reduces disease transmission and enhances overall health (Fadilah et al., 2023). Mixing water quality with community health teaches us that the line is drawn beyond simple quick fixes. In general, when individuals become more aware of making water safe, communities become resilient. Community leaders, healthcare workers, and community members mobilizing together hold the key to establishing long-term solutions that protect both a pure water supply and a healthier setting. As individuals navigate environmental transitions and periodic sanitation glitches, education on an ongoing basis and taking matters into one's own hands truly empower people to manage their own health. With time, these initiatives can result in incremental improvements in public health and highlight just how much water education matters to the community (Endale et al., 2016; Fadilah et al., 2023).

Water management is key to how our communities stay healthy, it's funny how something as basic as water can affect everything from our local ecosystems to our own bodies. Research has shown, in a sort of eye-opening way, that contamination levels in water are way higher than what we'd like to see, and that's hurting both nature and people. One of the studies in a small region along the Pachanlica River detected disquieting levels of heavy metals and fecal coliforms, which are problems that largely result from negligent industrial and agricultural processes. Discoveries of these types tend to indicate the requirement for simple, robust wastewater plans that reduce contamination and leave water cleaner. Public awareness campaigns and ecologically friendly agriculture practices continue to come up as crucial steps—yes, they contribute towards safeguarding our water and, indirectly, our well-being. Ultimately, when community groups support water policies that prioritize the well-being of the environment as well as human life, everyone gets to live in a safer world (Procel-Silva et al., 2025). Safe drinking water is a pressing issue, and arguments over community water fluoridation (CWF) underscore that. With time, developments in how we blanket communities with CWF have indicated some significant strides toward improved local health (Hamilton et al., 2023). An examination of data refinements from the Centers for Disease Control and Prevention demonstrates that, since 2012, the methods have tended to be refined to expose trends more accurately. Despite the fact that overall numbers did not dramatically change, more precise adjustments to the percentages provide a truer representation of how many individuals are receiving fluoridated water. In a majority of instances, such fine-tuning refines our health objectives and allows individuals to make better choices regarding water fluoridation policies. When such initiatives are based on stable, evidence-informed bases, communities are likely to better address the health disparities associated with water quality concerns (Erin et al., 2023). Apart from addressing the immediate problem of contamination, considering how we treat water implies planning for the future as well. Studies not only caution us about the threat of dirty water but, in more casual terms, they also tell us that we require broad-stroke environmental agendas that fit local circumstances. These agendas blend scientific water quality testing with local, community-based solutions that encourage people to participate. For instance, relaxed community events can make individuals realize how significant it is to conserve water sources and maintain habits that keep pollution in check—even if it requires repetition of the issue a couple of times. When scientists, policymakers, and local residents collaborate (despite the efforts sometimes seeming rough around the edges), they form a more consolidated defense against water-borne health issues, with water quality remaining a high priority in all health actions (Procel-Silva et al., 2025).

KEY TERMS FROM THIS CHAPTER

- Clean water
- Community health
- Environmental fluctuations
- Rainwater harvesting
- WASH strategies
- Mental health
- Water stress
- Waste management
- Complex sanitation
- Filthy water
- Sanitation infrastructure
- Waste management
- Public health
- Aerobic mesophilic bacteria
- Educational campaigns
- infectious diseases
- Spectrophotometry
- Water issues
- Waterborne disease

CLOSER LOOK

CLEAN WATER IN DISEASE PREVENTION

Clean water is necessary for disease prevention because it helps to destroy unwanted pathogens that induce diseases such as cholera, typhoid, and dysentery. Having access to clean water and sanitation, in addition to practicing hygiene, is effective in significantly minimizing the prevalence of waterborne diseases and ensuring good health. Having access to safe drinking water and sanitation improves overall health and well-being directly by preventing disease.

Here's how clean water contributes to disease prevention:

1. **Eliminates Pathogens**: Clean water, free from bacteria, viruses, and other pathogens, prevents their entry into the body and the subsequent development of waterborne diseases.
2. **Facilitates Hygiene**: Having access to clean water allows for proper hygiene practices like handwashing and bathing, which are essential for preventing the spread of microbes and infections.
3. **Reduces Diarrheal Diseases**: Safe water has tremendous potential for reducing diarrheal diseases, the main killer especially among children, by excluding pathogens from infected water and food.
4. **Improves Overall Health**: Having access to clean water results in healthier outcomes because it avoids a vast array of waterborne illnesses and enables better hygiene, resulting in a healthier and more resilient population.
5. **Supports Sustainable Development**: Clean water and sanitation play a significant role in sustaining development because they enhance well-being in terms of health, livelihoods, and education of people.

REFERENCES

1. Al-Daim SA. Virological Water Quality. Food Sci Nutr The. 2025;11(1):001-013. Available from: https://dx.doi.org/10.17352/jfsnt.000054 (accessed on 14 May 2025).
2. Alengebawy, A., Abdelkhalek, S. T., Qureshi, S. R., & Wang, M. Q. (2021). Heavy metals and pesticides toxicity in agricultural soil and plants: Ecological risks and human health implications. *Toxics, 9*(3), 42. https://doi.org/10.3390/toxics9030042.
3. Alghamdi, A. A., Mohammed, H. A., Alzahrani, R., Battayah, S., Alshahrani, S., & Almualled, Z. A. (2024). Fluoride and caries prevention: A scoping review of public health policies in Saudi Arabia. *Fuel Cells Bulletin*. https://www.semanticscholar.org/paper/1d747f82d71228b8f82d8da30a81a6e8888503c8 (accessed on 14 May 2025).
4. Alvernia, P., Soesilo, T., & Herdiansyah, H. (2021). Social impacts of oil spills towards the people living in coastal areas. *IOP Conference Series: Earth and Environmental Science, 802. OP Conf. Ser.: Earth Environ. Sci.* **802** 012001. https://www.semanticscholar.org/paper/c547cc42c3c83616a2e6de07f58d8cf3d4e4fa4f (accessed on 14 May 2025).
5. Andesgur, I. ., Hartono, Setyono, P. ., & Gravitiani, E. . (2025). Estimated health impact and economic loss from river water pollution. *International Journal of Innovative Research and Scientific Studies, 8*(2), 1715–1728. https://doi.org/10.53894/ijirss.v8i2.5532 (accessed on 14 May 2025).
6. Appadurai, A. N., Dinshaw, A., McGray, H., Rangwala, L., Chaudhury, M., Ginoya, N., & Srivatsa, S. (2015). Scaling success: Lessons from adaptation pilots in the rainfed regions of India. https://core.ac.uk/download/75782099.pdf (accessed on 14 May 2025).
7. Arasi, M. J. A., Brar, K., Nitika, Nancy, N., P., P., et al. (2022). A descriptive study to assess the knowledge and practice regarding domestic waste management and its effects on health among homemakers in selected urban areas of Yamuna Nagar District, Haryana. *Journal of Nursing Science Practice, Research and Advancements*. https://doi.org/10.46610/JNSPRA.2023.v05i01.001. https://www.semanticscholar.org/paper/caf880b66bd8b31d135309722355c9c50beb3bdc (accessed on 14 May 2025).
8. Batley, R., & McLoughlin, C. (2009). State capacity and non-state service provision in fragile and conflict-affected states. This report was prepared for DFID by Richard Batley (International Development Department, University of Birmingham) and Claire Mcloughlin (Governance and Social Development Resource Centre). https://core.ac.uk/download/103644.pdf (accessed on 14 May 2025).
9. Beatley, N. (2011). *Green Housing = Improved Health: A Winning Combination., Green Housing = Improved Health: A Winning Combination.* https://core.ac.uk/download/71345591.pdf (accessed on 14 May 2025).
10. Berg, S. (2021). *Conceptual and Practical Aspects of Water Regulation in Developing Countries.* https://www.semanticscholar.org/paper/9c362e0370985c1c7fb7a09b92ee8cbdc31e05b6 (accessed on 14 May 2025).
11. Broyles, L. M. T., Pakhtigian, E. L., Rosinger, A., & Mejia, A. (2022). Climate and hydrological seasonal effects on household water insecurity: A systematic review. *Wiley Interdisciplinary Reviews: Water, 9*. https://www.semanticscholar.org/paper/c4f8126d7066a02353b3960dc4b5f325090e747f (accessed on 14 May 2025).

12. Bugg-Levine, A., & Brandenburg, M. (2010). Impact investments: An emerging asset class. J.P. Morgan Global Research. https://core.ac.uk/download/71352133.pdf (accessed on 14 May 2025).

13. Bull, F., Al-Ansari, S. S., Biddle, S., Borodulin, K., Buman, M. P., Cardon, G., Carty, C., et al. (2020). World Health Organization 2020 guidelines on physical activity and sedentary behaviour. *British Journal of Sports Medicine, 54*, 1451–1462. https://doi.org/10.1136/bjsports-2020-102955.

14. Caputo, A., Tomai, M., Lai, C., Desideri, A., Pomoni, E., Méndez, H. C., Castellanos, B., et al. (2022). The perception of water contamination and risky consumption in El Salvador from a community clinical psychology perspective. *International Journal of Environmental Research and Public Health, 19*. https://www.semanticscholar.org/paper/33dd37dfd29c37687fb3094c20bdf5ac92f36c7c (accessed on 14 May 2025).

15. Hendra Cipta, Muslim, Rahmad Julianto, Rosnidawati, Teuku Maulana, Ambia Nurdin, Harri Santoso, & Aisy Al-Khansa. (2025). COMMUNITY-DRIVEN HEALTH STRATEGIES FOR PREVENTING DISEASE OUTBREAKS AFTER THE 2004 ACEH TSUNAMI. *Jurnal Penelitian Progresif, 4*(1), 16-31. https://doi.org/10.61992/jpp.v4i1.204 (accessed on 14 May 2025).

16. Corbett, A., Fuse, E., Hodge, J., & Scanlon, M. (2012). Legal review concerning the use of health impact assessments in non-health sectors. Pew reports. https://www.pew.org/en/research-and-analysis/reports/2012/04/04/legal-review-concerning-the-use-of-health-impact-assessments-in-nonhealth-sectors (accessed on 14 May 2025).

17. Elmadani M, Kasmai Kiptulon E, Klára S, Orsolya M. Systematic Review of the Impact of Natural Resource Management on Public Health Outcomes: Focus on Water Quality. *Resources*. 2024; 13(9):122. https://doi.org/10.3390/resources13090122 (accessed on 14 May 2025).

18. Endale, H., Faris, K., Legesse, W., Tiku, et al. (2016). Factors affecting drinking water quality from source to home in Tehuledere Woreda, Northeast Ethiopia. https://core.ac.uk/download/478439289.pdf (accessed on 14 May 2025).

19. Fatunmibi, I. (2024). Sustainable Development Goal-Six (SDG-6) water and sanitation, impact on Nigeria, assessing the intersection with public health and globalization: A systematic literature review. *International Journal of Research and Innovation in Social Science*. **https://dx.doi.org/10.47772/IJRISS.2023.7012060** (accessed on 14 May 2025).

20. Gatta, P. P. (2022). *The State of World Fisheries and Aquaculture 2022*. FAO eBooks. https://doi.org/10.4060/cc0461en.

21. Grover, S. A., Williams, C. J., Co-Dyre, A., Malkin, D., & Whitlock, J. (2024). Abstract B069: ACCESS: Advancing childhood cancer experience, science and survivorship in Canada. *Cancer Research*. https://www.semanticscholar.org/paper/be6cd03296e998e0cd43ea7d684d4eac1f45f066 (accessed on 14 May 2025).

22. Hamilton, E. K., Griffin, S., & Espinoza, L. (2023). Effect of CDC adjustment of state-reported data on community water fluoridation statistics. *Journal of Public Health Dentistry*. https://www.semanticscholar.org/paper/75fc8a62230d66ea181eeca632965b115c0bb162 Hamilton, E. K., Griffin, S. O., & Espinoza, L. (2023). Effect of CDC adjustment of state-reported data on community water fluoridation statistics. *Journal of public health dentistry, 83*(3), 320–324. https://doi.org/10.1111/jphd.12579 (accessed on 14 May 2025).

23. Intergovernmental Panel on Climate Change. (2023). *Climate Change 2022–Impacts, Adaptation and Vulnerability*. https://doi.org/10.1017/9781009325844.

24. Izah, S. C., Etim, N. G., Alaka, O. O., Nwachukwu, B. C., & Joshua, G. (2024). Public health interventions for cholera control and prevention: Water, sanitation, and hygiene (WASH) perspective. *Greener Journal of Epidemiology and Public Health.* ISSN: 2354-2381. Vol. 12(1), pp. 1-15, 2024. DOI: https://doi.org/10.15580/gjeph.2024.1.102024145 (accessed on 14 May 2025).

25. Juarez, R., Le, B., Bond-Smith, D., Bonham, C., Sanchez-Johnsen, L., & Maunakea, A. K. (2025). Socioeconomic determinants of mental health outcomes among Hawaii adults. *Frontiers in Public Health, 13.* https://www.semanticscholar.org/paper/854ae50153153234de046d64f0cdc89f5ee6d23a (accessed on 14 May 2025).

26. Karasaki, S., Goddard, J., Cohen, A., & Ray, I. (2023). Environmental justice and drinking water: A critical review of primary data studies. *Wiley Interdisciplinary Reviews: Water, 10.* https://www.semanticscholar.org/paper/0212a5e5c549bd794f415dbc26e0d2b92b88d6c1 (accessed on 14 May 2025).

27. Chishti DK, A study to assess the knowledge and practice regarding sanitation and hygiene among women in parts of Delhi, India, Journal of Drug Delivery and Therapeutics. 2023; 13(9):28-32 (accessed on 14 May 2025).

28. Khant, N. A., Lumongsod, R. M., San, A., Moon, J., Namkoong, S., & Kim, H. (2025). Navigating the complex landscape of waterborne disease research. *Journal of Water and Health, 23*(2), 168–189. https://www.semanticscholar.org/paper/d094a14718f4624afb797c8e1724738b007941c3 (accessed on 14 May 2025).

29. Mancia, G., Fagard, R., Narkiewicz, K., Redón, J., Zanchetti, A., Böhm, M., Christiaens, T., et al. (2013). 2013 ESH/ESC Guidelines for the management of arterial hypertension. *European Heart Journal, 34*, 2159–2219. https://doi.org/10.1093/eurheartj/eht151.

30. McGranahan, G. (2013). *Community-driven sanitation improvement in deprived neighbourhoods.*. Available at https://www.iied.org/g03615 (accessed on 14 May 2025).

31. Moallemi, E. A., Malekpour, S., Hadjikakou, M., Raven, R., Szetey, K., Moghadam, M. M., Bandari, R., et al. (2019). Local Agenda 2030 for sustainable development. *The Lancet Planetary Health, 3*, e240–e241. https://doi.org/10.1016/s2542-5196(19)30087-7.

32. Moore, C., Nichol, A., & Taylor, H. (2023). Supporting Solidarity: Public Health's Role in Achieving Social Justice. Voices in Bioethics, 9. https://doi.org/10.52214/vib.v9i.11758 (Original work published October 31, 2023) (accessed on 14 May 2025).

33. Morales, D. O., Ramos, K., Jauregui, E., Duenas, M., Rumaldo, N., Gogia, S., Lecca, L., et al. (2024). Perceptions of water security and climate change in Lima, Peru: Qualitative study of mothers and healthcare providers. medRxiv 2024.07.10.24309904; doi: https://doi.org/10.1101/2024.07.10.24309904 (accessed on 14 May 2025).

34. Mouteyica, A. E. N., & Ngepah, N. (2025). Exploring health outcome disparities in African regional economic communities: A multilevel linear mixed-effect analysis. *BMC Public Health, 25.* https://www.semanticscholar.org/paper/d6ac6e3fb64ec0f5e84cce9d1a713fe6a0352efd (accessed on 14 May 2025).

35. Murray, C. J. L., Ikuta, K. S., Sharara, F., Swetschinski, L. R., Robles Aguilar, G., Gray, A. P., Han, C., et al. (2022). Global burden of bacterial antimicrobial resistance in 2019: A systematic analysis. *The Lancet, 399*, 629–655. https://doi.org/10.1016/s0140-6736(21)02724-0.

36. Mwale , Memory, Teema Biko, Fatmata Sesay, and Omar Osman Omar. 2025. "Assessing Water Quality in Malawi: Contamination Sources, Public Health Impacts, and Sustainable Management Strategies". *Journal of Geography, Environment and Earth Science International* 29 (1):89-105. https://doi.org/10.9734/jgeesi/2025/v29i1858.(accessed on 14 May 2025).

37. Mwale, M., Chipimo, P., Kalubula, P., Mulima, S. M. C., Kapema, K., Mwangilwa, K., et al. (2025b). Building resilience against cholera: Lessons from the implementation of integrated community strategy for cholera control in Zambia. *BMJ Global Health, 10*. https://www.semanticscholar.org/paper/46931a0a182b532a1454f4f611d7b6cdf2568fee (accessed on 14 May 2025).

38. Kate Tulenko . (2007). *Analysis of Research on The Effects of Improved Water, Sanitation, And Hygiene on The Health of People Living with HIV and Aids and Programmatic Implications*. https://core.ac.uk/download/71345778.pdf Original review by Kate Tulenko (WB/WSP), with further expansion and revision by Renuka Bery and Julia Rosenbaum (USAID/HIP). Prepared by the USAID /Hygiene Improvement Project with the Water and Sanitation Program/World Bank. October 2007 (accessed on 14 May 2025).

39. Marije Broekhuijsen Edited by Nicholas Parrott, TextualHealing.nl Petterik Wiggers front cover photo and photos on pages 6, 29, 51, 61 Benno Neeleman photo on page 65 (2009). *Towards a Resilient Future: Experiences with Community Managed Disaster Risk Reduction and Climate Change Adaptation*. https://core.ac.uk/download/75781838.pdf (accessed on 14 May 2025).

40. ICAI (2016). *Assessing DFID's Results in Water, Sanitation and Hygiene: An Impact Review*. https://core.ac.uk/download/75761590.pdf (accessed on 14 May 2025).

41. Ngugi Mwaura J. (2024). Preventive Measures for Diarrhea in Communities Lacking Clean Water Supply: A Scientific Review. RESEARCH INVENTION JOURNAL OF BIOLOGICAL AND APPLIED SCIENCES 4(3):39-43. https://doi.org/10.59298/RIJBAS/2024/433943 (accessed on 14 May 2025).

42. Onifade, A. M. (2024). Wastewater infrastructure in Nigeria and the USA: A tale of two nations and their pathway to sustainable development. *International Journal of Multidisciplinary Research and Growth Evaluation*. https://www.semanticscholar.org/paper/c469fbd53c4b66d253295fa38e17990a9d3773c7 (accessed on 14 May 2025).

43. Pradhan, S., Pradhan, B. & Joshi, A. Leveraging geographic information systems (GIS) in water, sanitation, and hygiene (WASH) research: a systematic review of applications and challenges. *Spat. Inf. Res.* **33**, 11 (2025). https://doi.org/10.1007/s41324-025-00613-4 (accessed on 14 May 2025).

44. Procel-Silva, M., Moyano-Vallejo, H., Granizo-Espinoza, X., Cabezas, L., Godoy-Ponce, S., & Montenegro-Zambrano, Y. (2025). Environmental impact assessment and management strategies for the Pachanlica River micro-watershed, Ecuador: Addressing water pollution and its alignment with the Sustainable Development Goals (SDGs). *Journal of Lifestyle and SDGs Review*. https://www.semanticscholar.org/paper/09b781b2292bd112804d780c6b0cab3d3f40e934 (accessed on 14 May 2025).

45. Kathy A Seabrook, PL09 CONNECTING THE DOTS: THE VALUE OF PEOPLE AT WORK AND THEIR HEALTH, SAFETY AND WELL-BEING, *Occupational Medicine*, Volume 74, Issue Supplement_1, July 2024, Page 0, https://doi.org/10.1093/occmed/kqae023.0010 (accessed on 14 May 2025).

46. Setyaningsih, D., Handasah, R. R., Mamma, A. T., Krobo, A., Olua, E., & Iryouw, V. (2024). Fostering Eco-literacy and Naturalistic Intelligence through Environmentally Based Education in Coastal Preschool . *JPUD - Jurnal Pendidikan Usia Dini, 18*(1), 251–269. https://doi.org/10.21009/JPUD.181.18 (accessed on 14 May 2025).

47. Sylva Qamara Nur Fadilah, Rizqa Auliyah Shifah Sagala, Zahwatul Hasanah Siregar, Mega Rahmadani Siregar, Muhammad Ridwan, & Putra Apriadi Siregar. (2023). Description Of Community Knowledge And Attitude On Clean Water Sanitation In Flood Prone Areas On Pasar V Tembung Street Percut Sei Tuan District Deli Serdang District. *Journal of Educational Innovation and Public Health, 1*(3), 53–65. https://doi.org/10.55606/innovation.v1i3.1475 (accessed on 14 May 2025).

48. Soetikno, R., Teoh, A. Y. B., Kaltenbach, T., Lau, J. Y., Asokkumar, R., Cabral-Prodigalidad, P. A., & Shergill, A. K. (2020). Considerations in performing endoscopy during the COVID-19 pandemic. *Gastrointestinal Endoscopy, 92*, 176–183. https://doi.org/10.1016/j.gie.2020.03.3758.

49. Stoiber, T., Temkin, A. M., Andrews, D. Q., Campbell, C., & Naidenko, O. V. (2019). Applying a cumulative risk framework to drinking water assessment: A commentary. *Environmental Health, 18*. https://doi.org/10.1186/s12940-019-0475-5.

50. Tamene, A. (2021). A qualitative analysis of factors influencing household water treatment practices among consumers of self-supplied water in rural Ethiopia. *Risk Management and Healthcare Policy, 14*, 1129–1139. https://doi.org/10.2147/rmhp.s299671.

51. Tillett, T. (2013). Summit discusses public health implications of fracking. *Environmental Health Perspectives, 121*, a15. https://www.semanticscholar.org/paper/a53660fee303d83b3d74da6d10c934d5fc29fa59 (accessed on 14 May 2025).

52. Vizzarri, F. (2024). Central and Eastern European research and innovation scenario: Partnering for the future. *Slovak Journal of Animal Science*. https://www.semanticscholar.org/paper/fd63b3ba358c15f5bec4a8d8e4beac9514cddb4b (accessed on 14 May 2025).

53. Walther, A., Shaheen, A., Zubeidat, H., Shakhshir, G., & Hajat, S. (2025). Water insecurity in the Jordan Valley: Community perspectives on its impacts on maternal and child health. *International Journal of Environmental Research and Public Health, 22*. https://www.semanticscholar.org/paper/b32b110f6ccb679d465da36408870384dd240f23 (accessed on 14 May 2025).

54. WSP (2011). Political economy of sanitation: How can we increase investment and improve service for the poor? Operational experiences from case studies in Brazil, India, Indonesia and Senegal World Bank, Water and Sanitation Program (WSP), USA

55. Yuniarti, E., & Raharini, H. (2024). The relationship between healthy behavior and environmental sanitation with water quality in stunting occurrence work area of Sikabu Community Health Center Padang Pariaman. *IOP Conference Series: Earth and Environmental Science, 1317*. https://www.semanticscholar.org/paper/c535f84a43b38ffdecb616d2e14c2815bb246221 (accessed on 14 May 2025).

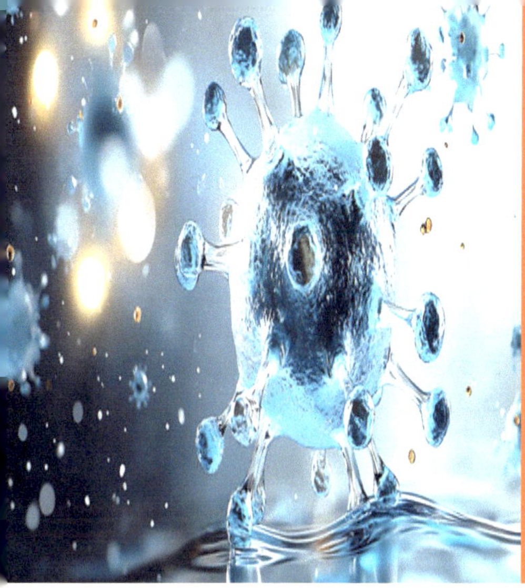

Chapter 2

WATERBORNE DISEASES AND THEIR IMPACT

Contents

Introduction

Waterborne illnesses are a worldwide problem, they affect more than just personal health. When pathogens infiltrate our water, whole communities, local economies, and natural environments take the hit. As cities expand and our environment is harmed, polluted water can ignite acute illnesses as well as chronic health issues. Pinpointing which bugs, whether bacterial, viral, or even protozoan, are causing these problems is important; in most instances, that simple understanding paves the way for more intelligent interventions. The methods through which these small perpetrators are transmitted can be fairly diverse. Contaminated water, scurvy sanitation, and even slips in common hygiene all provide channels for infections, frequently perpetuating a persistent cycle of health issues. It happens that poor or otherwise disenfranchised communities tend to suffer the most. Basic public health measures to sanitize water supplies and sanitation could, on the whole, reduce rates of sickness and death. Understanding precisely how these infections spread is important too, it assists with tracking outbreaks and informing effective, worldwide responses. Going a little deeper, you notice that the impact of waterborne diseases extends far past an individual's suffering. Communities tend to experience declines in productivity, lost school time, and increased health expenses, all of which can enslave individuals in vicious cycles of poverty that are difficult to escape. Addressing the problems requires a combination of approaches in health care, education, and environmental change. New concepts, such as applying sophisticated probiotics to attack certain pathogens, suggesting the potential for combining new scientific imagination with established public health practice. Overall, these challenges are not merely an emergency solution; it's a step in the direction of establishing sustainable improvement, particularly in regions where waterborne risk seriously undermines day-to-day well-being (Chen et al., 2024; Singh et al., 2024).

Definition of Waterborne Diseases

Waterborne illnesses tend to begin with a mess of variables—socio-economic, environmental, and biological—tending to leave populations more vulnerable to illness. Pathogenic microbes can find their way into water supplies through farm runoff, sewer spills, or simply plain old poor sanitation. Areas that lack much access to clean drinking water and proper sewer systems really bear the brunt. In certain areas where farming increases rapidly, new illnesses can even form. In general terms, more than 25% of the infectious diseases that have appeared since the 1940s have been attributed to farming practices, which indicates just how closely related water quality and public health are argued by Jason et al. (2019).

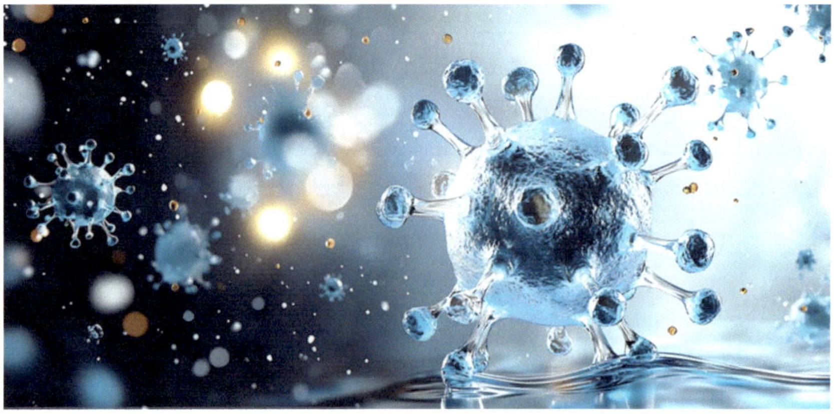

Source: Adobe Stock. (n.d.). *Abstract Water Sanitation Image.*

When water systems become contaminated, numerous health issues can ensue. Pathogenic bacteria, for example, are responsible for diseases like cholera, typhoid, and hepatitis A, and individuals typically acquire these by consuming or ingesting things that are already contaminated. You may see episodes of gastrointestinal discomfort, or worse, in some cases, even death. Notably, the problems usually have their roots in greater infrastructure issues; poor sanitation and lax waste management allow pollutants to seep continuously into the water. Thus, communities dependent on these degraded systems are exposed not only to waterborne microbes but also other hazards born out of environmental degradation and erratic public services (Stéphane et al., 2019). Apart from the direct health impacts, the ripple effects of waterborne diseases strike economic and social life severely. It's not uncommon for affected individuals to experience higher healthcare expenses, lost work or school days, and overall decreased opportunities for advancement. Recently, governments and organizations have come to realize the merits of investing in water and sanitation infrastructure, enabling communities to develop the resilience that makes recovery a less cumbersome task. In most instances, strengthening these systems can assist in countering the challenges presented by such diseases. Finally, addressing waterborne concerns requires a blended strategy that incorporates health care, improved sanitation practices, and even adjustments in farming procedures to make communities safer (Stéphane et al., 2019).

Importance of Studying Waterborne Diseases

Waterborne illnesses and the condition of our natural sources of water are inextricably bound together – they truly count when we consider public health. At times a decline in the quality of water, for instance, due to pollution, triggers an explosion of microbes that damage both humans and the environment. It happens that dealing with such problems effectively may even keep biodiversity intact, as infections can quietly alter the manner in which species compete and interact. There's even some research suggesting that certain pathogens may allow competing species to coexist by manipulating these competitive interactions (Chen et al., 2024). In a healthy ecosystem, a combination of various species typically develops natural immunity to infections, so monitoring this entire process is rather important if we need strategies to balance human requirements with nature's health. Waterborne disease doesn't only strike at health directly – it tends to ripple out to touch community life in unexpected ways. Ongoing illness can overwhelm local medical care, depress how much individuals accomplish on the job, and heap economic strain upon families and governments, generally. In addition, investigating how these waterborne pests play with other infections sometimes reveals unsuspected connections among diseases. For instance, STH may disrupt the immune system in a manner that exacerbates other prevalent infections, making decisions about treatment all the more difficult (Lebu et al., 2023). If you step back and look at it, it is obvious that investigating these relationships from a wider perspective is critical to informing the types of health policies and interventions that are effective. Excavating waterborne illness through investigation reveals opportunities to pinpoint specific preventive strategies and initiate public health campaigns that emphasize clean water and hygiene education. With millions struggling with these concerns globally, research investment is well-nigh inevitable for improving the resilience of communities and overall welfare. Collecting together public health, environmental science, and even socio-economic professionals may just be what the doctor ordered to create the plans that address all aspects. Bringing together health initiatives with improvements in water, sanitation and hygiene (WASH) can truly reduce disease transmission, resulting in improved overall community health (Lebu et al., 2023). By focusing on water-related diseases, we address the short-term problems as well as set the foundation for long-term community support and sustainability.

2.1. Types of Waterborne Diseases

Pathogens in contaminated water do present a serious threat to public health. Bacteria such as those responsible for cholera and typhoid fever strike hardest at communities when water is not of high quality. Vibrio cholerae, which causes cholera, typically appears where there is poor sanitation and water that is less than pristine. Typhoid fevercaused by *Salmonella typhi*, is commonly associated with fecal contamination. Social and environmental problems blend together here, so when a community doesn't have proper infrastructure, these bacterial issues just accumulate. Viruses pile on another layer of difficulty. Norovirus, for instance, spreads quickly when contaminated food or water is part of the mix—usually igniting outbreaks in schools or cruise ships. In the majority of instances, hepatitis A, which is caused by its eponymous virus, also enters through contaminated water and can contribute to liver inflammation and other systemic complications. As a general rule, wherever clean water is scarce, these viral dangers appear to lurk on every corner. And then there are the parasites (Figures 2.1 and 2.2).

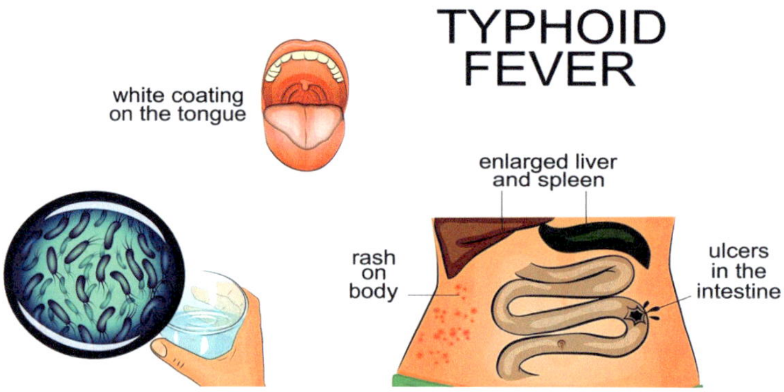

Figure 2.1. Typhoid fever.

Source: Touchwood Pharmacy. (2021). *What is Typhoid Fever and How do you Treat it?.*

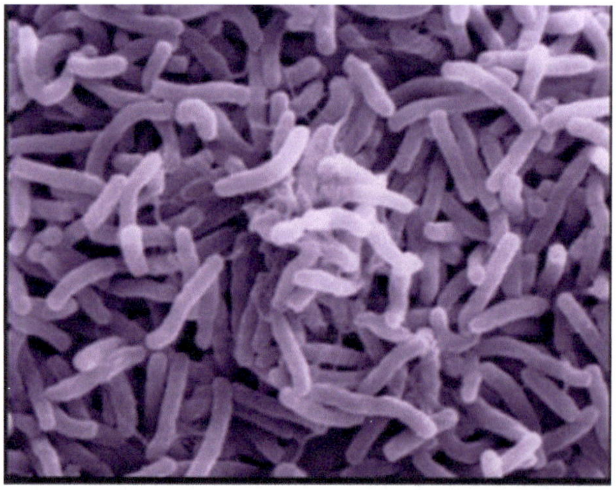

Figure 2.2. Structure of *V. cholera* bacteria.

Source: Kumar, P. (2018). *Structure of V. cholera Bacteria*. ResearchGate.

Giardiasis, resulting from *Giardia lamblia*, may produce uncomfortable stomach and bowel complaints that can wreak havoc on normal life. Alternatively, cryptosporidiosis—caused by *Cryptosporidium* species—is a resistant parasite able to withstand treatment of water through normal means and can be of additional risk for individuals with impaired immune systems. This type of parasitic misfortune suggests additional, more ingrained, ecological problems and socio-economic concerns within many marginalized social groups. Addressing these challenges involves integrating efforts in environmental health, education, and direct interventions to enhance water quality and protect public health (Cavicchioli et al., 2019; Rahman et al., 2020) (Figure 2.3).

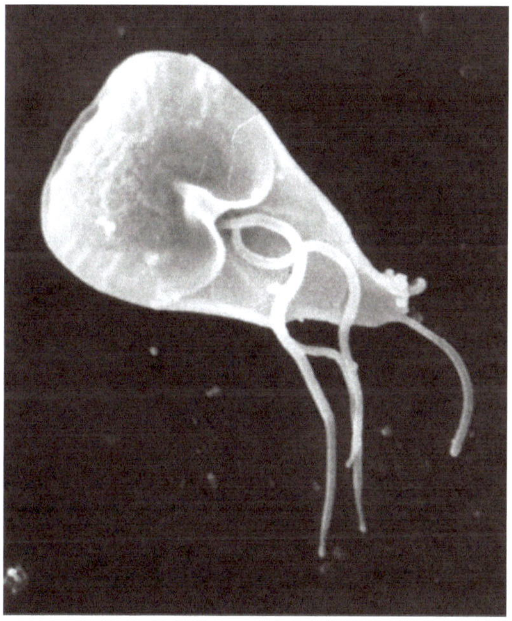

Figure 2.3. Giardiasis.

Source: https://en.wikipedia.org/wiki/File:Giardia_lamblia_SEM_8698_lores.jpg

2.1.1. Bacterial Diseases

Bacterial water contamination is a massive issue today, particularly where sanitation simply isn't adequate. Contaminated water can quickly become some kind of breeding ground for any number of bacteria, which in turn leads to diseases that affect vulnerable populations disproportionately. Densely populated cities, urbanization, and careless water treatment—these all combine to exacerbate the problem. Insects such as *Escherichia coli* and *Salmonella* spp. they tend to bring with them complex, nasty infections such as gastroenteritis and dysentery. Consider Nigeria, for instance; most homes wind up with water supplies that are nothing more than bacterial hotbeds, highlighting the necessity for improved sanitation and hygiene. It is not merely a question of keeping individuals healthy in isolation; improved water and sanitation serve to reduce healthcare expenses and enhance community output (Okafor, 2024). Bacterial illnesses have a habit of appearing in ways that are far from simple. A confusion of environmental conditions, such as changing temperatures and spasmodic rainfall, can alter the speed at which these infections take hold, and occasionally even the social setting inadvertently fuels the flames. And then there's the complication when bacteria join forces with viral illnesses, making it all that much more complicated, and usually more sinister. This type of mix-and-match activity between microbes compels us to consider layered, multi-faceted approaches to monitoring and managing outbreaks. In general, comprehending these complex transmission dynamics is central to informing public health measures that seek to interrupt the cycle of infection (Yano et al., 2024). The consequences of bacterial disease extend beyond illness, it erodes the economic and social fabric of communities. Disease from contaminated water too frequently translates into lost work hours, children absent from school, and increased health costs, all of which radiate outward to undermine community resilience and even kill local economic growth. Frequently, this creates a cycle that perpetuates poverty. That is why public health initiatives must focus on providing individuals with secure access to safe drinking water, adequate sanitation facilities, and strong hygiene education. Success here depends upon an occasionally rough, always significant cooperation between government agencies, medical practitioners, and community organizations. When these actors collaborate, there is a potential to reduce the heavy load of waterborne bacterial illnesses and make communities live healthier, more resilient lives (Okafor, 2024) (Figure 2.4).

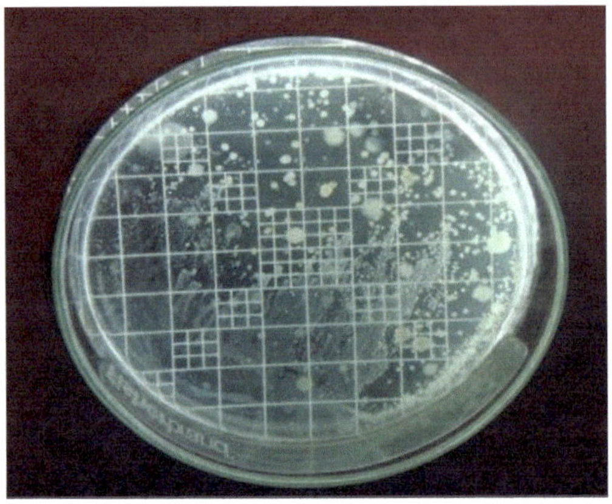

Figure 2.4. This figure shows the presence of pathogenic bacteria in one of the bottled water sample. This causes the contamination of water and this causes water borne diseases.

Source: Thallapalli, B. (2016). *Presence of Pathogenic Bacteria in Bottled Water*. ResearchGate.

2.1.2. Viral Diseases

Waterborne disease and virus pathogens blend together in a formula for disaster, particularly for neighborhoods already on their knees. Hepatitis A, norovirus, and similar diseases tend to creep into our lives via dirty water, sparking sudden outbreaks that can strain neighborhood clinics and hospitals. In most instances, the reaction is immediate: shots are administered and sanitation is improved.

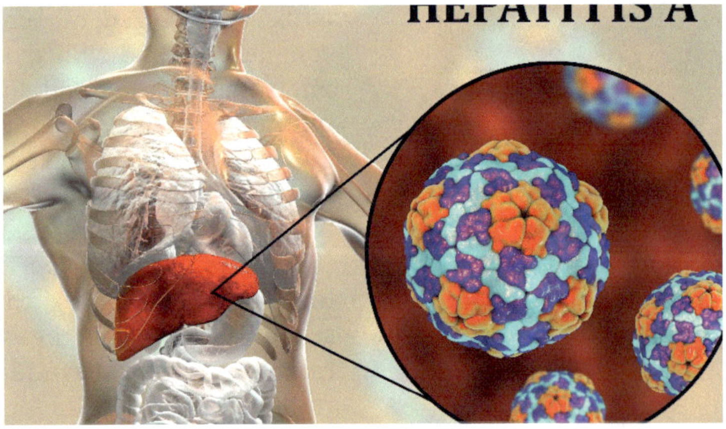

Figure 2.5. Hepatitis A.

Source: Mayo Clinic. (2019). *Hepatitis A.*

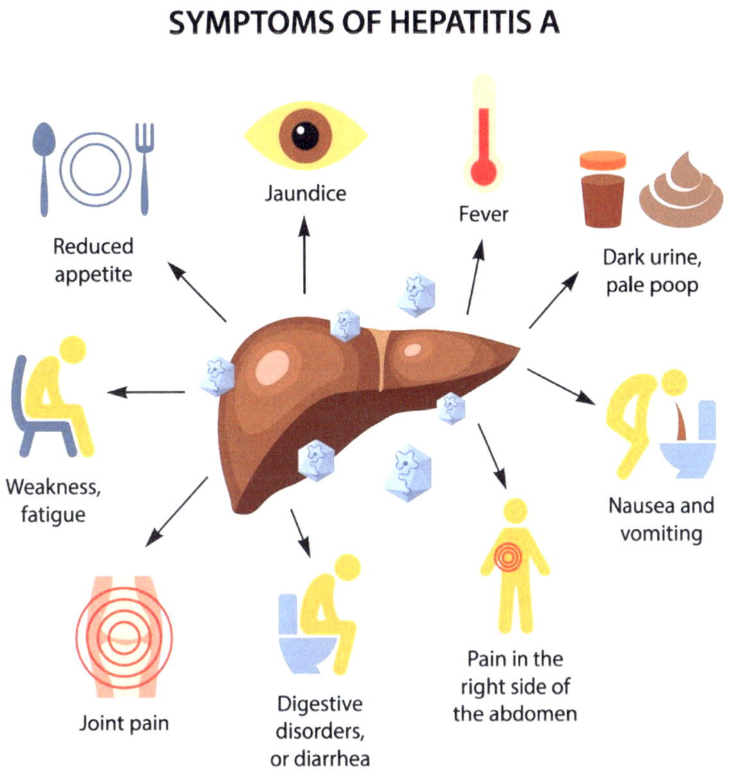

Figure 2.6. Symptoms of hepatitis A.

Source: Continental Hospitals. (n.d.). *Symptoms of Hepatitis A.*

Yet an enduring solution entails investing consistently in access to clean water. Fascinatingly enough, even our natural protectors—probiotics—may soften the impact of these viral blows, suggesting a type of synergy between our body's micro-population and our attempts to keep infection at bay (Singh et al., 2024). Occasionally, things only become more complicated. Virus outbreaks caused by rotavirus and enteroviruses show the actual necessity for stronger watch systems. These microorganisms are hardy and evolve rapidly, tending to make what we imagine were established prevention strategies challenging again. Science, as a whole, has attempted to decipher the puzzle of how these viruses navigate the water infrastructure and find refuge in nature's own reservoirs. On top of that, global warming—with its flooding and wobbly rain cycles—makes it even simpler for these microbes to find their way into our drinking supplies. The connection between human, animal, and environmental health stands out starkly, especially when our previous clearance techniques simply lag behind without a sweeping One Health approach to oversee the situation (Aguanno et al., 2022). A look back at previous outbreaks provides a rough outline for good public health policy. For example, organizations such as the Global Influenza Surveillance and Response System (GISRS) could very well expand their scope to include waterborne viral threats, as well. It's obvious that when populations aren't in on the risk of these infections, the situation only continues to deteriorate. That's one reason involving locals with straight talk and education appears to be important. We require policies that combine tough epidemiological evidence with local, everyday expertise to make our health systems sustainable (Aguanno et al., 2022; Singh et al., 2024) (Figures 2.5 and 2.6).

2.1.3. Parasitic Diseases

Parasitic illnesses just appear out of all kinds of challenging ecosystem interactions and are a significant component of the waterborne disease picture. These animals don't have a simple recipe to them – they employ kinky lifecycles and make use of everything nature and our daily routines provide. For example, *Giardia* and *Cryptosporidium* hang around in contaminated water and get into our bodies when we drink it, often leading to troublesome gut issues. Heavy rain or sudden floods can really overwhelm sanitation systems, and several literature reviews have pointed out that such weather extremes often come bundled with spikes in these gastrointestinal problems (Latendresse, 2023). Examining why these infections happen reveals that both human behaviors and local infrastructure conditions are significant determinants. Following a rain shower or heavy storm, numerous vulnerable populations are left with degrading WASH systems, and that degradation is only beneficial for parasites to gain traction. In such cases, people may end up using untreated water, for drinking, cooking or both—which increases the risk of infections. Recent statistics even suggest that changes in the climate are rewriting the maps and seasons when these insects emerge, making the entire transmission process a constantly changing puzzle. Research tends to show that temperature and rainfall shifts not only influence how long these pests linger but also how they travel between hosts, causing more outbreaks in infested territories (Fenta et al., 2019). With parasitic illness increasing—even among communities that have weathered their fair share, it's apparent that incorporating climate-conscious public health strategies is key. This involves strengthening surveillance systems and providing a true boost to WASH infrastructure so the communities are better equipped against outbreaks. Predictions indicate that severe weather is only going to become more frequent, so proactive measures are essential to combat the multi-layered risks these diseases pose. And, in addition, word-of-mouth about safe water habits is critical if we are to reduce transmission and enhance overall health. Once we understand how climate-influenced drivers determine the spread of these parasites, we can create wiser, more targeted interventions that safeguard public health and enable communities to recover stronger in the future (Fenta et al., 2019; Latendresse, 2023).

2.2. Common Pathogens Associated with Waterborne Diseases

Polluted water contains all sorts of toxic microbes, and people in regions with questionable sanitation typically suffer the most. Bacteria such as *Vibrio cholerae, Escherichia coli*, and *Salmonella typhi* are typically responsible for the worst stomach issues, they're almost exclusively transmitted when one consumes water or food that has come into contact with feces. It's no mystery that when water isn't sanitary, these microbes just continue to circulate, spreading illnesses even more widely. Easy solutions like treating water properly, cleaning up local sanitation systems, and spreading basic health information can greatly reduce these bacterial fiascos. Monitoring local water sources is important if we don't want to experience sudden outbreaks that can greatly affect at-risk communities. Not only bacteria, but small protozoan parasites also join in the trouble, creating such problems as giardiasis and cryptosporidiosis. These small nuisances can survive rough conditions and linger in water that is not filtered to its best. Their infections creep up gradually; symptoms arrive late, making it a nightmare to track down the source and often resulting in chronic disease. Places with less access to clean water and sanitation find it tougher since these parasites simply breed uncontrolled. A combination of hands-on sanitation education, regular water testing, and prompt treatments can prove to be a big help in combating these infections (Divyashri et al., 2024). And then there's the issue of fungal and viral pathogens, which pose another level of difficulty for public health. Certain fungi, for example, can spit out aflatoxins when drinking or food water becomes contaminated—a risk no one would want to take. Viruses such as norovirus and hepatitis A can also ride in contaminated water, sometimes causing outbreaks that disrupt community well-being. There's even increased buzz about how some probiotics can assist by reducing toxin levels and boosting our immune systems against these viral attacks (Singh et al., 2024). Although researchers are still working on learning all the ins and outs, it's certain that combining a number of approaches is our best option in combating the many faces of waterborne diseases.

2.2.1. Escherichia coli (E. coli)

Microbes in water are a big problem, and an understanding of how they move is a big part of solving waterborne diseases. *E. coli*, for instance, isn't any ordinary bacterium, it's a warning sign for fecal contamination in water. Its presence may be an indication that other bad bugs or viruses might be lurking in the background, waiting to trigger nasty stomach issues. Certain strains, such as Enterohemorrhagic *E. coli* (EHEC), are renowned for producing toxins that, in the majority of cases, can initiate extreme complications such as hemolytic uremic syndrome. Monitoring *E. coli* in drinking water assists health authorities in acting quickly and preventing communities from suffering, and it's essential to learn how these bacteria interact in water systems to better prevent sudden outbreaks that could cause disruptions to day-to-day life. The pathways through which *E. coli* ends up in our water aren't simple; they're complicated by multiple causes such as improper sanitation, farm runoff, livestock waste, and even botched sewer systems. Farm runoff and animal waste, together with a broken sewer installation, all contribute to a complex concoction where environmental forces and human behavior come together in odd ways. Recently, research has highlighted how antibiotic-resistant strains of *E. coli* are appearing particularly in agricultural areas—most notably because widespread livestock antibiotic use sometimes transfers resistance genes to microbes that infect humans (Mounsey et al., 2023). Overall, this turn makes it harder for public health groups to treat, says even more pressure on them to fortify surveillance and control efforts. Of even deeper concern beyond immediate health threats, *E. coli* contamination comes with a plethora of social and economic problems. Communities affected by waterborne diseases may endure lost hours of work, escalating healthcare costs, and long-term illnesses, particularly among the most susceptible, such as children and the elderly.

In communities already affected by scarce resources, these economic costs can really mount up, courtesy of slower response during crises. As mentioned in some research, public health officials are not always adequately ready to detect and manage such threats, leaving a sort of hush-hush relationship around such key issues (Jalali et al., 2021). Meeting this challenge involves devising general strategies that combine public education, improvements in infrastructure, and improved training for the officials responsible for health—so that, ultimately, communities have a better opportunity to succeed against the dangers posed by *E. coli* and other waterborne insects (Figure 2.7).

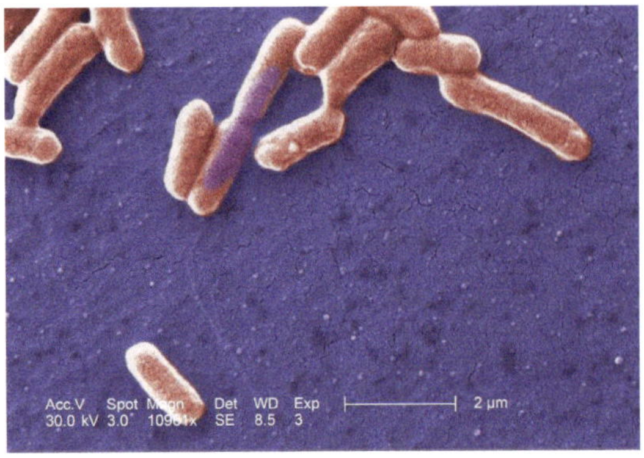

Figure 2.7. Schematic of *Escherichia coli* structure.

Source: By Photo courtesy CDC/Janice Haney Carr. - Original CDC image is herePhil Moyer https://www.flickr.com/photos/hukuzatuna/2536878015 Photo courtesy CDC/Janice Haney Carr., Public Domain, https://commons.wikimedia.org/w/index.php?curid=57721205

2.2.2. Giardia lamblia

Waterborne illnesses are quite a headache for communities with very little clean water, and small pathogens such as *Giardia lamblia* make things even worse. This protozoan pest, which is responsible for causing giardiasis, wreaks havoc with digestive processes. It primarily lurks in nature as resilient cysts that can survive in lakes, rivers, or other water sources. When these cysts get into human bodies, they tend to introduce ugly symptoms, diarrhea, bloating, and crampy aches that, with time, disrupt nutrient absorption. Recently, increased giardiasis cases have been broadly attributed to poor water treatment and water sources becoming contaminated with fecal material from infected individuals or animals, an indication that our water safety protocols seriously need improvement (Hoseinzadeh et al., 2021). The modes of transmission of *Giardia lamblia* truly highlight the grim interaction between the environment and human activity. Most often, contaminated drinking water is the primary causative agent of giardiasis. It usually results from a lack of sanitation or breakdown in water purification since regular filters are at times unable to trap these small 10–15 µm cysts. For instance, routine chlorination may not completely remove them, so they can remain in water sources during outbreak times. When you think about its occurrence in both surface and groundwater everywhere, it's obvious the parasite is adaptable and tenacious. In most instances, better monitoring combined with more sophisticated filtration technology is needed to keep this hardy pathogen under control (Todd et al., 1991).

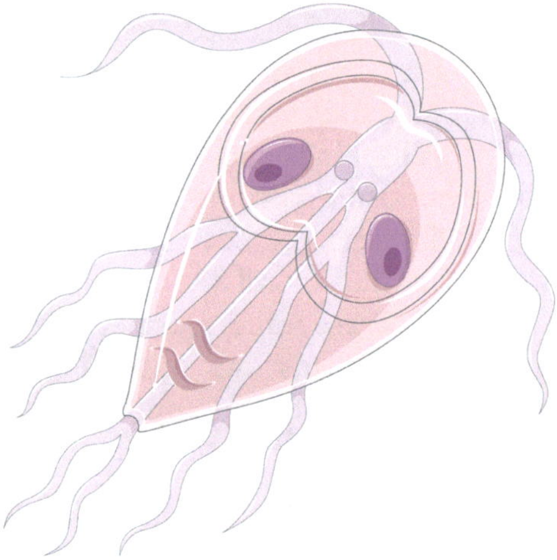

Figure 2.8. *Giardia lamblia*.

Source: By Laboratoires Servier - This file was made available with support from the Helpdesk at the Content Partnerships Hub. The Helpdesk provides hands-on support to community members working with content partnerships. Smart Servier website: Infectiology, CC BY-SA 3.0, https://commons.wikimedia.org/w/index.php?curid=128145855

Giardia lamblia's influence does not stop at a mere upset stomach, its influence can persist and result in long-term health issues, particularly in risk groups such as young children and those who have weakened immune systems. It has been reported by the World Health Organization that protozoan parasites such as *G. lamblia* are, on average, major contributors to disease and even premature death where healthcare facilities are already compromised. This situation creates a great workload for medical centers, not only in terms of the actual expenditures to treat giardiasis but also for lost productivity and reduced quality of life in patients. With increased awareness of waterborne threats around the world, an integrated strategy combining education, infrastructure development, and public participation is essential to mitigate the threats from *Giardia lamblia* and other pathogens (Hoseinzadeh et al., 2021) (Figure 2.8).

2.2.3. Norovirus

Norovirus is a well-known waterborne virus that transmits quickly and appears to linger in any kind of setting. It typically appears when individuals experience episodes of gastroenteritis—much vomiting, diarrhea, and abdominal cramps. You typically hear about it in busy places where sanitation and hygiene are not a priority. The virus survives on surfaces for extended periods, making contaminated food and water ordinary suspects. Understanding how norovirus spreads is important, particularly for vulnerable populations in communities; its capacity to spread through water systems only exacerbates health inequalities, so increasing water safety measures become imperative (Nichols et al., 2018). In most rural communities, where clean, safe drinking water is scarce, the risk of norovirus infection increases exponentially. Research tends to indicate that such communities experience a higher incidence of excreta-related disease due to inadequate sanitation and poor awareness of good hygiene. Surveillance data in the majority of instances tend to indicate increased risks of infection when water supplies are compromised, with norovirus and other such pathogens lingering in areas affected by water shortages (Peres, 2017).

This combination of water quality problems and health concerns makes it apparent that specific solutions; targeting improved sanitation and enhanced community education—are critically required.

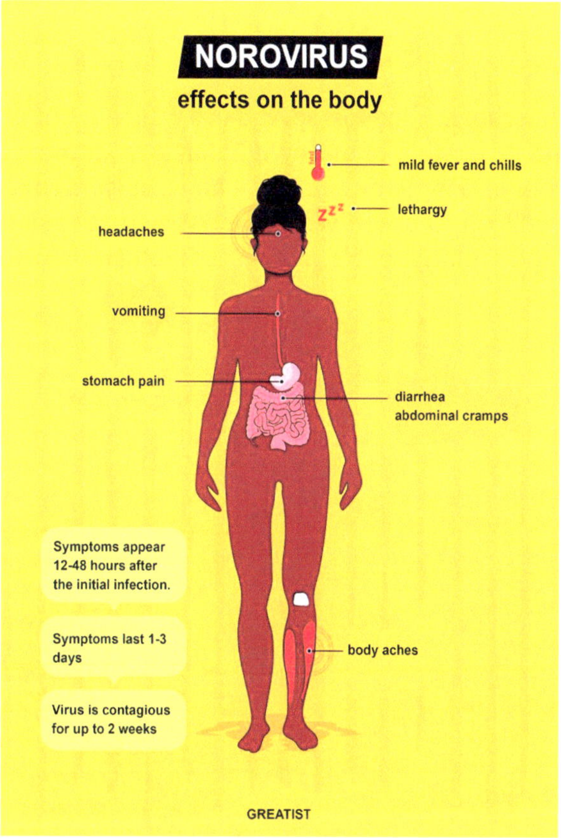

Figure 2.9. Norovirus: Effects on the body.

Source: Medium. (n.d.). *Norovirus: Effects on Body.*

Norovirus's effect isn't merely a matter of personal health, it has a ripple effect, impacting community productivity and taxing local healthcare resources. Hospitalizations are more likely to increase during outbreaks, which is an added burden for clinics that are already operating on lean budgets. Increased levels of sickness tend to cause absenteeism from schools and workplaces, hard-hitting local economies. Additionally, recurring outbreaks can make people in communities anxious and even distrustful of their food and water safety. Addressing these challenges requires a combination approach, one that combines public health measures with community education and robust infrastructure improvements to minimize the risk of norovirus (Nichols et al., 2018). Good water safety plans and reliable WASH procedures will be crucial in reducing the weight of this illness across the world (Figure 2.9).

2.3. Mechanisms of Transmission

Waterborne illnesses spread in a way that tends to be complex, weaving together natural circumstances with the effect of our own behaviors. In most societies, water becomes contaminated by pathogens from ill people or animals – an issue compounded when sewage systems and trash disposal simply aren't up to snuff. When infrastructure fails, the opportunity for toxic microbes to find their way into drinking water increases, typically increasing the likelihood of an outbreak.

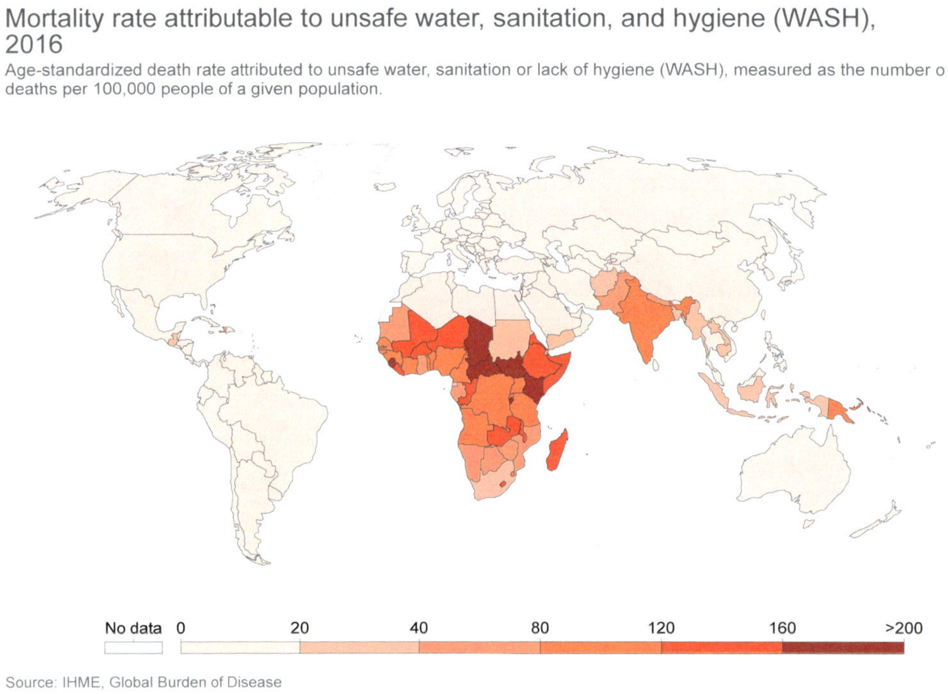

Figure 2.10. Schematic presentation of waterborne diseases transmission in human beings.

Source: By Our World In Data - https://ourworldindata.org/grapher/mortality-rate-attributable-to-wash, CC BY 3.0, https://commons.wikimedia.org/w/index.php?curid=86953269

This scenario strikes particularly in developing countries where both access to water and sanitation facilities are typically substandard. Climate change, through the disruption of rainfall patterns and the occurrence of unanticipated floods, can facilitate these pathogens to reproduce, thereby exposing community health to higher risks. Overall, the impending specter of outbreaks requires a firm emphasis on improved sanitation habits and tougher public health policies for safeguarding water quality (Angelos et al., 2017). Routine habits quite literally determine the spread of waterborne diseases. Inadequate handwashing, improper food handling, and overall breakdowns in personal hygiene facilitate the growth of pathogens and facilitate their spread. Sometimes water stored or transported in makeshift, unclean containers ends up collecting extra contamination along the way. Social setups, economic conditions, and cultural beliefs all mix together, making the picture even more complicated. In many cases, communities that lack access to clear health education remain unaware of simple ways to minimize these risks. Increasing awareness locally regarding hygiene and sanitation is primary, allowing communities to become active managers of their water health and the prevention of these illnesses (Angelos et al., 2017). Climate and environmental shifts are also contributing more heavily to how these diseases travel through populations. Increased temperatures in combination with changing rain and flood patterns leave reservoirs where pathogens can thrive. Severe weather events , such as flash floods – can strain sanitation systems, at times allowing untreated wastewater to contaminate drinking water sources. This type of feedback loop results in the fact that as climate change exacts its costs, the threat of waterborne outbreaks rises even higher, driving more public health issues. It's usually prudent to comprehend these environmental connections if we're to develop effective prevention measures. Current surveillance systems will need to be aligned with these emerging trends; with large-scale climate changes on the horizon, water management planning on a comprehensive level and readiness for community health becomes absolutely essential (Nichols et al., 2018) (Figure 2.10).

2.3.1. Contaminated Drinking Water

Clean potable water is a right that each person has, but dirty sources remain gigantic problems globally. In most locations, human activities and the surroundings tend to blend together in uncontrollable fashions that thrust waterborne diseases into the limelight. Climate change, for instance, has the tendency to disrupt natural water cycles and our supply systems, occasionally in manners we hardly anticipated. Places that do not receive adequate treatment or sanitation bear the brunt, leaving dirty bugs such as cholera and typhoid lingering. In general, rapid responses do make a difference; a combination of social and environmental variables results in no one-size-fits-all solution (Nichols et al., 2018). When individuals are left with dirty water, the impacts reach far beyond the mere speedy episode of illness. More often than not, it is not only immediate outbreaks such as increased gastrointestinal distress and cholera but also long-term health conditions that, with time, alter the fabric of the entire community. Such repeat water quality problems impose a major burden on health systems, making it more difficult for hospitals to attend to other needs. The families themselves can be financially hurt due to the constant health expenses, and local economies are sometimes affected by lost productivity, adding to the issues. In Massachusetts, for example, scientists have linked public health problems to water quality concerns (Das & Dorner, 2007). Saving water is not just a matter of running a filter; it requires strong infrastructure, sound investment, and genuine community commitment. Measurements must integrate both technological solutions and finance plans to enhance water quality, control sewage disposal, and enhance sanitation, particularly where climate change is expected to hit hardest. Research has demonstrated that when local authorities integrate hydrologic information with public health issues, the risk associated with water issues can be substantially lowered. A glimpse at how Massachusetts developed models to determine water vulnerabilities is a tidy instance of creative planning, allowing communities to better prepare for epidemics and take care of their people (Das & Dorner, 2007) (Figure 2.11).

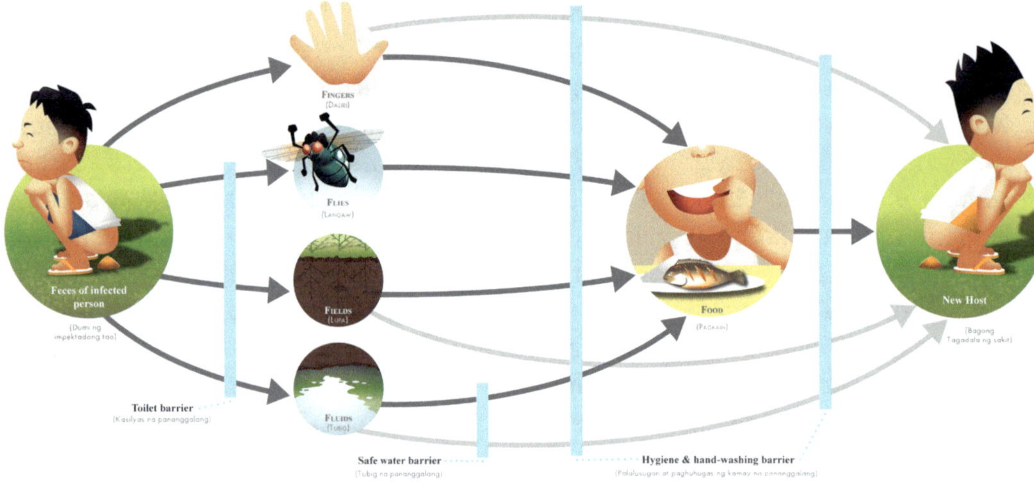

Figure 2.11. Potential impact of drinking contaminated water.

Source: By UNICEF Philippines and Luis Gatmaitan / 2014 / Gilbert F. Lavides - https://www.flickr.com/photos/gtzecosan/17125224489/in/set-72157648282032913, CC BY 2.0, https://commons.wikimedia.org/w/index.php?curid=39856655

2.3.2. Recreational Water Exposure

We love water sports without considering the unsuspected dangers—splashing about could leave you vulnerable to microbes. When people swim, surf, or water ski, particularly in nature areas that aren't regularly cleaned, those nuisance pathogens get a free ride. Pathogens like *Giardia, Cryptosporidium*, and some types of bacteria thrive in such environments, creating stomach illnesses that can really clog local healthcare systems. The incidence of these diseases usually relies on the quality of how well the water is maintained and managed, so frequent checks for these unwanted visitors are a necessity. Clean water for play isn't only a local problem; it's a wide-ranging public health issue, especially in regions where human activity or changing climates have compromised water quality (Nichols et al., 2018). Research now identifies unpredictable weather—imagine freak floods or downpours, often exacerbated by global warming, as a significant contributor to the spread of waterborne disease in recreational areas. A hard downpour or flood at times overwhelms sewage systems, leaving water tainted and unsafe for anyone wanting to take a plunge. Evidence indicates that during these events, agricultural and urban runoff has a tendency to deposit a range of pathogens into recreational waters, which lead to outbreaks of gastroillness and other diseases (Latendresse, 2023). Most times, combining erratic weather with low water quality is something we must reconsider when monitoring and managing areas where individuals take it easy and enjoy themselves. It's evident that the effect of contaminated recreational water is more than personal health, it can also be hard on local economies, particularly in areas where tourism is common. When there are outbreaks, they don't just overwhelm hospitals; they can also keep tourists away, hurting businesses and jobs. Public education, raising awareness, and maintaining facilities in reasonable condition all promote safer water recreation. Taking proactive measures such as frequent water quality testing and replacing aging infrastructure can reduce the health hazards associated with these environments. As communities struggle with altered climates and emerging microbes, it is imperative that a collective effort between government agencies, health professionals, and average citizens is taken to make our favorite splash areas safer (Nichols et al., 2018) (Figure 2.12).

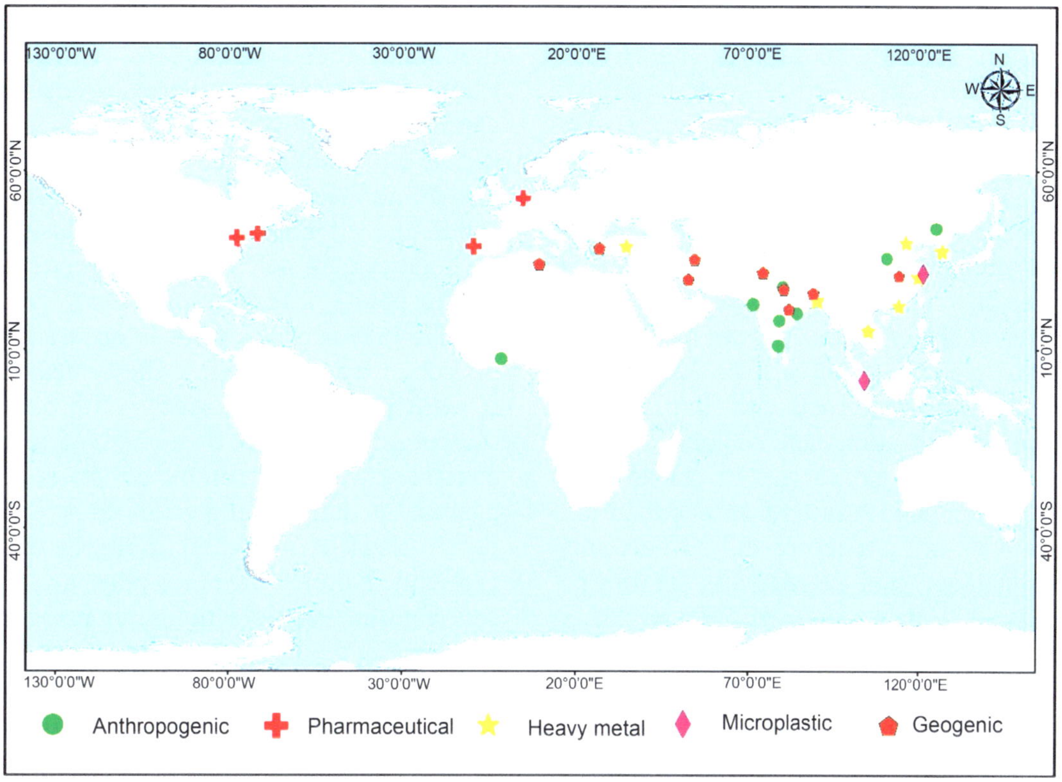

Figure 2.12. Number of waterborne disease outbreaks associated with recreational water.

Source: Babuji P, Thirumalaisamy S, Duraisamy K, Periyasamy G. Human Health Risks due to Exposure to Water Pollution: A Review. *Water*. 2023; 15(14):2532. https://doi.org/10.3390/w15142532

2.3.3. Foodborne Transmission

Foodborne illness owes much of its power to a complex combination of perps. Bacteria, viruses, and even those annoying parasites can creep into our food through several, usually unforeseen, stops on the farm-to-table journey. At other times, such incidents as contaminated water, careless kitchen cleanliness, or undercooked food become the prime sources of these illnesses. International trade, for instance, at times mixes around bad food around the world so quickly that tracing an outbreak's source becomes really difficult. The more hectic the world's markets become, the more likely widespread outbreaks start to enter the picture as well, which indicates a definite necessity for stricter checks and round-the-clock vigilance. How these foodborne microbes travel is not random, it is entwined with changes in our environment and lifestyle. Climate change, urbanization, and contemporary industrial agriculture are all pushing food supplies toward greater exposure. Rainwater runoff, transporting its incidental cargo of pathogens into production systems, illustrates how important water quality is. And then there's the reality that our changing travel patterns and local practices can sometimes introduce new, unfamiliar microbes to communities. All of these things are interconnected so that a wide-ranging, all-of-government strategy for evaluating risks and safeguarding public health becomes a need. When addressing foodborne transmission directly, it is sensible to take a One Health approach that brings together human, animal, and environmental health. This concept seems particularly apt when you realize that more than 60% of the known microbes that infect humans originate from animals (Rahman et al., 2020). In most instances, the solution lies in getting veterinarians, environmental scientists, and public health officials to join forces and keep these diseases under control. Strong food safety regulations, combined with simple public guidance on food handling and cooking, can do a great deal to reduce public health hazards. And, frankly, directing investments into education and improved infrastructure aligns perfectly with the broader goal of reducing foodborne hazards in our health systems (Morawska et al., 2021).

2.4. Risk Factors for Waterborne Diseases

Environmental and public health appear to be more interconnected than ever, particularly with regard to waterborne diseases. Climate change, which we tend to associate with global warming and erratic weather, sometimes gets our water systems in a twist, leading to problems such as tainted drinking water and epidemics of diseases like cholera and giardiasis. Flooding, droughts, and temperature fluctuations throw things out of whack erratically. More often than not, regions in developing areas are struck even harder because there is not sufficient access to clean water or adequate sanitation. All of this confused situation indicates that a sweeping, adaptable strategy, one that increases infrastructure and addresses environmental health, is required in areas with exceptional geographic and socio-economic challenges (Cianconi et al., 2020). Microbial responses are a further complication to this entire scenario. As our climate shifts and ecosystems change (usually in surprising ways), bacteria can grow and even intensify their resistance to treatment. A little warmer water, for example, may provide just the right conditions for pests such as Vibrio cholerae to thrive and multiply in aquatic environments. Short of it, these microscopic creatures—the so-called unseen majority—have a massive impact on health outcomes from waterborne diseases. Public health interventions, then, truly need to take into account what is occurring on the microbial front as well as the typical methods by which we monitor disease outbreaks. These bio-complexities may be addressed in order to construct wiser and more effective strategies against the dangers of unsafe water (Cavicchioli et al., 2019). And then there is the socio-economic factor, which also plays an important contribution. People with limited resources tend to reside in areas where infrastructure may be quite poor, so they're more likely to encounter issues with dirty water. In poor communities, the challenge is two-fold: not only is there difficulty accessing clean water and decent sanitation, but poor education and awareness can also retard proper hygiene. It's apparent that these social and economic determinants are large segments of the overall risk picture. As community health initiatives continue to grow, they need to consider economic hardship and increase educational initiatives so that long-term solutions for health equity, and a healthier community, can truly materialize (Cianconi et al., 2020).

2.4.1. Poor Sanitation and Hygiene

Sanitation is not only clean water, it's an important aspect of community health. In most areas, when good hygiene and cleanliness of water take a backseat, dangerous microbes have an opportunity to grow. Individuals become exposed to bacteria that live in unclean environments, which tends to cause outbreaks.

You can observe this with insects such as *Escherichia coli* and *Salmonella* spp.; research in Nigeria (Okafor, 2024) has indicated that where clean water and proper hygiene are absent, such pathogens wreak havoc. In the absence of sound sanitation, raw water is the frequent perpetrator of extreme cases of dehydration, malnutrition, and even death. Essentially, good sanitation habits are the way to minimize these hazardous health threats and establish true community resilience. Challenging hygiene measures practically invite all sorts of infections in. It's not a single problem—sometimes it is the absence of personal hygiene, poor food handling, or simply ignorance of the fundaments of secure practices. In most situations, unsanitary conditions provide viruses and bacteria with a free avenue to propagate, particularly those that are associated with food and water. Consider hepatitis A viruses of the Picornaviridae family, for example; these small mischief-makers appear to have just the right sort of neglected sanitary conditions to thrive in. Research has revealed that the complicated webbed production chains in food supply networks make it difficult to identify where contamination begins, something which only exacerbates the issue. Where hygiene education has not gained traction, outbreaks occur more frequently than they ought to—something that might be largely avoided through improved sanitation practices and focused public health campaigns (Simões et al., 2024). Sanitation and elementary hygiene problems radiate far past direct health issues. They reach far beyond to economic stability, and even the social cohesion of communities. When diseases caused by water infections attack, it's not merely a question of sickness and death; healthcare becomes over-extended and overall productivity suffers. A consistent pattern of illness can even drive children out of school and keep adults inactive. On top of that, the expense of treating preventable disease only adds to the economic burden. Solving such an involved mess of issues isn't simple, it requires a combination of intelligent infrastructure investment, mass hygiene education, and really hands-on community participation. In most cases, collaboration among governments, NGOs, and local stakeholders is absolutely vital if we're going to keep these pathogens in check and boost overall health outcomes (Okafor, 2024) (Figure 2.13).

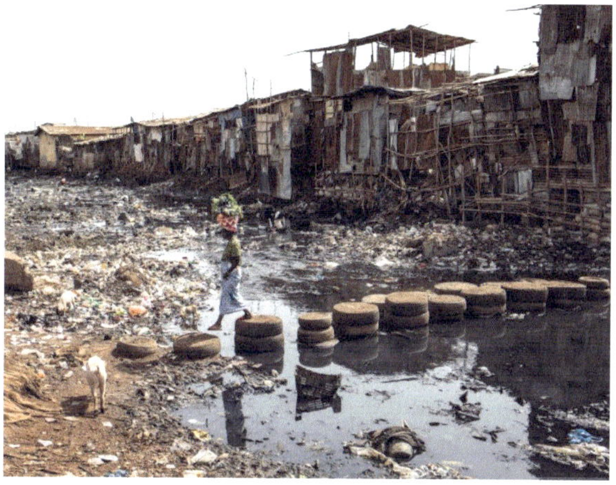

Figure 2.13. Poor sanitation causes disease and death.

Source: Getty Images. (2023). *Poor Sanitation Causes Disease and Death*. Jacobin.

2.4.2. Climate Change and Environmental Factors

Climate change is really shaking up our health landscape – we're seeing waterborne diseases pop up more and more as our environment shifts. Global warming brings on crazy weather, like floods that end up wrecking basic infrastructure and mucking up water supplies. When water gets contaminated, it turns into a perfect breeding ground for microbes such as *Vibrio cholerae*. In states such as Borno State, Nigeria, recurrent floods have had a devastating impact on water and sanitation infrastructure, causing massive surges in diseases such as cholera and diarrhea among displaced individuals. This all points to a glaring need for robust adaptation strategies that not only improve our health systems but also address the flood mess and malnutrition (Aborode et al., 2025). Meanwhile, bizarre changes in weather are driving disease carriers into new territory, making it much more difficult to manage outbreaks of waterborne illnesses. For instance, as temperatures rise, mosquitoes – you know, the ones responsible for malaria and dengue fever – are expanding their territories, threatening even more people. This spread has opened up the field of play for these pathogens and seriously complicated efforts to monitor and control them. In areas where the fundamental infrastructure is not up to par, the risk of cholera outbreaks and similar just increases. Public health interventions have to adapt, integrating nimble monitoring systems able to respond to climate fluctuations; investment in such more general methods is fairly vital if we wish to stay in front of the developing menace posed by infectious illness related to climate change (Zhang, 2024). Overall, the complicated combination of climate change, environmental stressors, and waterborne disease does present a dire public health issue that cannot be disregarded. People everywhere are now confronted with not only extreme weather conditions but with a quicker transfer of infectious disease – so it's now self-evident that an integrated strategy for health interventions must be attempted. Improving infrastructure and increasing public health education (and, sure, some international collaboration on what works) appear to be the way to stem the tide of such diseases. Ultimately, understanding how climate change affects our health is entirely critical to safeguarding communities and enhancing their resilience against future hardship (Zhang, 2024; Aborode et al., 2025).

2.4.3. Socioeconomic Status and Access to Clean Water

Clean water is not only a health issue, it's inherently connected to how resources are distributed in society. In a lot of developing regions, securing a stable water supply is not a simple task, and that compounds existing class disparities. Too often, richer households access superior water through investment in such items as better piping and filtering, while the poor suffer more from water-borne diseases that ultimately damage health as well as livelihood. As illness spreads this way, working opportunities diminish and even rudimentary health care becomes less accessible. Handling these water problems, therefore, truly demands policies that consider economic disparities, shattering a vicious cycle that traps many communities in bad health. Climate change also intensifies those challenges, affecting marginalized communities particularly badly because they're typically the least prepared to handle unanticipated weather changes. Rainfall becomes more unpredictable and severe events, such as unexpected floods or prolonged droughts, are frequent, which strains vulnerable water supplies, especially in the poor areas. Certain studies even observe that waterborne diseases, as well as emerging threats such as dengue and chikungunya, disproportionately affect people who are not well-off because they have less to spend on preventive measures or access to clean drinking water (Ahmed et al., 2020). In the majority of instances, measures to better the quality of water need to go hand-in-hand with adjusting to these changes in climate, reflecting that the combination of economic and environmental determinants requires one policy to ensure public health. The emerging challenge of AMR presents another level of complexity to communities that already face water that is not safe for consumption. In low and middle-income economies, AMR has commonly been attributed to inappropriate sanitation and unpurposeful sources of water (Fouz et al., 2020). Impure water turns into an abode of non-treatment susceptible bacteria that contribute to difficulty in eliminating the disease. Such an extra load goes disproportionately to underprivileged classes that lack adequate access to the right medical treatment. Consequently, the health disparities that arise from economic inequalities become further compounded when problems such as water quality and antibiotic-resistant microbes compound each other. To address this complex mess, a combination of measures—infrastructure upgrades, enhanced hygiene education, and equal access to medical treatment, are necessary to alleviate the overall burden of waterborne diseases in communities with varied economic problems (Figure 2.14).

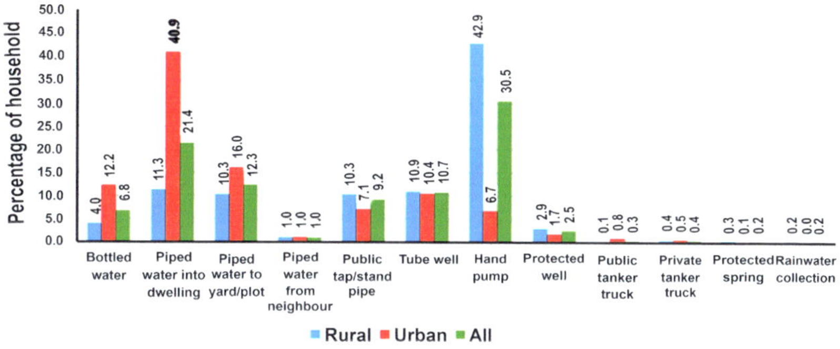

Figure 2.14. Percentage of households with access to principal sources of safe drinking water in India with resident type, 2018.

Source: Biswas, S., Dandapat, B., Alam, A. *et al.* India's achievement towards sustainable Development Goal 6 (Ensure availability and sustainable management of water and sanitation for all) in the 2030 Agenda. *BMC Public Health* **22**, 2142 (2022). https://doi.org/10.1186/s12889-022-14316-0

2.5. Health Impact on Communities

Waterborne disease strikes communities with vengeance, bringing with it a myriad of health issues that extend far beyond isolated incidents. All too frequently, these problems arise because water is not clean and sanitation is poor and thereby impact those who are already vulnerable even further. For instance, children aged four and below usually bear the worst of diarrhea, which in most instances, contributes to malnutrition and slows overall development. Households incur additional medical costs and lost income when sickness prevents individuals from going to work; occasionally, it even appears that the entire community's impaired healthcare system simply can't keep pace, eroding social cohesion and regional prosperity. Taking a step back, however, you can clearly understand how environmental conditions combine with waterborne disease transmission. Climate change, urbanization at lightning speed, and boorish water management all contribute to the increase of pathogens such as cholera and typhoid fever. Under unstable infrastructure in some regions, even a smidgen of rain or flood can cause systems to become overwhelmed, contaminating drinking water supplies; while warmer temperatures may even awaken poisonous algal blooms (Nichols et al., 2018). In general, these stressors inform us that preventing the spread of disease isn't just about health care, it's about paying attention to the natural world as well, combining ecological care with human well-being. Education is an important tool in combating the effects of these waterborne diseases. Educating people on simple safe water practices and good hygiene makes a big difference in infection reduction. Training programs that provide hands-on experience in sanitation and healthy practices, based on the One Health frame of mind, assist in building a more educated public (Angelos et al., 2017). When individuals are better informed, they begin to take responsibility for their own health, and collaborations between government, NGOs, and local organizations can mobilize the resources required for improved access to water and effective prevention (Angelos et al., 2017). These partnerships frequently result in early-warning systems and a faster response to outbreaks. Overall, consistent community involvement and education can soften the heavy burden of these diseases and assist in creating a healthier future.

2.5.1. Acute Health Effects

People tend to get hurt when their water isn't pure. Unclean water seriously strikes a blow—weak sanitation and contaminated resources create infections that spread quickly and become significant issues. Microorganisms such as *Escherichia coli*, as well as cholera and rotavirus, naturally reproduce in dirty environments, spreading quickly with immediate symptoms like gastrointestinal infections. Such a case doesn't only test our health services; it also affects routine, particularly for individuals who are already vulnerable.

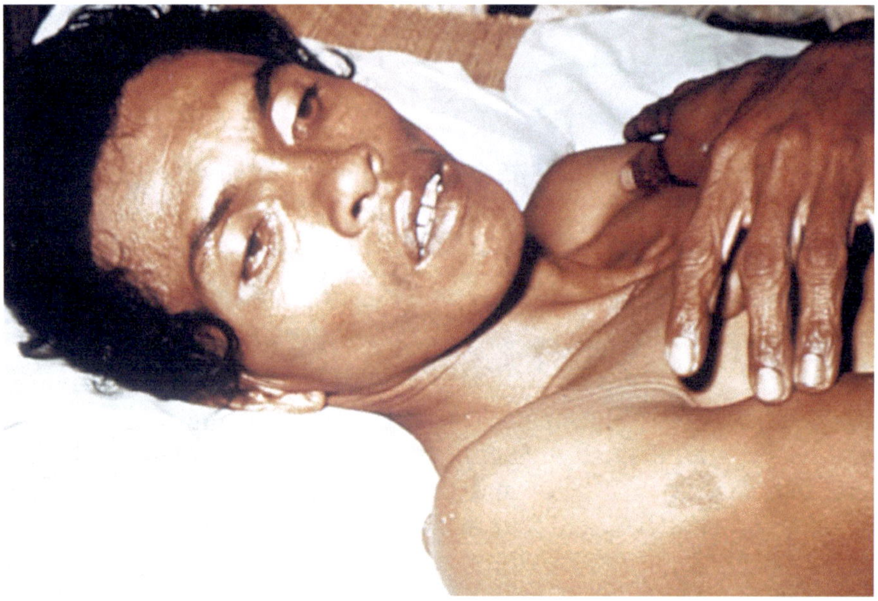

Figure 2.15. A person with severe dehydration due to cholera, causing sunken eyes and wrinkled hands and skin.

Source: Wikimedia Commons. (n.d.). *Adult Cholera Patient.*

Understanding how they work and how they spread is usually paramount to establishing public health action that holds immediate threats at bay. Illness from contaminated water usually manifests itself almost instantly and reaches beyond the individual to society as a whole. Local hospitals and clinics tend to become besieged with the sudden flood of waterborne illnesses, and in most low-resource settings, delays in treatment only serve to aggravate the situation, occasionally resulting in unnecessary losses among children and the elderly. Improved natural resource management appears to be inextricably linked with better water quality, which in itself reduces the incidence of these acute illnesses. A number of studies, such as one examining strategic watershed management and pollution control (Elmadani et al., 2024), suggest that these interventions can contribute to reducing the steep incline of water-related health ailments and enhancing the overall wellbeing of communities. Disease management related to water involves looking deeply into how a community works when there are unexpected health problems. Environmental circumstances, economic hardship, and the public health support available all interact to determine how people cope with these emergencies. When disease is rampant, it can create a cycle of sickness and poverty—making it all the more important that policymakers prioritize short-term relief as well as long-term care of the ecosystem. In the majority, studies indicate that even in instances where several competing microbe species exist side by side (Chen et al., 2024) highlight how intricate the connections between our well-being and the environment are. In addressing these interfused issues, communities can better negotiate the unforeseen effects of waterborne pathogens, setting the path towards a healthier future (Figure 2.15).

2.5.2. Long-Term Health Consequences

Waterborne illnesses strike communities in ways that extend far beyond a brief bout of illness. They do more than usher in short-term sickness; they also initiate long-term consequences that have the power to truly alter someone's day-to-day existence and stress out entire neighborhoods. Being repeatedly exposed to the insects that cause cholera or typhoid commonly ignites chronic belly problems, keeps kids from getting proper nutrition, and even stunts their development. Individuals who already have compromised immune defenses are likely to become trapped in a cycle of additional infections and ongoing health issues.

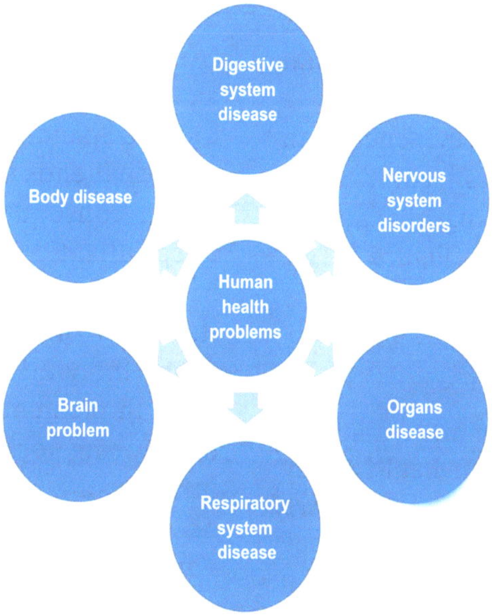

Figure 2.16. Long-term health impact of biological contamination in drinking water.

Source: ResearchGate. (2022). *Health Impact of Biological Contamination in Drinking Water.*

All this places additional pressure on our healthcare systems, diverts money away from other pressing requirements, and tends to disrupt the economic balance their overall (Vosa et al., 2025). It's not just the physical body that's harmed—there is also a psychological one, which tends to go unnoticed. Most who struggle with these illnesses find themselves battling not only the surprise of acute disease, but also the crushing burden of social shame, loneliness, and even economic loss from medical expenses or lost income. In communities struck by recurring cholera outbreaks, the psychological consequences can accumulate, appearing as worry, episodes of depression, and even decreased school performance in children. These conditions combine in such a way that they often keep individuals caught in a cycle of poverty and disease (Omoregie, 2024). Being able to control these long-term effects appears key to writing policies that are genuinely preventing waterborne diseases. In most instances, making sure everyone has clean water, improved sanitation, and basic hygiene education is step one. It is also reasonable to integrate mental health support directly into our current care arrangements—this gives us a more complete view of what individuals require. The complex interlinking between bodily illness and mental distress clearly highlights the necessity for a wide range of strategies, based on evidence from multiple disciplines, to establish community resilience and assist in achieving a healthier future for all (Vosa et al., 2025) (Figure 2.16).

2.5.3. Economic Burden on Healthcare Systems

Waterborne diseases strike us on more than one front. They do not only threaten health; they also push additional expenses onto healthcare systems. Epidemics compel individuals to pay for things such as treatments, hospitalization and even normal prevention. In most developing regions, where hospitals and clinics usually have weak support, the effect is even more severe—more get infected, and unfortunately, death rates increase. Extreme weather, such as sudden heavy rainfall, can spur a spike in cases. More often than not, such events overwhelm already strained facilities, causing additional funds into action. One systematic review even attributed these heavy precipitation events to disease spikes, quietly highlighting the financial burden on public health activities (Latendresse, 2023). On top of this, waterborne outbreaks have a lasting economic impact. Long-term conditions that result from these illnesses aren't merely individual losses, they reduce efficiency and even erode the economic health of a community. Absent workdays are an added expense, accumulating on top of direct treatment costs.

Repeatedly affected communities tend to have government and NGO budgets redirected toward immediate response rather than sustained improvement. In this complex feedback loop, even the resilience of a whole community can suffer if affected. Generally, by recognizing these blended financial impacts, policymakers could develop more intelligent investments in stronger healthcare systems (Nichols et al., 2018). Prevention does provide an attractive way out of this vicious cycle, though. Spending on WASH infrastructure really pays dividends by decreasing disease episodes, which consequently saves on treatment and hospitalization requirements. For instance, having clean water available to everyone lowers the level of pathogens that are present, so fewer individuals end up requiring expensive care. Implementing measures such as disease monitoring locally and rapid-response teams further enhances preparedness when outbreaks occur. Furthermore, if local communities are educated on what to watch for, they will automatically take precautions that relieve pressure on health services. In the majority of instances, the combination of simple economic reasoning with public health interventions creates a smoother road to lessening the ripple impacts of waterborne diseases on society (Latendresse, 2023).

2.6. Prevention and Control Measures

Waterborne illness is threatening public health in a significant manner, and firm prevention procedures are crucial immediately. Enhancing water quality and developing sanitation infrastructures are the first things to consider. With effective wastewater treatment systems and easy access to potable water, the quantity of threatening pathogens can be reduced dramatically. For instance, establishing regular water testing, even if it only provides coarse early alerts, can assist in signaling possible outbreaks and prevent people from exposure to harmful microbes. Public health campaigns stressing sound hygienic practices can also have an effect by pushing communities towards safer habits. And, by and large, as AMR is putting our health care systems to the test more today, these simple measures are more critical to combating both waterborne illnesses and their connection to AMR (Tang et al., 2023). As well as increasing water safety, it's also important to engage communities. Often, local-led projects—from educational initiatives to organizing local health professionals—aid in word of mouth about how these illnesses spread. When you look at human, animal, and environmental health connections, it's obvious that approaches must change following local threats. The One Health Approach is not theoretical mumbo-jumbo; it braids together various disciplines, particularly in locations where urban development is altering and climate change could allow zoonotic pathogens to go unnoticed (Md. Rahman et al., 2020). Collaborating, either from the agriculture or public health sides, can reduce immediate outbreak risks while constructing long-term resilience and improved local health understanding. Protecting our water assets for the long term is another important part of the equation. Policies promoting responsible water usage, protection, and equitable access to a safe water supply need to be top priorities to prevent health hazards. Regulations on wastewater discharge along with assistance for water purification technology can have a significant impact on the number of individuals who become exposed to harmful microbes, especially among vulnerable groups. International partnerships, in the majority of instances, pave the way for the exchange of know-how and enhancing local water management capabilities. As waterborne disease tends to disproportionately affect the communities that are already most vulnerable, providing everyone access to clean water and proper sanitation is nothing but a fundamental right. Finally, combining these preventative measures with large-scale public health interventions can treat waterborne ailments while improving the general health and quality of life of communities (Rahman et al., 2020; Tang et al., 2023).

2.6.1. Water Treatment and Purification Methods

Waterborne illness provides us with good reason to be concerned, so efficient water purification techniques are essential. Rather than depending on a single process, most treatment systems employ multiple. Begin with filtration—substances such as sand, carbon, or membranes trap particles and even small microbes. Follow that with disinfection, in which chemicals such as chlorine or more modern alternatives such as ultraviolet (UV) light (which disrupts pathogens' DNA, basically making them inactive) are employed. This step-by-step process generally prevents bugs such as *E. coli* and viruses like norovirus from spreading, a method that assists in safeguarding those most vulnerable. In most instances, acquiring a good grasp of these methods can reduce the incidence of waterborne disease. Beyond the standard physical and chemical solutions, recent water treatment developments trend toward more sustainable options. For instance, bio-filtration employs natural bacteria to degrade organic pollutants, minimizing the use of additional chemicals and maintaining the ecosystem in better balance. Such creative systems enhance water quality while addressing broader health concerns, illustrating how human health and environmental stewardship so frequently go together. Local people become involved as well; with training and education initiatives that enable individuals to better manage water resources (Figure 2.17).

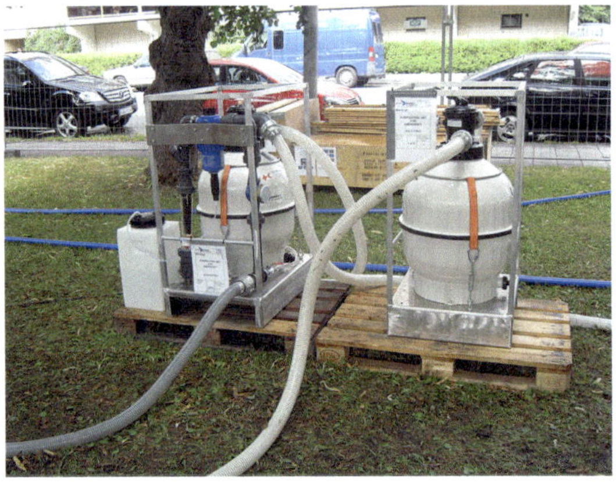

Figure 2.17. Portable water purification unit.

Source: Wikimedia Commons. (n.d.). *Water Purification Unit.*

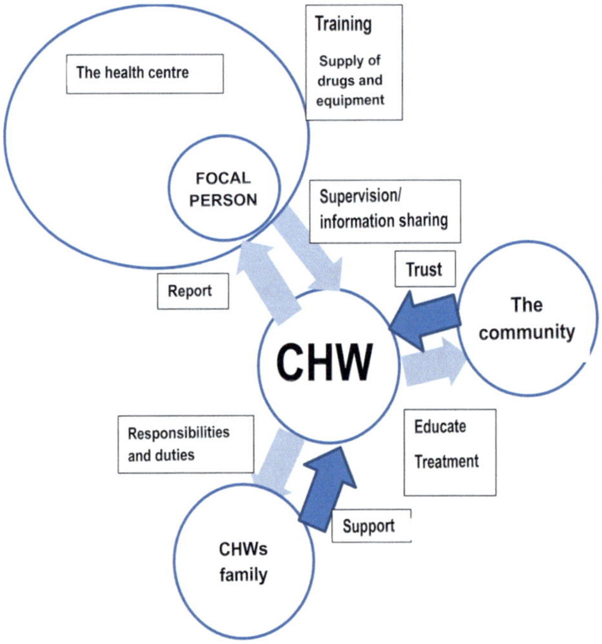

Figure 2.18. An adopted conceptual map of the CHW framework.

Source: Journal of Global Health Reports. (n.d.). *An Adopted Conceptual Map of the CHW Framework.*

Interventions that deploy community health workers (CHWs) and provide on-the-job training ensure the safe handling of water; where CHWs are adequately resourced, they provide good-quality health care and promote community confidence in water safety programs (Smith Paintain et al., 2014). Examining further, education for water safety seems to be an integral component of the picture. Public policy now tends to check the One Health box by connecting water treatment with larger environmental and health issues. Curriculums even now occasionally incorporate water safety, sanitation, and even food security content, making for a more informed populace. Underpinning educational systems (Angelos et al., 2017) have aided in the development of programs targeting water quality and other determinants of community health. Supporting these educational interventions with communities will enable them to be resilient against the numerous challenges presented by waterborne disease. In plain language, increased awareness and active water management can result in a significant enhancement of overall public health and a decrease in waterborne illness cases (Figure 2.18).

2.6.2. Public Health Education and Awareness

Public health education is more than a set of facts, it provides individuals with an actual chance to prevent waterborne diseases before they spread. When people learn the skill to recognize early indications and track where these pests begin, they can act quickly, and of course, reduce the odds of outbreaks. Certain programs blend in day-to-day advice on being clean, safe drinking habits, and right sanitation in a manner that is accessible to all; like, keeping it simple with boiling water or opting for a good filter can make a significant impact. Even identifying where these lethal microbes originate, such as those zoonotic agents mentioned by Rahman et al. (2020), contributes to a fundamental knowledge base that can lead to faster, wiser solutions. And, besides that, when people are educated, they will be more likely to demand cleaner systems and infrastructure to keep their water clean. It also makes a huge difference to understand how these uglies get around. Consider it: tainted drinking water, poor sewage removal, and just plain complex sanitation are all avenues these pathogens can take. And if you add in some externalities—climate change, say, as suggested in Cavicchioli et al. (2019)—the scene gets even more complicated (and, uh, a little complex). When individuals start connecting the dots between our warming planet and water quality problems, they tend to start reconsidering daily habits and become more conscientious about what they consume and how they process their water. Public health campaigns that use simple, earthy language have a way of reaching into daily life, pushing people in the direction of healthier habits without being too textbook. Ultimately, addressing waterborne illnesses requires a collaborative effort. Government agencies, nonprofits, and community members all have their role in implementing strategies that can reach everyone. Such collaboration not only reduces the effect of epidemics but also develops resilience to more profound social issues that allow these diseases to persist. By emphasizing the dissemination of useful information on microbes, their modes of transportation, and prevention, communities gain a form of collective expertise that makes them stronger even when things become slightly volatile. To summarize, mixing practical tips with community advocacy helps everyone move toward a healthier, safer future.

2.6.3. Policy and Regulatory Frameworks

Waterborne illnesses hit us on many levels, and the need for solid policies shows up as more than just an afterthought. We're talking about putting together rules that not only keep an eye on water quality but also wrap public health into one neat package. Governments can lower risks from nasty bugs like bacteria, viruses, and protozoa by setting up broad regulations that cover water testing, treatment, and distribution. It's fascinating how international collaboration is increasing as well – you find projects that align with the UN's Sustainable Development Goals (SDGs) to enhance water safety. When many individuals and organizations are involved, it really supports the notion of remaining proactive about accessing clean water and reducing disease transmission (Tang et al., 2023). Learning how our water systems interact with public health is another giant chunk of the puzzle. Consider this: our water and sanitation systems are at the core of both our well-being and economic security. Without proper systems, such as proper wastewater management or safe drinking water, communities become more vulnerable to dangerous pathogens. Therefore, regulations need to take into account whether or not our infrastructure can handle nature's accidents or other issues that may tamper with water safety (Stéphane et al., 2019). Evidently, combining robust infrastructure with effective health policies is essential to the creation of a system that holds waterborne illnesses at bay. While doing that, ensuring all get the word out is no less critical. Clear, simple communication can give individuals the power to identify dangers and take measures to prevent them. When campaigns educate people on simple water safety and sanitation practices, they can be effective in stopping disease transmission. It's convenient when policies allow people to report issues directly so that they can participate in the decision-making process in making these regulations. This dialogue back-and-forth not only keeps in check those in authority but also creates stronger, more resilient communities that can more effectively resist health dangers (Tang et al., 2023).

SUMMARY

Environmental factors and waterborne disease come as a package, calling on us to re-imagine how we deal with public health. Heavy flooding and rains disrupt water infrastructure and sanitation in a way that makes outbreaks more probable, and studies indicate that these severe weather conditions create the door through which pathogens can propagate in our communities. More often than not, it would appear that carefully examining how climate influences disease transmission is the way forward to developing savvy, effective interventions. This confluence of nature and disease highlights the fact that our previous models of preventing disease might no longer be sufficient (Latendresse, 2023). A closer examination reveals that waterborne illness tends to affect poor inner-city neighborhoods disproportionately. Individuals who reside in areas where the availability of clean water and good sanitation is limited are likely to be at greater risk. Social behavior and underlying vulnerabilities then further compound the issue, making a cycle such that ecological problems and low socio-economic status (SES) fuel each other. It is not so difficult to see why certain communities end up with an increased disease burden when all these elements are intertwined. Shoring up infrastructure, and even schools, can interrupt this vicious cycle, although the answers may not always be simple (Eisenberg et al., 2007). Ultimately, addressing waterborne illness requires a multi-layered game plan that combines environmental stewardship, social justice, and strong public health strategies. Essentially, constructing a framework that integrates all those disease-causing factors might lead to more effective, better-tailored responses. When ecology intersects daily social realities, decision-makers are able to tailor interventions to meet the actual needs of various communities. In addition, continued studies on how climate change reconfigures microbe behavior are paramount in creating future policies. Through collaboration across disciplines, in an at times chaotic but necessary manner—health officials can address these issues directly, opening the way to healthier, more sustainable communities (Eisenberg et al., 2007; Latendresse, 2023).

If you take a look at the complex combination of various microbes in our water, one sees that sweeping health plans are required. Most times, these little mischief-makers—bacteria, viruses, and protozoa—find a place to live in water that's less than sparkling clean. Their impact isn't experienced by one individual; they can turn entire communities upside down and even disrupt local economies. It's worth understanding how these diseases operate, from infection to spread, if we ever hope to end them. Identifying who's most vulnerable—typically people without consistent access to clean water—allows health workers to target their efforts where they'll be most effective. And when you look at those massive, sometimes staggering, figures of sickness and death, you get a sense of just how critical this problem truly is. Water is a primary route for microbes, revealing just how important good quality water and good sanitation are to preventing outbreaks. The fecal-oral route, for instance, reveals the connection between dirty water and the health dangers that strike poor communities hardest. Some recent research even implies that wastewater could be a breeding ground for these microbes, which makes control efforts even more complex. Finding fragments of viral RNA, such as from SARS-CoV-2, in wastewater creates the potential for expanded tracking techniques (Ruiz et al., 2020) that can monitor both waterborne and respiratory disease. It is obvious that educating individuals regarding regular hygiene and the safe use of water is important, and the combination of environmental science with public health is also becoming regarded as a fundamental instrument in limiting these problems globally. Addressing the harm of waterborne illnesses requires the combination of public health, environmental science, and social policy – an interdisciplinary approach many believe is required. Outbreaks do damage to more than just health; they increase healthcare costs, decrease productivity, and impose long-term social disturbance (Kitajima et al., 2020). In general terms, low-resource communities end up bearing most of these effects, further exacerbating already present inequalities. Global health systems and local authorities do need to work together in implementing sanitation and water treatment initiatives. Not only do these programs enhance water quality, but also reduce the transmission of many pathogens, with implications for broader public health objectives. Balancing prevention alongside treatment is imperative if we wish to construct enduring, healthier futures for those afflicted by these repeat problems.

KEY TERMS FROM THIS CHAPTER

Bacterial hotbeds	Bacterial water contamination	Clean potable water
Climate change	Community health workers	Dehydration
Disease outbreaks	Disease transmission	Environmental change
Environmental health	Excreta-related disease	Fecal contamination
Filtration technology	Gastroenteritis	Giardiasis
Hemolytic uremic syndrome	Hygiene education	Local healthcare systems
Malnutrition	Mental health support	Pathogenic microbes
Personal health	Public health interventions	Transmission dynamics
Typhoid fever	Water purification	Water safety protocols

CLOSER LOOK

CHOLERA

Cholera is a bacterial infection commonly transmitted by dirty water. Cholera results in severe diarrhea and dehydration. Cholera is lethal within hours if it goes untreated, even for healthy individuals. Severe cholera has been all but eradicated in developed nations by modern sewage and water purification. Cholera remains present in Africa, Southeast Asia and Haiti. The danger of a cholera epidemic is greatest when poverty, war or natural disasters compel individuals to reside close to one another under unsanitary conditions. Cholera is readily treatable. Severe dehydration can be avoided, thus preventing death, by using a simple and inexpensive rehydration fluid.

Symptoms:

- Most individuals infected with the cholera bacterium (*Vibrio cholerae*) remain symptom-free and unaware that they have been infected. However, since they pass cholera bacteria in their stool for seven to 14 days, they can transmit the disease to others through contaminated water.
- Most instances of cholera that result in symptoms create mild or moderate diarrhea that's frequently difficult to distinguish from diarrhea from other issues. Others develop more severe signs and symptoms of cholera, generally within a few days of contracting it.

Symptoms of Cholera Infection Can Include:

- **Diarrhea:** Cholera diarrhea is sudden and can result in rapid loss of dangerous amounts of fluid — up to a quart (approximately 1 liter) per hour. Cholera diarrhea usually has a watery, milky color that looks like rice rinsed from water.
- **Nausea and Vomiting:** Vomiting occurs especially in the early stages of cholera and can last for hours.
- **Dehydration:** Dehydration can occur within hours of the onset of cholera symptoms and is mild to severe. Severe dehydration is evidenced by a weight loss of 10% or more.

Symptoms and signs of cholera dehydration are irritability, tiredness, sunken eyes, dry mouth, intense thirst, dry, and wrinkled skin that doesn't quickly spring back when pinched into a fold, minimal or no urine output, low blood pressure, and abnormal heart rate.

Dehydration may cause a sudden loss of minerals in your bloodstream that help regulate the balance of fluids in your body. This is referred to as an electrolyte imbalance.

- **Electrolyte Imbalance:** An electrolyte imbalance can lead to serious signs and symptoms such as:
- **Muscle Cramps:** These result from the rapid loss of salts such as sodium, chloride, and potassium.
- **Shock:** This is one of the most severe dehydration complications. It follows when decreased blood volume leads to a reduction in blood pressure and a reduction in the level of oxygen in your body. Severe hypovolemic shock, if left untreated, may lead to death in minutes.

REFERENCES

1. Aborode, A. T., Otorkpa, O. J., Abdullateef, A. O., Oluwaseun, O. S., Adegoye, G. A., Aondongu, N. J., Oyetunji, I. O., Akingbola, A., Scott, G. Y., Kolawole, B. O., & Komakech, J. J. (2025). Impact of Climate Change-Induced Flooding Water Related Diseases and Malnutrition in Borno State, Nigeria: A Public Health Crisis. *Environmental health insights, 19*, 11786302251321683. https://doi.org/10.1177/11786302251321683(accessed on 14 May 2025).
2. Aguanno, R., Al Ariqi, L., Elkholy, A.A., Gardner, E., Grant, R., Pavade, G., von Dobschuetz, S. & D. Van Kerkhove, M. 2022. Global technical meeting on MERS-CoV and other emerging zoonotic coronaviruses – Virtual meeting 15–16 November 2021. FAO Animal Production and Health Report No. 16. Rome, FAO, Geneva, WHO and Paris, WOAH. https://doi.org/10.4060/cc1677en (accessed on 14 May 2025).
3. Ahmed, T., Zounemat-Kermani, M., & Scholz, M. (2020). Climate change, water quality and water-related challenges: A review with focus on Pakistan. *International Journal of Environmental Research and Public Health, 17*, 8518. https://doi.org/10.3390/ijerph17228518.
4. Eisenberg, J. N., Desai, M. A., Levy, K., Bates, S. J., Liang, S., Naumoff, K., & Scott, J. C. (2007). Environmental determinants of infectious disease: a framework for tracking causal links and guiding public health research. *Environmental health perspectives, 115*(8), 1216–1223. https://doi.org/10.1289/ehp.9806
5. Angelos, J. A., Arens, A. L., Johnson, H. A., Cadriel, J. L., & Osburn, B. I. (2017). One Health in food safety and security education: Subject matter outline for a curricular framework. *One health (Amsterdam, Netherlands), 3*, 56–65. https://doi.org/10.1016/j.onehlt.2017.04.001
6. Smith Paintain, L., Willey, B., Kedenge, S., Sharkey, A., Kim, J., Buj, V., Webster, J., Schellenberg, D., & Ngongo, N. (2014). Community health workers and stand-alone or integrated case management of malaria: a systematic literature review. *The American journal of tropical medicine and hygiene, 91*(3), 461–470. https://doi.org/10.4269/ajtmh.14-0094 (accessed on 14 May 2025).
7. Cavicchioli, R., Ripple, W. J., Timmis, K. N., Azam, F., Bakken, L. R., Baylis, M., Behrenfeld, M. J., et al. (2019). Scientists' warning to humanity: Microorganisms and climate change. *Nature Reviews Microbiology, 17*, 569–586. https://doi.org/10.1038/s41579-019-0222-5.
8. Chen Y, Liu Y, Liu X, Zhang Z, Zhang F. The Effects of Infectious Diseases on the Consequences of Interspecific Competition in Grassland Communities. *Diversity*. 2024; 16(4):231. https://doi.org/10.3390/d16040231 (accessed on 14 May 2025).
9. Cianconi, P., Betrò, S., & Janiri, L. (2020). The impact of climate change on mental health: A systematic descriptive review. *Frontiers in Psychiatry, 11*, 74. https://doi.org/10.3389/fpsyt.2020.00074.
10. Das, Debalina and Dorner, Sarah M., "Waterborne Diseases: Linking Public Health and Watershed Data" (2007). 2007. Paper 54. http://opensiuc.lib.siu.edu/ucowrconfs_2007/54 (accessed on 14 May 2025).
11. Divyashri G, Harini H, Likitha V, Lalitha Prasanna MV, Mahima ED, Shreya M. Traditional and Novel Foods as Vectors for Human Parasitic Diseases. J Biomed Res Environ Sci. 2024 May 28; 5(5): 474-487. doi: 10.37871/jbres1917, Article ID: JBRES1917, Available at: https://www.jelsciences.com/articles/jbres1917.pdf(accessed on 14 May 2025).

12. Elmadani, M., Kiptulon, E. K., Klára, S., & Orsolya, M. (2024). Systematic review of the impact of natural resource management on public health outcomes: Focus on water quality. *Resources.* https://www.semanticscholar.org/paper/b01c1455f01d739cf1de01d67d4012549a8bf5b6 (accessed on 14 May 2025).

13. Fenta, L. (2019). Effect of climate change on food and water borne diseases outbreak: A mini review. https://core.ac.uk/download/234684923.pdf (accessed on 14 May 2025).

14. Fouz, N., Pangesti, K. N. A., Yasir, M., Al-Malki, A. L., Azhar, E. I., Hill-Cawthorne, G., & Abd El Ghany, M. (2020). The contribution of wastewater to the transmission of antimicrobial resistance in the environment: Implications of mass collecting settings. *Tropical Medicine and Infectious Disease, 5*(1), 33. https://doi.org/10.3390/tropicalmed5010033.

15. Hallegatte, S., Rentschler, J., & Rozenberg, J. (2019). *Lifelines: The Resilient Infrastructure Opportunity*. Washington, DC: World Bank eBooks. https://doi.org/10.1596/978-1-4648-1430-3.

16. Nichols G, Lake I, Heaviside C. Climate Change and Water-Related Infectious Diseases. *Atmosphere.* 2018; 9(10):385. https://doi.org/10.3390/atmos9100385 (accessed on 14 May 2025).

17. Hoseinzadeh, E., Rostamian, A., Razaghi, M., & Wei, C. (2021). Waterborne transmission of protozoan parasites: A review of water resources in Iran—An update 2020. *Desalination and Water Treatment, 213*, 91–105. https://www.semanticscholar.org/paper/a45e84765496aee9920f00226231c0fa97d97298 (accessed on 14 May 2025).

18. Jalali FM, Gheibi M, Aghlmand R, Takhtravan A, Kian Z. Assessment and sensitive analysis of biological water risks in water resources with application of classical mass transfer computations. Ann Biomed Sci Eng. 2021; 5: 015-024. (accessed on 14 May 2025).

19. Kitajima, M., Ahmed, W., Bibby, K., Carducci, A., Gerba, C. P., Hamilton, K. A., Haramoto, E., et al. (2020). SARS-CoV-2 in wastewater: State of the knowledge and research needs. *The Science of the Total Environment, 739*, 139076. https://doi.org/10.1016/j.scitotenv.2020.139076.

20. Latendresse, Claire, "Drivers Of Global Waterborne Disease Transmission Following Extreme Precipitation Events: A Systematic Review" (2023). *Public Health Theses*. 2285. https://elischolar.library.yale.edu/ysphtdl/2285 (accessed on 14 May 2025).

21. Lebu, S., Kibone, W., Muoghalu, C. C., Ochaya, S., Salzberg, A., Bongomin, F., & Manga, M. (2023). Soil-transmitted helminths: A critical review of the impact of co-infections and implications for control and elimination. *PLOS Neglected Tropical Diseases, 17*. https://www.semanticscholar.org/paper/97566b06654bb31c75ca058d5ba87f4a5e5b9c37 (accessed on 14 May 2025).

22. Morawska, L., Allen, J. G., Bahnfleth, W. P., Bluyssen, P. M., Boerstra, A., Buonanno, G., Cao, J., et al. (2021). A paradigm shifts to combat indoor respiratory infection. *Science, 372*, 689–691. https://doi.org/10.1126/science.abg2025.

23. Mounsey, O., Marchetti, L., Parada, J., Alarcón, L. V., Aliverti, F., Avison, M. B., Ayala, C. S., Ballesteros, C., Best, C. M., Bettridge, J., Buchamer, A., Buldain, D., Carranza, A., Corti Isgro, M., Demeritt, D., Escobar, M. P., Gortari Castillo, L., Jaureguiberry, M., Lucas, M. F., Madoz, L. V., ... Pellegrino, M. (2024). Genomic epidemiology of third-generation cephalosporin-resistant *Escherichia coli* from Argentinian pig and dairy farms reveals animal-specific patterns of co-resistance and resistance mechanisms. *Applied and environmental microbiology, 90*(3), e0179123. https://doi.org/10.1128/aem.01791-23(accessed on 14 May 2025).

24. Okafor, C. A. (2024). Impact and interventions of waterborne and foodborne illnesses caused by bacterial pathogens in Nigeria: A review. *Food and Health*. https://www.semanticscholar.org/paper/81aa4514c66ceffe6413f3c40e43fe753e3124c2 (accessed on 14 May 2025).

25. Omoregie, J. (2024). The growing prevalence of Mpox and the impact on mental health: A public health emergency. *The American Journal of Social Science and Education Innovations*. https://www.semanticscholar.org/paper/a0881602740b2ae999ebedda268b29dd622356b3 (accessed on 14 May 2025).

26. Peres, M. R. (2017). Risk-based tools to prevent excreta-borne disease transmission in semi-arid rural communities. A document submitted in partial fulfilment of the requirements of the University of Brighton for award of the degree of PhD December 2017 School of Environment and Technology University of Brighton. https://core.ac.uk/download/379729155.pdf (accessed on 14 May 2025).

27. Rahman, M. T., Sobur, M. A., Islam, M. S., Ievy, S., Hossain, M. J., El Zowalaty, M. E., Rahman, A. T., et al. (2020). Zoonotic diseases: Etiology, impact, and control. *Microorganisms, 8*(9), 1405. https://doi.org/10.3390/microorganisms8091405.

28. Rohr, J. R., Barrett, C. B., Civitello, D. J., Craft, M. E., Delius, B. K., De Leo, G. A., Hudson, P. J., et al. (2019). Emerging human infectious diseases and the links to global food production. *Nature Sustainability, 2*, 445–456. https://doi.org/10.1038/s41893-019-0293-3.

29. Ruiz-Hitzky, E., Darder, M., Wicklein, B., Ruiz-García, C., Martín-Sampedro, R., del Real, G., & Aranda, P. (2020). Nanotechnology responses to COVID-19. *Advanced Healthcare Materials, 9*. https://doi.org/10.1002/adhm.202000979.

30. Simões, R. S. Q. (2024). Environmental virology linked to waterborne diseases and foodborne pathogens: Human and animal food viruses. *International Journal of Frontiers in Biology and Pharmacy Research*. Article DOI: https://doi.org/10.53294/ijfbpr.2024.5.1.0031. https://www.semanticscholar.org/paper/fa69ce9c1ec7472adebffe2b0fa68320ed94141e (accessed on 14 May 2025).

31. Singh, A., Mazumder, A., Das, S., Kanda, A., Tyagi, P., & Chaitanya, M. (2024). Harnessing the power of probiotics: Boosting immunity and safeguarding against various diseases and infections. *Recent Advances in Anti-Infective Drug Discovery*. DOI: 10.2174/0127724344308638240530065552. https://www.semanticscholar.org/paper/b04c7e7a70c739f83d7c8ff0e53248b572fa621e (accessed on 14 May 2025).

32. Tang, K. W. K., Millar, B. C., & Moore, J. E. (2023). Antimicrobial resistance (AMR). *British Journal of Biomedical Science, 80*. https://doi.org/10.3389/bjbs.2023.11387.

33. Todd, S., Phillips, M., Marchin, G., & Upton, S. J. (1991). *Cryptosporidium* and *Giardia* in surface waters in and around Manhattan, Kansas. *Transactions of the Kansas Academy of Science, 94*, 101. https://www.semanticscholar.org/paper/ac6b849403a74f223b4eb6de0bfb8121e5f7cea1 (accessed on 14 May 2025).

34. Vosa , O., Salibi, G., & Tzenios, N. (2025). Water pollution and its impact on human health in Nigeria. *Special Journal of the Medical Academy and Other Life Sciences., 3*(2). https://doi.org/10.58676/sjmas.v3i2.110(accessed on 14 May 2025).

35. Yano, T. K., Afrifa-Yamoah, E., Collins, J., Mueller, U., & Richardson, S. (2024). Mathematical modelling and analysis for the co-infection of viral and bacterial diseases:

A systematic review protocol. *BMJ Open, 14*. https://www.semanticscholar.org/paper/bf9845dd1a16d6fa356bbbf5302f4e881c8deedd (accessed on 14 May 2025).

36. Zhang, Y. (2024). Impact of Climate Change on Transmission Patterns of Infectious Diseases and Public Health Responses. *Highlights in Science, Engineering and Technology*, *123*, 71-76. https://doi.org/10.54097/p7328k87 (accessed on 14 May 2025).

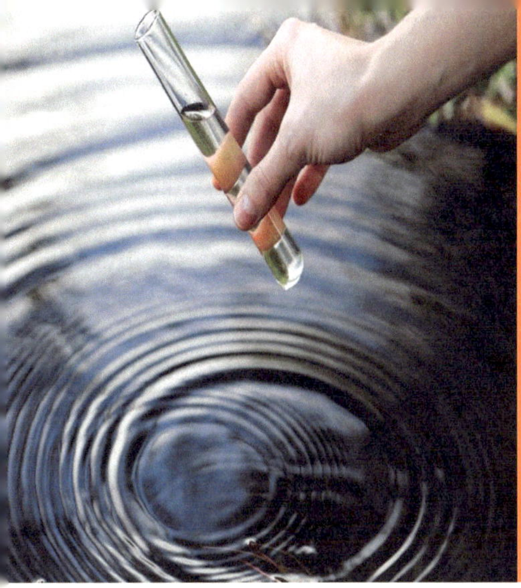

Chapter 3

WATER QUALITY: PARAMETERS AND TESTING

Contents

Introduction

Water quality is important—a big keeps our bodies alive but also keeps nature in check. Recently, however, water's consistently been threatened by all manner of things: heavy industry pumping out pollutants, chemicals raining down from agriculture, and cities sprouting up overnight. We genuinely need to monitor things such as pH levels, how cloudy the water becomes, the amount of bugs that swim about, and any unwanted chemicals. Research, in most situations, confirms that good testing practice serves as our initial barrier; by ensuring whether water complies with national standards, we protect those who cannot readily access safe water from illnesses (Intergovernmental Panel on Climate Change, 2023). Water quality standards are in place to inform us how safe water is and what levels we should adhere to. Consider, for example, United States Environmental Protection Agency (EPA) guidelines. Their regulations stemmed from mounds of research and changing data regarding how water pollutants affect our health. As a general rule, combining science results with policy-making is essential—community opinion is sometimes part of these discussions, too. Several evaluations even highlight that when water is not cleaned up, it tends to worsen existing social divisions because marginalized communities are usually most affected by pollution and the scarce availability of clean water. In essence, adherence to strong water quality measures is paramount to ensuring equitable health outcomes and developing resilient communities (Percie et al., 2020). There is a definite connection between water testing and the general well-being of our communities. Combining together different types of tests allows us to anticipate issues before they become full-blown crises, and that initial response can be a lifesaver. The information we obtain from those tests also informs policy and determines where resources are directed—making sure areas of greatest risk receive their share. Local public health initiatives, such as campaigns encouraging individuals to become educated about water safety and even contribute to testing, only reinforce this cycle of good. Ultimately, a hands-on, thorough knowledge of water quality, underpinned by sound testing and rigorous standards, truly empowers communities to take care of themselves and create a stronger future (Percie et al., 2020).

Definition of Water Quality

Water quality is not simply a matter of appearance; there is an entire combination of biology, chemistry, and physical indicators that collectively inform us about what's happening in our water systems. Rather than relying on appearances alone, you must consider things like pH, dissolved oxygen (DO) levels, and even the presence of toxic chemicals. In most instances, seasonal changes can throw these factors out of whack, disturbing aquatic life in ways that may not necessarily be immediately clear.

For instance, when scientists looked closer at Herohalli Lake, they discovered that various sampling locations had different tales to tell, with some places being in relatively better ecological health than others, which really underscores the value of monitoring on an ongoing basis (Raj & Philip, 2025). Water quality doesn't just impact the environment, it directly impacts our own health and the way communities grow. Access to clean drinking water is basic not only for preventing waterborne illnesses but also for improving daily life. It's widely acknowledged, and several studies attest, that where water is clean, infant mortality decreases and overall health problems are reduced, as a byproduct of which social and economic development ensues. Across much of the world, dirty water continues to drive diseases such as diarrhea and typhoid, and the importance of having assured safe water supplies should be self-evident (Sani et al., 2023). Having good standards and reliable testing protocols in place is entirely essential when it comes to water quality. Organizations such as the World Health Organization provide guidelines that assist communities and policymakers in determining what is "safe," and these regulations inform how we monitor everything from physical characteristics to chemical and biological constituents. Typically, intense testing serves as something of a checkpoint—a standard that keeps water management procedures in line. Through promoting sustainable habits and adhering to regular checks, it is evident that comprehensive water quality testing is essential to preserving public health and ensuring everyone can access clean water (Raj && Philip, 2025) (Figure 3.1).

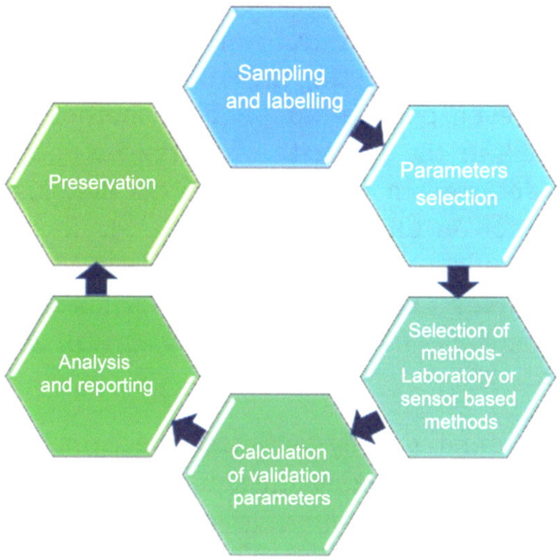

Figure 3.1. The water quality measurements.

Source: Geetha M, Bonthula S, Al-Maadeed S, Al-Lohedan H, Rajabathar JR, Arokiyaraj S, Sadasivuni KK. Research Trends in Smart Cost-Effective Water Quality Monitoring and Modeling: Special Focus on Artificial Intelligence. *Water*. 2023; 15(18):3293. https://doi.org/10.3390/w15183293

Importance of Water Quality in Public Health

Water quality is close to home when dirty water carries sickness all through a community. When water is dirty, it can cause a whole variety of issues, ranging from stomach cramps to chronic illness and even death. Most often, the most susceptible, children and seniors who are not as resilient against bugs, are the ones who feel the worst of these effects. It's obvious that maintaining water quality isn't merely a matter of compliance; it's a fundamental necessity for a healthy community. Different local initiatives, such as integrated management practices, cooperate in tandem to safeguard public health, even when they falter in implementation. Studies around places like Lake Sentani (Suhartawan, 2025) remind us that watching water quality closely and balancing nature with our needs is something everyone ultimately depends on. Securing a steady supply of clean water stands out as a game changer for public health services. In most instances, adding sustainable water systems to health centers improves the overall provision of care—from maintaining sanitation to standard to improved patient care. Consider the effort at the Bonggo Health Center, which demonstrates that mixing systematic methods with good old community wisdom makes all the difference. Cooperation between local populations and service teams, occasionally with a few teething issues—assists in determining precisely what the water requirements are and how they are best addressed. Adhering to health and safety rules, these ventures not only repair short-term problems but also lay the ground for future improvement in public health (Joni et al., 2024). It's a reminder that when health and clean water join forces, the benefits multiply in unexpected ways. Testing water quality is a key step in keeping our communities safe. Regular checks, for things like total dissolved solids (TDS), pH levels, and even tiny biological material, often catch hazards before they balloon into crises. This type of proactive strategy allows issues to be addressed early on so they don't end up becoming full-scale emergencies. When the proper testing strategies are implemented and guidelines are observed, it helps instill confidence that the water is indeed safe to consume. These steps go beyond simply checking off on health regulations; they instill public confidence and promote a broader culture of health awareness. Ultimately, regularly assessing water quality provides the firm information required for informed resource decisions and community planning.

3.1. Key Parameters of Water Quality

Water quality is not one measurement—rather, it's a mixture of variables that collectively determine whether water is suitable for drinking and safe for the environment. Microbial contamination is a major concern; bacteria, viruses, and protozoa can appear in water systems through sources such as agricultural runoff or even sewage discharge. These small intruders can disrupt community health, so testing must be comprehensive. New techniques, polymerase chain reaction (PCR) and even culture-independent methods, are now employed for faster, more accurate checks. Studies, in the majority of instances, indicate a concerning increase in antibiotic-resistant bacteria detected in water, a scenario that makes one wonder about public safety (Intergovernmental Panel on Climate Change, 2023). Chemical contaminants are another piece of the puzzle in this complex picture. Heavy metals, pesticides, and pharmaceuticals silently percolate into water resources until their presence is hazardous. Hexavalent chromium and lead, for example, are most notorious for carcinogenicity as well as the residual health damage they cause.

Researchers usually need instruments such as gas chromatography and mass spectrometry in order to trace these stealthy contaminants in an intricate mixture of water, and standards prescribed by the Environmental Protection Agency (EPA) are adamant about quantitative limits. Generally, adhering to these standards is imperative, particularly in societies that may rely on water sources that are susceptible to tainting (Dorothée et al., 2019). And then there are the simple, physical qualities of water such as temperature, turbidity, and pH, which, although simple, do make a difference. Temperature isn't merely an issue of comfort, it also determines how gases are absorbed and even affects metabolic levels in aquatic animals. Turbidity could suggest suspended solids that do not only restrict light but could also protect harmful microorganisms. And pH values, which adjust the chemical activity of contaminants and nutrients and metals' availability, feature prominently in water treatment. Regular monitoring of these variables offers a kind of early warning system, enabling communities to identify problems before they become inflated, and ensuring a more equitable approach to water safety overall (Intergovernmental Panel on Climate Change, 2023).

3.1.1. Physical Parameters (e.g., Temperature, Turbidity)

Temperature and water clarity give away a great deal about water conditions. Hot water is not merely a matter of a drop in oxygen; it also makes aquatic life work harder, and this can, in the long term, reduce the range of life below the surface. Observe how turbidity—usually caused by eroded land or pollution—reduces sunlight plants require. These small hints, when combined, really reveal what's happening under the surface and provide us with clues about our surroundings and public health. In most urban or industrial locations, the combination becomes even more complicated. Heavy water turbidity almost always indicates that undesirable pollutants are part of the mix, even if you can't immediately see them. Research overall indicates that industrial waste can increase turbidity and allow toxic metals to seep into aquatic ecosystems (Okereafor et al., 2020). Typically, performing routine turbidity tests, along with other water parameters, provides critical information for decision-makers in a local context. This data assists policy individuals and public health officials to determine how secure the water is. Typical methods for testing these characteristics are important to maintaining safety in our communities. Organizations have made regulations on what is acceptable as far as the warmth and cloudiness of water, whether it's used for drinking or recreational purposes. Adhering to these figures is important not only for water quality control but also for repelling waterborne illness, especially in at-risk areas. Newer testing methods have made it simpler and quicker to monitor these changes, reducing the risks associated with contaminated water. Overall, prioritizing these tests ensures communities stand a better chance of safeguarding their water and, by proxy, their overall health, reflecting continued efforts toward fighting pollution and climate change (Gonzales et al., 2019) (Figure 3.2).

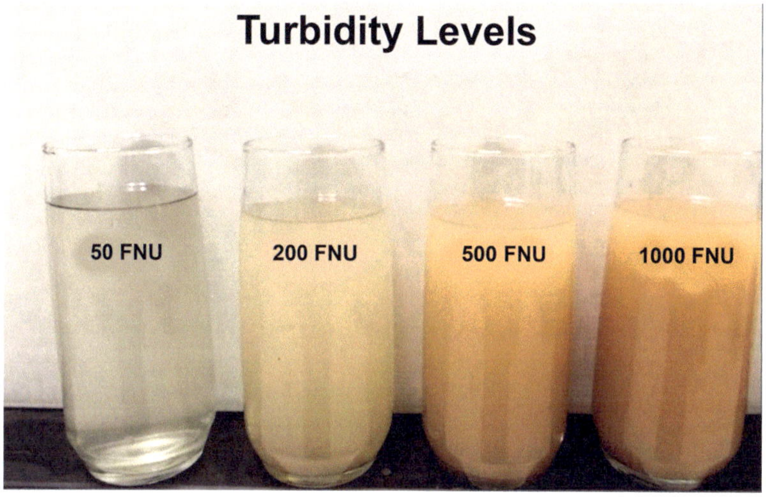

Figure 3.2. Turbidity levels.

Source: GCDAMP. (n.d.). *Turbidity Levels.*

3.1.2. Chemical Parameters (e.g., pH, Dissolved Oxygen)

Water quality impacts our day-to-day health more than we may recognize. pH, to take a specific instance, regulates the way nutrients and metals interact in water – a minor deviation out of that cozy neutral range (around 6.5–8.5) can ruin things. When the pH becomes too high or low, it can induce metal toxicity or deprive plants of essential nutrients. For the most part, excess acidity or alkalinity prevents plants from growing normally and then carries this effect through the food chain. Routine pH tests, honestly, provide safe swim areas and general well-being within the community, keeping the water critters and us in line. DO is another large component of water's wellness. Water animals rely on it to breathe – similar to how we use air. DO levels are not constant; they can fluctuate with changes in temperature, the rate at which organic matter decomposes, or even a stray pollutant. Low DO usually indicates problems such as eutrophication, which creates areas with little to no oxygen and threatens marine life.

For fishing communities or people who just like to hang out by the water, decreases in DO can trigger fish kills and even damage local economies severely. It is essential to check DO regularly if we're committed to maintaining our watering holes healthy and safe. Incorporating these chemical tests into daily water checks is important for intelligent environmental decision-making. As you observe how pH and DO communicate with other water chemistry indicators, you can intercept problems before they become worse. At other times, thorough testing even reveals industrial contaminants or unexpected changes in metal content—problems that could otherwise surprise individuals. In general, firm and sound testing procedures are not only about legislating; they cause industries to be accountable while reminding all of us just how important clean water is to our health and the health of our communities (Figure 3.3).

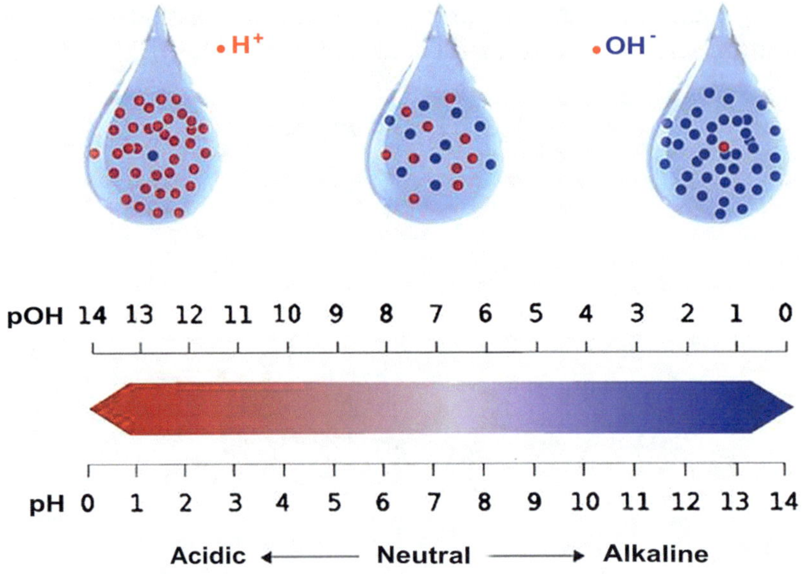

Figure 3.3. pH of water.

Source: Hassan Omer, N. (2020). Water Quality Parameters. IntechOpen. doi: 10.5772/intechopen.89657

3.1.3. Biological Parameters (e.g., Pathogens, Nutrients)

Biological processes in water quality are a significant thing, they give us a true sense of how healthy our water systems are and even suggest threats to public health. Pests such as bacteria, viruses, and even small protozoa are major indicators. Their occurrence in water usually indicates problems, sometimes materializing as stomach flu or other challenging waterborne diseases. Testing techniques that monitor these small creatures allow communities to detect contamination early and respond, sometimes utilizing such as fecal coliform bacteria as a proxy for even more vile pathogens. This method of testing water not only safeguards our drinking water; it also plays a role in caring for where people swim (Dadlani et al., 2023). Nutrient concentrations, like those from nitrogen and phosphorus, put yet another spin on the water quality tale. Even though these nutrients are necessary for aquatic life, excess can cause a wrench in the system, leading to eutrophication that can trigger toxic algal blooms. Those blooms then create toxins that disrupt human health and wildlife; they can even disrupt whole ecosystems. Monitoring nutrient loads is central to supporting communities in controlling runoff from cities and farms equally , and by doing this, it reduces the adverse consequences of nutrient pollution. Undoubtedly, water analysis must include nutrients as well, providing a complete picture with environmental and human health in mind (Alengebawy et al., 2021). The interaction between pathogens and nutrients only adds another layer of complexity to the entire picture of water quality. Oftentimes, these microbes can change the movement of nutrients through water, and in most situations, too much of an excess of nutrients may snuggle up with pathogens, enhancing their survival rate and reproduction. For instance, nutrient-rich water can cause pathogens to linger longer, which, of course, makes it more complicated to keep individuals safe. Identifying these connections can assist in informing management approaches that suit the unique challenges of each water body. When tests examine a broad spectrum of biological indicators, communities are more capable of establishing water quality standards that not only meet regulatory targets but also promote a healthier environment for all (Dadlani et al., 2023) (Figure 3.4).

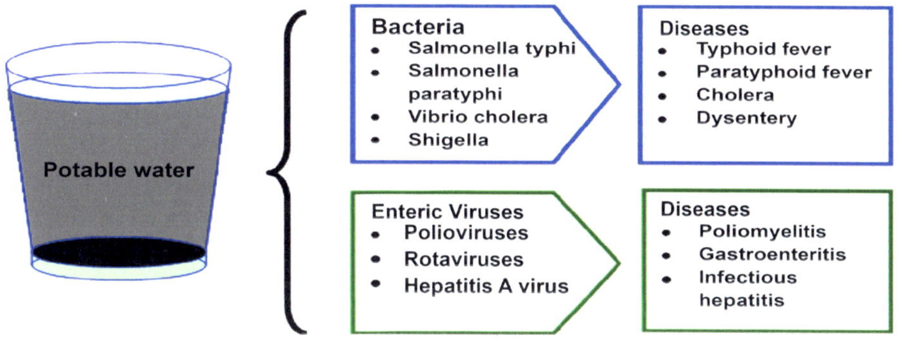

Figure 3.4. Common pathogens and relevant diseases in drinking water.

Source: Ewaid, S. (2016). *Common Pathogens and Relevant Diseases in Drinking Water*. ResearchGate.

3.2. Testing Methods for Water Quality

Safety from water is a delicate matter. The detection of contamination is a vital part, particularly identifying evidence of fecal material through the detection of *E. coli*. This small pest tends to warn that other pathogens may be present in the water, and that is why recommendations by entities such as WHO/UNICEF emphasize its detection. Individuals also fear excessive levels of arsenic and fluoride, considering their poisonous impact on community health. It's fascinating when you think that nearly 2 billion people globally still lack access to properly managed water, a statistic reiterated time and again by initiatives like the Joint Monitoring Program for Water Supply, Sanitation, and Hygiene. There have emerged new methods in water testing because communities require trustworthy and quick responses, particularly where resources are scarce. Standard lab tests are fine in a couple of respects, but they tend to encounter problems such as logistics, expense, and delay, which isn't really ideal when prompt action must be taken. As a stopgap measure, people have begun utilizing culture-based field tests that can be performed in the field, with room temperature incubation kits (Palou et al., 2022). Even better, synthetic biology is being prodded as a means to rapidly screen various water quality variables (Palou et al., 2022). These options are not only promising but also make testing much more accessible, even if they sometimes feel a little rough around the edges. Having a set of reliable testing protocols is just as vital as determining how to test in the first place. Regulatory bodies struggle to compile easier and more pragmatic standards that can be followed by all, which generally translates to improved evidence for public health policy. In the majority of instances, adherence to national and international standards isn't so much a regulation, it's how we marshal resources to assist areas most impacted by waterborne conditions. Test best practices end up linking with broader objectives, such as universal access to safe drinking water, which is something many organizations such as WHO and UNICEF continue to make the point about (Palou et al., 2022). All of it may be a little complex sometimes, but it is evidence that despite flaws, every step is one closer to safer water for all (Figure 3.5).

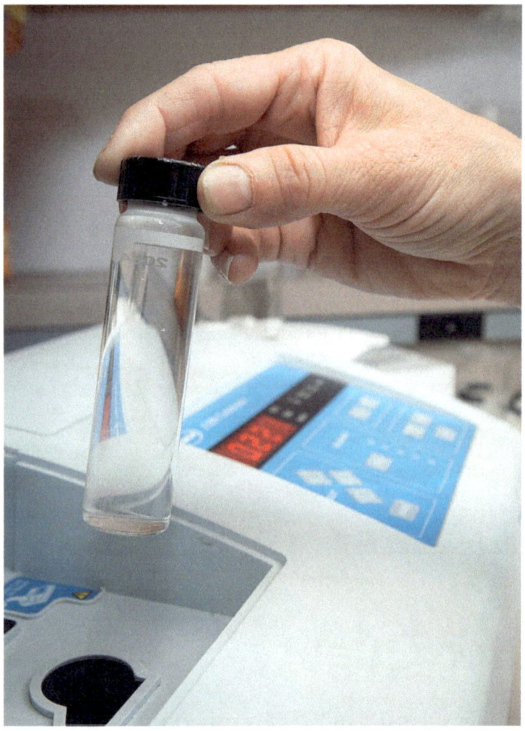

Figure 3.5. Drinking water testing.

Source: By U.S. Department of AgricultureLance Cheung/Photographer/USDA photo by Lance Cheung - 20150409-RD-LSC-0080, Public Domain, https://commons.wikimedia.org/w/index.php?curid=64976496

3.2.1. Field Testing Methods (e.g., Portable Kits)

Water quality matters a great deal, particularly when you factor in just how many communities are still struggling to access safe drinking water. Research continues to highlight that being able to have consistent, on-the-spot testing—that is, portable kits that will function even in extreme conditions in rural or remote areas— makes a significant difference. These kits allow people to test water without having to wait a long time for lab reports, so any potential issues can be addressed a little quicker. However, though they provide access, there's always the caveat that they must deliver up to certain standards for finding dangerous microbes. In the majority of instances, closing these availability and technology gaps is essential to getting long-term sustainable health solutions into low-income environments. When considering present-day portable testing technology, being able to meet thresholds such as the UNICEF target product profile (TPP) becomes a prerequisite. Currently, most testing kits for detecting *Escherichia coli* have serious drawbacks—usually they require their own power source and take between 18 and 24 hours to produce results, which is a very long time when every minute matters. It's ironic, really: these kits guarantee quick solutions, but none of them fully meet the TPP requirements.

This strongly indicates a crying need for innovation in the shape of low-cost, power-free substitutes that can still maintain accuracy and reliability. Overall, doing this properly would considerably enhance community health monitoring, particularly in resource-constrained areas. Although water quality testing field kits are slowly becoming more popular, there still exists a perceptible disconnect between what they can do and how often they are used in the field. They tend to be more expensive than the recommended 6 USD by UNICEF, and this discourages many communities from embracing them. It's not so much the price tag, however, conventional lab techniques are still the standard legally, making it more difficult to incorporate these handheld alternatives into daily health tracking. By lifting standards slightly, reducing costs, and attempting to make these technologies more accessible, portable testing really can revolutionize local health programs. Ongoing projects Pichel et al. (2023) seem to be taking on this challenge, pushing for safer water solutions one step at a time (Figure 3.6).

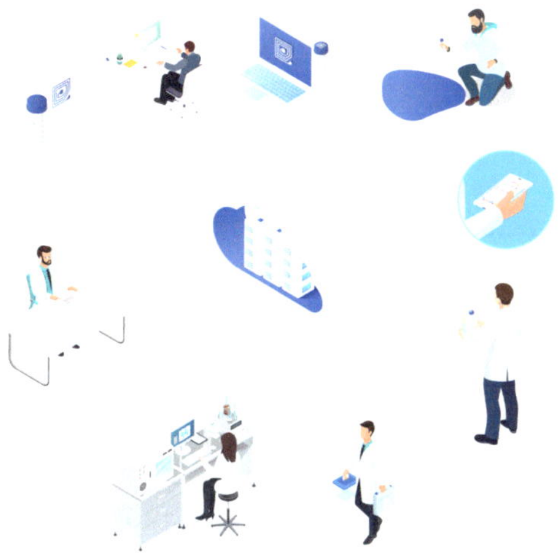

Figure 3.6. Field test kit diagram.

Source: ELICO Ltd. (2020). *Field Test Kit Diagram.*

3.2.2. Laboratory Testing Methods (e.g., Spectrophotometry)

Assessing our water's quality relies on a combination of laboratory tests that provide important information regarding environmental health. One of the best methods is spectrophotometry—a versatile technique that tests the amount of certain compounds by detecting light absorption at different wavelengths. This method, in general terms, allows scientists to detect contaminants such as heavy metals, nutrients, and organic contaminants; its accuracy is such that trace levels of pollutants are detectable, which is rather important when monitoring environmental changes and health issues around communities. Due to its ability to fit various types of samples, spectrophotometry is an in-demand method for furthering knowledge about water quality (Ali et al., 2021). Spectrophotometric testing not only detects pollutants but also casts some illumination on the microbial composition of the water. Recent research indicates that the community composition of microeukaryotes is subject to seasonal variation, thus affecting nutrient cycles and general water quality. By combining high-throughput sequencing with these light-based assays, scientists can track spatiotemporal patterns in microbial communities, seeing how environmental factors influence these ecosystems in a sometimes capricious manner. For instance, nutrient level fluctuations captured by spectrophotometry can complement shifts in diversity and biomass, providing a richer, if sometimes complicated, image of water dynamics. It is crucial to understand these relationships not only for compliance with regulations but also for informing sustainable water management strategies that safeguard community health (Chen et al., 2019).

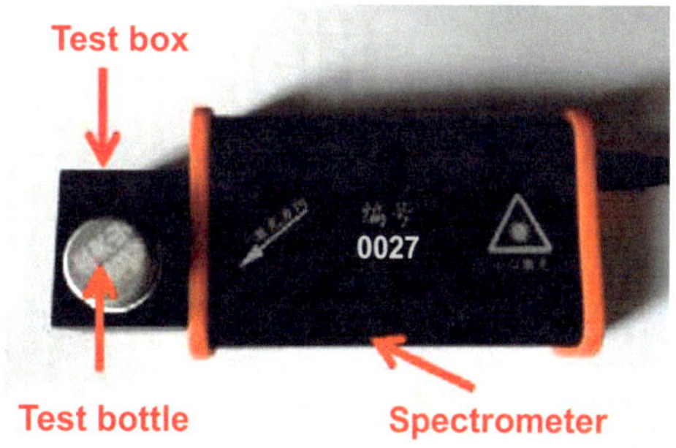

Figure 3.7. Water quality testing by the spectrometer.

Source: ResearchGate. (2020). *Water Quality Testing by the Spectrometer.*

Apart from light-based analysis, novel nanoparticle technologies are also stirring the waters of water testing. Magnetic nanoparticles (MNPs), for example, have been promising by enhancing the sensitivity and specificity of different testing processes. When functionalized to bind to specific contaminants, they essentially act as targeted biosensors that can monitor critical water quality parameters in real time. The combination of versatility and practicality in the application of MNPs to produce multifunctional materials represents a tremendous step towards advanced water testing techniques—a progress that ultimately aids community health programs. Despite challenges, continued research into creative laboratory techniques is poised to play an increasingly vital role in providing safe and sustainable water sources for all of us (Ali et al., 2021) (Figure 3.7).

3.2.3. Remote Sensing Technologies

Remote sensing has truly revolutionized the game for water quality monitoring. Today, people are realizing just how essential good water data are, so accessing satellite pictures and airborne sensors now captures all sorts of information on lakes, rivers, and ponds virtually on the fly. It monitors all sorts of things, including turbidity, chlorophyll concentrations, and even detects residues of unwanted chemicals. This method not only extends both the time and space reached but also reduces the heavy labor and expense that accompany traditional field sampling. In most instances, as neighborhoods strive to achieve water quality goals, this technology can identify potential hotspots, prompting authorities to take pre-emptive measures and, in so doing, protecting public health (David et al., 2020).

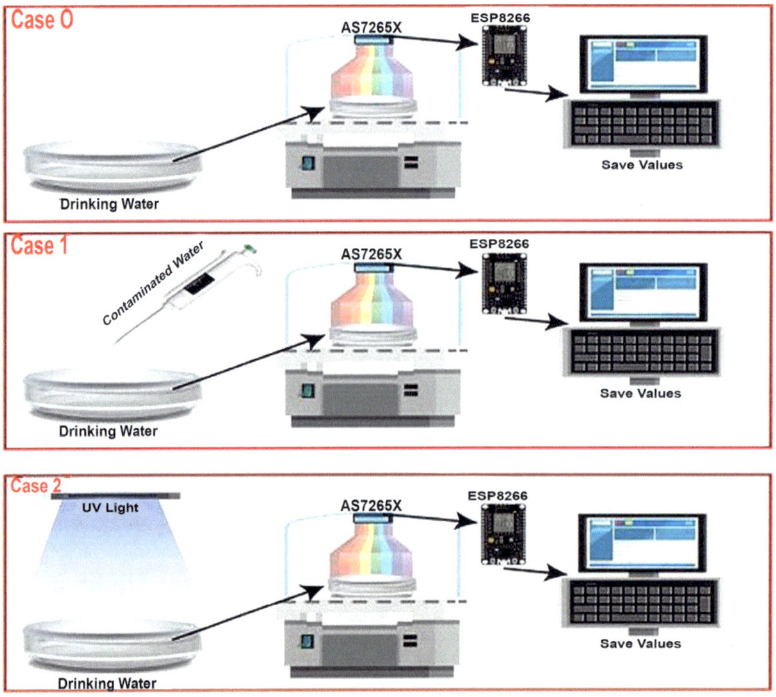

Figure 3.8. Remote sensing has really changed the game for monitoring water quality.

Source: Elsevier. (2024). *Remote Sensing Has Really Changed the Game for Monitoring Water Quality.*

Apart from basic monitoring, remote sensing is increasingly being utilized to predict how human endeavors and climate shifts may impact the quality of water. Rather sophisticated computer programs, usually regarded as state-of-the-art, are run on satellite images to simulate water movement, connecting everything from land use to the movement of water and pollution. For those communities that rely on neighborhood water to drink, cook, and even play, these observations are preliminary warnings for weaknesses that may require immediate repairs. At times, merging these technologies with local health programs even creates opportunities for study projects so that individuals can more readily engage to address water concerns. Data-driven strategies allow for customized reactions that fit every individual environmental condition, making the overall water degradation resilience greater (Rasheed et al., 2020). Remote sensing is not only a convenient tool for monitoring water quality; it is also part of a larger trend toward digital openness in environmental science. This technology revolution, borrowing concepts such as digital twins, enables stakeholders to see live water data in a virtual environment—a kind of digital viewfinder that can inform decisions. Policymakers and leaders in communities can experiment with modeled scenarios of prospective interventions, testing results before ever setting foot in the field. Overall, this ability to predict gives remote sensing its role as a cutting-edge tool in advancing wiser, more sustainable measures in water management. As societies continue to face intricate environmental issues, adopting these technologies remains central to ensuring high standards of water quality, and it ultimately ensures public health protection (David et al., 2020) (Figure 3.8).

3.3. Standards for Water Quality

Keeping our water safe isn't a luxury item to possess, it's entirely indispensable if you think about it. How often our health and local ecosystems are threatened by our very environment? Health authorities write government regulations establishing limits for undesirable material in our water, such as extreme pH, cloudiness (turbidity), and even tiny organisms colloquially known as pathogens. When our water surpasses these standards, it reduces waterborne sickness risks and enhances public health. Routine testing and looking out help go a big way toward providing people with access to water that's safe and reliable, which leads to better public health and quality of life. New test techniques are turning the industry on its head. Recently, smart devices such as handheld microfluidic tools have appeared, which allow individuals to test for toxic materials such as phosphates on the spot. This isn't about saving money, though, it's a step ahead that brings water safety testing within reach. While conventional methods tend to demand expensive lab equipment and skilled hands, these new machines bring possibilities for communities in developing countries to test water on-site without requiring special training. By doing this, they enable locals to look after their own health and facilitate awareness about water pollution problems (Miura et al., 2017). Meanwhile, the challenge of effectively utilizing rainwater and other unconventional water sources illustrates why strict standards are so necessary. In rain-abundant regions such as Indonesia, harvesting rainwater provides special opportunities to optimize water utilization. But if you cut corners on quality inspections, that same water might be a health error—a study, for example, showed a pH of 4.4 with overall coliform counts of about 6.1 CFU/100 ml, indicating it is not safe to drink without treatment. These types of mismatches truly emphasize why populations must test their water on a regular basis in accordance with public health regulations, such as Indonesia Health Minister Regulation No. 32 of 2017, to ensure that what they're drinking or washing with is safe (Asnaning et al., 2019).

3.3.1. National Standards (e.g., EPA Regulations)

Water quality regulations in the US are sort of complex—most of the knots come from standards established by the EPA. These standards aren't just about keeping lakes and streams under control; they help to protect individuals from dangerous contaminants too. Laws such as the Safe Drinking Water Act, for instance, drive heavy testing of everything from metals and microbes to organic chemicals. Since pollution sources continue to shift, it should be pretty apparent that the demand to revise and review these standards is essential. Consider PFAS, sometimes referred to as "forever chemicals" , and how well they illustrate how shifting threats compel the EPA to continuously rework its strategy in safeguarding public health (Wang et al., 2017). National standards not only establish compliance but function as guideposts for state and local agencies. These communities are going out to test water regularly and have EPA standards as their point of comparison to be able to provide everyone with safe drinking water. Local institutions are able to detect even minute concentrations of contaminants using equipment like spectrometry and chromatography, ensuring that their findings are in line with what the national standards anticipate. This is particularly crucial in the most impacted areas of pollution, where ongoing monitoring can identify potential health hazards early—allowing for tackling larger water quality problems (Wang et al., 2017). Public health policy hinges on the extent to which EPA regulations blend with community initiatives. When national standards are integrated into local practice, it's not merely clean water, it also empowers citizens to initiate advocacy and awareness initiatives based on freely shared information. That combination of high-level guidelines with grassroots efforts is particularly important in addressing health disparities brought about by environmental factors. And, while research continues to associate long-term exposure to low-level toxins with severe health consequences, even more COVID-19-linked deaths, an evergreen debate to toughen such standards is demonstrably necessary (Wu et al., 2020). For this alone, it's generally prudent to continue reviewing and adding muscle to these regulations in order to make them remain as effective as the next challenge, keeping our public safe (Figure 3.9).

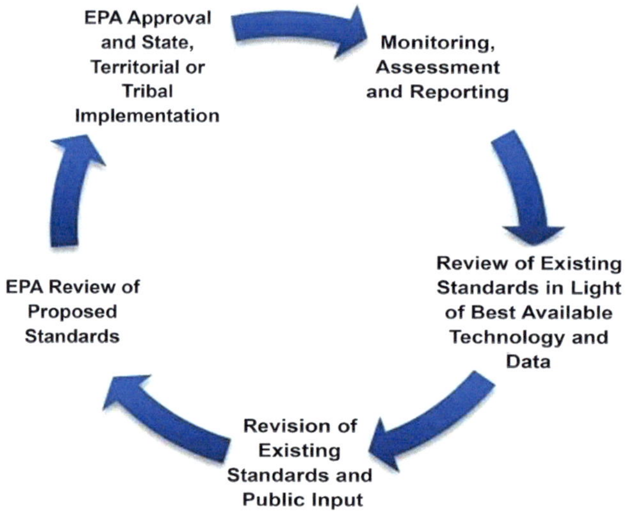

Figure 3.9. EPA regulations.

Source: U.S. Environmental Protection Agency. (2014). *EPA Regulations.*

3.3.2. International Standards (e.g., WHO Guidelines)

Guaranteeing our global health really comes down to how we take care of something as simple as clean water. We depend on initiatives that at times are a little disorganized but, fundamentally, all work towards safeguarding community well-being. The World Health Organization has truly come to be associated with laying down the guidelines for the safety of drinking water, which is central to avoiding waterborne diseases. Their recommendations – based on a combination of systematic reviews, expert discussions, and robust scientific evidence – run the gamut from chemical and physical issues to microbiological issues. These are not idle recommendations but significant standards against which countries can revise and refine their own water testing protocols in order to identify risks and assume any risks to public health, in general. In addition to this, there is the added twist of fighting antimicrobial resistance (AMR) alongside water safety. Inadequate water quality sometimes makes it easier for resistant microbes to spread, presenting yet another complication to public health. The WHO has, in many instances, underscored how much of a burden AMR can be, with things such as contaminated water having a significant factor to play. This constant interplay between water quality and AMR encourages policymakers to revisit water treatment practices and develop improved, more efficient solutions. An example is prioritizing safe sanitation and hygiene that isn't merely clean water, it's also about containing risks from persistent, drug-resistant pathogens; little strides that ultimately translate into larger community health projects. Regular checks on water quality are also heavily emphasized. The theory is that regular monitoring—by the newest testing technology—allows local health teams to collect accurate information and act fast when things go wrong, even when at times the process seems a little unbalanced. Ongoing such assessments not only keep communities adhering to international norms but also create confidence among people. The more people get to understand why it is important to keep water safe, the more likely the chances are that everyone will contribute to taking care of their own health. In the end, these standards take a prime position in improving community resilience and the fact that access to safe water is still a human right (Figure 3.10).

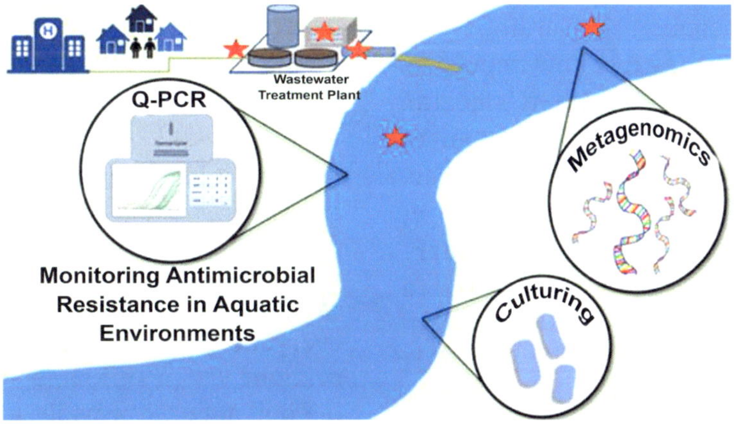

Figure 3.10. Antimicrobial resistance monitoring of water environments.

Source: ACS Publications. (2021). *Antimicrobial Resistance Monitoring of Water Environments.*

3.3.3. State and Local Regulations

State and local regulations play a tremendous role in the purity of our water, and they determine everything from the way we sample it to whether or not we are meeting health standards. They play a large role like the backbone of safe drinking water and appropriate wastewater management. Consider the EPA, for instance, its regulations establish what concentrations of contaminants are permissible in our water, in general safeguarding public health. Concurrently, local governments tend to modify these regulations to address issues such as industrial contamination or agricultural runoff. Other times, though, enforcement is not even, and that results in water quality problems that damage community health—as studies have demonstrated through frightening levels of pollution through industrial wastewater discharge (Zarate-Cáceres et al., 2025). Routine testing and public disclosure are truly key to keeping everyone informed, but not all water refill stations adhere to the complete testing regime; indeed, one study even reported that only around 50% complied with local water quality guidelines (Boston et al., 2024).

Such hit-and-miss practice leaves little confidence in consumer protection and undermines faith in local regulation. For the most part, though, if state authorities and local governments collaborated more effectively, testing would be better. Stricter regulations and improved follow-through would enable early detection of problems, safeguarding water sources and demonstrating just how important sound supervision is to a community's health. Community expertise plays a great deal of importance in water quality regulation, too. When grassroots campaigns and education get people in the know and engaged, they're more apt to demand better water testing and more effective pollution control if details fall through the cracks sometimes. Refill stations Boston et al. (2024) research reveals that when people know the danger of dirty water, they demand better practices. By participating in monitoring and reporting, communities not only make the entire system accountable but also ensure that the system becomes more responsive to actual needs. Ultimately, a little more local involvement can quite well close the gap between strict rules and what the community needs, ensuring our water remains safe for all.

3.4. The Role of Testing in Community Health

Testing water is a game-changer for the health of a community, it's the first line of defense against waterborne disease. Even a quick, complete scan could detect strange peaks in pollutants, allowing one to act fast on cleanup. Just look at Binji. A detailed analysis of their groundwater showed several chemical tests that not only surpassed Nigeria's drinking water requirements but also exceeded what the World Health Organization deems safe. That type of local analysis reveals concealed risks and pushes officials toward more intelligent public health decisions. Regular monitoring, in turn, establishes a rough benchmark, allowing neighborhoods to respond when water quality abruptly changes due to natural fluctuations or human activities and keep citizens safer and the water purer. Engaging local residents in such testing procedures is equally crucial. It sensitizes people to water issues and in fact improves the data collected, with the resulting findings feeling more grounded. One in North Carolina, where ordinary citizens participated in sampling private wells, discovered that variations in sampling techniques could warp the levels of lead reported a significant risk. By incorporating community members into the sampling process, the oddities in how samples were collected jumped out, enhancing everyone's understanding of the lead risks in drinking water. This hands-on, somewhat untidy method not only provides locals with a voice but also creates stronger community bonds, creating a patchwork base for both health activism and environmental stewardship. Sound water testing also ensures that safety standards intended to safeguard public health are indeed achieved. The changing lead levels observed in the North Carolina study demonstrate that unless tests are standardized, communities could wind up with a misleading perception of safety in their water, placing vulnerable populations, particularly infants, at higher risk. By and large, when individuals adhere to clear regulations and systematic testing protocols, they can reduce the adverse impacts of unwanted contaminants. Regular, science-driven checks not only tick the compliance box but also create trust in the individuals operating the water supplies. Over time, such tests can reveal seasonal changes and long-term trends, paving the way for improved water planning and healthier communities to come.

3.4.1. Identifying Contaminants and Health Risks

Water quality and public health are intertwined in a manner that compels us to see contaminants – those sneaky substances that tend to infiltrate our water. Chronic exposure to pollutants has been associated with everything from acute stomach problems to more chronic conditions such as kidney disease. Heavy metals and an array of microbial pathogens can insidiously accumulate in water over time. Rather than just depending on technical definitions, routine testing attempts to find these harmful chemicals, but the techniques we typically rely on , such as detecting fecal pollution using fecal indicator bacteria (FIB) – sometimes fail to follow the trail back to its origin (Intergovernmental Panel on Climate Change, 2023). Current research, for the most part, suggests our conventional strategies must have a less rigid, multifaceted approach if we wish to truly grasp the whole situation. Innovation gradually is retooling how we monitor these toxins. DNA diagnostic tools, for example, are gaining some attention.

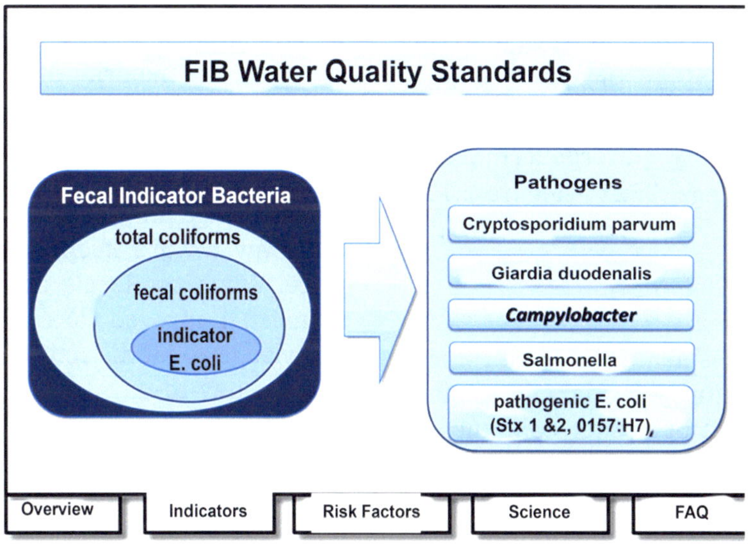

Figure 3.11. FIB water quality standards.

Source: UC Davis. (n.d.). *FIB Water Quality Standards.*

Tools such as quantitative polymerase chain reaction (qPCR) and high-throughput DNA sequencing have begun to marry science to pragmatism, particularly when it comes to unraveling the origins of fecal contamination. In a lot of rural towns – where simple FIB tests may not reach all the nooks and crannies – these technologies provide a much better view. Consider the example of a Wainfleet, Ontario study; what they found was that traditional methods couldn't identify the contamination sources, leaving health advisories lingering in the air. When scientists used microbial community profiling, however, they were able to track back pathogens to sources such as farm runoff and septic tank leaks and find out the dirty, intertwined nature of groundwater contaminants (Naphtali et al., 2019). Knowing how various contaminants wreak havoc with public health is central to establishing smart regulations and community health measures. It is not only about the pollutants themselves; there is an additional, complex layer present in the form of AMR. In most instances, resistance infections exacerbate health risks, causing severe illness and even death, particularly in settings with limited resources. The worldwide burden of AMR reinforces how many lives are involved, implying that detecting what contaminants contribute to resistance and regulating to counter this is imperative to the point of being absolutely critical. This more comprehensive, multi-faceted strategy not only reduces the transmission of infectious disease but also promotes a well-informed, proactive public reaction to water safety (Intergovernmental Panel on Climate Change, 2023) (Figure 3.11).

3.4.2. Monitoring Compliance with Water Quality Standards

Water resource management involves keeping a very close watch on things – regular checks must be done to ensure that our water continues to satisfy the quality standards laid down by various authorities. Governments and international agencies are generally responsible for determining these limits, controlling pollutants to safeguard people and nature. Periodic look-overs assist in identifying potential problems, which subsequently becomes simpler to correct issues before they become unmanageable. Through systematic sampling and testing, the authorities can trace significant factors such as chemical contaminants, microbial traces, and even certain physical characteristics of the water. Adhering to these quality standards is not merely about obeying rules, it is an integral aspect of protecting communities, particularly in areas where infrastructure is not the best or the population is more vulnerable. In this regard, monitoring water quality is a progressive move, making it possible for water to remain safe to drink, enjoy, or farm. The precision and reliability of testing methods are a big concern when it comes to monitoring water safety. There's a combination of methods available—from traditional lab tests to more recent on-the-spot methods—that have been developed to detect dangerous substances. The method you use should complement the particular problem at hand, as some pollutants are more difficult to detect than others. For example, detecting heavy metals may require some pretty sophisticated equipment, whereas microbe testing may use fast detection instruments. New technology just keeps coming along, sharpening our measurements and accelerating how quickly we can get results out, which is just really crucial for quick public health action. In the majority of instances, investment in solid testing isn't necessarily about checking boxes for compliance, it adds greater transparency and a degree of responsibility to water quality control. Engaging local communities comes a long way toward keeping water standards in place. When the locals are part of it, it tends to mean improved data collecting and more knowledge about the actual impact water quality has on day-to-day health. Open discussions among government organizations, NGOs, and citizens can result in more active involvement in monitoring the water. Community members may observe unusual changes, exchange notes, and collaborate on strategies to address any risks that arise. And when community-driven projects start, water quality information becomes clearer, which enables people to demand cleaner sources. Overall, combining rigorous scientific methods with active public participation not only serves to keep us all on track with safety regulations, but also creates a common agreement to improve health and an improved quality of daily existence (Figure 3.12).

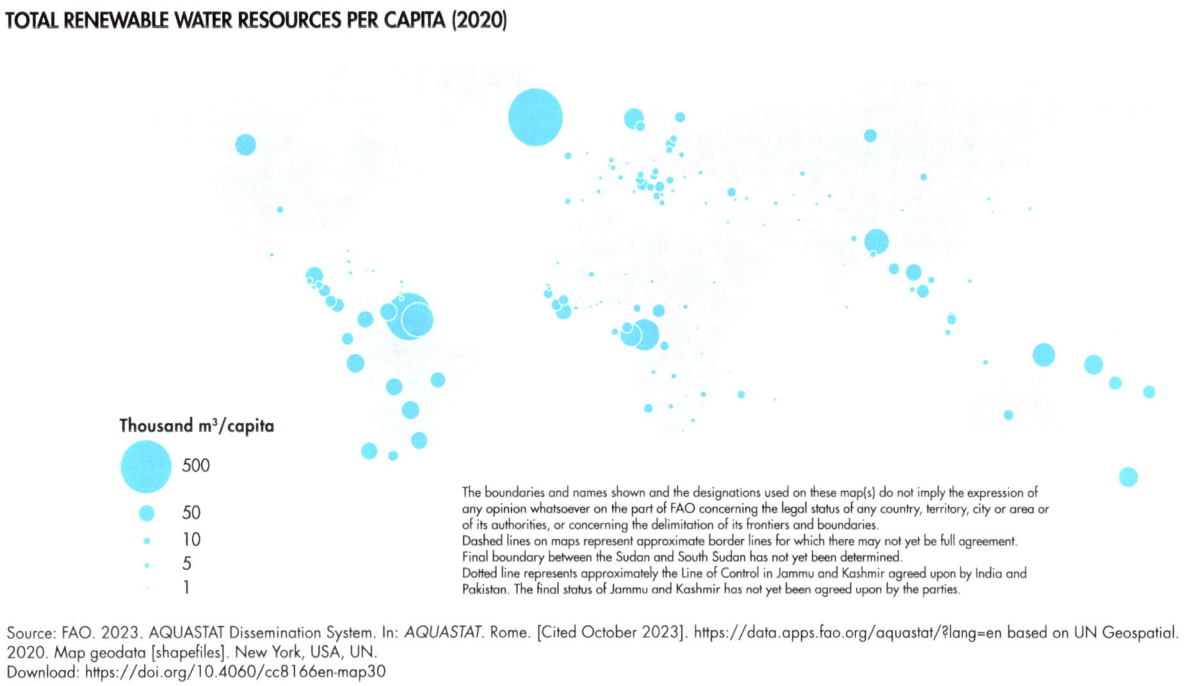

Figure 3.12. Water quality monitoring system infography.

Source: By FAO - https://www.fao.org/documents/card/en/c/cc8166en , File:World Food and Agriculture - Statistical Yearbook 2023.pdf, CC BY-SA 3.0 igo, https://commons.wikimedia.org/w/index.php?curid=142156187

3.4.3. Educating the Community About Water Safety

Water quality is important—a big deal—to how we feel on a daily basis, whether we're drinking it or just playing in it. It's strange the way something as fundamental as water can have such a significant influence on community health, huh? We do know that if bad chemicals, unwanted bacteria, or natural poisons get in, our health could really suffer. That's why it is reasonable to conduct workshops, distribute flyers, and even make school programs a means of transmitting what we have to learn regarding water safety. On most occasions, these steps assist individuals in comprehending the risks and advocating for frequent check-ups on the water, even instigating day-to-day discussions about how to keep our environment safe. You may not consider it initially, but determining such aspects as pH levels, water cloudiness, or if obnoxious microorganisms are lurking is important. Local health offices, teaming up with the water companies, can create simple-to-obtain materials that illustrate what occurs when water quality goes astray. By and large, talking simply and skipping over all the science jargon is a game-changer, it allows everyone to grasp why maintenance and testing matter so much. If you distill complicated concepts into easy components, it quite obviously encourages more people to engage with and back stronger water regulations. And there's testing in and of itself, which plays an actual backbone role in protecting our water. Routine tests—everything from basic at-home kits to more advanced lab work—make mysteries out of what's happening with our water. As citizens gain more knowledge about these techniques (and believe me, every little bit counts), communities will establish their own tiny checks, preventing potential dangers in their tracks. This type of local, grassroots effort, perhaps in collaboration with neighboring neighbors or local experts, truly promotes ownership of water safety and public health; a small but significant step toward a healthier community (Figure 3.13).

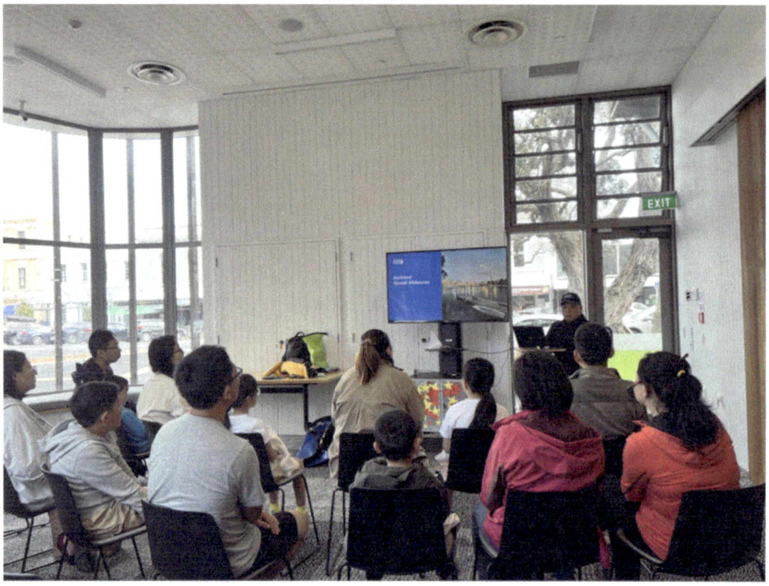

Figure 3.13. Bridging communities for water safety.

Source:. https://openandconnect.org.nz/wp-content/uploads/2023/10/Screenshot-2023-10-30-at-4.47.15-PM-1024x750.png.

3.5. Challenges in Water Quality Testing

Precise water testing makes a big difference. Populations worldwide are now relying on water from all types of sources that could be unclean, so ensuring we're aware of what's in the water is imperative. Clean drinking water has been classed as an essential human right, which implies that we should have reliable testing equipment in place. But too many locations continue to lack sufficient data, usually due to local systems not being at par with adequate water tests. In the absence of wide, representative data, it is challenging to monitor sustainably managed drinking water services (SMDW) as set out in international aims such as the United Nations' Sustainable Development Goals (SDGs). These lost pieces not only render it difficult to evaluate water quality accurately but also cause response lags to contamination, posing a threat to public health and safety (Robert et al., 2020). There are also more than enough technical challenges that make water testing unreliable. Laboratory practices, although generally accurate, are costly, time-consuming, and difficult to control particularly when resources are limited. At times, the lengthy drive to a laboratory and the requirement to handle sensitive equipment only serve to compound the clutter when in a rush to quickly identify contaminants. Often in such instances—in areas such as sub-Saharan Africa where urbanization outstrips testing facilities—the demand for intelligent, low-budget field techniques gains immediacy, targeting microbial and chemical contaminants (Xu & Braune, 2009). Water quality itself is liable to change immensely between various regions and socio-economic levels; too often, poor communities end up depending on water that is not safe. Local testing has even revealed that contamination consistently appears at the point-of-use, indicating that issues extend beyond the main supply. The actual problem is establishing community-based systems that allow locals to contribute to monitoring and analysis. These local initiatives can increase local awareness and start filling in the gaps left by unstable national surveillance, typically setting the stage for improved public health outcomes (Robert et al., 2020) (Figure 3.14).

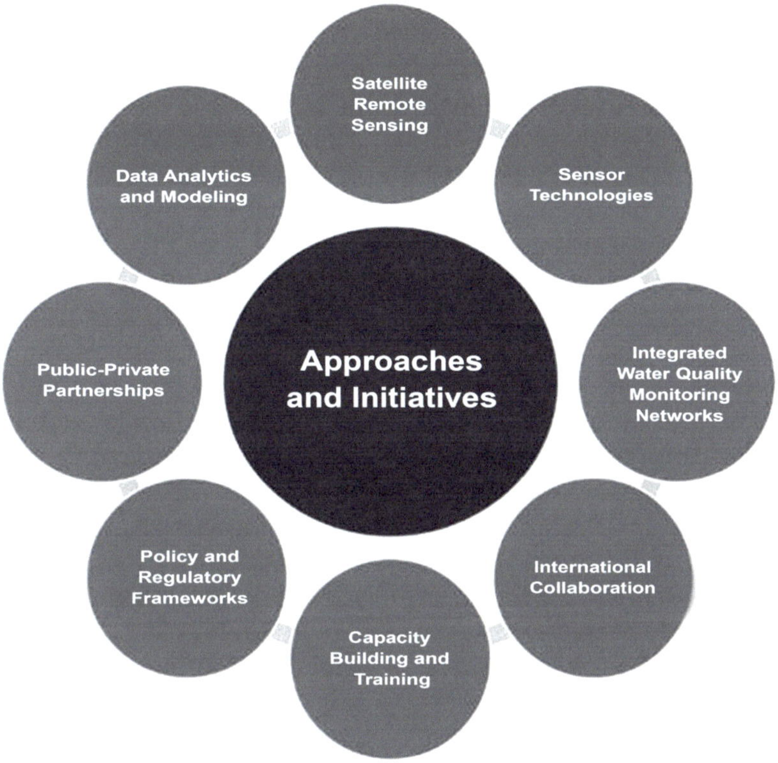

Figure 3.14. Various approaches and initiatives are being undertaken globally to address the challenges associated with water quality.

Source: ResearchGate. (2024). *Various Approaches and Initiatives are Being Undertaken Globally to Address the Challenges Associated with Water Quality.*

3.5.1. Accessibility of Testing Resources

Water quality testing usually falters because the right equipment isn't so readily available. Too often in most areas – particularly where there simply aren't enough resources – it is difficult to locate sophisticated laboratory equipment and skilled hands. Outdated techniques, which are also quite costly, consume resources and time, thus being less suitable for daily testing. Yes, lab tests generally find the target with accuracy, but their involved procedures and high costs often deter members of the community, who have more pressing health concerns, from using them. For instance, research on field tools such as colorimetric test strips indicates that though such kits are inexpensive and easy to implement, they may be too subjective and sensitive to variations in the environment. These concerns, in a large majority of cases, bring out the importance of new concepts that integrate modern methods with real access so that additional people can contribute to water quality monitoring (McCarty et al., 2025). Technology today presents new avenues for simplifying and making water quality analysis more accessible. IoT-driven solutions, for example, enable individuals to track important parameters such as pH, turbidity, and total dissolved solids (TDS) in real-time – no need to wait for laboratory reports. An array of sensors connected to platforms like the Blynk cloud enables communities to monitor water quality remotely, minimizing laborious manual sampling and intricate equipment (Karan et al., 2024). These systems not only simplify the process significantly but also provide real-time data, which facilitates quick feedback on any contamination issue. Remote monitoring, being flexible, is particularly suited to remote or poorly equipped areas where conventional approaches simply are not up to it. In reality, employing smart technology such as this can truly enhance access to the critical tools necessary to protect community health and water safety. Bridging resources is even more successful when government organizations, non-profits, and local communities collaborate. When collaborations offer training sessions and even some funding, locals acquire both the expertise and the equipment to conduct effective water quality monitoring. Sometimes that involves hosting workshops that show individuals how to apply simple, accessible test kits or implementing citizen-initiated projects that rely on genuine community feedback. Engaging the public not only makes people more aware of water concerns but create a sense of personal stake ; people care more about what they have a hand in creating. As numerous successful projects have indicated, if communities become responsible for monitoring their own water, then the health gains can be more sustainable and extensive. Ultimately, addressing resource issues collectively can result in outcomes that span long beyond quick solutions, fostering long-term environmental stewardship and increased public participation (Karan et al., 2024; McCarty et al., 2025).

3.5.2. Variability in Water Sources and Conditions

Various sources of water cause significant differences in water quality from one region to another, so it's challenging to ensure safe drinking water. We obtain water from various means – sometimes we pump it from the ground, sometimes it moves along the surface or is collected from the rain , and each is vulnerable to something." For instance, groundwater usually ends up absorbing chemicals from surrounding farms and industrial processes, which let inodorous things into our water; meanwhile, surface water can catch more biological contaminants, particularly in areas where sanitation is not really up to standard. Due to the fact that every source has its own combination of risks, testing techniques and standards must adapt accordingly. Without a clear understanding of the specific microbes and chemical composition present in each source, implementing proper community health strategies becomes an actual challenge (Palou et al., 2022). The interaction between sources of water and their environment also plays a major role in determining how clean or dirty the water ends up being. Weather changes, seasonal fluctuations, and general climate trends can suddenly reverse things such as water clarity, pH levels, and nutrient content. It may produce a lot of runoff through heavy rains that sweep pollutants into drinking water rivers and lakes and, in periods of drought, whatever water is left can be further concentrated with pollutants. In general terms, these volatile fluctuations require constant checking and a few adjustments in testing patterns so that policies remain effective throughout the year since water quality has a direct relationship with public health impacts (Palou et al., 2022). Social and economic considerations introduce yet another level of complication. In most instances, less resourceful communities use water that is not as well treated, and thus there is a higher incidence of waterborne diseases. Even the method with which water arrives at one's home may introduce additional contaminants that taint the quality of treated water. Urban development and industrial processes also introduce unintended impurities that may need specialized tests to identify. All these concerns imply that public health policies must rely on local information regarding water quality and associated health effects. Ultimately, the combination of various sources of water, environmental idiosyncrasies, and socio-economic issues leaves little doubt that a strong, flexible system of water quality testing is essential for protecting communities (Robert et al., 2020) (Figure 3.15).

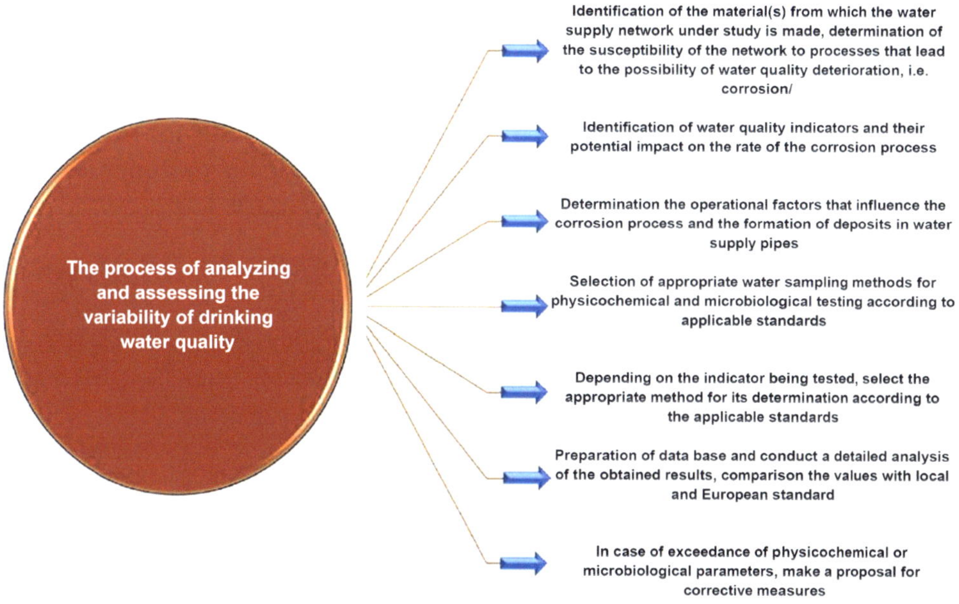

Figure 3.15. Steps of analyzing and assessing the process of the variability of drinking water quality.

Source: Piegdoń I. Variability of Drinking Water Quality on the Basis of Analysis of Qualitative Monitoring from a Selected Water Supply Network Located in South-Eastern Poland. *Water*. 2024; 16(23):3355. https://doi.org/10.3390/w16233355

3.5.3. Public Awareness and Engagement

Working on water quality problems engenders a wave of change within communities and, by and large, raises public health. There is a kind of complex dynamic going on: stress on resource distribution creates a shared sense of responsibility while an open vision for the effects of bad water moves people to do something. Most often, once communities understand bad water equals serious trouble, they plunge into environmental protection and embrace sustainable practices. Campos et al.'s (2025) study indicates that well-educated citizens can demand improved monitoring and even upgraded wastewater treatment—actions that enhance overall water management. Even specially focused educational initiatives, by sparking local engagement in determining water standards, have a tendency to link community efforts to a broader combination of government and non-government initiatives. At times, gaining knowledge on water quality alters daily habits more than anticipated.

Individuals come to realize that polluters such as heavy metals and microbial contaminates aren't merely theoretical concepts, but real dangers associated with their local water supply. Consider the Ichu River basin—there, anthropogenic contamination so seriously disrupts water quality that it is rather important to know the dangers to community well-being (Zarate-Cáceres et al., 2025). Educational campaigns make it possible to communicate how pollution works, getting residents to demand stronger regulations on factory runoff and advocating improved wastewater treatment. Most often, that increased awareness turns around and produces a culture within industries and communities alike that demands accountability. When citizens engage in the minutiae of water quality discussions, even local governance and policy begin to change. Getting involved in the dialogue and projects tends to fuel strategic modifications in the manner that resources are allocated toward water safety (Campos et al., 2025). It is not unusual for local officials, NGOs, and residents to collaborate and craft water management plans that suit particular regional imperatives—mixing bottom-up understanding with official planning. Public participation in water quality evaluations may enhance transparency and, in a slightly unconventional manner, accountability as well. As they come together as communities, their voice collectively not only calls for increased monitoring and increased standards but also pushes governance towards a more participatory, if not ideally streamlined, direction to protect public health and resources (Figure 3.16).

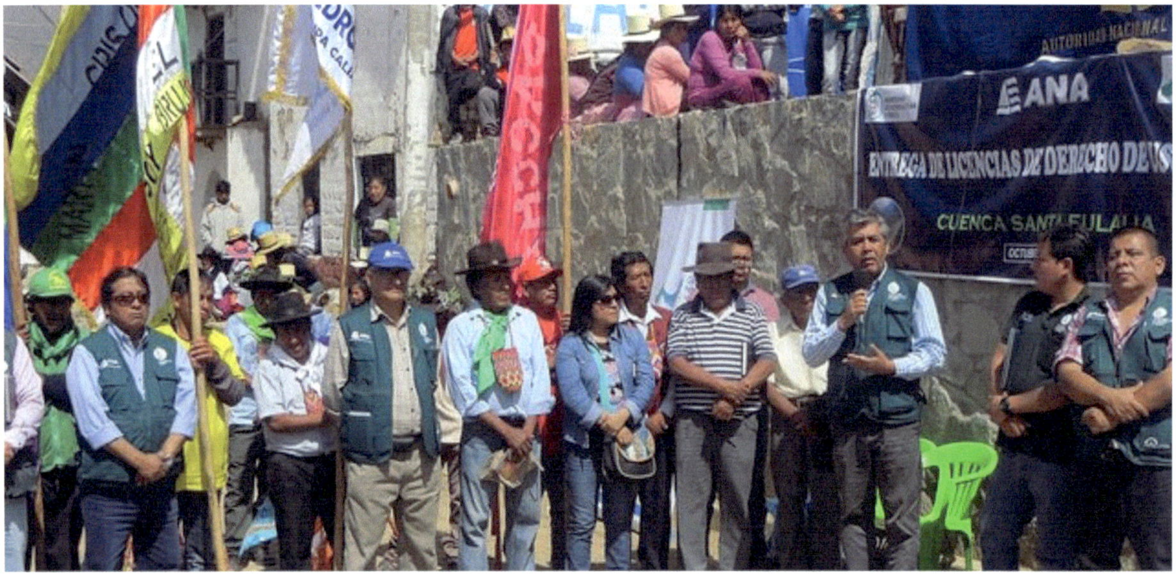

Figure 3.16. Raising public awareness.

Source: Global Water Partnership. (n.d.). *Raising Public Awareness.*

3.6. Innovations in Water Quality Testing

Tech innovations have revolutionized the way we monitor water quality nowadays. Handheld devices—equipped with sensors and onboard data processing, can provide you with fast, reliable measurements of different water parameters. They enable communities to monitor water in real time, which is extremely crucial when contamination occurs more than it doesn't. And when you connect these devices with smartphone apps, it means small groups or individuals can conduct their own tests. This move away from depending solely on labs allows individuals to identify potential dangers earlier and react in time enough to keep public health under control. On another level, there's a definite trend toward cleaner drinking water treatments. Continuing work, such as that technology scan conducted by the Scottish Government, is keeping itself busy searching out treatment approaches that might just suit small and medium-sized communities slightly better. Most of the time, these attempts not only provide a useful checklist of tech choices but also make up particular recommendations that align with local needs and sustainability objectives.

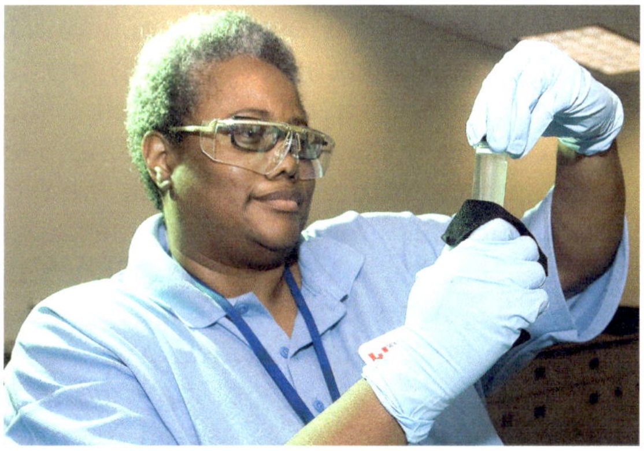

Figure 3.17. Clean water test. Schoolgirl doing a strip test to check water quality – this requires multiple, complicated steps.

Source: By USEPA Environmental-Protection-Agency - A scientist inspects a water sample., Public Domain, https://commons.wikimedia.org/w/index.php?curid=71595914

The findings from such research truly assist various stakeholders in making informed decisions, and they gradually develop a strategy that prioritizes local participation while adhering to wider health and environmental guidelines. And then there's the emergence of intelligent water management systems driven by Internet of Things (IoT) technology. These networks are essentially always online, constantly collecting information from various sources to provide a better indication of water safety and levels of pollution. They're designed to notify members of the community immediately if things get off track from set safety standards. The cool thing is that these data-sharing networks of communities tend to influence policy decisions at local, state, and even national levels. Overall, this experiential, holistic approach not only increases testing precision but also offers an essential tool for addressing larger challenges such as marine deoxygenation and nutrient runoff, as observed in ocean conservation efforts (Conservation X Labs, 2015). Combined, these developments ensure that community health remains well-supported and safeguarded (Figure 3.17).

3.6.1. Advances in Testing Technology

Water quality testing has come a long way these days, it's now one of the major players in making our communities safe. You see, new methods such as spectrophotometry and biosensors now test water for items such as pH balance, turbidity, and even indicators of microbial critters in an instant. These devices enable people to get into action quickly, keeping water safety on track and compliant with codes. Computer systems and certain intelligent automation have also streamlined the manner in which we collect and sift through data to make decisions instantly much easier. Quite a number of experts, as highlighted in microbiome debates of Berg et al. (2020), are of the opinion that employing rigorously refined testing techniques is quite important to address the complex problems that arise with human influences on our waterways. In short, these hands-on practices not only improve public safety but also make people feel more comfortable about what is emerging from their faucets. Nanotechnology has now entered the picture, rattling water testing in a huge way. Thanks to advances in nanomedicine and nano delivery systems, researchers have discovered new avenues to spot things like heavy metals and microbes that even previously managed to get past previous tests. By taking advantage of the special characteristics of nanomaterials, researchers have amplified conventional techniques so significantly that even minute contaminants—previously almost undetectable, can now be identified. This drive for accuracy in health diagnosis is right in line with the current trend toward precise, targeted treatment for public water systems. And in all sincerity, the precision of nanotech to target certain pollutants allows the community to direct their clean-up campaigns more specifically and not squander resources on the incorrect approaches (Patra et al., 2018). Normalized testing procedures still play a key part in our capacity to track water quality, something which only increases as the technology develops. Maintaining tests consistent means results become precise, comparable, and even reproducible—a trait that undoubtedly instills confidence in regulators and the public. Researchers in microbiome science have indicated (Berg et al., 2020) how important it is to take on a more consolidated testing paradigm that unites the most recent scientific advancements with the frequently complex interactions of microbes in water. As testing technologies become more sophisticated, they open the door to more robust means of assessing water quality, ultimately leading to healthier communities. By remaining open to these developments and continually implementing these innovations, public health workers can make informed decisions that best serve those who depend on these vital resources.

3.6.2. Citizen Science Initiatives

Community members becoming engaged in water monitoring provides a new opportunity to enhance environmental stewardship and public health simultaneously. Citizens tend to jump into citizen science activities, collecting readings of pH, turbidity, and even detecting microbial issues, in a very hands-on fashion. This type of activity, in most instances, organically brings attention to water issues while gradually enhancing the overall health of the community. Research tends to indicate that when people are involved in collecting and analyzing information, not only do they acquire important knowledge about their environment, but they also begin to have greater trust in science and government organizations a little more (Margaret et al., 2018). Once people know more, they're likely to demand policy reforms that can improve water quality and secure important assets. In areas where resources may be relatively constricted, particularly in low- and middle-income nations (LMICs)—citizen science frequently fills the bill as a primary resource. These initiatives enable ordinary individuals to make a tangible contribution toward scientific investigation, filling gaps in health and environmental information that formal monitoring may overlook. Not only does this give power to communities with the type of information they require to make decisions, but it, in a sense, also strengthens skills within local health systems. The information gathered from these efforts can fill critical gaps in our knowledge of water quality, setting the stage for timely interventions and overall improved health outcomes (Conservation X Labs, 2015). There is little doubt that governments and NGOs must support training initiatives teaching citizens the ins-and-outs of successful water quality monitoring, thus perpetuating a culture of continuous community engagement and scientific interest. The long-term viability of such water monitoring efforts ultimately depends on firm community commitment and strong governmental support. For these programs to work well, the folks in charge must ensure that the data is reliable and that the findings make their way into broader health policies. In most cases, aligning citizen-led efforts with key objectives, like the SDGs—gives communities a stronger voice in advocating for cleaner water and stronger public health measures. There's also a sort of feedback mechanism at work here: what the citizens tell us can inform policy choices that in turn direct additional sampling, a method that assist trust building even though it might at times be a bit unbalanced (Margaret et al., 2018). Overall, these citizen science initiatives can turn into a true pillar of community health, closing the distance between scientific studies and day-to-day public health practice (Figure 3.18).

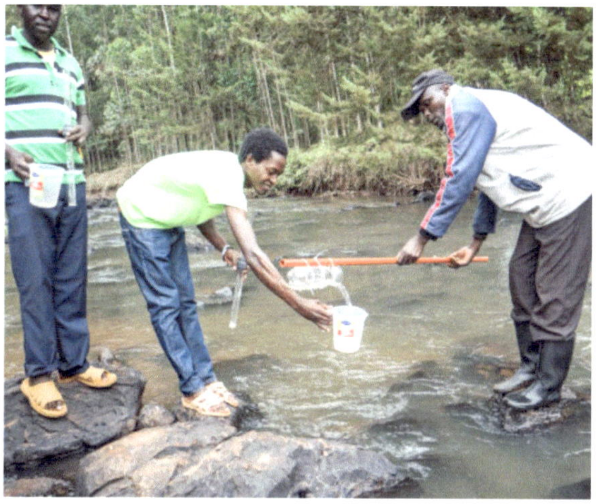

Figure 3.18. Citizen Scientists collecting water samples.

Source: https://encrypted-tbn0.gstatic.com/images?q=tbn:ANd9GcR6K7CZ8I_F_wsAGqzETLTznx0lyW25M5AzeWdkTKjyM7w4s9KvjoLXmXBxWg3LwIlkp1s&usqp=CAU.

3.6.3. Integration of Data Analytics in Water Quality Monitoring

Technology advancements have truly turned the page when it comes to water quality monitoring. Sensors nowadays do more than their predecessors did, it's not a matter of periodic check-ups anymore, but rather sensors that settle into IoT networks that continue to gather information from pH and turbidity all the way down to even nefarious contaminants. Mostly, that translates to us ditching ancient guesswork for streams of actual data, and honestly, it makes all the difference in speed and accuracy. Big data is not merely adding numbers; it's converting them into useful advice that guides decisions regarding water safety and achieving established standards. In most instances, possession of these intelligent analytics guides us towards a more forward-oriented, near-proactive approach to handling our precious water resources. But there's more to it. Data analysis in water monitoring also captures trends that would otherwise go undetected. Machine learning, say, processes vast mountains of data to identify anomalies and even presages problems—sometimes even before they develop in full. This preemption is particularly important where water sources are under constant attack like pollution or changing climate patterns. Using such technology as a backstop, agencies can then concentrate their efforts where things appear most perilous, and even stay ahead of the marks regulators set. The payoff? Safer, cleaner drinking water that gains public confidence naturally. And then there's the bigger picture. Plugging data tools into water tests has radiating effects far beyond mere instant health improvements. It provides us with a different perspective on how human activities, such as agricultural runoff—may be impacting water supplies. Data analysis now provides a means to quantify those effects so that communities can develop focused methods to reduce problems such as nutrient overload, something that has been mentioned in ocean conservation discussions (Conservation X Labs, 2015). This broader outlook doesn't simply address pressing health issues; it encourages us toward more sustainable methods that help maintain our water ecosystems. As environmental issues continue to escalate, resorting to innovative data approaches seems almost imperative for water management, ultimately strengthening our community's health and nature's equilibrium.

SUMMARY

Examining the quality of water at the Al-Dur Water Treatment Plant illustrates how crucial consistent, hands-on testing is for drinking water to be safe. They tested items such as pH, turbidity, and TDS — all measured differently — and pretty much had everything in accordance with the standards used normally. It appears that monitoring these aspects, even in surprise testing times, truly enhances public trust. You could say that knowing the state of water during various treatment steps assists in adjusting the process, eliminating pollutants more efficiently, and perhaps even reducing the risk of disease occurrence. In many situations, this information assists in planning that not only adheres to rules but also prioritizes the unusual health demands of the population, solidifying why continued water testing is important. Meanwhile, the relationship between water quality and public health is not merely a matter of short-term safety concerns; it even has wider social and economic dimensions. Water quality management frequently surprises us by averting waterborne illnesses that most affect vulnerable populations, and engaging the community in testing activities, in general, promotes awareness of accountability in matters of public health. The findings emerging from the Al-Dur plant can, in a very surprising manner, empower individuals to demand clean water rights — a combination of hard science and ordinary community action that sometimes feels strangely repetitive but real. Also, sharing and debating these findings in various circles, even with small discrepancies in how they get communicated, appears to promote a sense of ownership over one's own health. Ultimately, water quality is about more than checking off a list of requirements; it is a larger narrative about health equity and sustainability. Assessing the most important testing parameters is not just about regulatory compliance; it also moves public policy toward better safeguarding both our environment and human health. Regular testing, when brought into local health planning, can result in stronger outcomes and—if you consider it—a stronger future. Confronting the numerous challenges of our evolving world, the knowledge obtained from detailed testing can illuminate the path toward adaptable approaches that benefit both public well-being and the balance of nature. To summarize, a proactive attitude towards water quality stands as a cornerstone in our shared pursuit of healthier communities around the globe.

Water quality is important—period, and it has a significant impact on our health and well-being overall. We measure things such as pH, the clarity (or lack thereof) of the water, DO levels, and even test for heavy metals and bad microbes to determine whether or not the water is safe to drink. Frequent testing such as this, albeit seemingly mundane, goes a long way toward identifying latent hazards that can impact community health. When communities come on board and take comprehensive water testing seriously, they find themselves with information that unwittingly formulates public policy and determines the allocation of resources, pushing all parties toward the more active side of ensuring safe water. In the majority of instances, recent findings indicate that having such water information available not only supports health requirements but also encourages regional efforts to follow more sustainable routines in the ecosystem (Intergovernmental Panel on Climate Change, 2023). Methods for analyzing water have come a long way, as well. Those days are behind us when we were dependent only on traditional methods; today, instruments such as remote sensing and real-time monitoring systems emerge to capture anomalies almost as they happen. These new techniques increase our confidence in the information we collect, which—honestly, is quite crucial to adhering to health standards. And with standardized testing procedures at work, outcomes can be meaningfully compared between various regions and at various points in time, instilling confidence in the figures and providing regulators with the paperwork they require. Overall, this advanced testing strategy is an important component of efforts to prevent waterborne illness and assist in constructing healthier, more resilient communities (Percie et al., 2020). Ultimately, adhering to water quality standards accomplishes two great things: it keeps people safe and assists in creating a resilient community. These guidelines result from much scientific study and have certain thresholds for different kinds of pollutants, meant to ensure our drinking water and recreational waters are safe. Even so, part of the ongoing challenge is bridging the gap between standards-setters and the folks who live day-to-day with the water. Ongoing education and community conversations are required so that everyone receives what water testing is for personal health. When people have both the education and the resources within reach, they're more likely to demand improved practices and even summon local authorities where necessary, ultimately resulting in healthier results and a healthier relationship with this vital resource (Intergovernmental Panel on Climate Change, 2023).

KEY TERMS FROM THIS CHAPTER

- Antimicrobial resistance (AMR)
- Community health projects
- Dissolved oxygen (DO) levels
- Governmental support
- Nutrient pollution
- Organic chemicals
- Public health policy
- Target product profile (TPP)
- Turbidity tests
- Water management procedures
- World Health Organization
- Blynk cloud
- Community planning
- DNA sequencing
- Local governance
- Obnoxious microorganisms
- Polymerase chain reaction
- Safe Drinking Water Act
- Total dissolved solids (TDS)
- Volatile fluctuations
- Water quality monitoring
- Fecal indicator bacteria (FIB)

CLOSER LOOK

TESTING FOR WATER QUALITY

Testing the quality of water entails checking water for physical, chemical, and microbiological attributes to determine suitability for different uses. Physical checks analyze color, clarity, temperature, and turbidity. Chemical analysis checks pH, DO, TDS, and heavy metals. Microbiological analysis checks bacteria and viruses.

Physical Tests:

- o **Color:** Indicates the presence of dissolved organic matter, minerals, or algae.
- o **Clarity:** Measured as turbidity, which refers to cloudiness caused by suspended particles.
- o **Temperature:** Affects microbial activity and DO levels.
- o **Smell and Taste**: Can indicate the presence of organic matter, chemicals, or algae.

Chemical Tests:

- o **pH:** Measures acidity or alkalinity.
- o **Dissolved Oxygen:** Essential for aquatic life.
- o **Total Dissolved Solids (TDS):** Measures the amount of dissolved minerals and salts.
- o **Heavy Metals:** Such as lead, copper, and arsenic, are tested for their potential toxicity.
- o **Other Chemical Parameters:** Include alkalinity, chlorides, nitrates, and hardness.

Microbiological Tests:

- o **Bacteria:** Tests for indicator bacteria like *E. coli* and coliforms to detect potential fecal contamination.
- o **Viruses:** Detected using specialized techniques like membrane filtration.
- o **Protozoa and Worms:** May also be tested for, depending on the water source and intended use.

Testing Methods

- **Field Tests:** Portable digital instruments, colorimeters, and photometers can be used for on-site analysis.
- **Laboratory Tests:** Provide more comprehensive and accurate results, often using techniques like spectrophotometry, ion-selective electrodes, and titration.
- **Membrane Filtration:** A common method for detecting indicator organisms in microbiological tests.
- **Multiple Tube Dilution (MTD):** Another technique for detecting indicator bacteria.

References

1. Baidaa Khader Abdullah, Yassien Hussain Owaied Al-juboory et al. (2024). Physical and Chemical Analysis of Water Quality at Al-Dur Water Treatment Plant, Journal of Primeasia, 5(1), 1-9, 9766 (accessed on 14 May 2025).
2. Abdullahi, I. M., Abubakar, L., Saidu, G., & Yusuf, H. (2025). Hydrogeochemical characterization of groundwater using water quality index and multivariate statistical analysis in Binji town and environs, Sokoto Basin, Northwestern Nigeria. *Applied Water Science*. https://www.semanticscholar.org/paper/1c946aef9a05aac58e8f3a2f6cbea2b91117f02a (accessed on 14 May 2025).
3. Pichel, N., Hymnô de Souza, F., Sabogal-Paz, L. P., Shah, P. K., Adhikari, N., Pandey, S., Shrestha, B. M., Gaihre, S., Pineda-Marulanda, D. A., Hincapie, M., Luwe, K., Kumwenda, S., Aguilar-Conde, J. C., Cortes, M. A. L. R. M., Hamilton, J. W. J., Byrne, J. A., & Fernandez-Ibañez, P. (2023). Field-testing solutions for drinking water quality monitoring in low- and middle-income regions and case studies from Latin American, African and Asian countries. *Journal of Environmental Chemical Engineering*, *11*(6), Article 111180. https://doi.org/10.1016/j.jece.2023.111180 (accessed on 14 May 2025).
4. Asnaning, Aniessa R., et al. "Water Conservation with Rainwater Harvesting System in Lampung Province (Case Study in State Polytechnic of Lampung Campus Area)." *Journal of Science and Applicative Technology*, vol. 2, no. 1, 2019, doi:10.35472/281453. (accessed on 14 May 2025).
5. Alengebawy, A., Abdelkhalek, S. T., Qureshi, S. R., & Wang, M. Q. (2021). Heavy metals and pesticides toxicity in agricultural soil and plants: Ecological risks and human health implications. *Toxics, 9*(3), Article 42. https://doi.org/10.3390/toxics9030042.
6. Ali, A., Shah, T., Ullah, R., Zhou, P., Guo, M., Ovais, M., Tan, Z., et al. (2021). Review on recent progress in magnetic nanoparticles: Synthesis, characterization, and diverse applications. *Frontiers in Chemistry, 9*, Article 629054. https://doi.org/10.3389/fchem.2021.629054.
7. Amaral, D. G., & de Vries, P. J. (2020). COVID-19 and autism research: Perspectives from around the globe. *Autism Research, 13*(5), 844–869. https://doi.org/10.1002/aur.2329.
8. Ayilara, M. S., Olanrewaju, O. S., Babalola, O. O., & Odeyemi, O. (2020). Waste management through composting: Challenges and potentials. *Sustainability, 12*, 4456. https://doi.org/10.3390/su12114456.
9. Baaziz, A., Kleiner, A., Feigelson, E. D., Waller, M. A., Boyd, S., Vandermerwe, S., & Zhou, Z. (2015). *Big Data and the Internet of Things*. arXiv. http://arxiv.org/abs/1503.07092 (accessed on 14 May 2025).
10. Bain, R. E. S., Johnston, R., & Slaymaker, T. (2020). Drinking water quality and the SDGs. *npj Clean Water, 3*, 1–3. https://www.semanticscholar.org/paper/3e1d4fa65f42c5a4a9b51364b0dbfaf2aaff4d30 (accessed on 14 May 2025).
11. Berg, G., Rybakova, D., Fischer, D., Cernava, T., Champomier Vergès, M. C., Charles, T. C., Chen, X., et al. (2020). Microbiome definition re-visited: Old concepts and new challenges. *Microbiome, 8*, Article 103. https://doi.org/10.1186/s40168-020-00875-0.
12. Blackwood, D. J., Falconer, R. E., Gilmour, D. J., O'Keeffe, S., et al. (2016). An evaluation of water treatment technologies for sustainable rural communities. Conference: 13th International

Water Association Specialized Conference on Small Water and Wastewater Systems.At: Athens, Greece. https://core.ac.uk/download/228178252.pdf (accessed on 14 May 2025).

13. Boston, Cecil, Rajini Kurup, and Denise Beckles. 2024. "Analyzing Water Quality and Consumer Perceptions at Refill Stations in Guyana: Mixed-Methods Analysis". *International Journal of Environment and Climate Change* 14 (4):18-26. https://doi.org/10.9734/ijecc/2024/v14i44092. (accessed on 14 May 2025).

14. Bull, F., Al-Ansari, S. S., Biddle, S., Borodulin, K., Buman, M. P., Cardon, G., Carty, C., et al. (2020). World Health Organization 2020 guidelines on physical activity and sedentary behaviour. *British Journal of Sports Medicine, 54*(24), 1451–1462. https://doi.org/10.1136/bjsports-2020-102955.

15. Campos, J. D. S., & Campos, J. R. (2025). SDG6: The Interplay of Strategic Resources, Awareness, and Policy in Enhancing Water Quality and Health Outcomes. *Journal of Lifestyle and SDGs Review, 5*(1), e05039. https://doi.org/10.47172/2965-730X.SDGsReview.v5.n01.pe05039

16. (accessed on 14 May 2025).

17. Chandalwar, K. R., Barde, N. A., Pureddi, S. S., Uike, T., Yadgiri, N., & Dumbere, M. (2024). Water quality monitoring system based on IoT. *International Journal of Advanced Research in Science, Communication and Technology*. https://www.semanticscholar.org/paper/f7c489b1b614809fed53fb4df9f4a9368f11486e (accessed on 14 May 2025).

18. Chen, W., Ren, K., Isabwe, A., Chen, H., Liu, M., & Yang, J. (2019). Stochastic processes shape microeukaryotic community assembly in a subtropical river across wet and dry seasons. *Microbiome, 7*. https://doi.org/10.1186/s40168-019-0749-8.

19. Dadlani, M., & Yadava, D. K. (2023). Seed science and technology. https://doi.org/10.1007/978-981-19-5888-5.

20. Gatta, P. P. (2022). *The State of World Fisheries and Aquaculture 2022*. FAO eBooks. https://doi.org/10.4060/cc0461en.

21. Gonzales, W. V., Mobashsher, A. T., & Abbosh, A. (2019). The progress of glucose monitoring—A review of invasive to minimally and non-invasive techniques, devices and sensors. *Sensors, 19*, 800. https://doi.org/10.3390/s19040800.

22. Iskandar, M., & Sugiatini, T. E. (2024). The relationship between midwife performance with antenatal care (ANC) service satisfaction at Telagasari Community Health Center, 2023. *International Journal of Health and Pharmaceutical (IJHP)*. https://www.semanticscholar.org/paper/593353eb9a8aa105ec8cea1bfd396805a9e7b6eb (accessed on 14 May 2025).

23. Joni, J., Siregar, S., Ranteallo, O., Palamba, P., Tosuli, Y. T., Rantepulung, S., Giai, A., et al. (2024). Community assistance in constructing a clean water installation at the Bonggo Health Center, Armopa Village, Bonggo District, Sarmi Regency. *Abdi Dosen: Jurnal Pengabdian Pada Masyarakat*. https://www.semanticscholar.org/paper/14a887ad4cc27d6f6e02f507ccd9034d1922a242 (accessed on 14 May 2025).

24. Kruk, M. E., Gage, A., Arsenault, C., Jordan, K., Leslie, H. H., Roder-DeWan, S., Adeyi, O., et al. (2018). High-quality health systems in the Sustainable Development Goals era: Time for a revolution. *The Lancet Global Health, 6*, e1196–e1252. https://doi.org/10.1016/s2214-109x(18)30386-3.

25. Kumar, A., Kumar, A., Cabral-Pinto, M. M. S., Chaturvedi, A. K., Shabnam, A. A., Subrahmanyam,

G., Mondal, R., et al. (2020). Lead toxicity: Health hazards, influence on food chain, and sustainable remediation approaches. *International Journal of Environmental Research and Public Health, 17*(7), 2179. https://doi.org/10.3390/ijerph17072179.

26. Liebschner, D., Afonine, P. V., Baker, M. L., Bunkóczi, G., Chen, V. B., Croll, T. I., Hintze, B. J., et al. (2019). Macromolecular structure determination using X-rays, neutrons and electrons: Recent developments in *Phenix. Acta Crystallographica Section D: Structural Biology, 75*, 861–877. https://doi.org/10.1107/s2059798319011471.

27. McCarty, D. A., Kim, M., Jo, H., Yim, E., Yun, H., Sims, S., et al. (2025). Accessible water quality monitoring through hybrid human–machine colorimetric methods. *Environmental Monitoring and Assessment, 197*. https://www.semanticscholar.org/paper/9ff1a71b0d41c5761e7e3d75563360d13a9d2c1b (accessed on 14 May 2025).

28. Miura, B., Wagner, A., & Wu, P. (2017). Phosphate contaminant detection in water through a paper-based microfluidic device. https://core.ac.uk/download/127619787.pdf (accessed on 14 May 2025).

29. Murray, C. J. L., Ikuta, K. S., Sharara, F., Swetschinski, L. R., Robles Aguilar, G., Gray, A. P., Han, C., et al. (2022). Global burden of bacterial antimicrobial resistance in 2019: A systematic analysis. *The Lancet, 399*(10325), 629–655. https://doi.org/10.1016/s0140-6736(21)02724-0.

30. CONSERVATION X LABS (2015). Launching the grand challenges for ocean conservation. WWF, Working paper. https://core.ac.uk/download/84911929.pdf (accessed on 14 May 2025).

31. Naphtali, P., Mohiuddin, M. M., Paschos, A., & Schellhorn, H. E. (2019). Application of high-throughput 16S rRNA sequencing to identify fecal contamination sources and to complement the detection of fecal indicator bacteria in rural groundwater. *Journal of Water and Health, 17*, 393–403. https://doi.org/10.2166/wh.2019.295.

32. Okereafor, U., Makhatha, M. E., Mekuto, L., Uche-Okereafor, N., Sebola, T. E., & Mavumengwana, V. (2020). Toxic metal implications on agricultural soils, plants, animals, aquatic life and human health. *International Journal of Environmental Research and Public Health, 17*, 2204. https://doi.org/10.3390/ijerph17072204.

33. Palou, A., & Sánchez, J. (2022). Late-breaking abstracts for ECO2022. *Obesity Facts, 15*, 241–286. https://www.semanticscholar.org/paper/fe76ddf227502b447bffc194428a1a67890b6488 (accessed on 14 May 2025).

34. Patra, J. K., Das, G., Fraceto, L. F., Campos, E. V. R., Rodriguez-Torres, M. P., Acosta-Torres, L. S., Díaz-Torres, L. A., et al. (2018). Nano based drug delivery systems: Recent developments and future prospects. *Journal of Nanobiotechnology, 16*. https://doi.org/10.1186/s12951-018-0392-8.

35. Percie du Sert, N., Ahluwalia, A., Alam, S., Avey, M. T., Baker, M., Browne, W. J., Clark, A., et al. (2020). Reporting animal research: Explanation and elaboration for the ARRIVE guidelines 2.0. *PLOS Biology, 18*, e3000411. https://doi.org/10.1371/journal.pbio.3000411.

36. Raj, M. P., & Philip, R. S. (2025). Seasonal dynamics of Herohalli Lake in North Bangalore, Karnataka, India: A limnological study of water stations and its impact on a vertebrate biological system. *Journal of Environmental Biology*. 6, issue 1, pp. 47-57. DOI: 10.22438/jeb/46/1/MRN-5300. https://www.semanticscholar.org/paper/eee43e2fa7bf2279b55b702057c76ea70176db6b (accessed on 14 May 2025).

37. Rasheed, A., San, O., & Kvamsdal, T. (2020). Digital twin: Values, challenges and enablers from a modeling perspective. *IEEE Access, 8*, 21980–22012. https://doi.org/10.1109/access.2020.2970143.

38. Sani, M., Muazu, Z., & Dangaladima, H. (2023). An assessment of the physiochemical quality of drinking water from tube wells and its effects on human health in Sokoto metropolis. *Caliphate Journal of Science and Technology*. . 5. 132-139. 10.4314/cajost.v5i2.7. https://www.semanticscholar.org/paper/c5ba48b38701ce648f23631fa9e703144240662e (accessed on 14 May 2025).

39. Suhartawan, B. (2025). Application of the British Columbia Water Quality Index (BC-WQI) method to determine the water quality status of Lake Sentani in Jayapura. *Riwayat: Educational Journal of History and Humanities*. https://www.semanticscholar.org/paper/7167879df116411be8505783d4f8d42db8797519 (accessed on 14 May 2025).

40. Wang, Z., DeWitt, J. C., Higgins, C. P., & Cousins, I. T. (2017). A never-ending story of per- and polyfluoroalkyl substances (PFASs)? *Environmental Science & Technology, 51*, 2508–2518. https://doi.org/10.1021/acs.est.6b04806.

41. Wilson, L., Hayes, W., Jones, N., Eaves, L. A., Wait, K., George, A., Freeman, B., et al. (2024). Lead occurrence in North Carolina well water: Importance of sampling representation and collection techniques. *Environmental Research Letters, 19*. https://www.semanticscholar.org/paper/45eed4e35fdb9a9f43b949382bd98a61ca221b82 (accessed on 14 May 2025).

42. Wu, X., Nethery, R. C., Sabath, M. B., Braun, D., & Dominici, F. (2020). Exposure to air pollution and COVID-19 mortality in the United States: A nationwide cross-sectional study. *medRxiv*. https://doi.org/10.1101/2020.04.05.20054502.

43. Xu, Y., & Braune, E. (2009). *Sustainable Groundwater Resources in Africa: Water Supply and Sanitation Environment*. CRC Press. DOI: https://doi.org/10.1201/9780203859452. https://www.semanticscholar.org/paper/1803c90e406bf4d872e8081a07392a57e5a39947 (accessed on 14 May 2025).

44. Zarate-Cáceres, C.R.; Iparraguirre-Meza, M.; Pérez-Venegas, C.J.; Picoy-Gonzales, J.A.; Ordoñez-Ccora, G.; Lacho-Gutiérrez, P.; Riveros-Laurente, K.Y.; Diaz-Aranda, D.L.; Gutiérrez-Iparraguirre, G.G.; Huarcaya-Taype, R.; et al. Integrated water quality assessment and health risk analysis of heavy metal and microbial contamination in the Ichu River, Peru. *F1000Research* **2025**, *14*, 384, https://doi.org/10.12688/f1000research.162022.1. (accessed on 14 May 2025).

45. Zhong, R. Y., Xu, X., Klotz, E., & Newman, S. T. (2017). Intelligent manufacturing in the context of Industry 4.0: A review. *Engineering, 3*, 616–630. https://doi.org/10.1016/j.eng.2017.05.015.

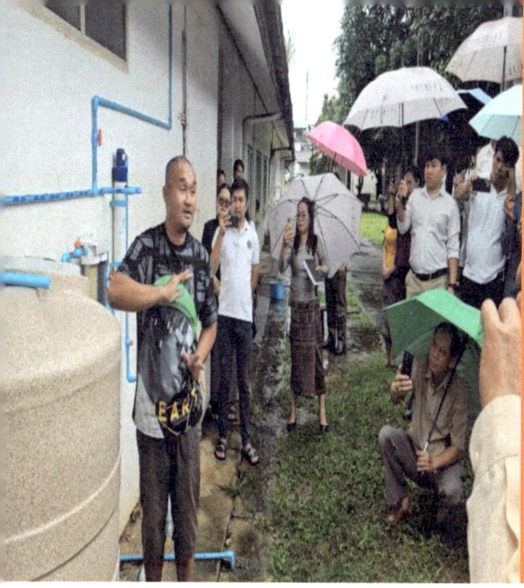

Chapter 4

WATER TREATMENT METHODS FOR COMMUNITY HEALTH

Contents

Introduction

Water is essential to our daily well-being, but so many communities do not have the necessary water treatment that could make a difference. Plenty of evidence exists that indicates that safe drinking water is associated with improved public health, but too many times the systems do not work. In most areas, inadequate or simply poor water treatment results in waterborne disease outbreaks—harming health, destabilizing economies, and shaving quality of life. Scientists, for instance, have long established that poor sanitation and unsafe water are closely linked to increased cases of diarrheal diseases, particularly in low- and middle-income regions (Wolf et al., 2014). Therefore, developing and implementing the correct treatment strategies isn't only crucial, it's necessary. Ineffective water treatment not only increases the risk of disease but traps communities in poverty and disparate health statistics. Individuals with waterborne diseases end up staying home from work and school, and this subsequently hinders economic development and academic advancement. In general, making sustainable water treatment is more than just technology; it needs to involve locals and take firm action. Surprisingly, new ideas such as output-based financing for sanitation services are becoming effective means of increasing how effectively and responsibly water services are provided (Evans et al., 2010a). It would appear to be obvious that as much as we need to maintain a watch over what is currently in operation, backing new policies is the essential factor in the mitigation of such health risks. In the future, addressing water treatment problems quite literally requires patchwork efforts on the part of government agencies, nonprofits, civic groups, and others. Where multiple sectors are contributing, you have more funds, improved public education, and grassroots efforts that advocate for quality water. From filtration to boiling or chemical disinfection, knowing the different methods influences solutions that cater to each community's requirements. Balancing the meticulous assessments of these methods with targeted actions can ease the burden of waterborne diseases, and, in doing so, further social equity and enable local folks to own up to their water sources.

Importance of Clean Water for Public Health

In South-Western Nigeria, in one study it was revealed that as few as 25% of schools received adequate drinking water points, with an estimated 40% missing simple gender-separated latrines—a deficiency seriously compromising the privacy and safety of older girls. Clean water is not a luxury; it's a necessity, and where it is lacking, communities will experience an outbreak of waterborne diseases that usually result in increased rates of disease and even premature death. Public facilities such as schools often experience deficits in water, sanitation, and hygiene (WASH) facilities, and the combined problems cause not only health damage but also interrupt educational advancement and gender balance, clearly demonstrating the close link between water quality and overall well-being of society (Olukanni et al., 2013). Understanding how people act in terms of water use—how they comport themselves around handwashing and sanitation, for example—tends to be most important in the task of improving water quality. Most researchers tend to indicate that combining several different advertising strategies, as opposed to the use of a single method, can change behaviors positively. A combination of approaches that considers local threats and enablers appears to enhance the effectiveness of water treatment programs. Once communities incorporate these behavioral elements, they can influence policies and programs that not only improve treatment processes but also public health. Innovative educational programs packaged with infrastructural improvement make clean water more accessible and promote healthier lifestyles (Musekiwa et al., 2017). Providing clean water to flow into a neighborhood isn't simply a matter of working past logistical barriers, it's a critical issue of public health. The moment that proper water treatment goes into effect, the payoffs are soon extended far beyond short-term health gains; lower healthcare expenditures and greater productivity allow individuals to positively contribute more to their neighborhoods. Improved health simply means that families ultimately spend less on healthcare, which saves them resources to spend on education and economic investments and hence halt poverty cycles. For all of these reasons, public policy regarding water treatment should be inclined towards holistic strategies that solve both the consistent supply of clean water and the development of safe hygiene habits, finally raising community health on every level (Musekiwa et al., 2017).

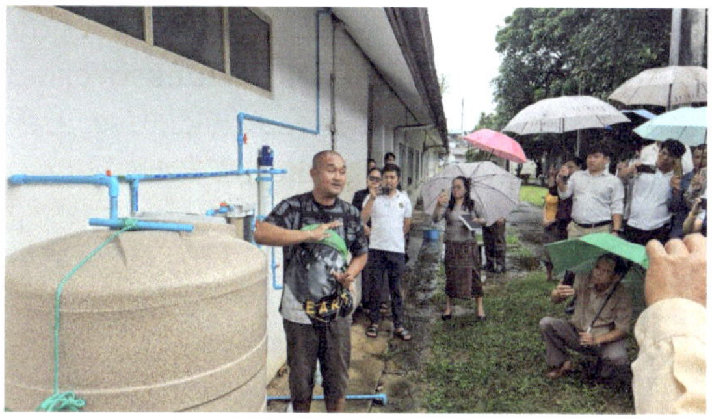

Source: NUS Saw Swee Hock School of Public Health. (2024). *Water Quality Initiative.*

4.1. Types of Water Contaminants

Water becomes contaminated in several ways, and these pollutants disrupt nature and our bodies as well. Organic chemicals—most times flowing in with farm waste or industrial runoff, can seep into our water and appear in wastewater as such items as phosphor organic flame retardants and musk scents. Research tends to indicate that most of these chemicals tend to harm small animals that act as living gauges for aquatic health. , orders such as Ephemeroptera and Plecoptera appear affected the most, and their decline makes the biodiversity wane and the urban rivers lose some of their natural integrity. The effects cascade beyond the water itself, as reduced biodiversity can disrupt food chains and the entire ecological balance, highlighting the necessity for improved cleaning practices (Borja et al., 2013). Heavy metals represent another tangible threat. They enter water primarily by way of industrial discharge and mining activities, accumulating gradually in sediments and gradually seeping into the food web. Heavy metals like lead, mercury, and cadmium, usually with long-term accumulation, are associated with neurological disorders and developmental conditions in several instances. Remediation may fall short if it does not penetrate the root of the pollution. Community health initiatives, therefore, need to address these metals with innovative filtration technologies and even bioremediation strategies to assist in making water safe. Only an integrated approach can face the complicated web of contaminants we have (Borja et al., 2013).

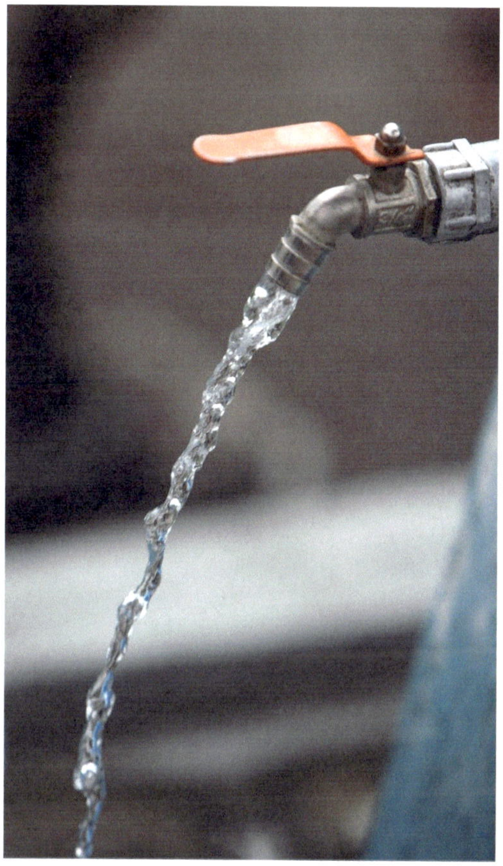

Figure 4.1. Contaminants in your drinking water faucet.

Source: By Josh Estey/AusAID, CC BY 2.0, https://commons.wikimedia.org/w/index.php?curid=32167621

Microbial invaders are another threat that can compromise water quality nearly instantly. Disease-causing organisms such as bacteria, viruses, and protozoa infiltrate through sewage spills, animal fecal matter, or even rain runoff, and tend to strike hardest at the most vulnerable—children and the elderly. A sudden outbreak of waterborne disease can rapidly escalate into a full-fledged public health emergency, reminding us that our monitoring and treatment infrastructure requires a serious overhaul. Although processes like chlorination and UV disinfection do serve to limit these risks, overuse of chemicals could ironically do even more damage to water quality. Finding the balance between effective pathogen removal and the preservation of the overall ecosystem is critical to ensuring long-term community health (Figure 4.1).

4.1.1. Biological Contaminants

Water infrastructure takes a beating from small biological intruders that disrupt both our well-being and nature's equilibrium. Bacteria, viruses, and protozoa, essentially the same suspects found in raw sewage and agricultural runoff—disrupt water quality and generally in novel and often unpredictable manners. When these microorganisms multiply, diseases emerge, sometimes targeting susceptible populations like children and elderly individuals particularly severely.

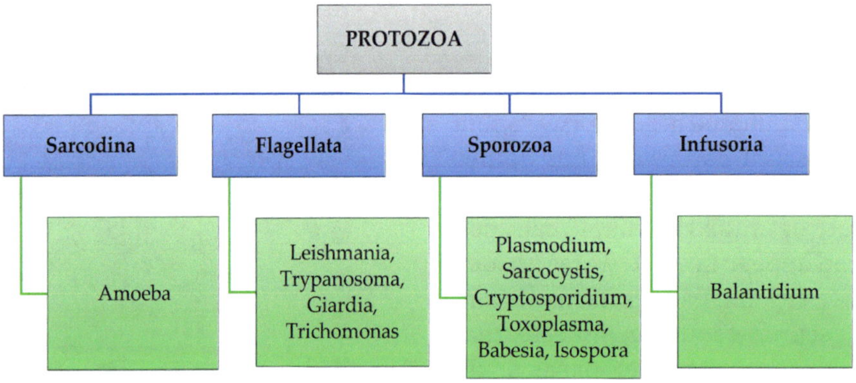

Figure 4.2. Parasitic protozoa.

Source: Omarova A, Tussupova K, Berndtsson R, Kalishev M, Sharapatova K. Protozoan Parasites in Drinking Water: A System Approach for Improved Water, Sanitation and Hygiene in Developing Countries. *International Journal of Environmental Research and Public Health*. 2018; 15(3):495. https://doi.org/10.3390/ijerph15030495

Typically, these health warnings alert us to the fact that rapid, effective treatments for water are required. Today, technologies such as membrane filtration or UV treatment are used more and more to knock these pathogens out of the way, rendering drinking water safer (even when the outcomes aren't ideal every time). Ultimately, determining the sources of these contaminants and how they act is the key to developing regulations that really do serve communities. Research has consistently demonstrated that aquatic environments can become disrupted once biological pollutants enter the scene. An examination of some sampling locations confirmed that organic contaminants, such as those from organic wastewater, can disrupt the balance for invertebrate populations, suggesting an overall ecological breakdown linked to human activities. In one case, it was documented that treated wastewater pollutants significantly rewrote species compositions, threatening biodiversity. In general, improved water treatment appears to hold out the prospect of a healthier aquatic atmosphere. That implies intelligent, well-targeted measures are necessary not only to reduce these pollutants but also to assist with the rehabilitation and conservation of the fragile systems we rely on. It is no simple balancing act between the demands of human beings and our surroundings; our waterways ought to be capable of sustaining a rich diversity of life. Communities that are honest with themselves need to invest in new fresh water treatment systems that balance efficiency with sustainability if they want to outsmart the danger of biological contaminants. Traditional chlorination may help to some extent, but it often leaves behind disinfection by-products that can cause further health issues. On the other hand, contemporary methods such as biofiltration and combined membrane systems appear to address an extensive spectrum of pathogens while minimizing ecological damage. Research, even though occasionally it produces variable outcomes—indicates that state-of-the-art activated sludge systems can take water quality to an entire different level. Real-time monitoring of the water and engaging the locals also greatly enhance treatment effects, even though the process is not entirely flawless. In short, adopting a multi-faceted, comprehensive strategy for managing water seems vital for maintaining public health in its place and keeping nature's equilibrium intact, allowing aquatic ecosystems to flourish (Figure 4.2).

4.1.2. Chemical Contaminants

Everybody should have clean water, but far too many communities continue to have to deal with drinking water contaminated by chemicals. More often than not, these intrusive chemicals seep in through farm runoff, industrial spills that are accidental, or simply bad waste disposal – a complex combination that includes heavy metals like lead, mercury, and arsenic, which have contaminated many water supplies and can interfere with health and human development. In remote locations like regions of the Amazon, where simple sanitation is just not there, waterborne diseases continue to crop up. Addressing this type of pollution is not easy; it requires innovative, new strategies that treat people's health and the environment with equal respect. Essentially, we require programs that treat to contain these hazardous substances while safeguarding vulnerable populations. Meeting this challenge, several new water treatment technologies are beginning to make their presence felt. Some of these compact systems rely on processes such as copper ionization and ultraviolet (UV) light to purify water, eliminating scores of biological and chemical contaminants in the process. One study examined an automated treatment system and discovered it reduced heavy metal levels , for example, iron and zinc in addition to cleaning out a lot of microorganisms. Naturally, the system is not flawless; its shortcomings serve as a reminder that there is continuous research and refinement necessary, particularly in areas with mercury pollution caused by mining activities (Nadia et al., 2025). As a whole, applying these types of technologies has the ability to cut down on the health hazards of contaminated water, typically improving public well-being and strengthening resistance to environmental decline. To that end, biosorption methods are becoming a green solution for industrial wastewater treatment. This method depends on natural, or in some cases, altered—biomass to behave similarly to a sponge for harmful contaminants such as heavy metals and organic pollutants. In a Panipat District Haryana case, biosorption was truly impressive: activated carbon (AC) achieved nearly 96% chromium removal, and agricultural residues removed approximately 95% of dye pollutants. These results underscore the fact that biosorption can be very practical, particularly in situations where conventional treatment options simply don't work. Combining such innovative concepts not only enhances water quality and safeguards aquatic environments but also ensures communities have a safe source of drinking water, thus proving biosorption to be a vital component in sustainable water treatment processes (Maan et al., 2024) (Figure 4.3).

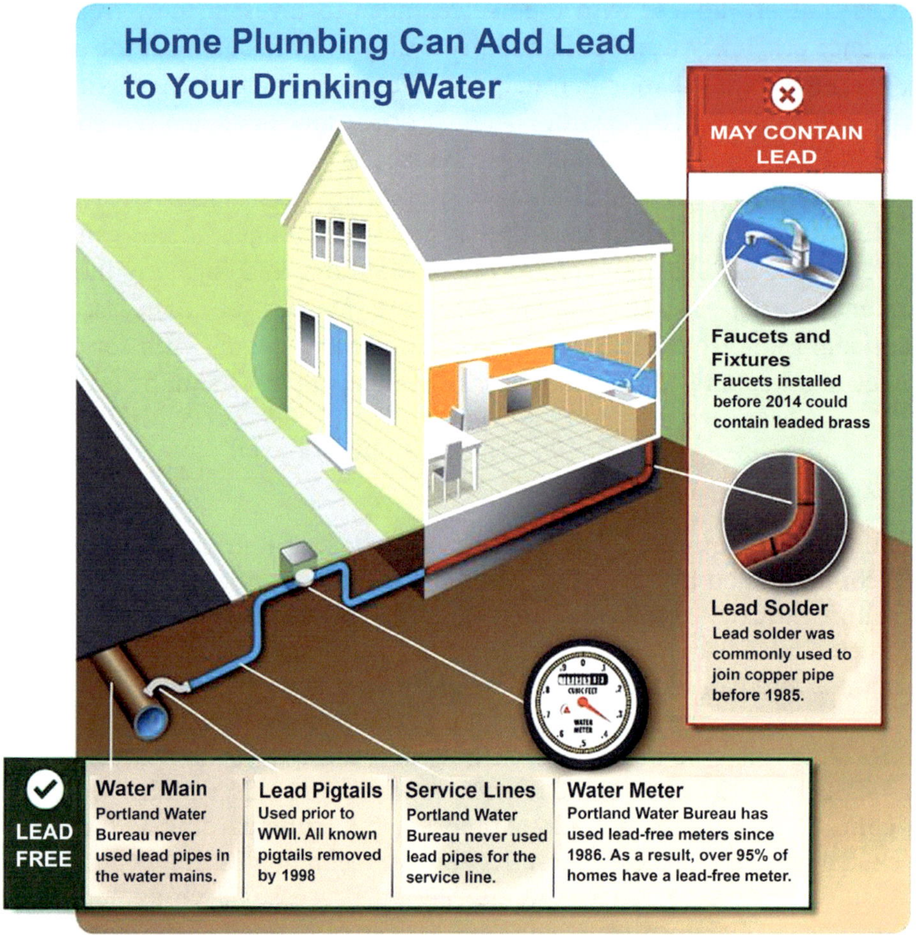

Figure 4.3. Lead and drinking water.

Source: https://files.mtstatic.com/site_4334/401669/0?Expires= 1745398291&Signature=UBieKI0xar6UUFzhYtU4aQ6ia6nDWj1p2SFQ2oX9JsNwuM30~Sdz3FRL8Cqey3OOg6EHxg4NSyFDW9hxtNsmscuHXj7LijWFI vstgJ0NxcadkVo7GWIv59X5BfM6S~5ddyh0Iwt5AHY1vxYT xfen7evzc7Byhf393-~oX~Z7tFE_&Key-Pair-Id=APKAJ5Y6AV4GI7A555NA.

4.1.3. Physical Contaminants

Contaminated water is a very real issue, and honestly, the starting point is trying to get your head around all the various pollutants that are out there. Physical material, such as sediments, plastics, and pieces of organic trash, can ruin water quality and even cause us harm in ways you'd never suspect. These pollutants usually originate from things such as urban runoff, factory spills, and agricultural methods. When they accumulate, freshwater and marine ecosystems suffer; aquatic ecosystems get disrupted, habitats become impaired, and it becomes simpler for pathogens to spread. Overall, drinking or even being exposed to such water is perilous, highlighting just how much we require improved means of ridding ourselves of these physical impurities. Traditional water treatment techniques struggle with these problems. Yes, filtration can catch the larger particles, but it tends to miss the smaller sediments and those annoying microplastics. The combination of organic waste, too, has a way of derailing chemical treatments so that disinfection isn't as effective as hoped. More often than not, a new, creative approach must be used. Consider biosorption, for instance, in this process, organic substances essentially grasp onto pollutants such as heavy metals and organic toxins, reducing their occurrence in wastewater. It assists in making water more drinkable and enhances the overall sustainability of treatment methods, which is instrumental in safeguarding community health and our environment alike (Maan et al., 2024). Technology continually alters the water treatment game. The recent advances are utilizing nanomaterials to boost filtration, and one of the techniques that are being considered increasingly is membrane distillation (MD). The method enables water vapor to separate in a selective way from the array of contaminants, so the water emerges much cleaner. It's regarded as an environmentally friendly method that's also scalable, providing a substitute to conventional strategies that tend to require heavy use of chemicals and may even generate toxic byproducts (Kakkar et al., 2024). Through the implementation of these sophisticated strategies, treatment systems can really shine at removing physical contaminants, which ultimately makes a significant impact for communities that rely on clean water.

4.2. Conventional Water Treatment Processes

Keeping the community healthy is mostly up to how well we take care of our water, and the process is not quite as simple as it seems. Traditional treatment typically starts by adding chemicals that cause impurities to stick together in a process called coagulation so that small particles and microorganisms clump into small masses or flocs. Gravity then comes in during sedimentation, pulling down these heavier clumps and reducing turbidity and pathogens, and a filter finally traps any wayward particles. However, although this initial protocol is effective for many types of contaminants, it is less effective when it comes to recalcitrant stuff like PFAS, which tends to resist these usual approaches. As Fernandes et al. (2025) suggest, these persistent chemicals pose actual health threats, prompting scientists and engineers to explore additional methods that could complement the normal measures. After a majority of particulates are removed from the mixture, disinfection takes over as an essential follow-up measure. In most cases, measures based on chlorine, UV radiation, or ozone are used to decontaminate the remaining pathogens in the water supply. Now, while chlorine is inexpensive and prevalent, it occasionally creates by-products that can potentially lead to long-term health issues. Current research in most instances has indicated the positives of new methods that can more effectively combat waterborne microbes while keeping risks under wraps. For instance, Chaudhry et al. (2017) illustrate that microbial risks in recycled water could exceed safety limits, highlighting the critical importance of strong disinfection measures not only in traditional but in reclaimed water supplies as well. Combining such state-of-the-art techniques with traditional installations can increase public health protection. Despite the firm foundation these traditional processes give, they are not without criticism as water quality issues continue to develop. There remains concern regarding both chemical and microbial pollutants that find their way past conventional treatment protocols. Ongoing innovation in water treatment technologies is thus necessary to address ongoing concerns such as PFAS and to remain compliant with health regulations. As communities make more and more communities consider alternatives such as reclaimed water, it becomes increasingly critical to balance risk considerations fully and work to reconcile health protection with the effective use of resources. The constantly evolving nature of water treatment requires continued study and a partnership among public health practitioners, engineers, and environmental scientists, efforts that will be central to ensuring the future stability of our water infrastructure and health of our communities.

4.2.1. Coagulation and Flocculation

Treatment of water usually begins with coagulation and flocculation. What these processes basically do is introduce a coagulant that causes small particles to clump together into aggregates—flocs, they're called, which you can then settle out or simply filter out. The goal is to reduce turbidity and meet important water quality targets. These days, there is a lot of interest in the use of natural products such as Moringa oleifera; not only do they work pretty well, but they also come with fewer environmental liabilities than conventional chemical agents. Numerous communities are turning to these more environmentally friendly alternatives as part of a general effort toward sustainable water treatment. In a number of tests—yes, even in strict pilot plant trials—*Moringa oleifera* has proven to have a penchant for lowering turbidity, at times averaging decreases as high as 96.9% when beginning with extremely high levels. In most instances, the process, which progresses from creating flocs to allowing them to settle, ultimately results in water with residual turbidity far below set limits. It's a sequential dance in which every step overlaps to some extent with the one that follows, all designed to improve quality and decrease dependence upon abrasive synthetic chemicals. The biodynamic nature and comparative ease of access to these coagulants made from natural products contribute to their popularity, particularly when public health issues hang heavily over polluted water supplies. There is also an increasing concern regarding the long-term dangers associated with synthetic coagulants. Research in general indicates that although effective, chemicals may harbor chronic toxicity and present environmental risks. Surprisingly, the combination of natural agents such as Moringa oleifera with conventional options like Alum has proved to be very effective—more like a synergistic loophole that enhances general treatment efficacy. For example, certain trials have shown outstanding turbidity and organic load removal rates when the two forms are used together. Admittedly, the cost may be slightly more, but the added cost frequently correlates with a decrease in public health hazards and an inclination towards sustainability. Consequently, coagulation and flocculation, when carefully incorporated into community water treatment systems, can not only enhance health outcomes but also promote environmental stewardship that serves future generations (Deswal et al., 2023; Mohammed et al., 2001) (Figure 4.4).

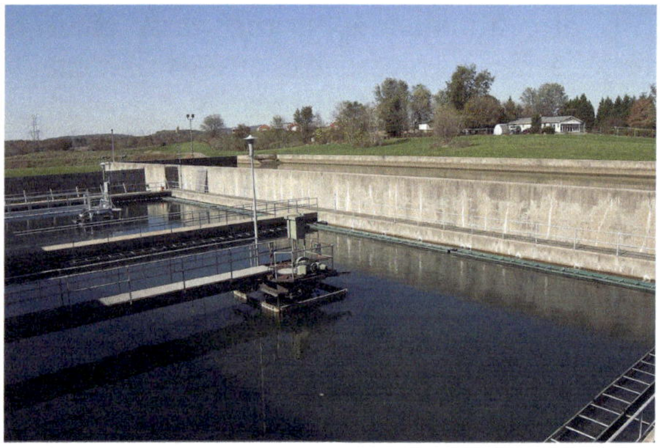

Figure 4.4. Coagulation and flocculation in water treatment.

Source: By USEPA Environmental-Protection-Agency - The coagulation and filtration processes at a drinking water treatment plant., Public Domain, https://commons.wikimedia.org/w/index.php?curid=51969765

4.2.2. Sedimentation

Water treatment makes communities healthy, particularly where safe water is not easily accessible. Sedimentation comes in handy here; gravity does all the work by allowing particles to settle naturally at the bottom of a tank. In most instances, this simple trick reduces turbidity and other contaminants. If researchers add coagulation (with chemicals such as aluminum sulfate or ferric chloride), the smaller pieces clump together, making it simpler to settle out (Mahdavi et al., 2024). Research has even confirmed that when they test for lower heavy metal content and reduced cloudiness, these techniques work well enough. Sedimentation is a low-cost method of improving water quality before additional treatment in certain rural or low-resource communities. Consider, for example, certain Amazonian villages where individuals blend sedimentation with domestic activities such as filtration and chlorination. You may assume that sedimentation is merely the process of solids removal, but it also reduces organic load, subsequently reducing microbes. In experiments, scientists observed that as much as 22% of turbidity was eliminated from river water samples, a finding that not only enhances the appearance of the water but also reduces possible dangers (Gomes et al., 2024). Such gains highlight the way, in most instances, this process is necessary when sophisticated purifying isn't feasible. Despite all its advantages, sedimentation isn't a magic solution for water safety. The last water quality relies on proper handling and subsequent treatment. Different studies, even those on isolated Amazonian villages—show that although sedimentation can lower turbidity, carelessness in subsequent processes such as chlorination may lead to recontamination. This indicates, quite evidently, the necessity for hands-on water safety education so that people can benefit fully from sedimentation while minimizing waterborne hazards (Gomes et al., 2024) (Figure 4.5).

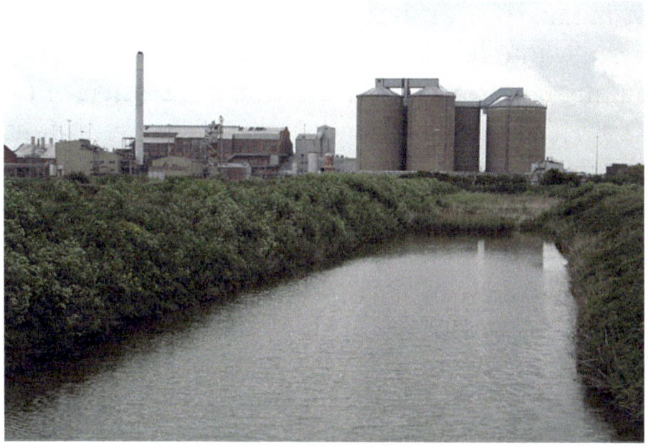

Figure 4.5. Sedimentation.

Source: By Alan Murray-Rust, CC BY-SA 2.0, https://commons.wikimedia.org/w/index.php?curid=12955326

4.2.3. Filtration

Filtration is the most common way of ensuring our drinking water is pure. Towns count on a combination of filter types—sometimes it's just plain sand or AC, other times membrane filters—to remove particles, organic material, and even unwanted microorganisms. For most people, this solution not only enhances overall wellness but also establishes a certain level of trust in community water systems, encouraging individuals to take more interest in community health. Particularly where waterborne disease represents a very real danger for vulnerable individuals, having some such filtration systems in place is absolutely critical. Meanwhile, filtration frequently intersects with the daily financial situation. Mostly, when families and local health systems are less plagued by waterborne diseases, everybody benefits—less money spent on medication and improved overall quality of life, some studies say. People using stable filtration systems report less sickness, and that means lower overall costs. And when local health practitioners become involved in maintaining the systems, clean water becomes even more reliable. A resident-centered installation such as this not only gives the local populace power, but also subtly pressures for a sustainable way of handling public health. Taking a step back, filtration is not sufficient by itself, it collaborates with other water treatment processes such as coagulation, sedimentation, and chlorination. Research has indicated that when all these methods are combined, pollutants get eliminated more effectively, creating healthier water and additional health benefits. What's cool is that filtration systems can be modified to meet local needs, addressing particular issues the community may have. Ultimately, filtration isn't merely some sort of high-tech solution; it's central to bettering community health, encouraging all to participate and have faith in their water supply safety (Figure 4.6).

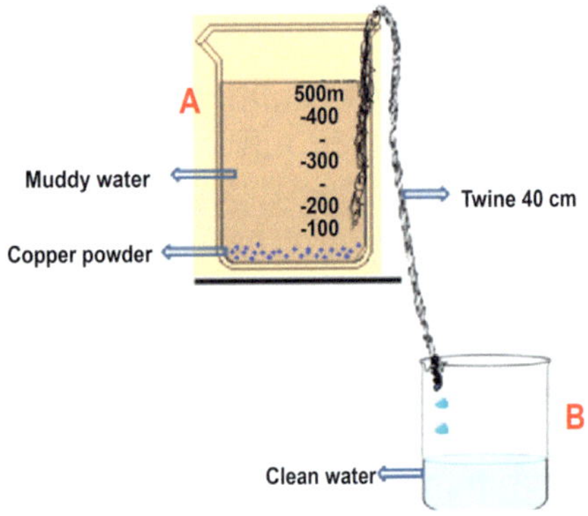

Figure 4.6. Filtration of contaminated water using cotton ropes.

Source: Banerji, A. (2017). *Filtration of Contaminated Water Using Cotton Ropes.* ResearchGate.

4.3. Advanced Water Treatment Technologies

Clean water demand is increasing, and this demand has prompted some rather significant jumps in how we process it. Small and mid-sized communities, especially, can't always count on the tried and true, so there's been an effort to experiment with new techniques. For instance, one study under the auspices of the Scottish Government examined various possibilities for purifying drinking water in rural communities. They conducted a wide assessment of existing technology—seeking not just to achieve health targets but also to make it sustainable. In most instances, such efforts allow communities to choose for themselves what works best, which makes the process more inclusive and better informed (Blackwood et al., 2016). By combining cutting-edge technologies with solutions tailored to local requirements, these actions assist in advancing improved health outcomes and increasing public confidence in water quality. A combination of challenging environmental problems and aging infrastructure has highlighted the shortcomings of conventional wastewater treatment. In areas such as New Hampshire's Great Bay community, increased levels of pollutants like nitrogen have overwhelmed facilities that previously coped adequately. This deterioration, in the majority of instances, threatens both our environment and public well-being. Scientists have been warning of the necessity to upgrade facilities, which has paved the way for innovative thinking on more innovative treatment concepts at lower costs. Local initiatives now target eradicating excessive nitrogen levels while recycling wastewater for other purposes. With assistance from emerging technology, communities are able to reduce pollution and achieve clean water for both immediate requirements and in the future (Kaczynski, 2015). Modern water treatment technology contributes directly to the health of a community by ensuring access to safe drinking water and keeping practices sustainable. When communities are prioritizing methods that boost treatment efficiency, they're in a stronger position to combat local problems such as pollution and scarcity of water resources. Occasionally professional workshops and roundtable discussions assist in paving the way to the selection of proper methods—such discussions naturally combine views and adapt to local circumstances (Blackwood et al., 2016). Finally, such strategies not only make water systems more resilient but also enable communities to flourish, even as problems continue to accumulate (Figure 4.7).

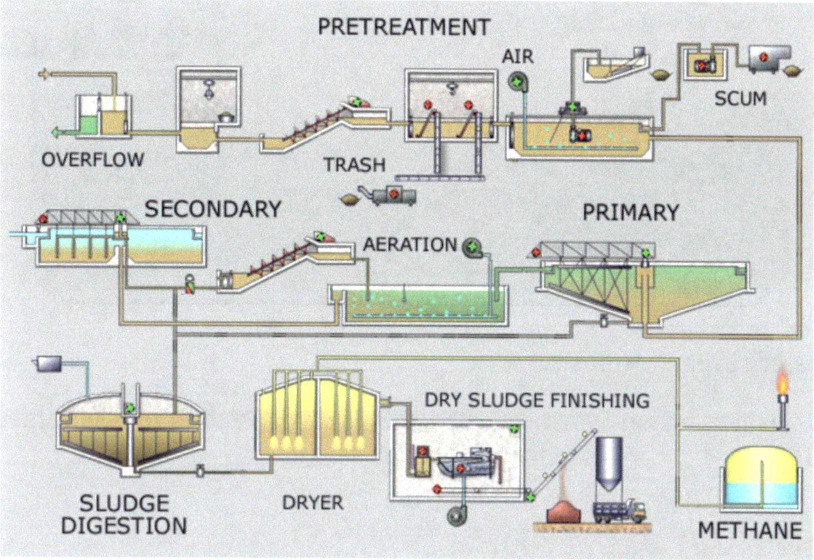

Figure 4.7. The most important water treatment processes.

Source: https://courses.lumenlearning.com/suny-mcc-microbiology/chapter/wastewater-treatment-and-water-purification/

4.3.1. Reverse Osmosis (RO)

Safe, clean drinking water is more necessary than ever before, and individuals are seeking out all sorts of treatment methods to provide this necessity. RO, or RO, has emerged as a favorite because it isn't merely about filtering, it removes water by forcing it through a semi-permeable membrane with pressure, allowing water molecules to pass while capturing dissolved solids, contaminants, and pathogens. This procedure does not simply purify the water; it will also make its taste and sensation better. More often than not, determining the environmental trade-offs is crucial in deciding whether RO should be utilized in public health measures. Rolling out RO in water treatment is not all sail though. An examination of some of the different treatment situations typically finds that although RO will enhance water quality, its energy requirements can cause more environmental impacts than traditional practices. Evidence indicates that water treated through RO in large plants has environmental impacts nearly double that of residential systems primarily due to the more substantial energy involved (Garfi et al., 2016). This raises the question naturally of how sustainable RO is in the long term, particularly in areas where energy is scarce. Otherwise, though, the possible health gains may offset the energy liabilities. Some evidence suggests that traditional sources of water—especially those receiving de facto reuse—have substantial microbial dangers associated with them, such as from *Norovirus* and *Salmonella* contaminants (Chaudhry et al., 2017). In crowded urban areas, where shortages and contamination of water are real threats, applying RO could prove vital to protecting drinking water. So while it's worth considering RO carefully in terms of its environmental impact, its ability to decrease microbial risk is an integral part of the overall water treatment discussion (Figure 4.8).

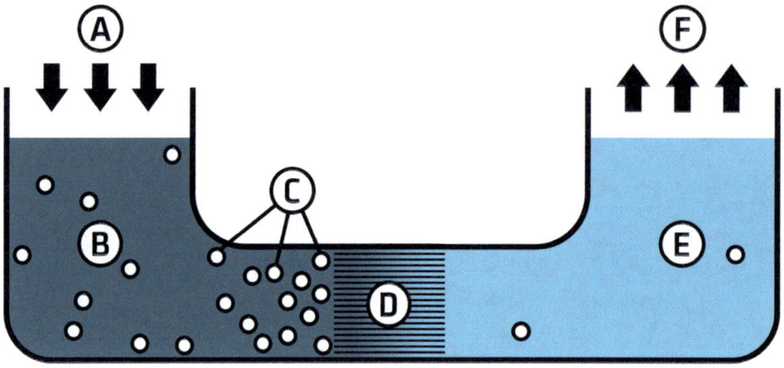

Figure 4.8. Stages of reverse osmosis.

Source: By Colby Fisher - Own work, CC BY-SA 3.0, https://commons.wikimedia.org/w/index.php?curid=25213532

4.3.2. Ultraviolet (UV) Disinfection

Waterborne diseases have been at the forefront of minds recently, compelling communities to look into alternative ways to treat water. UV disinfection, for instance, presents itself as a prime choice, it utilizes UV light to penetrate microbial cell walls and disrupt their DNA so that they can't replicate, all without the vile chemicals that traditional treatments frequently require. In small to medium-sized towns where chemical treatments may not be effective enough, adding UV systems to existing configurations can truly strike gold in terms of sustainability and health objectives. Its ability to clean water fast also makes it a good option in rural areas where conventional treatments sometimes fall behind demand. Getting up close and personal, UV disinfection flaunts its versatility in water reuse applications. In direct potable reuse or reclaimed water schemes, this treatment comes in to address both microbial trouble and chemical residues, thus providing a surefire next step after wastewater treatment. While concerns regarding certain recalcitrant microbes continue to arise, in most instances UV application trims those risks down, a factor that contributes to reconciliation with reclaimed water safety and increases public health efforts in most instances. This dual role of providing security and assisting in environmental objectives certainly makes it a player to watch in the context of new water treatment concepts. When you take a step back, incorporating UV disinfection into overall water treatment strategies really coheres with sustainability objectives, particularly in neighborhoods with special requirements. Recent research funded by government initiatives, for instance, highlights that choosing the right technology is crucial for rural areas aiming to improve resilience and overall health outcomes. Besides being effective, UV disinfection doesn't produce harmful byproducts like those chemical processes do. As various stakeholders continue to weigh their options, figuring out when and how to plug in UV systems is becoming essential. This approach not only maintains public health levels high, but it also engages the community, sometimes in a slightly rocky process, to make sure decisions about managing water take us to a cleaner, more sustainable future (Figure 4.9).

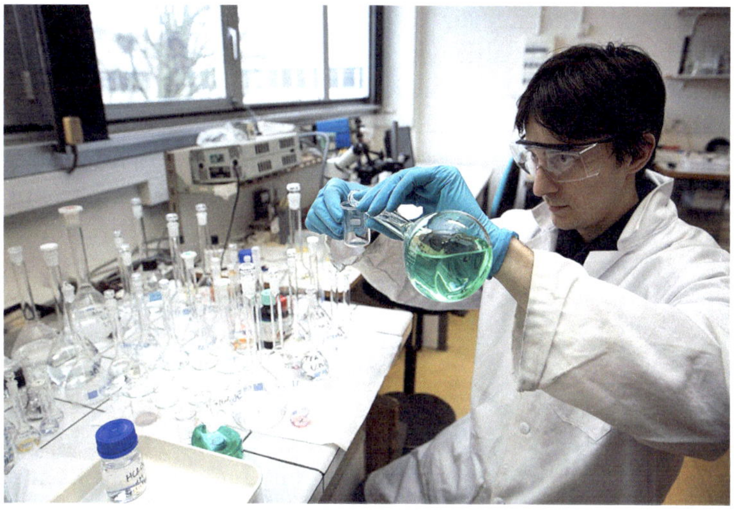

Figure 4.9. UV disinfection system for water treatment.

Source: By Ecole polytechnique / Paris / France - https://www.flickr.com/photos/117994717@N06/46078413375/, CC BY-SA 2.0, https://commons.wikimedia.org/w/index.php?curid=89609516

4.3.3. Advanced Oxidation Processes

Water networks are often filled with toxic contaminants that undermine public health and need new solutions for scrubbing them clean. One concept that's been making waves is advanced oxidation processes (AOPs), they involve using high-energy agents to degrade pollutants where traditional measures simply fail. These processes initiate the creation of hydroxyl radicals, those small, militant oxidizers that assist in breaking down complex organic substances into forms that are much less harmful. Adding AOPs to our water treatment regimen appears to be full of potential, in general, because when noxious substances are eliminated more efficiently, the entire community reaps the rewards through safer water and healthier environments. TiO_2 photocatalytic degradation, with titanium dioxide nanoparticles, is another avenue individuals are pursuing. With UV light, the nanoparticles get to work, initiating oxidizing reactions that facilitate breaking down of pollutants. However, there is still some concern as to whether the nanoparticles themselves are toxic, so caution must be exercised in most instances. Scientists are also experimentally examining replacements such as ultrasonic cavitation—a technique wherein small microbubbles are formed and they later collapse while delivering hydroxyl radicals along the way. With it sometimes becoming difficult to perfect the efficiency in using the prevailing ultrasonic tools, innovative set-ups like that of a targeted ultrasonic setup are emerging that are poised to accelerate the deterioration process. Overall, these innovations are truly contributing to changing the way we address persistent contaminants that resist treatment through conventional means. There is also an urgent need for improved treatments since standard wastewater treatment procedures tend to flounder with such pollutants as cytotoxic antibiotics and non-biodegradable dyes. Recent research shows that AOPs can degrade such substances that persist even after traditional procedures have had their way. For instance, how methylene blue is degraded under such systems indicates AOPs' capabilities in addressing industrial wastewater issues. Such recalcitrant dyes, resistant to normal treatment protocols, not only linger but also pose major ecological and health threats. Through the proper implementation of AOPs, communities are inching nearer to water of improved quality, a public health win and a step in the direction of more sustainable, environmentally sound practices that ultimately benefit overall health (Figure 4.10).

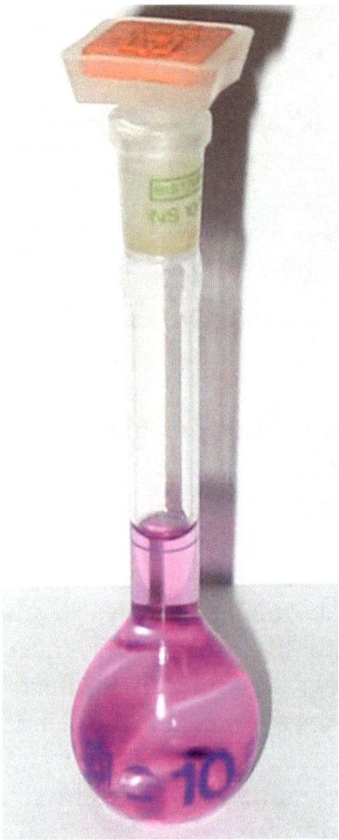

Figure 4.10. Advanced oxidation processes (AOPs) in water treatment.

Source: By David Mülheims (David Mülheims, Microbeany) - Self-photographed, CC BY-SA 2.5, https://commons.wikimedia.org/w/index.php?curid=1254767

4.4. Community-Based Water Treatment Solutions

Community water treatment systems are becoming more visible these days because they contribute to better public health, particularly in areas where resources are scarce. Locals utilize what nature has provided for them and blend in old-fashioned ingenuity in creating systems that suit their own requirements. Nature-based methods, for example, appear to play double-duty by providing individuals with clean drinking water while also keeping the environment under control. Recent assessments tend to suggest that such approaches bring additional benefits to human welfare and community resilience, hence being more effective and affordable than conventional systems. It's quite crucial, therefore, to engage local stakeholders from the very conceptualization stage; this way, projects end up feeling culturally appropriate and working well in actual environments, increasing the likelihood that everyone will remain committed to them (Cecchi et al., 2015). It also happens that education is a significant factor in the success of community-based water treatment initiatives. When locals are educated on water management and care, they are likely to adopt practices that safeguard their water sources for the long term. Workshops and even practical sessions that include activities such as rainwater harvesting and basic filtering serve to disseminate useful skills and instill a sense of individual responsibility towards water resources. Such learning tends to bring the community together. For the most part, studies have found that if individuals are informed of what is happening, they're more likely to get involved and assist with water management, which results in improved long-term outcomes and even better public health statistics (Nicolay & Fliessbach, 2012). Combining indigenous wisdom with these community-based arrangements really increases their effectiveness. Time-tested traditions often have clever insights into regional ecosystems, seasonal patterns, and resource management that may elude conventional technical approaches. By embracing such tried-and-true concepts, communities can brew water treatment solutions that are adaptable and attuned to their unique environments.

With urbanization and global warming causing water scarcity to become an increasing concern, such nature-based solutions are more relevant than ever before. They can reduce the threat of water scarcity while providing a boost to local ecosystem functions, ultimately enhancing community health and general sustainability (Cecchi et al., 2015).

4.4.1. Rainwater Harvesting (RWH)

Demand for clean drinking water is increasing in so many locations that new, innovative solutions simply can't be dismissed. RWH—literally harvesting rain and saving it for the future—has become an astute, eco-friendly solution, particularly where unpredictable weather or antiquated piping causes shortages. Studies of rooftop runoff systems, in general terms, when they are well taken care of, indicate that these configurations can produce an abundance of drinkable water. Nevertheless, quality issues emerge: microbial and chemical contaminants regularly exceed local health thresholds. Overall, upgrading these systems to consistently provide safe drinking water is considered essential for communities with the most severe shortages. Meanwhile, new ideas are fermenting to improve rainwater systems against both microbe and chemical threats. A study, for instance, highlighted the promise of incorporating silver ions in addition to conventional filtration systems—a strategy that looks especially promising for small-scale, rural applications. When these added systems were implemented, scientists found a significant decrease in indicator microorganisms, which highlights the approach's potential. Maintaining all surfaces as clean as possible proves to be the crucial factor, and in most instances, well-managed rainwater systems can help enable improved community health benefits. This all urges us to combine proven practices with emerging technologies in local water treatment programs. Knowledge of local conditions and user requirements is essential if rainwater projects are to find their target. Look at places such as the Cuvelai Basin in Namibia, where erratic rains and brackish groundwater call for a smart, demand-driven strategy. Far from a single-sized solution, these models are based on active community planning and participation, reminding us that technology solutions need to really align with social and cultural practices on the ground. By incorporating local knowledge early, the potential for success of a rainwater system can be appreciably increased, even at the cost of some additional stops along the way. This type of strategy facilitates mutual learning, advancing not only adoption of such systems but also general, sustainable improvement in community health, demonstrating that successful water treatment involves more than engineering to integrate social needs as well (Figure 4.11).

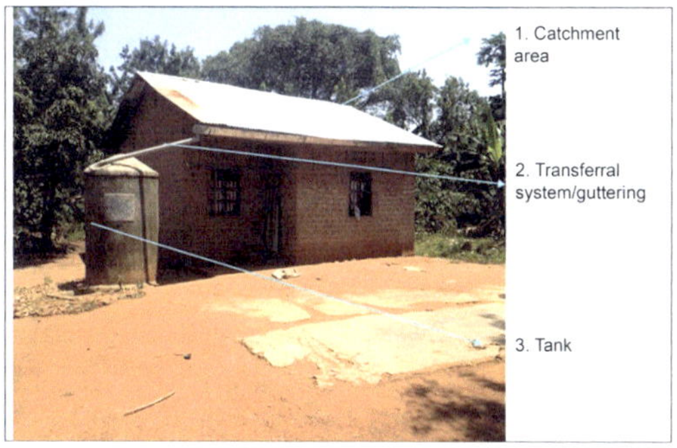

Figure 4.11. Rainwater harvest system.

Source: By Chad.staddon - Own work, CC BY-SA 4.0, https://commons.wikimedia.org/w/index.php?curid=116124741

4.4.2. Bio Sand Filters

Drinking water access in rural regions has become an increasing concern recently, prompting some fairly innovative solutions. Bio sand filters, henceforth referred to as BSFs, are garnering significant attention because they operate exactly at the point of use, which is wonderful for people without consistent water resources. Studies in general indicate they do a good job of removing pathogens and sediment, so a significant decline in waterborne disease that affects most vulnerable individuals the most. Yet their effectiveness truly depends on adequate training and local participation; when users are not instructed on how to use them appropriately, even smart technology isn't effective (Spowart, 2012). Just distributing the filters simply isn't enough, an across-the-board strategy with support follow-up is necessary. Take a look at the case study from Nkokonjeru, Uganda. In a collaboration between Engineers Without Borders and a local non-governmental organization, the project revealed some interesting gaps between what was expected of BSFs and what transpired in regular use. Indeed, the statistics revealed a satisfactory reduction in bacterial levels upon installing the filters, but most of them ended up being underutilized or even dysfunctional. It appears that user misinterpretation regarding maintenance and the absence of sustained support quite undermined their potential. In the majority of instances, this suggests that the health impacts of BSFs get considerably diluted if there is no concrete plan for training and empowering the users. Ongoing follow-ups and training not only increase the filter's performance but also assist in building a community with an interest in improved hygiene and general health (Spowart, 2012). And then there is the larger context when you think about various cultural and practical contexts. A study in certain rural Indian villages indicated that local water properties, personal taste, and customary health behaviors all determine whether technologies such as BSFs gain traction. Implementing these systems is not simply a case of fitting equipment; it requires a considered examination of what each community truly requires. In most cases, stakeholders need to adapt their strategy to suit local traditions and circumstances so that the filters are effective initially but still yield benefits in the long term. This type of adaptable, holistic approach can truly propel sustainable water management practices and leave a lasting beneficial effect on public health (Figure 4.12).

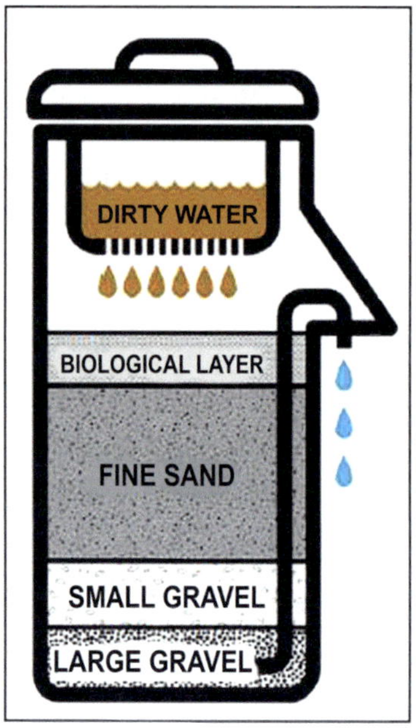

Figure 4.12. Basic diagram of a concrete bio sand filter.

Source: Wikimedia Commons. (n.d.). *Basic Diagram of a Concrete Bio Sand Filter.*

4.4.3. Community Water Purification Systems

Growing populations and the continually increasing demand for clean drinking water compel us to seek novel means of water purification, and local water infrastructure has emerged at the forefront of that effort. In much of the distant or underserved areas where conventional infrastructure simply does not exist, communities are receiving customized water solutions that match their very own needs. Scientists, for example, tested out using silver ions in combination with standard filters in rural areas of Mexico, and overall, the outcomes were quite remarkable, with these systems all but eliminating harmful microbes at around 99.9% effectiveness, although occasionally additional contamination from other sources made a difference. This indicates, in the majority of instances, that water purification must be modified to suit certain local conditions and community requirements (Adler et al., 2011). Individuals not only require water that's safe today but also a means to maintain it that way in the long term. Sustainability is an important consideration here. Designs inevitably favor low-maintenance and inexpensive technologies so that local people can readily assume the maintenance. Consider RWH, for instance. It's frequently promoted as a great method for collecting clean water, but it can't avoid problems of microbial and chemical cleanliness if safety is at all a concern. Research has identified that intelligent design paired with consistent servicing allows communities to retain water for more extended times without loss of quality. In all but a few exceptions, this sustainable configuration does more than solve short-term health concerns; it creates a feeling of ownership by community members, enhancing overall well-being in a natural, sometimes circular, rhythm of care (Adler et al., 2011). Regional areas also include their own challenges, though, Arctic regions, for instance, are a whole different ball game. In these cold climates, freezing conditions and remoteness compel engineers to reevaluate how water and wastewater infrastructure is constructed. Researchers have explored such uncommon challenges, identified breakdowns, and suggested potential design refinements that could boost reliability. Such analysis is necessary if we are to refine current practices and initiate the development of tougher, more robust purification systems that suit the remote villages' requirements. In general, these findings assist in guiding future developments, ensuring that as the environment changes, our water treatment solutions are able to keep pace (Adler et al., 2011) (Figure 4.13).

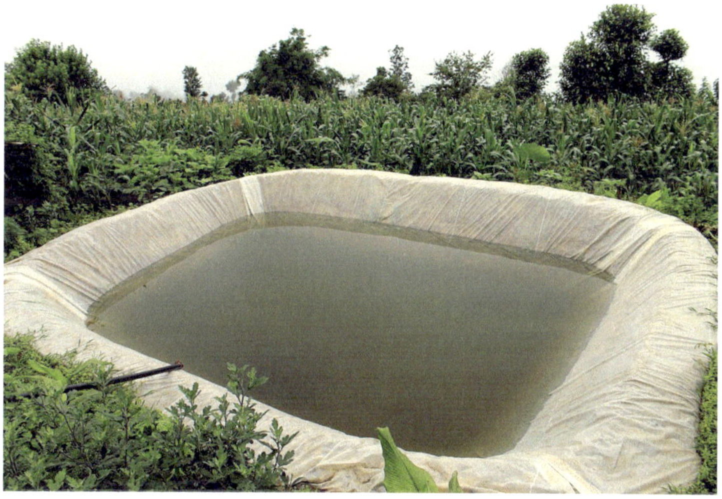

Figure 4.13. Mobile water filtration system.

Source: By Shree Krishna Dhital - Own work, CC BY-SA 3.0, https://commons.wikimedia.org/w/index.php?curid=28333385

4.5. Challenges in Water Treatment

Pure water is essential to the health of communities, but numerous hurdles still stand in the way of effective water treatment across large areas. In many areas, they just do not have the type of fundamental infrastructure that is required , consider treatment plants and good distribution networks , and this is a significant roadblock. On top of that, then there are problems such as corruption and patronage that wind up distorting equitable distribution of resources. Consider the Central Gonja District; research there tends to indicate that the consistent gap in access to safe drinking water is connected to faulty local governance that puts communities behind. In most cases, it takes fixing these ingrained issues to hold local authorities accountable so that communities are not sidelined for narrow, special interests. Such steps could even initiate wider debates on sustainable water management - an important step towards safeguarding public health and building community resilience to environmental hazards (Bazaanah et al., 2024). Financial concerns come into play as well, particularly in developing nations where budgetary limitations render the establishment and maintenance of efficient water treatment systems challenging. Others have explored output-based financing models as a realistic solution; these models emphasize funding centered on concrete, outcome-oriented results in community health. However, more frequently than not, such efforts meet bureaucratic red tape and a lack of trained human resources in contemporary water treatment techniques. In addition, skewed levels of funding can create uneven service provision, further exacerbating disparities in health among the resource-poor population. For the most part, the education and empowerment of locals so that they may assert their rights, and public-private partnership-building, may very well set the stage for more positive health outcomes and enhanced water access (Evans et al., 2010b). It's difficult to overemphasize the importance of involving communities in water treatment decision-making. When local individuals are allowed to express their individual needs and proposed solutions, water projects work a great deal better, creating an actual sense of ownership and responsibility. The evidence is fairly unequivocal that community engagement makes services more effective and responsive. Additionally, partnering with local government can increase transparency and result in faster action when things go wrong. This type of collaboration could even draw outside funding since it demonstrates a serious commitment to long-term, equitable solutions. Simply, centering community engagement may be the solution to surmounting the numerous challenges in water treatment and providing all individuals with access to safe, reliable water (Bazaanah et al., 2024).

4.5.1. Infrastructure Limitations

Community health usually suffers when water treatment systems simply cannot cope with aging or deficient infrastructure. Water systems in much of the developing world are not just scarce but are also badly maintained, which reduces water treatment practices' effectiveness. For instance, look at Indonesia's Water and Sanitation Hibah Program: utility companies there sometimes have extra capacity but lose out on the investment to upgrade their infrastructure. Essentially, this program bypasses typical infrastructure barriers by paying for confirmed water service connections, improving access without a large up-front cost (Nordiawan et al., 2011). It's an obvious indication that managing with what one has, even in the face of urgent requirements for improved investments, can influence community health outcomes. Regional environmental idiosyncrasies put another spin on the tale. In areas such as Namibia's Cuvelai Basin, erratic rains and brackish groundwater lead planners to really get down to the nitty-gritty of how communities utilize water. When infrastructure is constructed ignoring these physical quirks, the repairs come up short—sometimes even exacerbating the problems. Projects like CuveWaters demonstrate a surprising strategy by decentralizing water supply and sanitation; with a demand-responsive approach that encourages local participation in planning as well as maintenance, they develop systems that suit the local atmosphere (Deffner & Mazambani, 2010). More often than not, this type of community engagement helps build resilience and makes sure treatment practices complement local customs. Ultimately, coming up short on robust infrastructure has repercussions far beyond the quality of water, it reaches the larger public health landscape. Aging systems can bring a whole host of risks, from the return of waterborne disease to increased exposure when the climate changes. Effective water treatment isn't only about the latest technology; it must also take the state of infrastructure into account, acting sometimes as a gateway and other times as a stumbling block. Focusing solely on technical fixes, without addressing the shaky foundation beneath them, might mean missing the bigger problem embedded in community contexts. A well-balanced combination of tech, better infrastructure, and authentic community participation is, in all but a few instances, the solution to sustainable public health improvement (Figure 4.14).

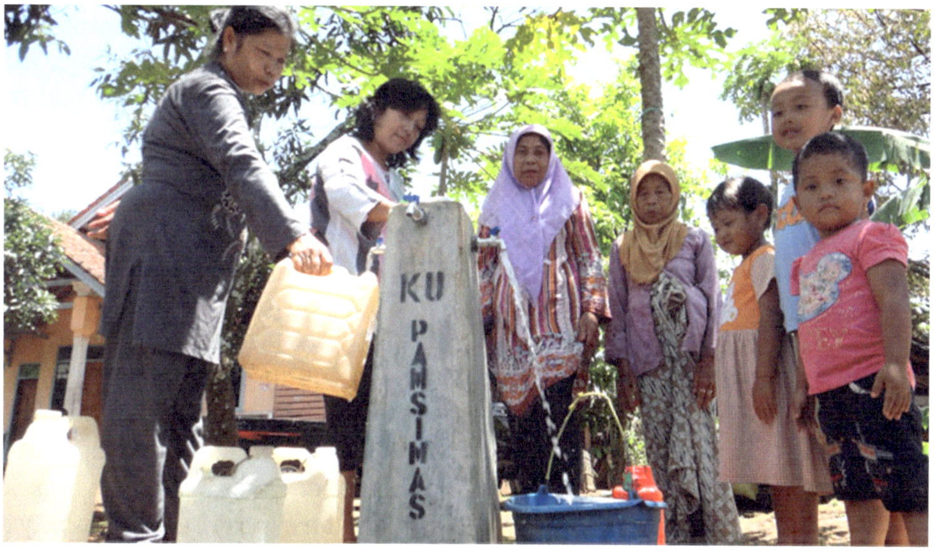

Figure 4.14. Access to clean water has helped Indonesian women and children put better use of their time since they no longer have to walk far to fetch water.

Source: World Bank. (2019). *Access to Clean Water has Helped Indonesian Women And Children.*

4.5.2. Financial Constraints

Financial matters hold back communities from implementing good water treatment systems. Local governments and organizations simply don't have enough money, so they can't spend money on the equipment they require , and that may compromise public health. It's not merely a matter of implementing high-technology treatment systems; maintaining older ones is equally daunting. Prices are as varied as can be based on the approach, and although some chemical or biological methods may look like they provide instant cost-cutting, they mostly rely on consistent funding support and hands-on administration—something that is difficult to find when budgets are strained (De Winton et al., 2013). In most instances, addressing these issues of money is important if water treatments are to function effectively and endure. Lacking sufficient funds also renders it difficult to conduct very extensive checkups on current water treatment systems. Reviews are imperative since they identify exactly what a community really needs, but without sufficient money, authorities tend to have ad-hoc remedies that merely scratch the issues of water quality. This problem is particularly obvious in some developing countries, where there has been a shortage of planned investment in sanitation and inadequate infrastructure, compelling individuals to use improvised means that fall below minimum public health standards. Output-based finance could appear to be a tidy solution, but then again, such models typically require a large initial investment that simply isn't on hand in cash-short locations (Evans et al., 2010a). Basically, the battle with scarce resources is constantly undermining attempts to improve community health with intelligent water treatment. To add insult to injury, preventive actions, usually the less expensive route tend to go unseen due to these budget constraints. Consider how easy measures such as promoting improved hygiene habits or running community workshops could decrease water contamination hazards at a minimal cost. Nevertheless, in times of constraint, these future-oriented alternatives take a back seat to crisis response. This priority of crisis prevention can pay more in the long term with greater healthcare expenditures and costly cleanup missions for waterborne diseases. It would make sense to invest some money into sustainable, prevention-oriented approaches (De Winton et al., 2013). Ultimately, addressing these financial challenges is crucial to constructing a water treatment system that truly prioritizes public health.

4.5.3. Public Awareness and Education

If individuals don't know how to handle water the right way, it can cause serious issues for all of our health. Most people just don't have the rudimentary know-how regarding keeping water clean—not for themselves, but for those around them, too. Surveys indicate that individuals tend to learn what they know from informal conversations or neighborhood meetings more than from reliable, research-based sources; this has a tendency to circulate confused concepts regarding waterborne diseases and how to address them. Increasing day-to-day water education may just close that gap between knowing and doing, enabling neighborhoods to take care of their water supplies better. Ultimately, increasing local learning can result in healthier people and communities better prepared to resist disease (Torres et al., 2025). Water treatment at home is a standout aspect of maintaining health. Where safe drinking water is not an expectation, simply knowing about simple things, such as boiling or chlorine treatment, can significantly reduce the risk of contracting waterborne pests. Despite all this, many families do not maintain any routine treatment course, even though they may have heard of them. Low educational levels and the absence of stable community bonding can make this worse.

A few studies, in general, indicate that health education targeted effectively can encourage individuals to treat water more consistently; programs emphasizing simple ways and providing hands-on training can enable even resource-constrained individuals to make a significant impact (Assefa, 2024). Sustaining the flame of water treatment consciousness over the long term requires community involvement. It's not a matter of throwing a method in and then walking away—continued support is what keeps people on course. Involving local groups, schools, and even community clinics has the effect of spreading the message more organically, in a down-to-earth way. Community leaders and educators tend to blend various approaches that suit the idiosyncrasies and requirements of their particular area, creating a wellness-first culture in the process. By sustaining the cycle of conversation and learning, communities are in a stronger position to respond to emerging new public health issues as they arise. Overall, this sustained emphasis not only serves to reduce waterborne diseases but also promotes a forward-thinking approach to controlling water safely and sustainably (Assefa, 2024; Torres et al., 2025) (Figure 4.15).

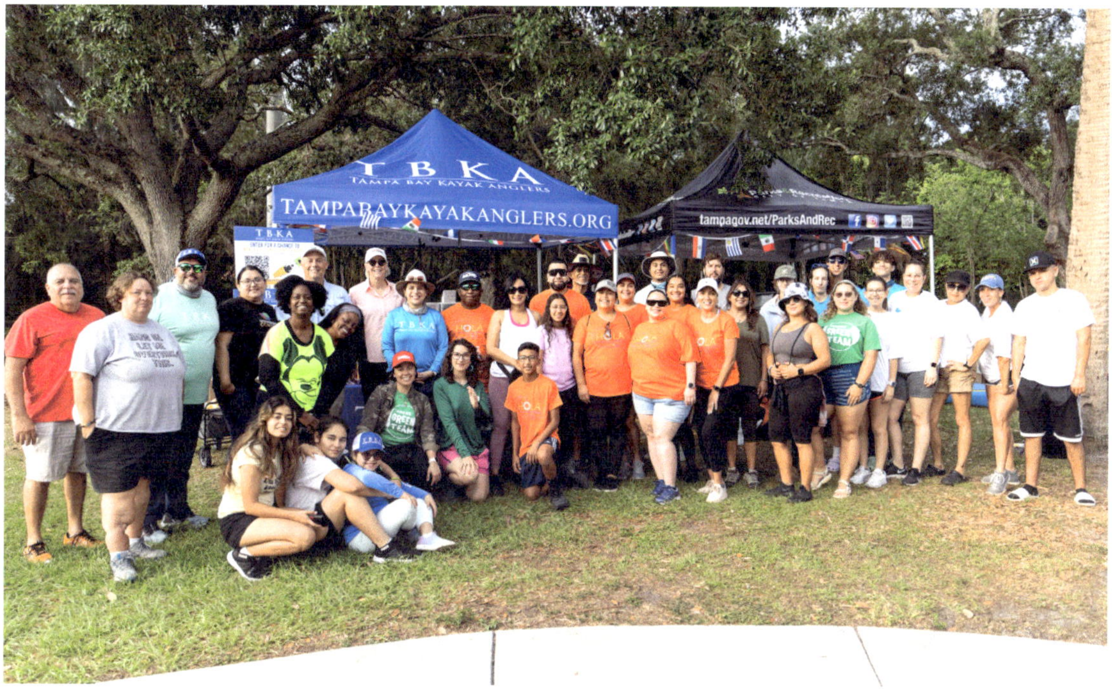

Figure 4.15. Public awareness program.

Source: Tampa Bay Water. (n.d.). *Public Awareness Program.*

SUMMARY

Clean water is not only a fundamental need, it's a lifeline to healthy communities. Everywhere around the world, a host of programs has emerged that guarantee water is both safe and sustainable, sometimes without rewriting the entire infrastructure playbook. The Indonesia Water and Sanitation Hibah Program, for example, drew on local utility know-how (without enormous new investment) to increase water service delivery. Program assessments, on the whole, suggest that even established systems might be adjusted in order to attain improved health effects. It looks like maximizing currently available resources and monitoring accountability seriously improves community wellbeing and prevents waterborne diseases. Various strategies promoting water and sanitation are scattered about everywhere. Some recent critiques note that no one trick will alter behavior around hygiene habits each time—you truly need a combination of approaches. In most instances, when communities are actively involved and receive a good introduction to safe hygiene, involvement naturally increases. Barriers and facilitators, which differ from location to location, must be accounted for in policy design. Community involvement, for instance, coupled side-by-side with education on sanitary practices, has been found to drive improved participation and adherence. It's a fascinating reminder that each community has its own beat, so interventions will need to be fine-tuned in real-time. Wrapping up, it seems water treatment success depends on both high-tech methods and grassroots community involvement. Assessments, from case studies such as the Indonesian pilot to behavior change systematic reviews, tend to find that meeting local needs is central to healthier results. Combining technical innovation with local expertise results in communities not only receiving cleaner water but also slowly developing habits that last. In the end, uniting technology and public spirit appears to be the key to fostering more equal public health and less waterborne disease in a variety of contexts.

Community health benefits when water treatment functions properly. Folks have observed that interventions like WASH can knock out disease, particularly among small children. Diarrhea and mother and newborn complications appear to decrease when water is purified more thoroughly. Taking care of water wisely even contributes to making food safer, sort of a double whammy, you see? Water safety, health, and nutrition all intersect, which is why solid water cleaning is so important. This combination tends to smooth out public health issues observed in areas where it is a true challenge to access clean water (Mills et al., 2016). In urban areas, new approaches to water management can disrupt both the environment and neighborhood health. Consider permeable pavements, for instance, they reduce stormwater runoff and improve water quality simultaneously. In cold weather, such systems can be particularly beneficial, addressing not only the amount of water that flows but also keeping it cleaner throughout winter. Some research indicates that installing these pavements in the most strategic locations not only retards runoff but also provides a boost to the health of the soil in the wintry months. It sort of indicates that combining water management with environmental concern can kill two birds with one stone; the people feel better and the environment gets some relief as well. Overall, playing with such ideas may be opening doors to long-term solutions to water treatment issues (Haselbach & Nassiri, 2017). Clean water is not only about battling disease, it touches every aspect of life. In most instances, if water is clean, children, particularly girls, tend to remain at school more frequently, with issues of menstrual hygiene leading the way. WASH initiatives appear to erode not just anxiety but even cases of violence in some groups. If water treatment is addressed on a broad level, communities become more cohesive and resilient. Melding these together suggests that water quality aligns with greater social strengths and potentialities. Using this, policymakers are able to create better schemes that move water treatment to center stage for public health activities (Mills et al., 2016).

KEY TERMS FROM THIS CHAPTER

Aquatic atmosphere
Biological intruders
Chemical agents
Cutting-edge technologies
Ecological damage
Flocculation
Invertebrate populations
Microorganisms
Organic contaminants
Recalcitrant microbes
Social equity
Urban areas
Bio sand filters
Biosorption
Community clinics
Deterioration process
Filtration
Heavy metals
Membrane distillation (MD)
Nature-based methods
Real-time monitoring
Safe hygiene habits
Sustainable water treatment
UV disinfection

CLOSER LOOK

ADVANCED WATER TREATMENT TECHNOLOGIES

New water treatment technologies seek to enhance water quality and sustainability by targeting more types of pollutants than conventional technologies, with advantages such as increased contaminant removal, lower energy use, and greater reuse potential. These technologies are membrane filtration, AOPs, biological treatment, and UV disinfection.

Membrane Filtration:

i. **Membrane Bioreactors (MBR):** Integrate biological treatment with membrane filtration for enhanced removal of nutrients, organic matter, and suspended solids.
ii. **Reverse Osmosis (RO):** Uses semi-permeable membranes to remove dissolved salts, organic matter, and microorganisms, producing high-quality purified water.
iii. **Other Membrane Technologies:** Ultrafiltration (UF), microfiltration (MF), and nanofiltration (NF) are also commonly used for various water treatment applications.

Advanced Oxidation Processes (AOPs):

i. **Ozonation:** Uses ozone gas to oxidize pollutants, making them more susceptible to removal or **transformation.**
ii. **UV Disinfection:** Uses UV light to inactivate pathogens and other microorganisms.
iii. **Chlorination:** Uses chlorine to disinfect water and remove microorganisms, although it can also produce disinfection byproducts.
iv. **Activated Carbon (AC):** Absorbs organic matter, dyes, and heavy metals, improving water quality.

Biological Treatment:

i. **Biological Treatment:** Includes use of microorganisms for breaking down organic matter and other pollutants, sustainable technology.

Other Advanced Technologies:

i. **Electrocoagulation:** Uses an electric field to remove contaminants by creating a charge-neutralized precipitate.
ii. **Enzyme Treatments:** Use enzymes to degrade specific pollutants, offering a targeted approach.
iii. **Algae:** Use algae in the treatment of wastewater to remove nutrients and as a possible source of biofuel.

References

1. I. Adler, K. A. Hudson-Edwards, L. C. Campos; Converting rain into drinking water: quality issues and technological advances. *Water Supply* 1 December 2011; 11 (6): 659–667. doi: https://doi.org/10.2166/ws.2011.117 (accessed on 14 May 2025).
2. Brooks, Norman H., Robert G. Arnold, Robert C. Y. Koh, George A. Jackson, and William K. Faisst. 1982. "Deep Ocean Disposal of Sewage Sludge Off Orange County, California: A Research Plan". California Institute of Technology. https://doi.org/10.7907/Z9HD7SKS.
3. Assefa SA. Assessment of Household Water Treatment Practices in Odaya Kebele at Dilla Town, Southern Ethiopia. J Water Resour Ocean Sci. 2024;13(6):158-165. doi: 10.11648/j.wros.20241306.12(accessed on 14 May 2025).
4. Bandaru, S.R.S.; Smesrud, L.; Majmudar, J.; Hernandez, D.; Wickliff, P.; Tseng, W.; Gadgil, A. Field Testing of an Affordable Zero-Liquid-Discharge Arsenic-Removal Technology for a Small-
5. Wolf, J., Prüss-Ustün, A., Cumming, O., Bartram, J., Bonjour, S., Cairncross, S., Clasen, T., Colford, J. M., Jr, Curtis, V., De France, J., Fewtrell, L., Freeman, M. C., Gordon, B., Hunter, P. R., Jeandron, A., Johnston, R. B., Mäusezahl, D., Mathers, C., Neira, M., & Higgins, J. P. (2014). Assessing the impact of drinking water and sanitation on diarrhoeal disease in low- and middle-income settings: systematic review and meta-regression. *Tropical medicine & international health : TM & IH, 19*(8), 928–942. https://doi.org/10.1111/tmi.12331 (accessed on 14 May 2025).
6. Prosper Bazaanah, Smangele Johanna Buthelezi, Dina Afua Kobe Oppong; Qualitative study of drinking water, sanitation, and hygiene access: perspectives from the Central Gonja District, Ghana, and Mtubatuba Municipality, South Africa. *Journal of Water, Sanitation and Hygiene for Development* 1 November 2024; 14 (11): 1043–1065. doi: https://doi.org/10.2166/washdev.2024.021 (accessed on 14 May 2025).
7. Beatley, N. (2011). *Green Housing = Improved Health: A Winning Combination*. Commissioned by NeighborWorks America® for the Symposium: Green Choices, Green Value, for the Families and Communities We Serve. https://core.ac.uk/download/71345591.pdf (accessed on 14 May 2025).
8. Blackwood, D. J., Falconer, R. E., Gilmour, D. J., & O'Keeffe, J., et al. (2016). An evaluation of water treatment technologies for sustainable rural communities. https://core.ac.uk/download/228178252.pdf (accessed on 14 May 2025).
9. Borja, A., Ginebreda, A., Magdeburg, A., Ricciardi, A., Laursen, A. E., Botzat, A., Magdeburg, A., et al. (2013). Do contaminants originating from state-of-the-art treated wastewater impact the ecological quality of surface waters? https://core.ac.uk/download/14529455.pdf (accessed on 14 May 2025).
10. Marianna Garfi', Cadena, E., Sanchez-Ramos, D., Ferrer, I. Life cycle assessment of drinking water: comparing conventional water treatment, reverse osmosis and mineral water in glass and plastic bottles. "Journal of cleaner production", Novembre 2016, vol. 137, p. 997-1003. (accessed on 14 May 2025).
11. Fernandes, Ricardo; Silva, A. R.; Cardoso, Beatriz D.; Coutinho, Paulo J. G.; Pereira, Luciana, Potential of photocatalytic nanomaterials for PFOA and PFOS degradation: challenges and opportunities. Journal of Environmental Chemical Engineering, 13(115201), 1, 2024 (accessed on 14 May 2025).

12. Cecchi, C., Egbert, R., Eva, M., & Mayerhofer, J., et al. (2015). *Towards an EU Research and Innovation Policy Agenda for Nature-Based Solutions & Re-Naturing Cities: Final Report of the Horizon 2020 Expert Group on Nature-Based Solutions and Re-Naturing Cities.* https://core.ac.uk/download/54517673.pdf (accessed on 14 May 2025).
13. de Winton M, Jones H, Edwards T, Özkundakci D, Wells R, McBride C, Rowe D, Hamilton D, Clayton J, Champion P, Hofstra D (2013). Review of best management practices for aquatic vegetation control in stormwater ponds, wetlands, and lakes. Prepared by NIWA and the University of Waikato for Auckland Council. Auckland Council technical report, TR2013/026 (accessed on 14 May 2025).
14. Chaudhry, Rabia M., Kerry A. Hamilton, Charles N. Haas, and Kara L. Nelson. 2017. "Drivers of Microbial Risk for Direct Potable Reuse and de Facto Reuse Treatment Schemes: The Impacts of Source Water Quality and Blending" *International Journal of Environmental Research and Public Health* 14, no. 6: 635. https://doi.org/10.3390/ijerph14060635 (accessed on 14 May 2025).
15. Deffner, J., & Mazambani, C. (2010). Participatory empirical research on water and sanitation demand in central northern Namibia: A method for technology development with a user perspective. https://core.ac.uk/download/14526924.pdf (accessed on 14 May 2025).
16. Deswal, S., Rawat, S., Kumar, S., & Sangwan, V. (2023). Potential of Moringa oleifera and Okra as Coagulants in Sustainable Treatment of Water and Wastewater. *Ecological Questions, 34*(4), 1–17. https://doi.org/10.12775/EQ.2023.045(accessed on 14 May 2025).
17. Evans, B. E., Peal, A. J., & van der Voorden, C. (2010a). *Hygiene and Sanitation Software: An Overview of Approaches.*
18. Evans, B. E., Shaub-Jones, D., & Trémolet, S. (2010b). *Output-Based Aid for Sustainable Sanitation.*
19. Nicolay, Gian L. and Fliessbach, Andreas (2012) Production of Innovations within Farmer–Researcher Associations Applying Transdisciplinary Research Principles. In: *International Conference on Research for Development (ICRD 2012). Research for Global Transformation, Theme 4: Enabling Research in Global Transformation Session 26: Integrated Development Research Approach*, NCCR North-South Dialogue, no. 44, p. 164.(accessed on 14 May 2025).
20. Mahdi, S., Moamar Shakir Mahmood, Shather Salah Mahdi, & Shaddan Salah Mahdi. (2025). PUBLIC AWARENESS OF ACUTE LEUKEMIA IN A SAMPLE OF IRAQI PEOPLE. *Global Journal of Public Health Medicine, 7*(1), 1–13. https://doi.org/10.37557/gjphm.v7i1.284 (accessed on 14 May 2025).
21. MCRL, de Andrade LC, Barbosa MP, Lopes BC and Mota Filho CR (2024) Performance of traditional household drinking water treatment methods used in rural Amazon. Front. Water. 6:1392800. doi: 10.3389/frwa.2024.1392800 (accessed on 14 May 2025).
22. González-Burciaga LA, Silerio-Vázquez FdJ, Antileo C, Rosales-Castro M, Núñez-Núñez CM, Proal-Nájera JB. A Review on Cytotoxic Antibiotics: Occurrence in Water Matrices, Degradation by Advanced Oxidation Processes, and By-Product Formation. *Water.* 2025; 17(5):628. https://doi.org/10.3390/w17050628(accessed on 14 May 2025).
23. Morse, Tracy and Nicholls, Rosely and Grimason, Anthony and Smith, Huw (2008) Epidemiology of cryptosporidiosis in rural Malawi. Environment & Health International. pp. 36-44. ISSN 1726-9210 (accessed on 14 May 2025).

24. Haselbach, L., & Nassiri, S. (2017). *Stormwater-Pavement Interface in Cold Climates*. Final Report: 05/2014 - 5/2017. https://core.ac.uk/download/286999888.pdf (accessed on 14 May 2025).

25. Jeffreys, K. G. (2012). *A Survey of Point of Use Household Water Treatment Options for Rural South India*. https://core.ac.uk/download/71422308.pdf (accessed on 14 May 2025).

26. Tilsworth, T., Justice, S. R., Smith, D. M., Zemansky, et al. (1977). *Cold Climate Water/Wastewater Transportation and Treatment–A Bibliography: Completion Report*. University of Alaska, Institute of Water Resources. https://core.ac.uk/download/162573813.pdf (accessed on 14 May 2025).

27. Kaczynski, Jessica I., "Waste Water Treatment in New Hampshire: Analysis of Nitrogen Treatment in the Great Bay Community" (2015). *Honors Theses and Capstones*. 213. https://scholars.unh.edu/honors/213 (accessed on 14 May 2025).

28. Kakkar, R., Kaur, D. P., & Raj, S. (2024). Investigations of nanomaterial-based membranes for efficient removal of contaminants from wastewater via membrane distillation: A critical review. *Zastita Materijala*. https://www.semanticscholar.org/paper/3cfecb54cbbffde1bdc31356d25338bc3544ca89 (accessed on 14 May 2025).

29. Kim, S. Y., Kim, I. Y., Park, S. H., Hwangbo, M., & Hwangbo, S. (2024). Novel ultrasonic technology for advanced oxidation processes of water treatment. *RSC Advances, 14*, 11939–11948. https://www.semanticscholar.org/paper/d919ede45c7cb56fde3221ff5c4509d39d8a63b8 (accessed on 14 May 2025).

30. López-Ejeda, N., Charle-Cuéllar, P., Samake, S., Dougnon, A. O., Sánchez-Martínez, L. J., Samaké, M., Bagayoko, A., et al. (2024). Effectiveness of decentralizing outpatient acute malnutrition treatment with community health workers and a simplified combined protocol: A cluster randomized controlled trial in emergency settings of Mali. *Frontiers in Public Health, 12*. https://www.semanticscholar.org/paper/fa28dbacedcdbefe184c6d9d88c369af973b2d3d (accessed on 14 May 2025).

31. Maan, R., Mathur, P., & Sharma, A. K. (2024). Impact of biosorption process on industrial wastewater treatment in Panipat District, Haryana. *International Journal for Research in Applied Science and Engineering Technology*. https://doi.org/10.22214/ijraset.2024.62201. https://www.semanticscholar.org/paper/a72c887d40813e2d8babc2f4006ee203c7ea100c (accessed on 14 May 2025).

32. Mahdavi M, Mahvi AH, Mohebbi M, Teimuri MH, Mamaghani Nejad M, Hoseinzadeh E, et al. Health

33. risk assessment for reused backwash water from Saveh water treatment plant. J Adv Environ Health Res. 2024; 12(1):46-51. doi:10.34172/

34. jaehr.1329 (accessed on 14 May 2025).

35. Mann, B. (2014). *Navigating The Water, Sanitation, And Hygiene (Wash) Sector: A Guide for Corporate Grantmakers*. http://water.issuelab.org/resource/navigating_the_water_sanitation_and_hygiene_wash_sector_a_guide_for_corporate_grantmakers

36. Mills, J. E., & Cumming, O. (2016). *The Impact of Water, Sanitation, And Hygiene on Key Health and Social Outcomes: Review of Evidence*. https://core.ac.uk/download/75761114.pdf (accessed on 14 May 2025).

37. Mohammed, A. H. B. (2001). *Pilot Plant Studies Using Moringa Oleifera (Kacang Kelor) Seeds as a Primary Coagulant in Surface Water Treatment.* https://core.ac.uk/download/43000740.pdf (accessed on 14 May 2025).

38. Molanes-López, E. M., Ferrer, J. M., Dougnon, A. O., Gado, A. A., Sanoussi, A., Ousmane, N., Lazoumar, R., et al. (2024). Cost-effectiveness of severe acute malnutrition treatment delivered by community health workers in the district of Mayahi, Niger. *Human Resources for Health, 22.* https://www.semanticscholar.org/paper/ab5f98d8336b4b72a294f88b1646f3615a313921 (accessed on 14 May 2025).

39. Musekiwa, A., Vande Veegaete, A., Avau, B., De Buck, E., Van Remoortel, H., Mosler, H. J., Hannes, K., et al. (2017). Promoting handwashing and sanitation behaviour change in low- and middle-income countries: A mixed-method systematic review. https://core.ac.uk/download/141922886.pdf (accessed on 14 May 2025).

40. Nordiawan, D., Gouy, J., Scally-Irvine, K., Averill, K., & Howard, M. (2011). Independent evaluation of the water and sanitation Hibah Program Indonesia. Indonesia Water and Sanitation Hibah: Independent review. https://core.ac.uk/download/71360953.pdf (accessed on 14 May 2025).

41. Olukanni, D. O. (2013). *Assessment of WASH Program in Public Secondary Schools in South-Western Nigeria.* Journal Article - Journal of Engineering and Applied Science. http://eprints.covenantuniversity.edu.ng/1948/1/Dr. Olukanmi 3.pdf

42. Torres, N. N. S., Borne , I., Souza, S. A. S. de, Frigo, J. P., & Ando Junior , O. H. (2025). Alternative Water Treatment System Using Ionization and Ultraviolet Radiation for Isolated Communities. Revista De Gestão Social E Ambiental, 19(1), e010890. https://doi.org/10.24857/rgsa.v19n1-085 (accessed on 14 May 2025).

43. Spowart, M. E. (2012). *Educational Concerns of Implementing Biosand Water Filters in Rural Uganda.* Submitted in Partial Fulfillment of the Requirements for the Degree Master of Science in Education School of Education and Counseling Psychology Dominican University of California San Rafael, CA December 2012. https://core.ac.uk/download/215554294.pdf (accessed on 14 May 2025).

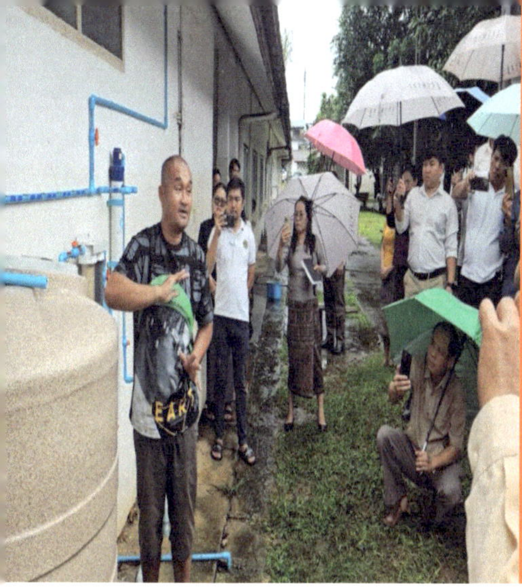

Chapter 5

SANITATION AND WASTEWATER MANAGEMENT

Contents

Introduction

Clean water and sanitation significantly contribute to public health, they profoundly impact how communities prosper and how our environment remains healthy. Sanitation can exacerbate the spread of waterborne diseases, which in most instances causes severe health problems and significant economic losses. In general terms, the World Health Organization emphasizes that a deficiency of safe water and adequate sanitation is responsible for almost 2 million deaths each year , and tends to affect children under the age of five particularly severely. The consequences of poor sanitation aren't just in the form of short-term health hazards; they also impact economic productivity and social equity. Grasping control of wastewater and sanitation serves not only to protect health but can also spark economic development and strengthen social stability. It's important to comprehend how sanitation practices are connected with public health, as this helps fuel the resource mobilization and political momentum necessary for more enduring solutions in sanitation infrastructure (Tortajada, 2016). Sanitation and wastewater issues become more complex as urbanization expands and populations cluster more densely. As cities grow, demand for clean water and secure waste disposal can soar, typically outpacing available systems. Developing countries in particular grapple with challenges such as limited resources, and technical expertise that is rare, and laws that simply haven't kept pace. At the same time, contamination from both identified (point) and diffuse (non-point) sources continues to erode water quality, pushing the need for sustainable management up the list of priorities. New wastewater treatment technologies need to be leveraged to reduce pollution and protect our precious water resources. In most instances, catalyzing innovation through public-private collaborations and investing in sustainable technologies can even convert waste into a productive asset, yielding benefits to local communities and the environment as well (Cunha et al., 2012). More still, the broader effects of poor sanitation extend to environmental health, economic performance, and day-to-day quality of life. When facilities fall short, nearby water bodies get impacted—making water shortage and environmental imbalance even more problematic. The cost of poor sanitation is colossal, not just putting pressure on healthcare systems but on individual livelihoods as well. It appears crucial, therefore, to implement efficient water management efforts that target reversing such unsustainable patterns. This may involve practices such as *in situ* remediation, which restores ecological equilibrium even as cities keep expanding. Ultimately, achieving sustainable sanitation solutions requires a holistic approach that incorporates technological advancement, people's participation, and intelligent policy adjustments to foster communities that are safe, healthy, and resilient (Tortajada, 2016).

Definition of Sanitation and Wastewater Management

Knowing the fundamentals of sanitation and wastewater management is important to addressing public health challenges and maintaining our ecosystem in balance. Sanitation is not merely a jargon term, it is simply collecting, treating, and disposing of wastes (primarily human excreta) in a manner that reduces health hazards and safeguards nature. In most instances, proper sanitation slows down the spread of disease and keeps drinking water safe, thereby improving community health. Wastewater management, however, involves cleaning and recycling water before it comes back into our environment—a process that, frankly, converts what could be harmful waste into beneficial resources for environmental health and conservation of resources. This is an approach that is more and more recognized as a foundation for building communities that can be self-sustaining. Failing sanitation and defective wastewater practices have negative effects rippling far beyond personal health concerns, they significantly compromise water sources and the varied life that they harbor. Polluted water may create declining ecosystems, particularly when it impacts freshwater areas. Wetlands, for instance, might take up little land, but they are vital in maintaining diversity. Sadly, these fragile environments are vanishing at a frightening rate, with freshwater vertebrate populations falling more than twice as precipitously as terrestrial or marine ones. It can be said that something coordinated is obviously in order here, with plans aimed at sprucing up the quality of water and safeguarding key habitats, initiatives discussed in emergency recovery plans prioritizing freshwater ecosystems (Tickner et al., 2020). With regard to innovation, new concepts in sanitation and wastewater management are holding significant promise for public health as well as our planet. The combination of intelligent technologies and digital systems is optimizing treatment processes, providing real-time monitoring and optimizing available resources. By leveraging these high-end systems, communities can gradually move towards sustainable practices that match, for instance, the United Nations Sustainable Development Goals (SDGs), providing clean water access and monitoring responsible consumption. Furthermore, encasing these efforts within a comprehensive plan can even help enable underserved communities to have control of their own sanitation and health gains. To summarize, the transformative potential of these innovations underscores just how important it is to focus on sanitation and wastewater management if we're to nurture healthier societies and safeguard key natural resources for future generations (Turner, 2018).

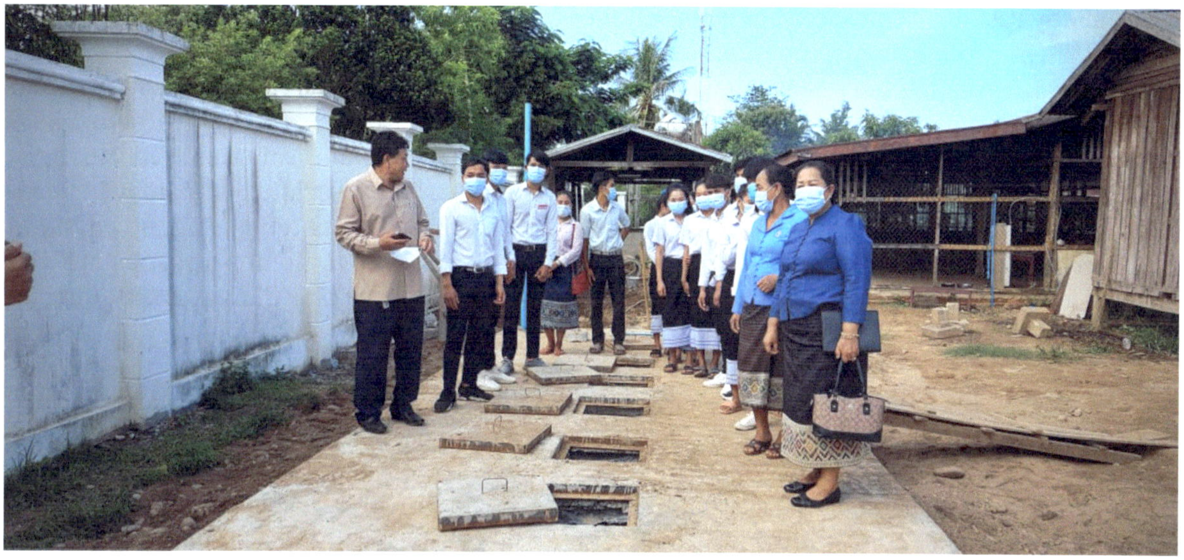

Source: SIWI. (2021). *Water and Sanitation DEWATS Project.*

Historical Context and Evolution of Sanitation Practices

Sanitation evolved with time as individuals realized that cleaning their environment could improve community health. Ancient communities in Rome and the Indus Valley constructed rudimentary water channels and waste management systems that, in a sense, initiated public health concepts. Then, during the 1800s—when epidemics like cholera ravaged society—individuals such as Edwin Chadwick in England took matters into their hands. He advocated full sewer systems and secure water supplies, turning sanitation from a mere necessity into a part of urban planning that connects day-to-day life with the general health. Science continued to advance ideas during the late 1800s and early 1900s. While scientists discovered that small pathogens, rather than dirty environments, caused diseases, attention turned to proper hygiene and waste management. At that time, the initial wastewater treatment arrangements were introduced, mixing natural processes and chemicals to reduce health threats. Governments began to realize, more or less on their own, their part in all this; they sponsored more research on waste management, even if it wasn't everyone who received equal access—pointing out ongoing social disparities that reverberate in today's communities. Recently, discussions on sanitation have expanded to incorporate green methods. Rather than simply dumping trash, there is now talk of recovering resources and even planning in terms of a circular economy. Studies such as the 12 challenge area analyses (WWAP report, 2012) highlight water concerns in various regions and demonstrate that local, hands-on solutions are required. Politically, there's a little give-and-take: some prefer tweaking the systems we already have, while others fantasize about totally reimagining how things get done (Ampe et al., 2019). Overall, sanitation continues to evolve—due to new technology, changing societal demands, and environmental concerns—so sustainable practices are a big deal for global health and resource management.

Importance of Sanitation in Modern Society

Urbanization and thriving industries have made it fairly evident—we require working sanitation systems. Poor sanitation, particularly in poor communities, places a great burden on health services and frequently results in the spread of diseases such as cholera and dysentery, impacting thousands annually. When water becomes polluted and refuse isn't removed suitably, the entire community suffers. Overall, investing in good wastewater management is a good decision that raises the public health and environment. Investing in improved sanitation infrastructure is not all about having cleaner water, it's about improving overall quality of life for people and communities. Most often, solid sanitation planning in cities can significantly decrease the risks associated with poor sanitation, establishing a healthier ground for all. Technologically driven solutions for managing wastewater are revolutionizing sanitation in numerous environments. Intelligent equipment, particularly those connected with IoT, introduce new avenues for monitoring and adjusting these systems such that the waste is dealt with effectively.

This sounds like science fiction, but these technologies assist farmers with access to safe, treated water for their crops—similar to how natural organic farming recycles nutrients. In others, the application of these advanced techniques not only streamlines everyday functions but reduces pollution and promotes a circular economy in which water cycles round and round in productive manners. The combination of technology and sustainability truly establishes a strong foundation for public health initiatives and a greener world. It's difficult to overstate how closely sanitation is linked to community health. Clean and pure water is not a luxury, but something that everyone needs for good health, justice, and even economic stability. When sewer systems fail, the consequences aren't isolated to one individual, it threatens our water supplies and the entire environment. Solving the problem means examining a broad array of options, from improved hygiene education to more intelligent management techniques. Digital tools today assist local teams in collecting helpful data that, in turn, makes it simpler to address what communities require. Climate change and increasing populations create new challenges, making it even more important to keep our sanitation approaches on their toes and innovative so that everyone has access to the clean, vital resources they are worthy of.

5.1. Overview of Public Health and Sanitation

Clean sanitation is regarded as central to healthy communities. When waste is not handled properly, a whole host of health issues will arise, and we usually find that there is a connection between poor practice and outbreaks of communicable diseases. There is a lot of evidence—broadly speaking, which suggests how failing sanitation causes water contamination and other problems. Improved sanitation reduces health threats, saves medical expenses, and even increases work performance, all of which are positive developments for daily life. Actual transformation, however, requires individuals of all stripes to dive in and build solutions that last. Technology advances in treating wastewater have proved to be an actual game-changer in terms of sanitation and public health. New treatment concepts, ranging from simple biological processes to some fairly sophisticated filtration systems, struggle to eliminate dangerous pathogens before the water reaches the environment. In most instances, communities can even recycle treated water, conserving valuable resources in the process. Nevertheless, implementing these innovations isn't easy, it requires meticulous planning, sound investment, and sufficient local expertise to keep things in motion. Research, for example, identifies that relying on available expertise is crucial when establishing sanitation programs that achieve health objectives (Gumbo et al., 2012). Politics and finance clearly have significant influences on how sanitation policies fall. Experiences across the world indicate that political initiatives and how finances are structured tend to define sanitation initiatives. Consider nations like Brazil and India, where excavating local political environments has resulted in targeted investments that assist the most vulnerable. In the majority of instances, pro-poor interventions ensure that even the underserved receive adequate access, which in turn makes a significant difference in health outcomes. All of this emphasizes the necessity for governments and institutions to collaborate, even if political waters can get a little rocky, to obtain long-term enhancements in public health (WSP, 2011) (Figure 5.1).

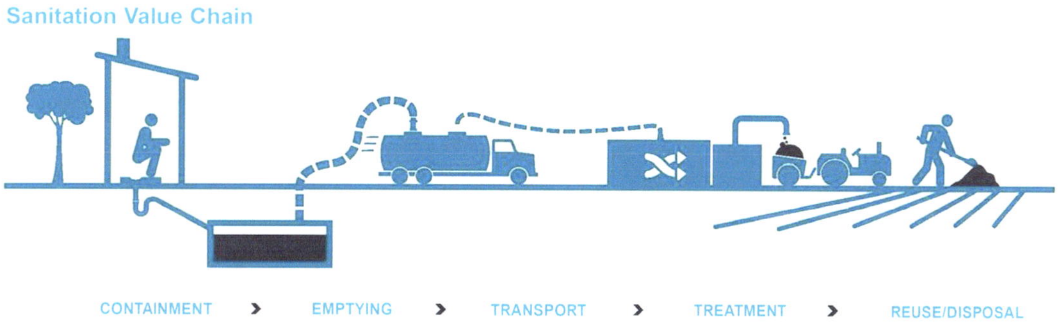

Figure 5.1. The sanitation system: collection, transport, treatment, disposal or reuse.

Source: Wikimedia Commons. (n.d.). *Sanitation Value Chain.*

5.1.1. Relationship Between Sanitation and Public Health

Cities that are overflowing today have a huge headache with sanitation systems that simply can't keep up. Proper waste management isn't just about relocating garbage, it prevents water sources from becoming contaminated and keeps susceptible people from getting waterborne pests. Consider Dar es Salaam, Tanzania; here, urban development has stretched the management of wastewater so thin that facilities strain and buckle under pressure, frequently releasing untreated sewage into adjacent streams, which increases health risks as well as environmental deterioration. Fixing this issue is not just about improved pipes and plants, for the most part, it also means engaging communities and investing in new, agile tech. Obviously, sanitation and public health go hand in hand, so firm regulation and consistent funding are essential (Azizi et al., 2025). Sanitation problems extend well beyond bricks and mortar; they're entwined with social and economic facts that dictate who receives safe facilities and who doesn't. Individuals in poorer communities frequently suffer most from inadequate sanitation, which can result in unpleasant epidemics of diseases such as cholera and dysentery. An abrupt microbial check of local water can be a bright red light indicating just how profound the problem is. In most developing areas, inadequate sanitation allows waterborne disease-causing organisms to wreak havoc, further taxing public health. Predictive modeling nowadays identifies contamination hotspots so interventions can be targeted precisely where they're required. With these cutting-edge tools to rely on, stakeholders can more effectively balance resources and increase public health initiatives, making the burden that poor sanitation imposes on communities less severe (Izah et al., 2025). Fresh concepts in wastewater treatment are turning the entire scene on its head, reinforcing the fact that sanitation is incredibly tied to general health. Methods such as Anaerobic Digestion (AD) aren't merely treating wastewater better—on the side, they're producing renewable energy. Those creative systems reduce environmental degradation and assist with a reduction in disease transmission associated with poor sanitation. It is about bringing tech solutions in concert with community involvement; one solution is not going to address all aspects. If you consider all the angles of sanitation, from broken-down infrastructure to social challenges, it becomes obvious that you need a balanced strategy. And by developing public-private partnerships and investing in resilient infrastructure, communities have a greater opportunity to safeguard public health and enhance the quality of life (Azizi et al., 2025) (Figure 5.2).

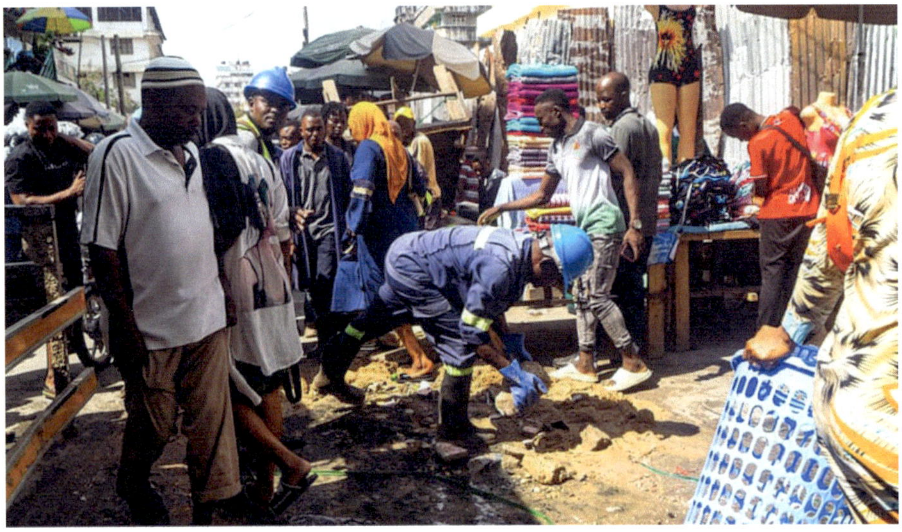

Figure 5.2. In Dar es Salaam, over 90% of residents depend on on-site sanitation systems like septic tanks and pit latrines, many of which are poorly maintained.

Source: Down To Earth. (2024). *Tanzania.*

5.1.2. Key Public Health Issues Related to Poor Sanitation

Sanitation is important—a lot. When systems fail, communities are inundated with all manner of waterborne issues that straight-up originate from contaminated sources. In other areas, unpleasant bugs like cholera, dysentery, and typhoid become established, which unfortunately increases sickness and even mortality rates, particularly among children and the elderly. Individuals may end up absent from work or school when such diseases spread, and local health facilities also end up bearing the brunt. It's like poor sanitation traps communities in a challenging cycle where clean water and proper facilities become a luxury few can afford. In most instances, addressing sanitation head-on is critical to reversing these trends (Vosa et al., 2025). Water sanitation and quality dance together, more or less, deciding just how healthy a community remains. Without an effective means of treating wastewater, nasty things filter into our water systems—increasing the risk for all of us. In much of sub-Saharan Africa, for example, the absence of effective wastewater management has resulted in high levels of toxic heavy metals and insidious disease-causing pathogens in the water. This type of contamination not only plays havoc with human health, sometimes resulting in long-term problems such as cancer or even neurological disorders but also endangers aquatic life. Rural women and children, where medical facilities are not always close at hand, usually bear the brunt. In general terms, increasing wastewater treatment processes and supporting them with strong legislations is crucial in reducing these health risks (Omohwovo, 2024) (Figure 5.3).

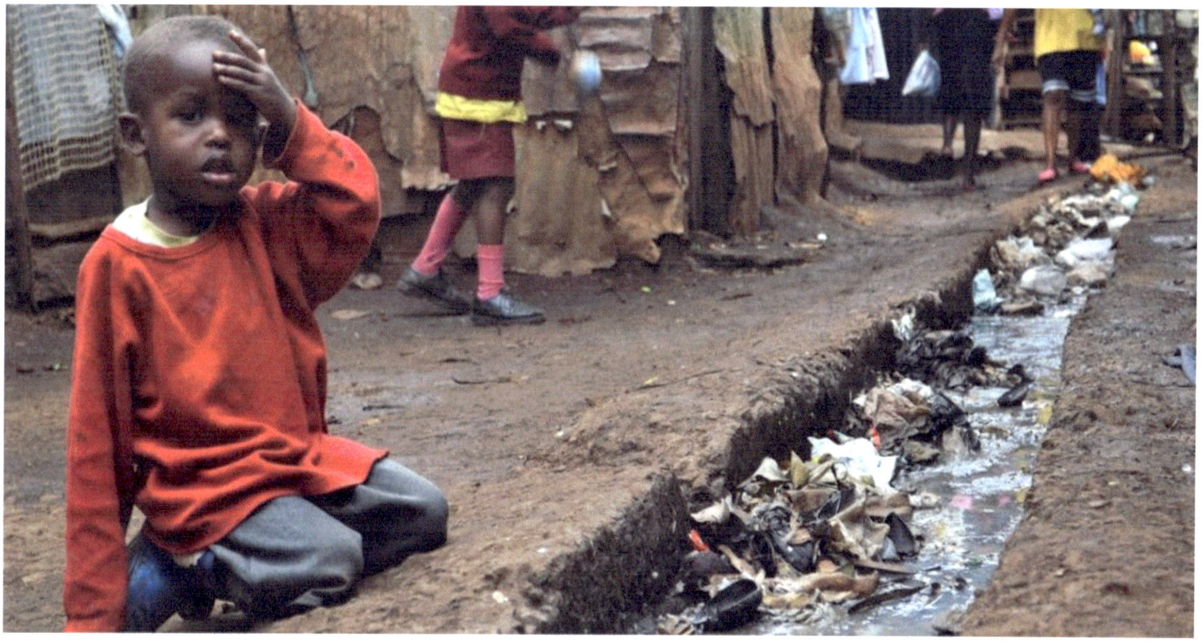

Figure 5.3. Sanitation woes cost Africa 115 lives every hour.

Source: LinkedIn. (2023). *Sanitation Woes Cost Lives in Africa.*

Sanitation issue isn't only a health issue, it overflows into how individuals live, learn, and work. Children in households where proper sanitation is absent frequently are absent from school because they're too ill or must assist with additional loads in the home, which delays their learning. This context further can ensnare families in poverty cycles, with little opportunity to improve over time. Local health systems become overwhelmed as well, so costs rise to the point where other essential services are compromised. A combination of outreach to communities, education about hygiene in ways that work, and upgrading water infrastructure can halt these cycles. Increased investment in sanitation usually lays the foundation for a healthier, more resilient community and even catalyzes long-term economic development (Omohwovo, 2024; Vosa et al., 2025) (Figure 5.4).

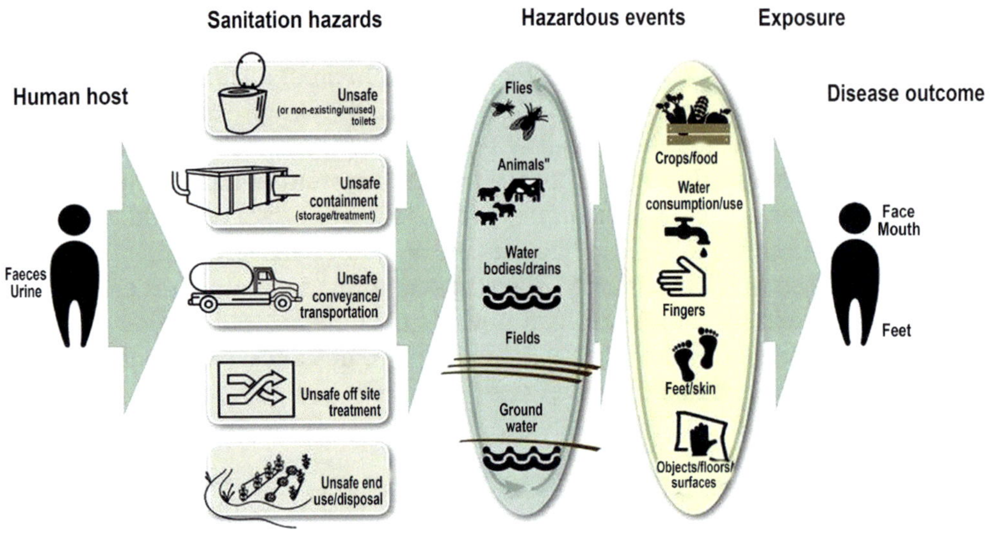

Figure 5.4. The health impacts from unsafe sanitation through various transmission pathways.

Source: Wolf, J., Johnston, R., Hunter, P. R., Gordon, B., Medlicott, K., & Prüss-Ustün, A. (2019). A Faecal Contamination Index for interpreting heterogeneous diarrhoea impacts of water, sanitation and hygiene interventions and overall, regional and country estimates of community sanitation coverage with a focus on low- and middle-income countries. *International journal of hygiene and environmental health, 222*(2), 270–282. https://doi.org/10.1016/j.ijheh.2018.11.005

5.1.3. Role of Sanitation in Disease Prevention

Good sanitation is important in preventing diseases. When societies lack adequate mechanisms for waste handling, it is not merely a matter of human waste but also public health in general. Clean water and properly treated wastewater can reduce the cases of outbreaks such as cholera, typhoid fever, and so forth, and research tends to find that low-quality sanitation not only affects individuals severely but also imposes a huge financial as well as systematic burden on our healthcare systems. Implementing infrastructure that both treats wastewater and promotes daily hygiene appears to be a logical, organic move in the direction of creating communities that can cope with health issues, even if the strategy does indeed seem somewhat haphazard at times. One escalating concern these days is antimicrobial resistance, referred to as AMR, which insidiously develops when antibiotics are overused and, frequently, when waste disposal simply isn't quite good enough. Leaving behind contaminated water or poorly disposed waste in most instances provides resistant bacteria with space to thrive, and as a result, it becomes extremely challenging for clinical interventions to be effective (Salam et al., 2023). It appears that suboptimal sanitation pushes pathogens to evolve in a manner that makes antimicrobials virtually ineffective. Brushing up on hygiene procedures and bolstering control over toxic waste could just serve to bust this cycle, providing something of a bulwark for communities from these pesky microbes. Innovative wastewater treatment concepts are disrupting our perceptions of sanitation, particularly in regions where clean water is not a certainty. Rather than simply treating sewage, these systems recycle water and take the pressure off of our shrinking freshwater resources. By embracing more sustainable methods, communities are able to watch healthier ecosystems develop nearly automatically. In a majority of instances, wise policies that blend these technologies with public health interventions work as initial buffers against outbreaks – a value strongly experienced by at-risk populations (Salam et al., 2023). When governments, NGOs, and local authorities coordinate (occasionally with a couple of coordination hiccups along the way), making sure they have equitable access to these amenities can greatly support community resilience while emphasizing the importance of adequate sanitation for ultimate well-being.

5.2. Wastewater Treatment Processes

New tech has revolutionized how we clean up wastewater. Nowadays, incorporating devices such as membrane bioreactors (MBR) and oxidation processes isn't merely hoity-toity, it reduces contaminants in ways beyond our wildest dreams. Smart equipment allows us to monitor systems in real-time, which is vital when things get nasty with complex installations. This type of digital spin, in general, goes hand in hand with sustainable objectives while saving resources and our environment. In the process, such methods not only improve water quality but also open the door to a cycle where useful components are salvaged and given new life (Turner, 2018). Understanding the steps of cleaning wastewater is central to why it is important for our wellbeing and the world. Normally, the procedure begins by allowing large particles to settle out in what is referred to as primary treatment. Microorganisms take center stage next, chomping on organics to reduce pollutant levels. Last is a polishing cycle—utilizing filters or even chemicals—to achieve rigorous safety marks. Every component, though it may appear straightforward by itself, contributes its share towards maintaining releases low and ensuring reused water is safe enough (WSP, 2011). When wastewater is not treated properly, the consequences can be quite severe. Challenging treatment can contaminate surrounding water sources and even ignite health emergencies by spreading waterborne diseases. Nature also suffers, with local ecosystems frequently disturbed and water bodies facing degradation. As our cities expand and more fill in, the demand for smarter sewage solutions grows even more urgent. Creative possibilities such as biogas capture and nutrient recycling provide avenues that can alleviate the strain of expanding populations and climate change. In the majority, these actions are able to enhance community health and protect water and keep it clean, remaining committed to the general goals of environmental care and public health (Turner, 2018) (Figure 5.5).

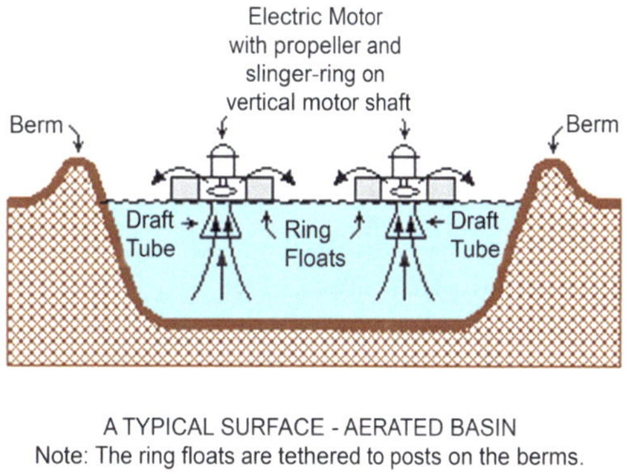

Figure 5.5. The wastewater treatment process.

Source: By Mbeychok - Own work, Public Domain, https://commons.wikimedia.org/w/index.php?curid=2930661

5.2.1. Primary Treatment Methods and Their Effectiveness

Successful primary treatment in wastewater treatment is an important initial barrier against pollution, safeguarding public health from the beginning. From the outset, operations such as sedimentation and flotation help remove larger solids and particles from the water. This simple process reduces the organic load that could prove to be too much for subsequent, more sophisticated treatments. In most developing regions where fancy technology is not always an option, these simple approaches tend to be the most convenient solution. Stopping contaminants at the beginning not only serves to keep close water safe but also relates to larger initiatives in terms of sanitation and hygiene. The effectiveness of these initial methods, particularly within countries with less capable infrastructure, highlights their functionality in applying to pressing public health issues (Drechsel et al., 2010). Addressing the numerous problems that accompany inadequate sanitation most certainly warrants a closer examination of how effectively such simple treatments work. Research indicates that sedimentation tanks can effectively reduce solid waste, which in most instances decreases the risks associated with waterborne diseases. Urban centers, where space is limited, occasionally find these simple methods indispensable because more elaborate treatment options simply are not possible. Nations that have incorporated rudimentary wastewater practices into everyday life tend to experience salient increases in public health; the connection between good sanitation and public well-being is difficult to ignore. Encouraging more extensive implementation of these effective treatments, particularly where availability is limited—not only reduces stress on water systems but also establishes the foundation for further, more sophisticated solutions (Tulenko, 2007). Considering beyond health, the economic perspective further emphasizes why beginning with good primary treatment is important. By getting rid of pollutants in the first place, cities are able to reduce the burden downstream, saving money and preserving resources in the process. Cleaner water can drive healthier communities and even shake the wheels of local economies, like agriculture, for example, which does well when reclaimed water is utilized. Research tends to indicate that investment in primary wastewater management yields important benefits through minimizing health risks and enhancing overall productivity and quality of life. As an important piece in the big picture of water management, a concentration on primary treatment not only safeguards public health but also reinforces the economic basis important for community development (Drechsel et al., 2010) (Figure 5.6).

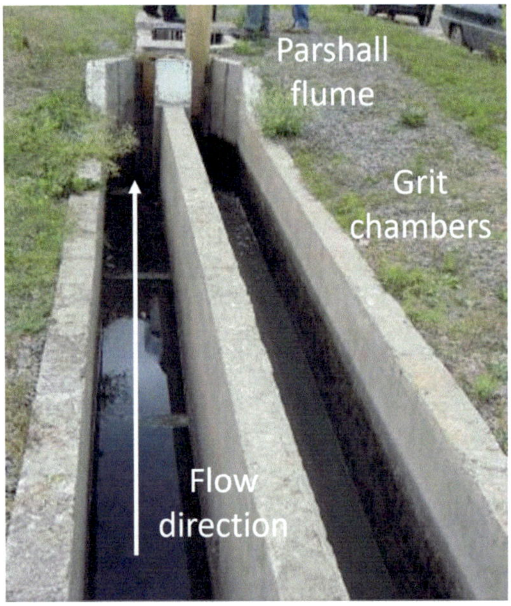

Figure 5.6. Primary treatment of wastewater.

Source: By Marcos von Sperling - Marcos von Sperling, CC BY-SA 4.0, https://commons.wikimedia.org/w/index.php?curid=110794478

5.2.2. Secondary Treatment Processes and Biological Treatment

Efficient wastewater handling relies a lot on the efficiency of secondary and biological treatment. You have these processes decomposing organic waste and trimming excess nutrients so that the water that is acceptable to the environment is within regulations; effluents should be clean. Microorganisms become industrious here – they essentially consume the toxins, which is a lot greener compared to producing it with chemicals. Processes such as activated sludge and biofilm reactors have been able to seriously increase the amount of pollutants removed.

Added to that, employing locally available bio-waste as adsorbents open a smart possibility: not only can wastewater be treated, but agricultural waste can also be minimized and its negative contribution to the environment lessened. Looking at it all in its totality, these combined approaches remind us that using natural resources can address ecological issues at the same time as maintaining treatment effectiveness (Nataša et al., 2021). Although biological treatment approaches appear promising, there are indeed still plenty of challenges when handling new pollutants, considering the recent global health concerns. Viruses like SARS-CoV-2 persist in wastewater – a serious public health issue , and normal facilities only partially eliminate these dangers, so additional disinfection truly is called for. In most instances, this entails an additional check and recheck to ensure pathogens don't get through. Periodic reviews of residual risks may well result in management systems that are custom-designed to allow the safe reuse and disposal of water. In general, the pandemic has demonstrated that secondary treatment can't simply be geared toward organic content and nutrients; it has to address viral invaders as well (Bogler et al., 2020). Advances in secondary treatment technology are proving to be an actual game-changer towards sustainable wastewater management. Recent innovations like MBR and even artificial wetlands come to the rescue to augment the natural acumen of biological processes; they utilize the capability of certain organisms to degrade pollutants, reducing the overall ecological footprint of treatment facilities. With urban sprawl increasing and environmental issues piling up, integrating high-tech interventions with nature's own processes is fast turning into a need rather than an extravagance. This combination not only assists in fulfilling more stringent regulatory requirements but also plays an important part in protecting public health by preventing treated water from damaging surrounding ecosystems (Nataša et al., 2021) (Figure 5.7).

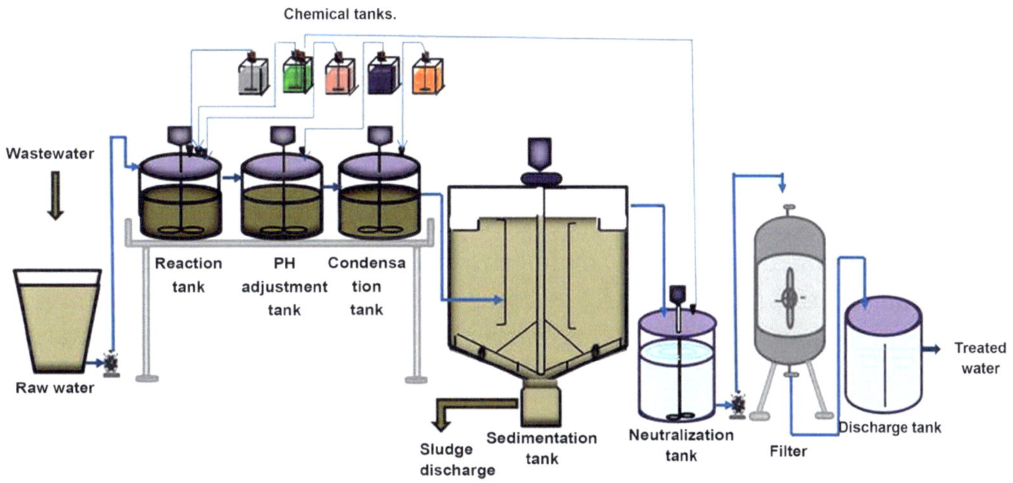

Figure 5.7. Secondary wastewater treatment methods.

Source: ResearchGate. (2023). *Secondary Wastewater Treatment Methods.*

5.2.3. Tertiary Treatment and Advanced Purification Techniques

Innovative wastewater treatment isn't an afterthought move; it's a paradigm shift. Tertiary processes stretch beyond primary and secondary treatment to address the recalcitrant portions; nutrients, pathogens, and organics that made it through. Facilities in most instances currently utilize processes such as MBR and reverse osmosis (RO), which, quite honestly, do wonders at eliminating micro-pollutants. Ozonation and advanced oxidation processes (AOPs) step in to decompose complex organic materials that previous steps may not catch. This added step of purification can render treated water safe for anything from watering crops to even (in some instances) drinking, an important consideration when water is limited.

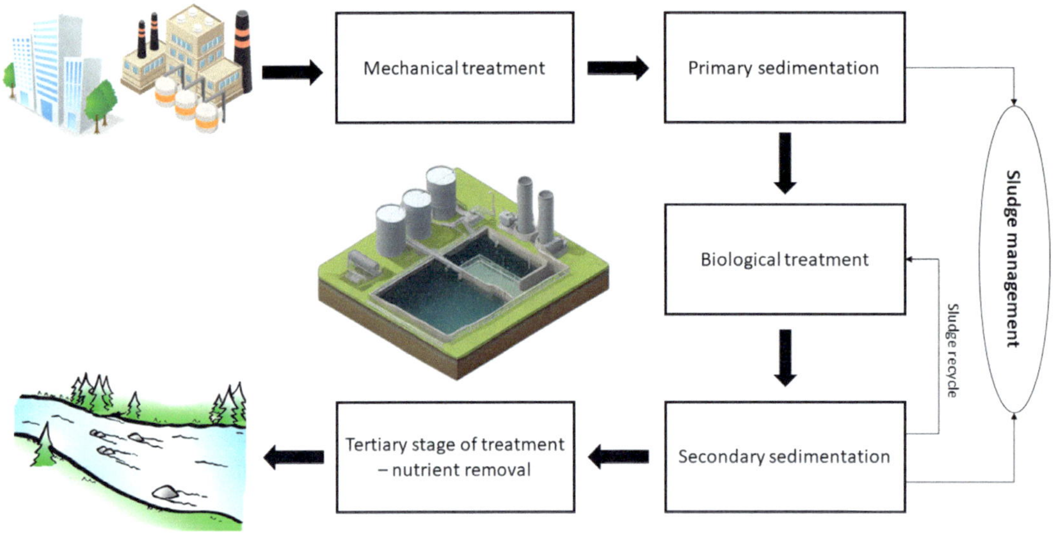

Figure 5.8. Schematic flowchart of the tertiary treatment step.

Source: Solcova O, Dlaskova M, Kastanek F. Challenges and Advances in Tertiary Waste Water Treatment for Municipal Treatment Plants. *Processes*. 2024; 12(10):2084. https://doi.org/10.3390/pr12102084

When sanitation is lacking, the consequences bleed over far beyond local ecosystems. Inadequately treated wastewater can contain a variety of pathogens, laying the groundwork for waterborne disease such as cholera and dysentery, particularly in areas where clean water is an amenity. Numerous communities have determined that targeting microbial reduction by means of tertiary treatment alleviates these risks. Research, in most cases, supports the concept of predictive modeling to identify hotspots of contamination, informing local efforts to where the intervention is required most. In most instances, by relying on these focused strategies and periodically utilizing information that is a little unconventional, communities can more effectively protect public health from the ravages of waterborne disease. Cutting-edge wastewater treatment isn't merely about tweaking vintage systems, it's also about adopting new, sometimes unconventional, solutions from nature. Constructed wetlands and biological nutrient removal systems allow nature to take care of part of the load, a solution that's resourceful and eco-friendly; these techniques are even frequently married to attempts that recycle valuable by-products such as biogas and reusable fertilizers. For example, research in places like Zambia's Copperbelt Province (Tortajada, 2016) has demonstrated that as mining discharges and sewage effluent blend together, these intelligent methods can mitigate the load on local water systems. By integrating findings from a range of disciplines, and yes, sometimes tolerating small imperfections in data and punctuation, stakeholders are developing wastewater management strategies that respond to public health requirements, defend ecosystems, and facilitate sustainable development (Figure 5.8).

5.3. Technologies in Wastewater Management

High population growth and industrialization have made wastewater management a nightmare, particularly in regions such as Africa where existing treatment facilities simply don't cut it. Untreated wastewater continues to get discharged, which disrupts water quality and compromises public health, particularly of the most susceptible. Dozens of recent reports indicate that wastewater treatment is not just a matter of keeping people healthy but also preserving aquatic life and the environment in general. It obviously demands new, locally adapted concepts. In all but a few instances, sustainable approaches, such as developing local technologies and adjusting how plants operate, can improve performance to levels adequate for regulators while producing healthier, more resilient communities and ecosystems. All of which play a pivotal part in meeting Sustainable Development Goal 6 (SDG 6), aimed at universal sanitation and clean water access (Omohwovo, 2024).

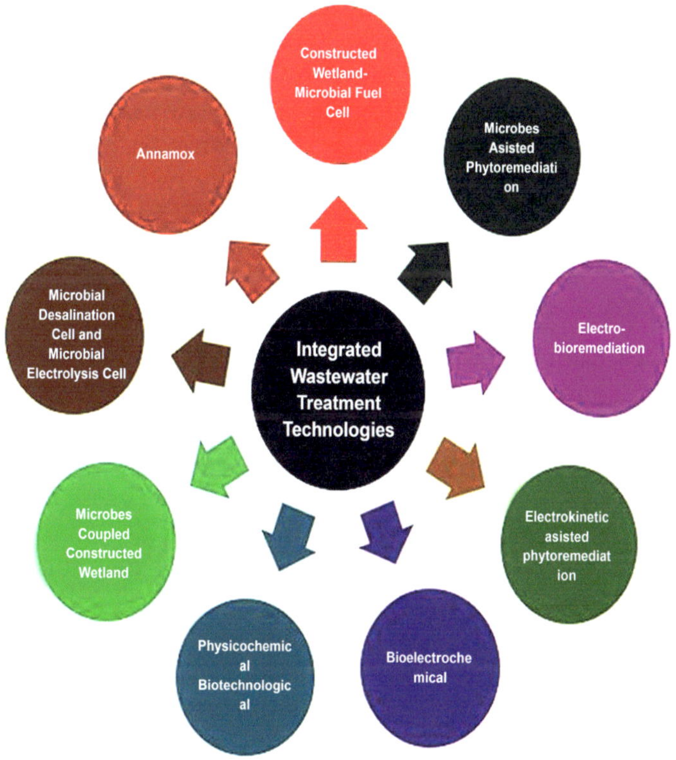

Figure 5.9. Various integrated environmental technologies used for wastewater treatment and management.

Source: Kumar V, Bilal M and Ferreira LFR (2022) Editorial: Recent Trends in Integrated Wastewater Treatment for Sustainable Development. Front. Microbiol. 13:846503. doi: 10.3389/fmicb.2022.846503.

Methods for wastewater treatment have evolved immensely, especially given the fact that more than 60% of the population lives life without clean sanitation services, meaning properly managed ones. Such a fact essentially accentuates the need for mixed solutions that couple new technology with socio-economic intelligence. Decentralized alternatives, when properly implemented, tend to increase local participation and management of resources, setting the stage for improved wastewater recycling and even nutrient recovery. There's a palpable shift these days—treatment for reuse is gaining traction—implying that wastewater is not necessarily waste to be discarded but a resource waiting to be exploited. Overall, an understanding of the root drivers of sanitation services and the advocacy of a more service-oriented model may usher in society gains that could secure investments. Numerous studies support that these new tech turns are capable of remedying short-term health risks as well as underpin greater sustainable development goals (Andersson et al., 2018).

Addressing wastewater management challenges is not a silver bullet solution, it requires a combination of tech enhancements, public participation, and better governance. The challenge tends to intensify with murky infrastructure and political instability, especially in disadvantaged regions. With greater government support and more grassroots-level community involvement, these creative solutions may be here to stay. Additionally, public-private collaboration can frequently trigger a chain reaction towards more reliable management systems. Quick fixes, such as low- or no-flush toilets and dividing waste flows, are stealthily cutting out a way for more environmentally friendly waste practice. Through taking inspiration from effective frameworks and adapting them to suit conditions on the ground, one is able to alleviate the public health burdens accompanying unsanitary conditions and water inefficiency – ultimately checking off key public health and environmental objectives (Omohwovo, 2024) (Figure 5.9).

5.3.1. Overview of Traditional Wastewater Treatment Technologies

Wastewater treatment technology has evolved far – it's revolutionized public health and our environment more than most folks know. In the past, people used simple methods such as sedimentation and lagoons to discharge coarse solids and reduce pathogens by natural processes. These processes were effective in part, but they weren't specifically designed for the complex, urban sanitation problems that arise today. As industrialization progressed, newer methods such as the activated sludge process came into the limelight. This method utilizes aeration and biological treatment to decompose organic matter much more efficiently, resulting in cleaner effluent. Yet, those traditional methods tend to consume lots of energy and chemicals, which can be a nightmare for cities that are already trying to cater to the needs of a burgeoning population. With the majority of instances, breaking away from basic, primitive practices to these sophisticated yet energy-consuming processes proved to be a turning point in the battle against wastewater issues (WSP, 2011). In the case of conventional wastewater treatment, there's a three-step system which may sound too tidy on chapter but is slightly more haphazard in reality. Leading the parade is primary treatment, where emphasis is placed on physical methods – screening and sedimentation remove the large solids. This phase sets the stage, but it barely addresses all pathogens or completely breaks down organic pollutants. Next, the system changes gear to secondary treatment, one that employs microorganisms to digest organic pollutants. You notice technologies such as trickling filters and activated sludge appearing here, each with its own spin on increasing microbial activity.

Last but not least, tertiary treatment comes along with high-tech filtration and disinfection methods. This phase may employ chemicals or even ultraviolet (UV) light to refine the water before discharge. While this multi-step method better addresses the degree to which the water becomes clean, its energy-intensive and other resource-heavy dependence makes it important to consider alternatives that are more cost-effective and sustainable (Choudhary & Ray, 2024). City populations are surging, and that really puts the squeeze on conventional wastewater treatment systems. Outdated systems tend to break under heavy operating expenses and environmental concerns ; the type that accompanies high energy loads and volumes of chemicals. It is no surprise that many cities are now in search of new ideas that combine technology with a pinch of nature. Consider Nature-Based Solutions (NBS), for instance; they offer some very promising possibilities. Through natural processes accessed via such things as constructed wetlands and green infrastructure, NBS not only enhances treatment effectiveness but also reduces environmental damage. Such combined approaches typically provide sanitation services while also supporting local ecosystem restoration by enhancing biodiversity and urban greening. Evidently, a transition to a combination of the old and the new is inevitable if sustainable sanitation and intelligent wastewater management in the future are to be achieved (WSP, 2010; Choudhary & Ray, 2024) (Figure 5.10).

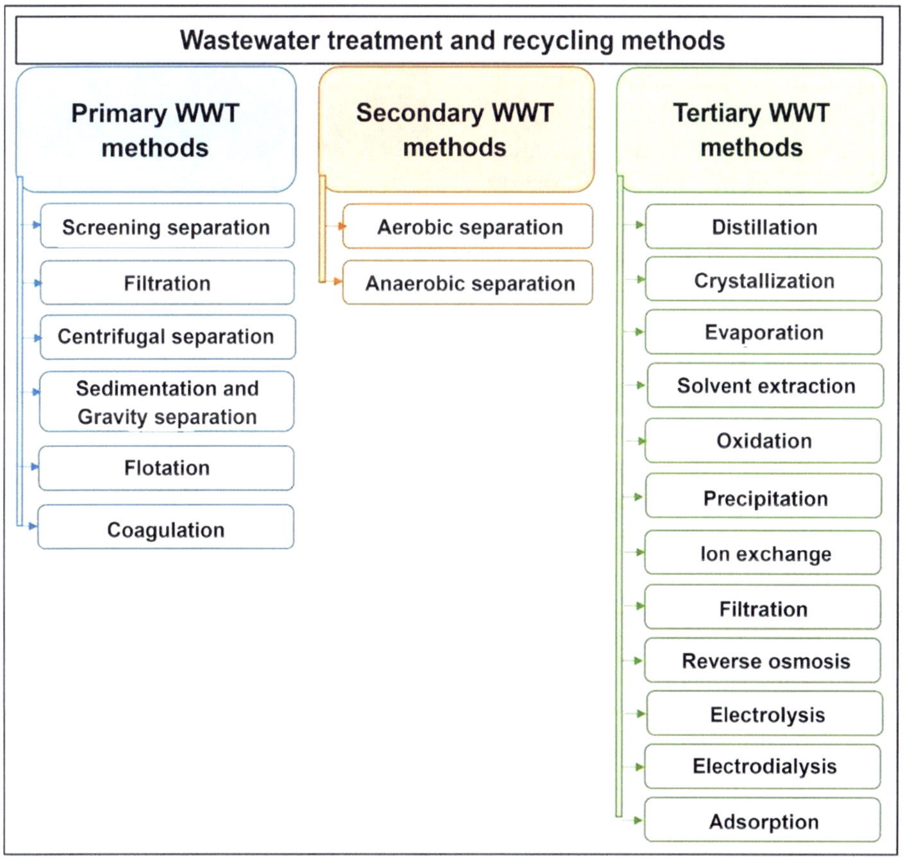

Figure 5.10. Traditional wastewater treatment methods.

Source: Sibali, L. (2020). *Traditional Wastewater Treatment Methods*. ResearchGate.

5.3.2. Emerging Technologies in Wastewater Treatment

Wastewater treatment technology has made great strides, urbanization and growing populations really made us jump into thinking about new ways of doing things. In the past, we primarily relied on traditional methods that just dealt with the waste without seeking out secret advantages. Then, as municipal health concerns and environmental harm began to cast larger shadows, some newer concepts emerged from the shadows. Then you have things such as MBR, various types of biogas recovery, and even AOPs taking over the industry. Combining these innovations with our traditional systems isn't always seamless; local conditions and accessible resources have much to do with whether these updates function well or not (Turner et al., 2018). Emerging technologies are converting wastewater from an absolute liability into a potential asset, and that aligns with the circular economy principle. Current research largely suggests the potential for upcycling wastewater into valuable products such as nutrients, energy, and even simple construction materials. This rethink isn't solely for saving the planet—there's an economic side to it as well. Business models based on these concepts are beginning to deliver, closing the gap between eco-friendliness and profitability. In most instances, participants in these conversations now recognize sanitation as not only treating waste but now they're picturing a time when wastewater infrastructure enhances community well-being and economic resilience (WSP, 2011). How individuals perceive these wastewater solutions also plays an important role. Typically, there is a gap that is easily apparent—most people are still pretty unaware of how wastewater treatment works. Studies have revealed that this general misinformation regarding the complete lifecycle of wastewater leaves room for a communication gap, hence a negative impact on public opinion. Interestingly, as awareness improves, concern about water pollution also increases, implying that education could be a way to convert people. Many appear willing to fund treatment center improvements, showing an emerging willingness to do something sustainable. In the end, incorporating community involvement into the equation seems critical to breaking past lingering reservations and effectively integrating these new solutions into current systems (Turner et al., 2018) (Figure 5.11).

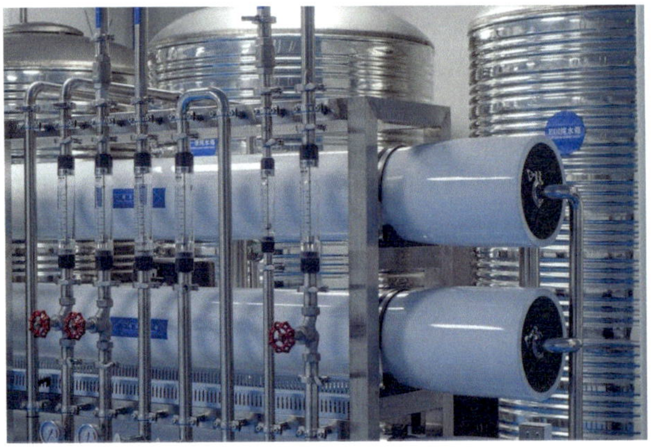

Figure 5.11. While low-pressure membrane filtration has been around for more than four decades, only now is it being utilized in wastewater treatment plants.

Source: Water Tech Online. (2025, February). *Low Pressure Membrane Filtration.*

5.3.3. Role of Digital Technology and Automation in Wastewater Management

Digital technology has transformed wastewater management in ways that aren't necessarily apparent at first glance. Today, utilities employ real-time monitors that allow them to monitor wastewater quality more easily – so even low-level contamination is detected quickly. IoT sensors, for example, stream data continuously that aids in treatment decision-making, and data analytics software tends to even anticipate system glitches before they become full-blown problems, reducing downtime and maintenance costs. The secret appears to be collecting data at various points of treatment, which makes the entire process more transparent and accountable. This pre-emptive approach, in the majority of instances, constructs a stronger template for regulatory checks, while safeguarding water sources and public health. Automation entered wastewater management and, in general terms, it streamlines the treatment process by aligning tech and human decision-making closer to each other. Automated systems now adjust treatment parameters in real-time according to the flow of incoming wastewater – producing a fairly consistent output quality. Concurrently, these systems lighten the load of cumbersome, time-consuming processes, such that personnel can engage in more difficult challenges. With machine learning and artificial intelligence added to the mix, projections regarding wastewater patterns assist in more intelligent utilization of resources. Education to work with these new systems is essential; the digital transition also serves as a catalyst for talent building, which is essential to maintaining a workforce that can mesh with rapidly changing technologies and handle the nuances of contemporary wastewater treatment. Digital technology isn't merely a matter of day-to-day efficiencies; it also comes into play when long-range planning of wastewater assets is being addressed. Take the case of digital twins, which are virtual representations of real systems. These allow utilities to test out scenarios from simple repairs to massive infrastructure overhauls, reducing the risks associated with large projects. Visualization tools provided by digital platforms are more likely to enhance public participation and trust, in a sort of relaxed but efficient way. As most utilities start their digital transformation, expertise from efforts such as the IWA Digital Water Program , intermixing university knowledge with field experiences – is a critical enabler. This all enables wastewater professionals to blend digital advancement with public health aspirations, eventually opening the door for a more resilient and sustainable water management arrangement (WSP, 2011) (Figure 5.12).

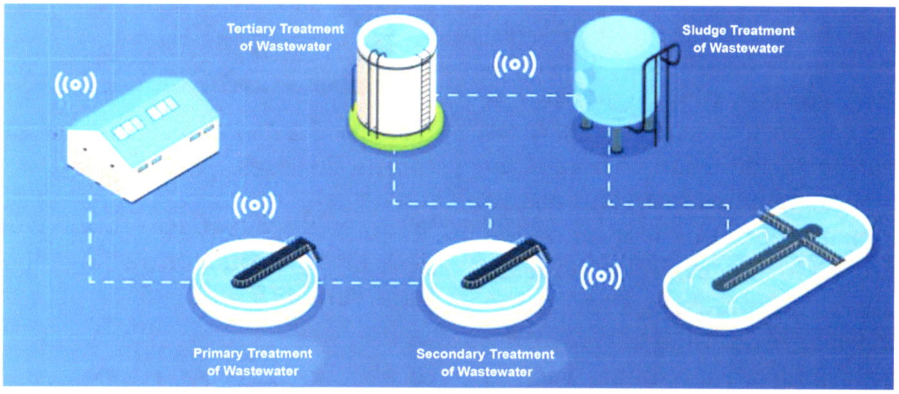

Figure 5.12. *Transforming wastewater treatment with IoT technologies.*

5.4. The Impact of Poor Sanitation on Water Resources

Bad sanitation truly ruins our water. When raw wastewater is simply dumped into nature, it has the effect of polluting lakes and rivers—basically inviting bad microbes to the party. You can usually see how uncontrolled waste flow allows ugly microorganisms to grow, and these little perpetrators can find their way into our drinking water and make health issues even worse. A population that is struggling with poor sanitation often experiences higher incidents of waterborne diseases that not only expose people to health risks but also overwhelm the local health system and reduce productivity. In general, the fact that more than 60% of the world's population lacks access to safe sanitation indicates how severely water quality and public health can be impacted (Andersson et al., 2018). Controlling our water effectively begins with grasping how bad sanitation creates huge issues. Despite the United Nations 2030 Agenda for Sustainable Development encouraging more effective water and sanitation management, most places lack the fundamental infrastructure for it. The economic, social, and environmental consequences, such as incessant water quality deterioration, require immediate, hands-on action. As populations expand and water demands continue to increase, neglecting sanitation problems only makes it more difficult to ensure clean water for all. Too often, local customs simply don't live up to those international aspirations, revealing a disconnect between high-minded policies and actual practice. In most instances, redirecting our attention to pragmatic, effective policies to manage water in response to sanitation failures is an imperative (Tortajada, 2016). There is no doubt that we require innovative solutions to reduce the detrimental effects of poor sanitation on water resources. Moving towards a model in which we recycle water for reuse can reduce the volume of wastewater in addition to recovering valuable nutrients. Innovative thinking, such as decentralized treatment systems and even low-flush toilets—provides viable alternatives that can significantly enhance sanitation outcomes. These solutions not only provide greater access to sanitation but also open the door to reusing treated water in activities such as irrigation, among other applications. Most importantly, a combination of initiatives by public agencies, private organizations and community groups is required to drive these concepts forward. More often than not, the integration of technological advances and intelligent policy shifts can produce an enhanced and stable system for water management and sanitation, ultimately providing healthier communities (Andersson et al., 2018) (Figure 5.13).

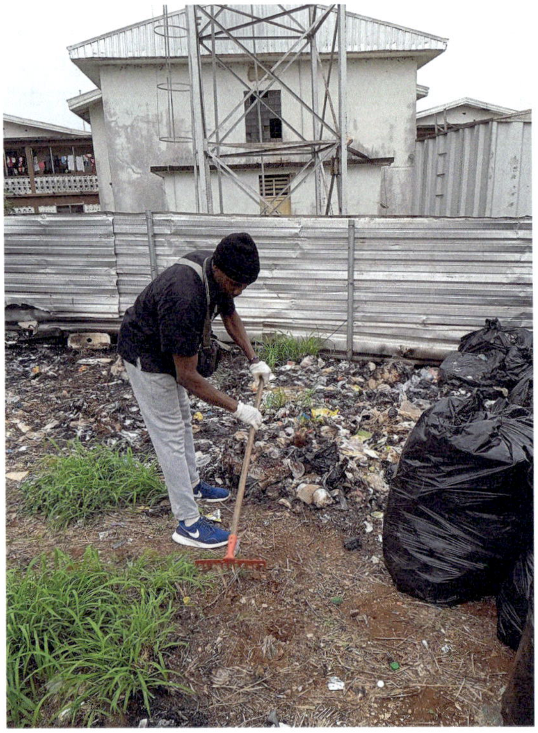

Figure 5.13. Poor sanitation breeds vector-borne diseases.

Source: By SusuGeo - Own work, CC BY-SA 4.0, https://commons.wikimedia.org/w/index.php?curid=151832395

5.4.1. Effects of Untreated Wastewater on Water Bodies

Untreated wastewater is a big concern for fish environments and for our own well-being. Wastewater discharged untreated from farms, factories, and cities comes with a complex cocktail of pollutants—consider heavy metals, excess nutrients, and even disease-causing agents—that taints water supplies in chaotic ways. In most instances, these toxins stew what is called eutrophication, where an overload of nutrients leads to unexpected occurrences of algal blooms. Such flowering sucks oxygen from the water and causes hypoxia and mass death among many aquatic organisms. Pathogens carried along in untreated wastewater can stray far, occasionally endangering human health while insidiously distorting biodiversity. In summary, confronting these environmental hazards is paramount if we are to maintain our aquatic systems in harmony and our populations safe, with effective wastewater management a pressing need. The consequences of untreated wastewater reach far beyond short-term ecological damage; they also strike communities on several fronts. People using these waters for drinking, bathing, or a little recreation risk more waterborne disease. For instance, exposure to a combination of pathogens and toxins can initiate gastrointestinal problems, and occasionally even play havoc with reproductive health. As water quality degrades, local agriculture and fisheries also suffer, which can escalate food insecurity and undermine livelihoods. Thus, the consequences of not treating wastewater are not merely a matter of nature out of balance, it resonates into social injustices and economic stability. In general, an even-handed strategy for treating wastewater must address both public health and economic issues if we ever want to create truly resilient communities. New wastewater treatment technologies and sustainable management practices have become critical solutions to these problems. Today, innovations combine biological, chemical, and physical methods to further screen out pollutants before water is returned to nature. One fascinating example is the application of bio-based sorbents derived from agricultural waste, which can capture pollutants efficiently—solving waste management and water purification simultaneously. Since certain studies are indicated Nataša et al. (2021), going for local solutions based on utilizing what is readily available can both save costs and be environmentally friendly. Furthermore, installing regulations to continually monitor wastewater output and making new treatment plant investments are critical moves toward the conservation of our water. In the majority of situations, providing clean water—as the SDGs emphasize, is adopting a balanced approach that integrates public health and environmental protection (Abascal et al., 2021) (Figure 5.14).

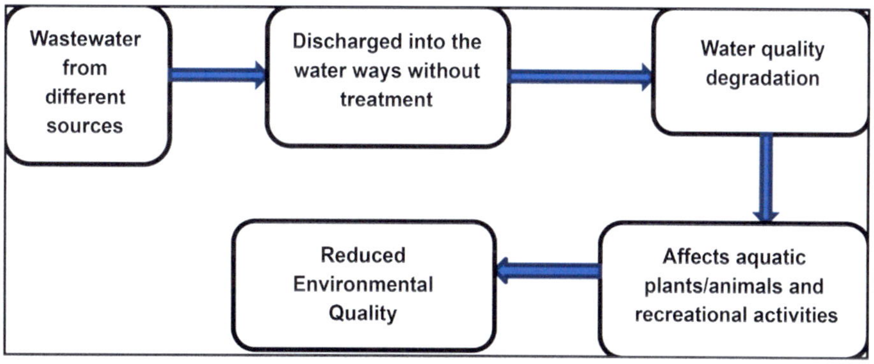

Figure 5.14. Impacts of untreated wastewater on the surface water.

Source: Ogueri, D. (2021). *Impacts of Untreated Wastewater on Surface Water*. ResearchGate.

5.4.2. Consequences for Aquatic Ecosystems

Releasing untreated wastewater into our rivers and lakes isn't simply an innocent mistake, it has an array of unforeseen, far-reaching issues. Quite often, too many nutrients, such as nitrogen and phosphorus, dumped in the waters result in an uncontrollable explosion of algae growth, commonly known as algal blooms. Such blooms have a tendency, in most instances, to absorb oxygen from the water, making aquatic life suffocate. And as the algae decay, oxygen levels fall even lower, creating those feared dead zones where life just can't exist. Delicate species are the first to disappear, which in turn disrupts the entire balance of the ecosystem. Overall, treating wastewater effectively isn't merely a matter of cleaner water; it's a matter of guarding the very foundation of aquatic health and resilience (Rodr JasíGuez, 2023). Clean water and sustainable development appear to be hand in hand, as noted by the United Nations SDGs, particularly those that work to promote water quality and lively ecosystems. If water is not well treated, the danger is not limited to fish or sea organisms; it overflows to touch communities depending on these bodies of water for drinking, recreation, or even small business undertakings. Occasionally, contaminants accumulate—heavy metals and toxins finding their way into aquatic organisms and, ultimately, being passed on to individuals further up the food chain, which can have serious health consequences. Overall, this entire scenario highlights the importance of an integrated strategy for wastewater management, one that brings together different SDGs to improve both community and environmental health. In some sense, this integration lays the path to ecological balance and environmental justice in the long run (Wang et al., 2022). The price tag of poor wastewater management goes well beyond harm to nature, it creeps into our socio-economic structures as well. When water quality is compromised, fisheries are harmed; these are not merely sources of food, but also significant pillars of economic stability for a large number of communities. Overfishing and dirty water can ignite a meltdown in neighborhood fisheries, exacerbating poverty and disrupting nutritional levels. Even recreational uses such as swimming and fishing could suffer, which would suppress local tourism and other economic prospects. Substituting modern wastewater treatment practices and more sustainable methods can reduce these escalating issues, laying the groundwork for healthier waters and more resilient neighborhood economies. Finally, achieving a balanced relationship between our daily chores and nature's requirements boils down to intelligent and efficient wastewater planning and sanitation programs (Rodr Jasí-Guez, 2023).

5.4.3. Long-Term Implications for Water Quality and Availability

Sanitation and water quality are closely interrelated in ways that impact our long-term health—large impacts that we observe in the environment and health. Poor sanitation, such as unsanitary facilities, tends to soil our clean water, gradually reducing its quality and availability. People depending on this dirty water are at greater risk for waterborne disease while their healthcare systems are strained to the limit. Gumbo et al. (2012) demonstrate some very smart combinations of water supply solutions with improved sanitation habits, which appear to allow communities to recover. Ultimately, our safe water relies on managing waste intelligently—prioritizing people's health and attempting to balance nature. Quality setup of sanitation can also relieve some of the pressures of cities on water. Busy urban areas, particularly following mass migrations, wind up overburdening their old water systems, as Mosello et al. (2016) observe. With more people, sanitation facilities usually get overwhelmed, hence waste isn't properly treated and additional runoff finds its way into local streams or ponds. Eventually, this gradual loss damages not just local aquatic life but also the safe water individuals require for consumption, cooking, and agriculture. More often than not, reconsidering the way we manage these systems and respond to urban pressures ends up being the key to keeping water cleaner in constantly changing urban landscapes. In the future, the issues created by poor sanitation systems extend beyond immediate health issues and begin to interfere with the broader social and economic equilibrium of communities. Clean water truly serves as the foundation for farms, factories, schools—name it. Thus, when water quality is compromised, its implications spread to all aspects of society, hampering economic growth and even occasionally increasing inequality. Building up our expertise in how to manage water resources, Gumbo et al. (2012) proposes, is important to ensure habits which enable communities to cope with these changes in the environment more effectively. Overall, investment in improved infrastructure and education on sanitation can initiate a self-reinforcing process which, in the long term, enhances both water quality and supply for generations to come (Figure 5.15).

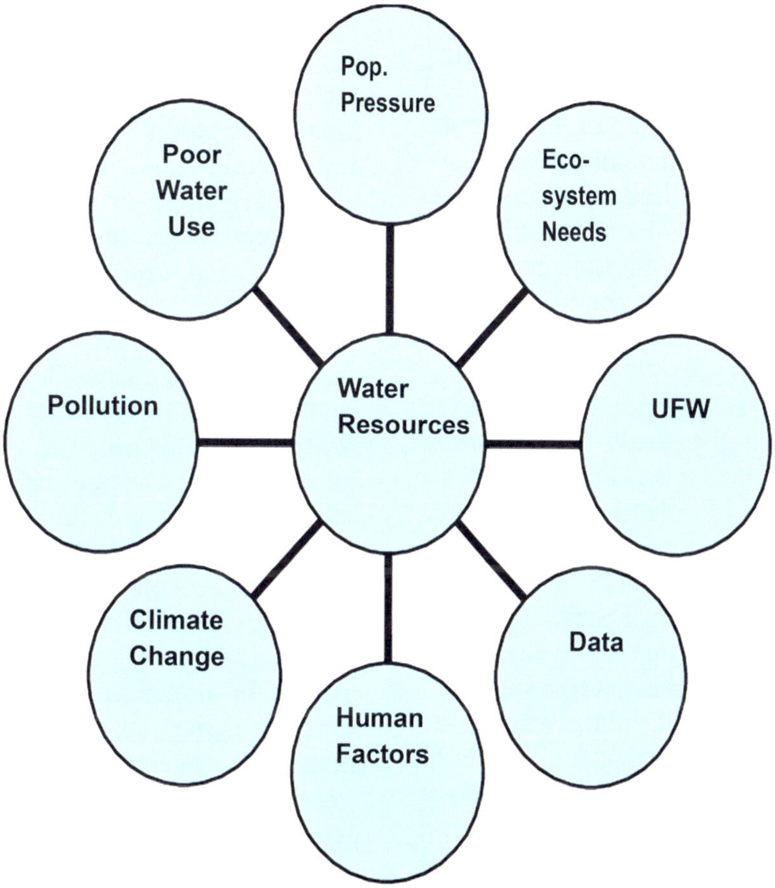

Figure 5.15. Interlinking of factors impacting water quality and availability.

Source: Zeman, C. (2011). *Factors Impacting Water Quality and Availability. ResearchGate.*

5.5. Community Health and Sanitation

Sanitation is at the very center of maintaining healthy communities. Proper waste cleanliness prevents disease by preventing contaminants from entering drinking water supplies—a problem that's particularly concerning in regions where basic infrastructure is inadequate. All too frequently, waterborne disease runs rampant in low-income areas, where inadequate sanitation puts people at risk. When communities implement improved waste management systems, the incidence of such diseases decreases significantly, and overall health improves. Good sanitation therefore not only safeguards health but also enhances social and economic conditions through cleaner living environments. Most often, integrating contemporary technology to ensure the use of resources in a sustainable manner converts sanitation into a real pillar of public health initiatives (María et al., 2021). Enhancing sanitation and wastewater treatment is also in tandem with universal SDGs. The United Nations SDGs primarily emphasize that all individuals—most especially marginalized communities without proper services—have the right to safe, accessible sanitation. Digital technology and sanitation technology innovation can come in and make data collection, monitoring, and management significantly more effective. For example, smart systems connected to the Internet of Things provide such detailed datasets that oftentimes, quite naturally, result in improved community health choices. These advancements tackle not only the immediate challenges of keeping areas clean but also broader environmental issues, carving a pathway toward fair and sustainable health outcomes. So, a focus on innovation in sanitation is pretty crucial for enhancing community well-being worldwide (María et al., 2021). Addressing the effects of poor sanitation on water resources requires a mix of policy reform, community input, and tech-driven solutions. When water infrastructure is contaminated due to poor sanitation, not only human health is threatened—but the native ecosystems are affected as well. Proper wastewater treatment is essential in order to resist environmental deterioration and end the disease-poverty cycle. Recently, technologies such as biological treatments and nutrient recovery have emerged as viable, sustainable alternatives. Through better management of wastewater, communities are able to conserve valuable water supplies while gaining benefits for agriculture, energy, and beyond. Overall, the convergence of community health and intelligent sanitation sets the foundation for healthy environments that facilitate today's and tomorrow's success for individuals all around the world (WSP, 2011).

5.5.1. Correlation Between Sanitation and Community Health Outcomes

Proper sanitation is an enormous community health factor and is receiving greater awareness today. Proper sanitation prevents disease and creates healthier daily environments, particularly in poverty-stricken neighborhoods, where poor facilities contribute to increased incidents of waterborne diseases such as cholera and dysentery. Studies generally confirm that investment in improved sanitation reduces healthcare expenditures and improves people's quality of life. Interventions in such locations as Brazil, India, Indonesia, and Senegal that consider sanitation politically and economically will generally produce the results to demonstrate that selective, deliberate intervention yields tangible effects on the most marginalized (WSP, 2011). It's quite literally as though investment in sanitation truly pays dividends on multiple fronts. In addition to the outright health advantages, sanitary practices also work into sustainable development and societal overall well-being. Poor sanitation is not just a risk to people's health but can also further degrade water quality, lead to pollution, and degrade ecosystems. That is why integrated wastewater management—where approaches take into account both health impacts and environmental impacts, is critical. Assessments from locations like Ghana and Sri Lanka show, in the majority of instances, that innovative wastewater treatment can increase resource recovery while addressing sanitation problems at the same time. If you examine these linkages, it becomes apparent that combining sanitation upgrading with wise environmental management is the key to long-term community strength (Merrey et al., 2020).

Sanitation even carries over into economic productivity and social equity. Communities with good facilities tend to have a healthier labor force, meaning fewer days lost to sickness and reduced transmission of disease—essential drivers that can increase economic output overall. Concurrently, poor sanitation tends to fall disproportionately on disadvantaged groups, uncovering underlying social disparities that must be fixed. In most instances, adopting more inclusive sanitation policy can assist in closing these gaps, with both health improvements and economic advantages being distributed more fairly. This overall strategy—tying health, economic development, and social fairness together—truly gets to the heart of why multifaceted strategies for sanitation are so very important to long-term community health (WSP, 2011) (Figure 5.16).

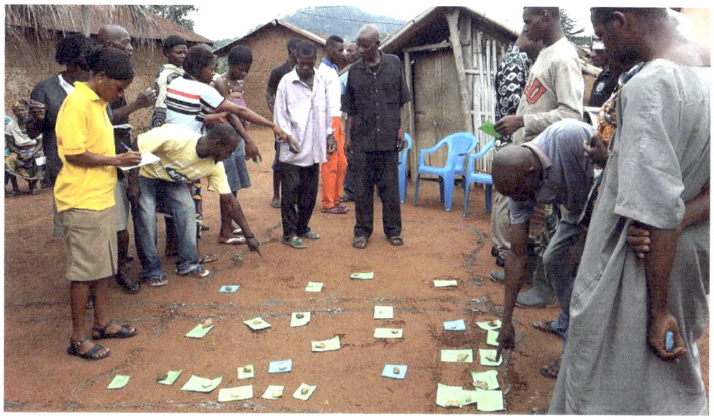

Figure 5.16. Community-led total sanitation (CLTS) triggering process: Community members in Ghana are drawing a map of open defecation for their community.

Source: Wikimedia Commons. (n.d.). *CLTS Triggering Process in Ghana.*

5.5.2. Vulnerable Populations and Sanitation Challenges

Vulnerable populations are left to bear the brunt when sanitation facilities are inadequate. Most communities in low- and middle-income countries have their needs severely impacted as cities grow—demand outpaces existing facilities. Rapid urban growth, in most instances, has marginalized groups with very little access to clean and safe sanitation, which subsequently leads to major health problems. Poverty, gender, and one's social status all combine to determine who gets served, with women and children usually bearing the greatest cost. Unremunerated care labor and safety concerns, for example, can turn something as mundane as accessing a safe restroom into a real trauma. This cycle even fosters mental tension, as trauma and persistent stress seep into the struggle for basic needs (Batra & Erbas, 2025). Evidently, policymakers must rely on new, diverse ideas if they have any hope of closing these gaps. Consider the case of Dar es Salaam, its burgeoning population, projected to reach 8.5 million by 2025, has pushed wastewater infrastructure far beyond its capacity. The growing numbers in the city have ultimately overwhelmed treatment facilities and, in most instances, allowed untreated sewage to flow into nearby waterways. This grim portrait is not merely about failed technology; it suggests a more profound connection between environmental degradation and widespread health crises that most harm the most vulnerable populations. Research tends to make the case for a fundamental rethink about how wastewater is handled. Promising solutions such as AD could enhance treatment effectiveness, though, only if these tech band-aids accompany engaged community action and consistent, sustainable financing (Azizi et al., 2025). Bypass these larger steps, and the poverty cycle for the vulnerable repeats itself. Sanitation is not merely a threat to individual health—deteriorating sanitation conditions can erode community ties and local economies, as well. In many cases, the ones who need good facilities the most find themselves in the ones without the minimum infrastructure, which is a recipe for disaster in the form of water-borne disease. If health suffers, then communities experience a loss in productivity, with limited resources going towards healthcare rather than other necessities. This issue illustrates, quite clearly, that a single-solution approach won't work; rather, some combination of tech breakthroughs and socio-economic solutions is required. Inserting a little mental health care into sanitation strategies could just smooth the way for recovery from failures and reduce the daily burden of poor infrastructure (Batra & Erbas, 2025). Ultimately, addressing these challenges from every possible direction isn't a nice-to-have, it's what's necessary to advance equity in sanitation access and safeguard public health for all, particularly those most vulnerable.

5.5.3. Case Studies of Communities Affected by Poor Sanitation

Inadequate sanitation most certainly leaves its stamp on communities in most unlikely manners. Different case studies reveal the numerous layers of influence on public health. In the Vietnamese countryside, for example, water operators and sanitation vendors have precipitous infrastructure hurdles and high cost operations that put them under grave financial threats. This tends to prompt a demand for donor-supported projects to support low-income families - something difficult to ignore. Interviews from surveys and focus group discussions with 15 suppliers in public–private partnerships indicate just how complex it can be to operate sanitation services. Erratic material prices, combined with tight household budgets, have a tendency to result in a perpetual cycle of bad access. Overall, targeted financial and policy interventions appear to be important here, as they vow to increase service accessibility without destroying market dynamics. Overall, these results emphasize that proper sanitation infrastructure is needed to protect public health and promote equitable access to water (Pham, 2025). Taking climate change into consideration puts an additional layer on the situation. As temperatures increase, communities that are already suffering from poor sanitation tend to have their systems overloaded, which contributes to an outbreak of waterborne diseases. Environmental degradation combining with tenuous sanitation arrangements worsens things even further—there's a distinct need for new, creative engineering solutions in urban design. Various strict studies, for instance, have revealed that when health programs and engineering solutions collaborate, populations tend to be better equipped to deal with climate-related challenges. Globally, effective interventions serve as reminders that the intermixing of public health concepts with intelligent engineering can reduce risks associated with failed sanitation systems as well as with climate changes. In most situations, interdisciplinary cooperation is essential in enhancing overall public health conditions where regions are hardest hit by sanitation failures (Irene, 2025). Certain specific cases truly highlight the broader, system-level issues at stake when sanitation fails. Consider one city settlement in a developing country where cholera is all too frequent, primarily due to the lack of appropriate wastewater treatment. The consequences do not remain at direct health issues, they overflow into economic insecurity and even impacts community bonds. Many families are burdened with significant medical bills, and lost income from disease only serves to complicate matters. And on top of that, that hovering stigma over poor sanitation can bring down social mobility and inclusion. These cases clearly demonstrate that the remedy isn't solely about enhancing wastewater infrastructure; it's also about coming to terms with the intricate link between sanitation, community health, and resilience. If stakeholders can guide efforts towards wiser, more efficient wastewater management innovations, they could be the ones who create healthier communities and reduce some of the public health loads that we experience in similar environments (Pham, 2025) (Figure 5.17).

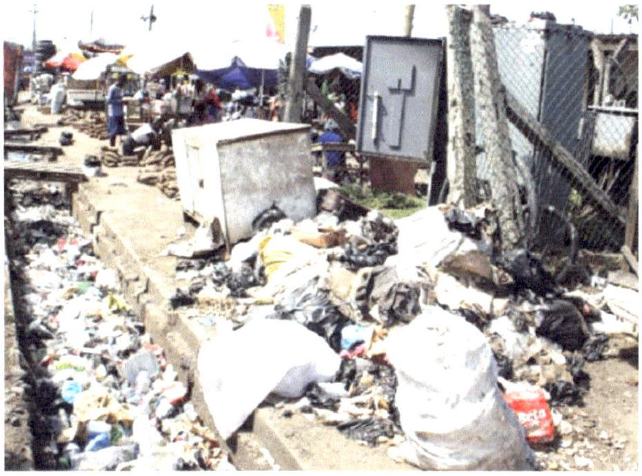

Figure 5.17. Poor sanitation in Ghana.

Source: Modern Ghana. (n.d.). *Sanitation Challenges in Ghana.*

5.6. Solutions and Innovations in Wastewater Management

Wastewater treatment today is receiving a new twist as grimy sewerage is addressed with a combination of newer technology and tried-and-tested concepts. Today, systems that combine physical-chemical treatment with biological remedies have resulted in significant improvements in the quality of water—yes, in several instances, the outcomes truly talk for themselves. Such practices not only render water more secure for recycling but also reduce pollution, particularly in urban locations. Looking more broadly, a comprehensive treatment of wastewater has the effect of reducing overall water consumption and lowering the cost of treatment, both without compromising on rigorous quality requirements (Amin et al., 2025). Ultimately, such hybrid approaches secure our water resources and, through the reduction in exposure to dangerous waste, even push public health in a positive direction. An important component of moving wastewater practice along has been, broadly put, the application of socio-technical systems theory. Consider the case of Dhaka City, for example, where hospital waste becomes a full-blown health scare if not contained. By getting into the day-to-day work and the behind-the-scenes activity at healthcare facilities, this methodology uncovers significant flaws in current treatment arrangements, such as shaky management, funding challenges, and a definite demand for improved employee training. There is a common thread: hospital administrators tend to prioritize patient care over wastewater problems, so targeted policy solutions are a necessity (Amin et al., 2025). More often than not, placing the emphasis on how humans and technology blend produces practices that are not just smarter but endure in the long term. Interagency collaboration between government, healthcare, and environmental agencies also keeps surfacing as a game-changer for wastewater regulations. When various groups negotiate policies together, it not only binds disparate interests but also ignites investment in innovative technologies. At times, decentralized systems provide neighborhood-scale solutions that truly appeal to local demands, improving sanitation in unconventional ways. And there's the increasing acknowledgment of green tech and nature-based solutions—consider constructed wetlands or bioreactors—a turn that tilts toward healing our environment as well as purifying water. As cities experience the pressure from urbanization and a constantly fluctuating climate, driving such innovations becomes increasingly necessary for both long-term water sustainability and public health (Kerpaci et al., 2024).

5.6.1. Sustainable Practices in Wastewater Management

Wastewater management is one of those complicated conundrums that intertwine environmental stewardship, public health, and economic development. Cities continue to grow, and as more individuals crowd in, our treatment plants are under increasing pressure, which requires new, and sometimes innovative—solutions to clean up and recycle what we can.

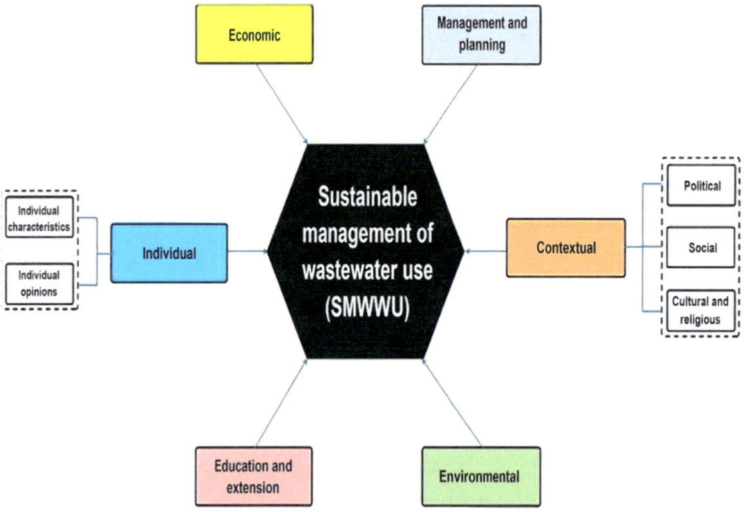

Figure 5.18. Sustainable management of wastewater use.

Source: Ghanbari M, Naeimi A and Bijani M (2024) Sustainable management of wastewater use in agriculture: a systematic analysis. Front. Sustain. Food Syst. 8:1409293. doi: 10.3389/fsufs.2024.1409293.

Treating wastewater is not merely a matter of reducing the amount of bad stuff going into nature; it's an opportunity to reclaim water, nutrients, and energy. Consider MBR or even constructed wetlands, they demonstrate that you can improve cleaning efficiency without disturbing the surrounding ecosystems. By adopting these less mainstream methods, communities may reduce water scarcity and environmental degradation, very much in harmony with broader sustainable objectives and health gains, as described in SDG 6 (Omohwovo, 2024). Throughout the world, particularly in developing regions, a shortage of adequate wastewater treatment continues to threaten both human health and wildlife habitats. Defective sanitation practices spill pollutants into water supplies, which only increases waterborne disease and affects vulnerable individuals the most. When wastewater is properly treated, before it's released back or reused, those threats decrease significantly. This becomes even more important in rural or under-served areas, where safe water and good sanitation aren't always a guarantee. Municipal authorities are able to make a tangible difference by installing strong treatment facilities and providing specific training to operators; sometimes, the answer is to join forces under public-private partnerships to help innovative processes take off (Tortajada, 2016). Ultimately, controlling wastewater is the key to safeguarding our health and that of the environment. Picture a plant that not only treats the water but also turns it into valuable products—generating biogas for power or even cranking out nutrient-packed fertilizers to sell to farmers. These types of systems literally close the loop back into the water-energy-food nexus in a tidy manner. When people come on board and take ownership in controlling their own water resources, it creates that all-important sense of ownership that leads to sustained success. Even modest education campaigns that highlight why good sanitation is important can encourage local advocacy for improved practices and policies. By adopting sustainable approaches, we are closer to cleaner water, healthier individuals, and a future that checks off global sustainability milestones along the way (Omohwovo, 2024; Tortajada, 2016) (Figure 5.18).

5.6.2. Role of Policy and Regulation in Improving Sanitation

Sanitation policies are at the center of maintaining healthy people and a sustainable environment. When governments negotiate well-defined, actionable regulations, waterborne diseases decrease—a signal that a nation's health is improving. It's fascinating how countries with sound frameworks have had fewer instances of disease and even lower death rates attributed to unsanitary environments. For most instances, prioritizing health allows governments to access funds for issues such as advanced wastewater treatment and then match them with on-the-ground monitoring to ensure everything functions as it needs to. All these actions contribute to increased public trust as well as initiating cross-border collaborations, pushing us toward a more concerted approach to global sanitation issues (Philip et al., 2020). Policy not only reduces short-term health threats, it also constructs our natural world in ways that aren't immediately apparent. Inadequate sanitation can decimate freshwater resources, causing habitats to collapse as wetlands vanish at a nearly frightening rate; this, naturally, leaves both wildlife and humans in a bind (Tickner et al., 2020). Stricter regulations on agricultural runoff, industrial spills, and loose sewage controls can reduce the impact of pollution and enhance the health of our water.

Making these policies work isn't a one-person show either—a combination of government, NGOs, and public input is necessary in order to truly make an impact, recalling that a healthy planet and healthy people are inextricably linked. Local participation is the final piece of the jigsaw. The most effective sanitation strategies tend to emerge when local knowledge combines with initiatives from public authorities, private companies, and community organizations, even if the strategy is a little bit scattergun at times. Getting everyone on board sets the stage for policies that hold up against distinctive local challenges and think outside the box. It is also beneficial when policies contain informational nuggets that share word on hygiene and intelligent sanitation technology—empowering individuals to take ownership of their health choices. Such inclusive, at times defective, collaborative work can yield bespoke local solutions that harmonize well with larger plans, ultimately creating a healthier society and a stronger environment (Philip et al., 2020).

5.6.3. Community-Driven Initiatives and Public Awareness Campaigns

Local ground-level movements are absolutely essential when it comes to resolving sanitation issues, particularly in bustling metropolises where outdated arrangements simply do not work. How they operate is by leveraging ordinary local expertise and mobilizing neighbors to take part—a step that quite significantly enhances public health. You may be witnessing a sanitation project run by the community, for example, designed by local organizations that focus on specific urban needs while opening the gates to safer facilities. In most cases, such initiatives motivate people to contribute to both constructing and maintaining sanitation systems, which creates a common sense of responsibility. In the majority of instances, this hands-on activity is central to changing behavior and even fortifying local governance—a perspective highlighted by some research (Bandyopadhyay et al., 2025). By molding solutions that align with the personality of each community, such projects highlight just how vital localized remedies are for long-term outcomes. Public awareness campaigns also add a critical boost to these community-based efforts, often shining a light on the finer points of sanitation issues and their broader health impacts. They tend to mix it up by using a variety of media channels to spread the word about the dangers of poor sanitation and the benefits of cleaner facilities. Breaking it down in plain terms, these campaigns illustrate the reasons why proper hygiene is important and how having good facilities can transform attitudes and impact everyday behavior. They even incorporate links between poor sanitation and larger issues such as environmental degradation and unstable economies—an angle that serves to rally the locals and institutions alike. Activities such as the 2008 World Water Week, for example, pooled different stakeholders with an emphasis that addressing sanitation requires joined-up action (WSP, 2011). Generally, the campaigns perform well in establishing a down-to-earth message that resonates with various audiences. In general terms, the success of such community-initiated projects and public initiatives largely depends on bridging gaps between different groups—whether government agencies, NGOs, or local residents. When resources, ideas, and true community feeling combine, the reach of sanitation initiatives can spread out. Consider, for instance, the concept of mobilizing informal sanitation workers—a strategy that some praise—of engaging those that are typically on the periphery and improving the way services are made available. Through collaboration, these efforts not only guide us toward more sustainable gains but also promote policies that ensure sanitation remains a public priority. The combination of grassroots mobilization and policy gentle pressure reminds us that equitable access to sanitation is essential to healthier communities and a cleaner world. In most instances, such collaboration opens the door to innovative, scalable solutions to both near-term and more profound, systemic sanitation issues (Bandyopadhyay et al., 2025).

SUMMARY

Sanitation and wastewater treatment are closely linked to maintaining healthy communities and our environment in harmony. Effective waste systems aren't merely a matter of infrastructure – they prevent the spread of disease, and research indicates that cleaner conditions reduce waterborne disease, which in turn improves community health. Cities are expanding rapidly everywhere, so it's increasingly clear that we need new, smarter approaches to treating wastewater. Combining old methods with new technology could be the key to results that benefit both public health and the environment. A number of long-term studies suggest that connecting infrastructure repairs, community mobilization, and even elementary education can pave the way for sustained sanitation success. Poor sanitation demands quick, firm action. When locations fall short on decent waste management, water resources are hit and public health declines – particularly for the most susceptible individuals. Cutting back on investment in sanitation and decent wastewater treatment can cause not only environmental deterioration but also precipitate economic downturns. Glancing at history, it would appear evident that a combination of methods, ranging from developing local competencies to engaging people in their own neighborhoods, can yield extraordinary changes on all fronts, allowing a healthier world. Glancing toward the future, incorporating emerging technologies and innovative methods into wastewater control will have an impact. There's a huge potential for these breakthroughs to change how communities deal with water—in many cases, strategies like the global Water and Development Strategy have already pointed the way. In spots where strong partnerships and even some market incentives are in play, we're beginning to see the early signs of a sustainable shift in sanitation. Generally speaking, putting governments, NGOs, and local groups together is key. With cooperative efforts and a little determination, we can alleviate the issues of inadequate sanitation and maintain public health in the limelight, leading the way to a more resilient future for everyone.

Sanitation and wastewater treatment is not merely an infrastructure issue, it has a strong relationship to how healthy our populations remain. Research continues to highlight that when our sanitation is inadequate, it tends to go hand-in-hand with an increase in health issues such as outbreaks of infectious diseases. By and large, studies, such as statistics from the World Health Organization, indicate that poor sanitation contributes to a remarkably high rate of deaths annually, particularly in the less developed world. It is as much a matter of moral imperative as health and safety to upgrade the basic waste handling systems. Addressing these issues requires new thinking, education at the community level, and a little bit of creative thinking—all of which gradually but surely push individuals toward improved habits. Wastewater treatment, for its part, occupies the center of maintaining our sanitation. You see, numerous different methods, ranging from MBR to biological nutrient removal-based approaches, are implemented in diverse environments. These technologies attempt to cut back on environmental damage while also reclaiming valuable resources. In addition, these are supplemented by an increasing buzz about smart city concepts; in most instances, IoT equipment now assists in monitoring and adjusting the treatment processes in real-time. This combination of high-tech equipment with traditional wastewater methods allows cities to sometimes make spontaneous choices to increase efficiency as well as sustainability (Bellini et al., 2022). On a separate note, the consequences of poor sanitation extend far beyond short-term health concerns. Polluted water sources can cause long-term harm, affecting not just the drinking water but also the plants and animals that rely on it. When sanitation is not up to par, communities come together—local governments, NGOs, and residents all get into the mix to clean up the mess. Solutions such as decentralized wastewater systems are showing to be bright spots in contexts where one-size-fits-all don't cut so well. Literature largely appears to concur that when sanitation systems and policies communicate more effectively together across sectors, the benefit of improved public health and environmental attention is not an easy option to overlook (Huovila et al., 2022).

KEY TERMS FROM THIS CHAPTER

Advanced oxidation processes (AOPs)
Biological processes
Construction materials
Ecosystem
Environmental protection
Green infrastructure
Human excreta
Local participation
Membrane bioreactors (MBR)
Modern wastewater treatment
Nature-Based Solutions (NBS)
Oxidation processes
Public awareness campaigns
Anaerobic digestion (AD)
Climate change
Ecological footprint
Environmental degradation
General health
Health crises
Hygiene education
Mainstream methods
Micro-pollutants
Natural resources
Organic materials
Poverty cycle
Public health initiatives

CLOSER LOOK

WASTEWATER TREATMENT PLANT PROCESS: SAFEGUARDING OUR ENVIRONMENT

Wastewater treatment plants are essential for ensuring environmental sustainability and safeguarding public health. With the world's population increasing and the activities of industries on the rise, wastewater generation grows exponentially, and effective treatment processes become more important than ever before. In this article, we will discuss the process of a wastewater treatment plant, outlining the steps used to convert dirty water into clean, safe effluent.

1. **Preliminary Treatment: The First Line of Defense:** Wastewater treatment commences with initial treatment, which is the first line of defense for large trash and contaminants. Incoming wastewater is screened for solid objects like plastic, twigs, and leaves to avoid damaging equipment in the treatment plant. Grit chambers are also used to remove heavy inorganic materials like sand and gravel to enable smoother flow through the system.
2. **Primary Treatment: Settling for Clarity:** After initial treatment, the partially treated wastewater is pumped into primary settling tanks, where gravity works its magic. The heavier solids and organic material sink to the bottom and form a sludge layer, while the lighter material floats to the top and forms a scum layer. Mechanical scrapers carefully remove the sludge and scum, leaving the water ready for the next step.
3. **Secondary Treatment: Unleashing the Power of Microorganisms:** The centerpiece of the wastewater treatment process is the secondary stage, where biological means are used to further clean the water. The most prevalent process is the activated sludge process, where the wastewater is mixed with a microorganism culture named activated sludge. The microorganisms dine on organic material in the water and digest it into harmless byproducts such as carbon dioxide and water.
4. **Aeration: Breathing Life Into Treatment:** In order to keep a healthy population of aerobic bacteria that can degrade organic pollutants effectively, the wastewater is aerated. Oxygen is supplied into the treatment tanks, giving vital oxygen to the microbes, enhancing their metabolic process, and making for an ideal performance of the treatment.
5. **Secondary Clarification: Separating the Wheat from the Chaff:** Following the biological treatment, wastewater goes into secondary clarifiers where activated sludge drops to the bottom and forms a sludge blanket. The water that has been clarified goes up to the top and is drained for subsequent treatment. A part of the settled sludge is returned back to the aeration tanks to maintain the microbial community, while excess sludge is harvested for subsequent treatment.
6. **Tertiary Treatment: The Finishing Touch:** If a more advanced level of water quality is needed, tertiary treatment can be used. Tertiary treatment involves further filtration, chemical treatment, and more advanced techniques such as UV disinfection or chlorination to filter out the remaining contaminants and pathogens. This process guarantees that the effluent is within the strict environmental requirements and safe for discharge or reuse.

References

1. Abascal, E., Gómez-Coma, L., Ortíz, I., & Ortiz, A. (2021). Global diagnosis of nitrate pollution in groundwater and review of removal technologies. *Science of the Total Environment, 810*, 152233. https://doi.org/10.1016/j.scitotenv.2021.152233.
2. Ampe, K., Asveld, L., Block, T., & Osseweijer, P. (2019). A transition in the Dutch wastewater system? The struggle between discourses and with lock-ins. https://core.ac.uk/download/237011598.pdf (accessed on 14 May 2025).
3. Andersson, K., Otoo, M., & Nolasco, M. (2018). Innovative sanitation approaches could address multiple development challenges. *Water Science and Technology, 77*(3, 4), 855–858. https://www.semanticscholar.org/paper/2731ed063de61cfc43876a953492febffb3c67e3 (accessed on 14 May 2025).
4. Pay Drechsel, Christopher A. Scott, Liqa Raschid-Sally, Mark Redwood, and Akiça Bahri (2010)
5. *Wastewater Irrigation and Health: Assessing and Mitigating Risk in Low-Income Countries.* Publisher(s) Earthscan, IWMI, IDRC
6. ISBN 9781844077953. https://core.ac.uk/download/pdf/6405282.pdf (accessed on 14 May 2025).
7. Bandyopadhyay, K. K., Bharti, M., Das Gupta, S., & Dasgupta, R., et al. (2025). *Social Innovations in Urban Sanitation in India.* https://core.ac.uk/download/637926675.pdf (accessed on 14 May 2025).
8. Batra, M., & Erbas, B. (2025). Extreme Weather, Vulnerable Populations, and Mental Health: The Timely Role of AI Interventions. *International journal of environmental research and public health, 22*(4), 602. https://doi.org/10.3390/ijerph22040602(accessed on 14 May 2025).
9. Bellini, P., Nesi, P., & Pantaleo, G. (2022). IoT-enabled smart cities: A review of concepts, frameworks and key technologies. *Applied Sciences, 12*(3), Article 1607. https://doi.org/10.3390/app12031607.
10. Bogler, A., Packman, A. I., Furman, A., Gross, A., Kushmaro, A., Ronen, A., Dagot, C., et al. (2020). Rethinking wastewater risks and monitoring in light of the COVID-19 pandemic. *Nature Sustainability, 3*, 981–990. https://doi.org/10.1038/s41893-020-00605-2.
11. Choudhary, M., & Ray, S. (2024). Sustainable wastewater management: Exploring nature-based treatment. *International Journal on Environmental Sciences.* IJES 15(2): 63-69 (2024) • ISSN: 0976-4534. https://www.semanticscholar.org/paper/1a4ea406678e33dca0eaf2608803e61a91c8d958 (accessed on 14 May 2025).
12. Davi Gasparini Fernandes Cunha, Maria Do Carmo Calijuri, Doron Grull, Pedro Caetano Sanches Mancuso, Daniel R. Thevenot. In situ Remediation Technologies Associated with Sanitation Improvement: An Opportunity for Water Quality Recovering in Developing Countries. Voudouris, Kostas. Ecological Water Quality - Water Treatment and Reuse, InTech - Open Access Publisher, pp.255 - 272, 2012, 978-953-51-0508-4. ffhal-00709477(accessed on 14 May 2025).
13. WWAP (World Water Assessment Programme). 2012. The United Nations World Water Development Report 4: Managing Water under Uncertainty and Risk. Paris, UNESCO. The United Nations World Water Development Report 4: Managing Water under Uncertainty

and Risk (Vol. 1),Knowledge Base (Vol. 2) and Facing the Challenges (Vol. 3). (accessed on 14 May 2025).

14. Gamage, A., Gangahagedara, R., Gamage, J., Jayasinghe, N., Kodikara, N., Suraweera, P., & Merah, O. (2023). Role of organic farming for achieving sustainability in agriculture. *Farming System, 1*, 100005. https://doi.org/10.1016/j.farsys.2023.100005.

15. Gumbo, B., Indij, D., Coates, D., Lentini, E., Sewilam, H., Liebe, J., Bernaudat, L., et al. (2012). *Water in the Green Economy: Capacity Development Aspects.* https://core.ac.uk/download/71360162.pdf (accessed on 14 May 2025).

16. Huovila, A., Siikavirta, H., Antuña Rozado, C., Rökman, J., Tuominen, P., Paiho, S., Hedman, Å., et al. (2022). Carbon-neutral cities: Critical review of theory and practice. *Journal of Cleaner Production, 341*, 130912. https://doi.org/10.1016/j.jclepro.2022.130912.

17. Izah, S. C., & Ogwu, M. (2025). Modeling solutions for microbial water contamination in the global south for public health protection. *Frontiers in Microbiology, 16.* https://www.semanticscholar.org/paper/ad7f76dcd051943f4aab4a532bc0e383b0b5b2d2 (accessed on 14 May 2025).

18. Karić, N., Maia, A. S., Teodorović, A., Atanasova, N., Langergraber, G., Crini, G., Ribeiro, A. R., et al. (2021). Bio-waste valorisation: Agricultural wastes as biosorbents for removal of (in) organic pollutants in wastewater treatment. *Chemical Engineering Journal Advances, 9*, Article 100239. https://doi.org/10.1016/j.ceja.2021.100239.

19. Kerpaci, A., & Lako, A. (2024). Integrated water supply and sanitation management: Environmental impact assessment and wastewater and stormwater treatment. *Grassroots Journal of Natural Resources.* https://www.semanticscholar.org/paper/7d75075681e19555b8442882a9e5fa16d90b35a7 (accessed on 14 May 2025).

20. Landrigan, P. J., Stegeman, J. J., Fleming, L. E., Allemand, D., Anderson, D. M., Backer, L. C., Brücker-Davis, F., et al. (2020). Human health and ocean pollution. *Annals of Global Health, 86*(1), Article 151. https://doi.org/10.5334/aogh.2831.

21. Md. Abdus Salam, Md. Yusuf Al-Amin, Moushumi Tabassoom Salam, Jogendra Singh Pawar, Naseem Akhter, Ali A. Rabaan, & Mohammed A. A. Alqumber. (2023). Antimicrobial resistance: A growing serious threat for global public health. *Healthcare, 11*(13), Article 1946. https://doi.org/10.3390/healthcare11131946.

22. Merrey, D., & Sally, H. (2020). *Outcome Evaluation of Research for Development Work Conducted in Ghana and Sri Lanka Under the Resource, Recovery and Reuse (RRR) Subprogram of the CGIAR Research Program on Water, Land and Ecosystems (WLE).* https://core.ac.uk/download/288633572.pdf (accessed on 14 May 2025).

23. Mondéjar, M. E., Avtar, R., Baños Díaz, H. L., Dubey, R. K., Esteban, J., Gómez-Morales, A., Hallam, B., et al. (2021). Digitalization to achieve sustainable development goals: Steps towards a smart green planet. *Science of the Total Environment, 794*, 148539. https://doi.org/10.1016/j.scitotenv.2021.148539.

24. Mosello, B., Cummings, C., Doczi, J., & Matoso, M. (2016). *Sanitation Under Stress: How Can Urban Services Respond to Acute Migration?* https://core.ac.uk/download/75760980.pdf (accessed on 14 May 2025).

25. Msuya, A. S., Bojang, O. A., Nyika, S. H., & Amara, E. (2025). Wastewater Management Challenges

and Solutions in Tanzania: A Case Study of Dar es Salaam City. *European Journal of Ecology, Biology and Agriculture, 2*(2), 68-82. https://doi.org/10.59324/ejeba.2025.2(2).07(accessed on 14 May 2025).

26. Mutika, R., Tun, S. Z., & Tembo, F. M. (2024). Review of Mining and Sanitation Waste Water Management and Their Contribution to Water Contamination in Zambia. *European Journal of Theoretical and Applied Sciences, 2*(3), 745-759. https://doi.org/10.59324/ejtas.2024.2(3).58 (accessed on 14 May 2025).

27. Original review by Kate Tulenko (WB/WSP), with further expansion and revision by Renuka Bery and Julia Rosenbaum (USAID/HIP). Prepared by the USAID /Hygiene Improvement Project with the Water and Sanitation Program/World Bank. October 2007 . *Analysis of Research on the Effects of Improved Water, Sanitation, and Hygiene on the Health of People Living with HIV and AIDS and Programmatic Implications.* https://core.ac.uk/download/71345778.pdf (accessed on 14 May 2025).

28. WSP (2011). Political economy of sanitation: How can we increase investment and improve service for the poor? Operational experiences from case studies in Brazil, India, Indonesia and Senegal World Bank, Water and Sanitation Program (WSP), USA(accessed on 14 May 2025).

29. Nagawa Jackline Irene (2025). Impact of Climate Change on Public Health: Engineering Responses. RESEARCH INVENTION JOURNAL OF PUBLIC HEALTH AND PHARMACY 4(1): 24-28. https://doi.org/10.59298/RIJPP/2025/412428(accessed on 14 May 2025).

30. Nuhu, A., Foster, T., Tabassum Shimki, N., Hasan, M. R., Sarkar, S., Adnan, S. D., Rahman, A., et al. (2025). Inadequate wastewater management in Dhaka's major hospitals: A socio-technical systems analysis of leadership, policy, and technological challenges. *PLOS Water.* https://www.semanticscholar.org/paper/ed2281183db3d4eda055aeb5f67bc13571983c5b (accessed on 14 May 2025).

31. Omohwovo, E. (2024). Wastewater management in Africa: Challenges and recommendations. *Environmental Health Insights, 18.* https://www.semanticscholar.org/paper/8ae263be32fe44dd82708eccf607cc13c5eb7939 (accessed on 14 May 2025).

32. Pham, L. (2025). Balancing financial risks with social and economic benefits: Two case studies of private sector water, sanitation, and hygiene suppliers in rural Vietnam. *Journal of Risk and Financial Management.* https://www.semanticscholar.org/paper/50639d3dc949b130d35b1c11ec98ae82a9f76d03 (accessed on 14 May 2025).

33. Silva Rodríguez de San Miguel, J. A. (2023). Wastewater treatment and reuse for sustainable water resources management: A systematic literature review. *Sustainability, 15*, 10940. https://doi.org/10.3390/su151410940.

34. Tickner, D., Opperman, J. J., Abell, R., Acreman, M., Arthington, A. H., Bunn, S. E., Cooke, S. J., et al. (2020). Bending the curve of global freshwater biodiversity loss: An emergency recovery plan. *BioScience, 70*, 330–342. https://doi.org/10.1093/biosci/biaa002.

35. Tortajada, C. (2016). Editorial. *International Journal of Water Resources Development, 32*, 817–818. https://www.semanticscholar.org/paper/a36eb6ee87cf33ca5cf8328cd4cc57739f4a85d0 (accessed on 14 May 2025).

36. Turner, S. S. (2018). *To Treat or Not to Treat: The Evolution of Wastewater Treatment Management Approaches.* Colorado State University. https://hdl.handle.net/10217/193085

37. https://core.ac.uk/download/354462454.pdf (accessed on 14 May 2025).

38. Vosa , O., Salibi, G., & Tzenios, N. (2025). Water pollution and its impact on human health in Nigeria. *Special Journal of the Medical Academy and Other Life Sciences.*, *3*(2). https://doi.org/10.58676/sjmas.v3i2.110(accessed on 14 May 2025).

39. Wang, M., Janssen, A. B. G., Bazin, J., Strokal, M., Ma, L., & Kroeze, C. (2022). Accounting for interactions between Sustainable Development Goals is essential for water pollution control in China. *Nature Communications, 13*, Article 685. https://doi.org/10.1038/s41467-022-28351-3.

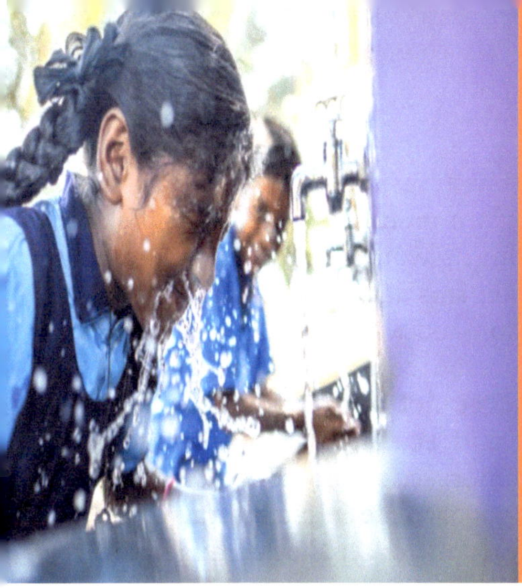

Chapter 6

SAFE DRINKING WATER ACCESS AND DISTRIBUTION SYSTEMS

Contents

Introduction

Safe water is an innate human right and an integral part of public health, yet millions worldwide still lack an adequate water supply system. Inequalities in access to water are mainly due to geographic, socioeconomic, and infrastructural inequalities that exist in the urban and rural environments. Water supply systems based on community provide promising alternatives that usually have their roots in local government and participatory methods. These systems not only increase the efficiency of water supply but also enable communities to use their resources more sustainably. As highlighted during the UN COP26 conference, local initiatives could be complemented by technological interventions in the guise of monitoring mechanisms that are community-responsive and responsible, supporting the case for the importance of local participation in ensuring equitable access to water (Birnbaum et al., 2021). However, obstacles to universal access to clean water are multifarious and complex. Foremost among these obstacles are, in the case of such populations as women, children, and the poor. They usually face added hurdles with regard to existing social norms and poor infrastructure. According to the WHO/UNICEF JMP, ongoing inequalities in sanitation and water access compound health burdens, with vulnerable groups taking the brunt of unsafe resource management (Macura et al., 2021). Reduction of these inequalities is one of what is required not just to enhance public health benefits but also for the realization of gender equality and economic empowerment. Attenuating these disparities is therefore central to determining the intersectionality of access issues in planning effective water supply interventions. The role of local governance in facilitating equal access to potable water cannot be overstressed. There is a well-developed governance arrangement that guarantees the needs of the community come first in making decisions, as well as entrenches accountability and transparency. Participation of the community in managing and planning the water supply system is also empowering and gives citizens a feeling of responsibility and ownership. By incorporating the voice of the community into the system of governance, local governments can then respond to the specific needs of individual communities. Overall, the connection between governance and community participation is at the heart of crafting inclusive models of drinking water that are responsive to specific social and infrastructural contexts of communities. These issues will keep shedding light on the future of improving water supply networks across the world.

Definition of Safe Drinking Water

Not only is safe and accessible drinking water of vital importance but also involves guaranteeing that water meets a specific health and safety level. Safe drinking water is water that does not contain harmful contaminants, pathogens, and pollutants to ensure it is safe for human consumption without posing adverse health impacts. Issues such as turbidity, chemical content, and the presence of microbes must be carefully regulated in a manner that guarantees assurance. Moreover, drinking water also has to abide by regulatory standards set by regulatory bodies like the World Health Organization that set parameters for the acceptable limits of most contaminants. The regulations point towards a critical acknowledgment that water may not always be safe for consumption. Thus, quality control measures must be integrated within community-based water supply systems for the protection of public health and safety. The problem of demarcation and providing safe drinking water is a miniaturization of larger system problems in water distribution systems. The majority of the world does not have the facilities to ensure the quality of the water, such that there is a large segment of the population without access to clean drinking water. Research quotes USAID in pointing out the need for coordination across sectors to construct sustainable water management systems. This coordination is what serves to play the central role in identifying and correcting water quality and accessibility differences. In addition, less-developed areas are also afflicted with pollution by runoffs or ruptured pipes, which requires stringent monitoring and upkeep procedures in water networks. This is why local efforts and grassroots government are central to these solutions and equitable access to clean drinking water. Local government is a part of the determination, allocation, and upkeep of safe drinking water programs. Including the local population assures policies can be shaped to most effectively meet the specific needs and concerns of specific regions. When water supply decisions are taken through people's participation, it generates a sense of ownership and enhances the accountability of local government institutions. Sustainable capacity development, as suggested by Gumbo et al. (2012), is necessary for effective water resource management, both sanitation and supply. Community-based responses can contribute significantly towards the perception, utilization, and sustainability of safe drinking water systems and thus create culture of hygiene and health beyond timely access. This community-oriented approach places safe drinking water at the center of community health and environmental conservation, driving progress towards higher public health goals.

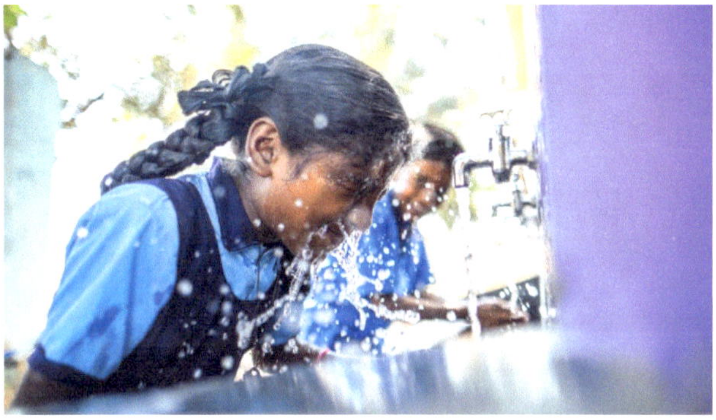

Source: WaterAid. (n.d.). *Safe Sanitation.*

Importance of Access to Clean Water

Access to clean water is the linchpin of human health and well-being, with an impact on communities across a variety of fronts. Clean water is a key factor in preventing waterborne disease, which falls hardest on vulnerable populations, especially children and the elderly. Research indicates that people living in areas that have access to proper water supply systems have fewer cases of diseases like cholera and dysentery. The costs of poor access are much broader than health, reaching into education and potential to a considerable extent. For instance, children will miss school due to disease or preoccupation with collecting water far away, robbing education and potential. Therefore, the place of proper water delivery systems should be at the top of the agenda to address resilience and development in communities, and access to clean water as a solution to sustainable growth. The equity of access to pure water is deeply enmeshed with other economic and social determinants, and will most likely perpetuate the inequalities already present. Disadvantaged groups are denied structurally access to clean drinking water, which leads to enormous health and opportunity gaps. Closing these gaps involves not only infrastructure upgrading but also targeted outreach to the communities to get these groups' voices into the decision-making process. Institutional building of local governments through participatory mechanisms can build transparency and accountability, which can make water supply facilities more responsive to all citizens' needs. Through various fields of evidence, including gender equality-based domains, equitable access to resources like clean water is essential in sustaining the ecosystem and community (Galizzi & Herklotz, 2012). Moreover, the intricacies of water distribution underscore the value of upholding the essence of community participation in the policy-making process. A collective effort between communities and local governments can optimize the efficiency of managing water, rendering infrastructures culture-friendly and sustainable. As seen in United Nations consultations, contributions from various individuals from young people to elderly people may assist in a more inclusive manner of resource management and distribution. Closing the policy-practice gap allows communities to advocate more effectively for their water rights and tackle neighborhood issues. Generally, active community engagement not only promotes direct access to safe water but also cultivates ownership and responsibility, ultimately leading to better health outcomes and social equality among communities (Figure 6.1).

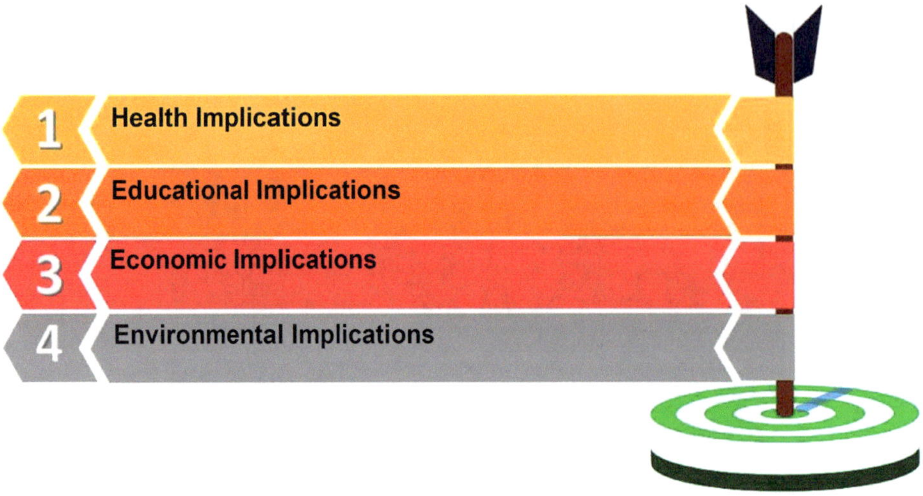

Figure 6.1. The importance of access to clean water.

Source: FasterCapital. (n.d.). *Water Provision: Quenching Thirst – The Essentiality of Water Provision – The Importance of Access to Clean Water.*

6.1. Community-Based Water Supply Systems

The meeting of water supply with technology is imperative, especially with regard to community-based initiatives. These tend to make use of local expertise, as well as resources, and these too are further enhanced via digital means from a perspective for increased efficiency as well as sustainability. For example, with machine learning algorithms in place, the management of water resources can be done more wisely, with coping with demand projection and supply maximization being addressed. Such a system is not just a fad; it is required so that the most vulnerable are provided with equal access to clean water. The cry for inclusive innovation is very strong, especially when societies are confronted with distinctive challenges defined by their particular socio-economic contexts (Rolnick et al., 2022). By making the convergence of technology and people a top priority, such water supply systems can have robust frameworks that promote resilience and flexibility in the face of ongoing environmental transformation. Community-based water supply systems are promising to provide equitable access but are equally challenged with infrastructure development and management. These programs are likely to rely on government mechanisms at the local level to implement and sustain programs, but discrepancies in levels of political will and resources may cross effective management. Successful interventions do not just require robust technical capabilities but also needs and local circumstances knowledge. Engaging stakeholders at the local level through participatory planning has a high likelihood of engaging more local solutions that solve individualized requirements and create ownership by residents. Such projects' sustainability, nevertheless, depends mainly on outside assistance and financing, which might be unreliable. The intricacies involved in infrastructure problems require a multi-faceted solution, emphasizing cooperation among residents and town councils in establishing robust water distribution networks

(Yogesh et al., 2021). Water supply system planning and management largely depend on people's participation because it has an important role in making them effective and sustainable. With the active participation of the people, these systems are also able to harness tacit information about adjacent sources of water and usage patterns. People are not only consumers but also guardians of their water supply, maintaining and adjusting the systems over time. Participatory engagement enhances accountability and transparency, aspects that are important for the building of stakeholder trust. Further, community empowerment to take control of water can help alleviate gender discrimination since women usually play leading roles in water management and harvesting in the majority of areas. Lastly, utilizing the full potential of community-based governance can attain an equal and resilient system of water distribution that attains timely availability and sustainability requirements (Yogesh et al., 2021; Rolnick et al., 2022) (Figure 6.2).

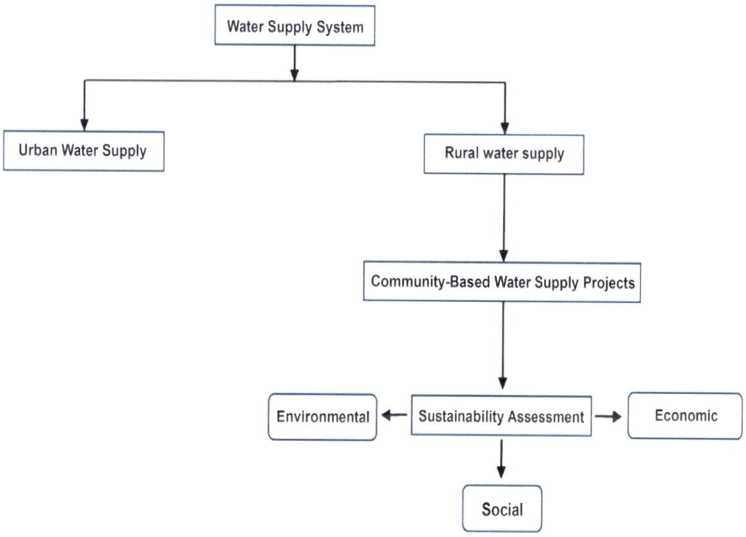

Figure 6.2. Water supply system.

Source: Elsevier. (2022). *Water Supply System.*

6.1.1. Characteristics of Community-Based Systems

The success of community-based systems in water supply depends on their inherent adaptability and sensitivity to local circumstances. In contrast to the centralized strategy with its predisposition to one-size-fits-all, community-based systems prioritize local engagement, enabling communities to design their water supply programs according to individual environmental, cultural, and socioeconomic realities. Local adjustment to these circumstances promotes community ownership and stewardship, increasing the potential for long-term involvement in the systems. From experiences recorded in different case studies, successful capacity development in the context of water resources management demonstrates that institutional and individual capacities can be developed through local-based strategies, resulting in more efficient results in water supply and sanitation (Gumbo et al., 2012). The focus on the local surroundings not only leads to enhanced water management practices but also promotes cohesion within communities as citizens work together to fulfill their water requirements.

Additionally, the community's engagement is of utmost importance in the preservation of fairness in accessing clean water. With community members involved in decision-making, they stand a chance to be more assertive about the fairness and equality of water allocation policies. Programs that involve community participation assist in determining barriers experienced by marginalized communities so that interventions will not favor a specific group over the other. Research based on sustainable municipal water practice highlights that the involvement of people fosters enhanced transparency and accountability and ultimately reinforces building trust between citizens and governments at the local level (DeFries et al., 2024). Community involvement has the potential to reduce historic inequalities in the availability of water and contribute towards the generation of greater accountability in the management of water resources, which is crucial when devising a resilient and equitable water distribution system. The sustainability of community-based water systems is also supported by their capacity to effectively utilize local knowledge and resources. Implementation of indigenous practices and use of local materials not only minimizes environmental effects but also instills a feeling of pride within the members of the community. Merging traditional knowledge with contemporary water management techniques can lead to innovative solutions particular to regional issues. Engagement of the community as co-owners of decision-making is what collaborative governance under equal involvement in decision-making can achieve. In countries where such participatory systems have been established, studies show substantial improvements in water quality and delivery service outcomes, demonstrating the potential of community-owned systems to meet essential infrastructure requirements while promoting responsible stewardship of shared water resources (Gumbo et al., 2012). Essentially, the feature of community-based systems not only improves access to water but also promotes fair and sustainable systems that serve whole communities (Figure 6.3).

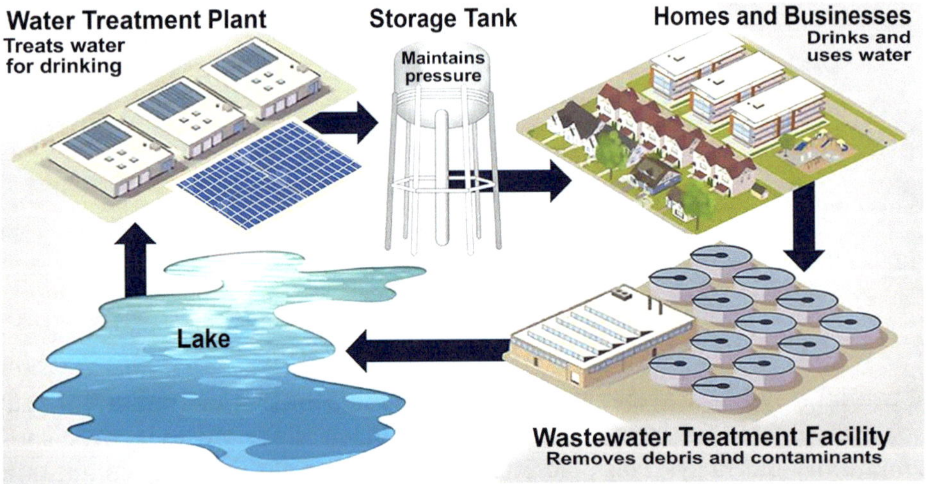

Figure 6.3. Element of the community drinking water system.

Source: FEMA. (n.d.). *Element of the Community Drinking Water System.*

6.1.2. Benefits of Local Management

Organized local management of water supply systems has been a top strategy for enhancing access to safe drinking water. Citizens to control and manage their own water resources not only provide for their own needs and interests but also create a sense of belongingness and responsibility among citizens. Such a community-focused approach can lead to enhanced maintenance and sustainability of water systems because community members have a better understanding of the problems and resources. Decentralizing decisions to involve local stakeholders enhances institutions' accountability and supports transparency in resource management and service delivery. Enhanced community involvement is needed, especially to end the inequities in access to water in different socio-economic contexts, as noted by the inequities in WASH services.

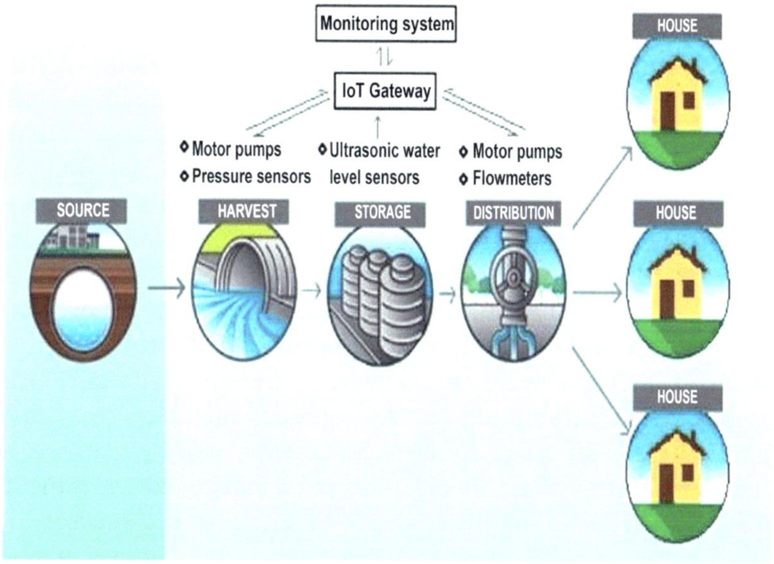

Figure 6.4. General outline of water management and distribution system.

Source: ResearchGate. (n.d.). *General Outline of Water Management and Distribution System.*

The local governance also offers an effective venue in which to utilize local knowledge and practices, hence providing more appropriate and culturally adapted water supply solutions. This is especially important in rural areas where local traditions and indigenous practices can inform improved solutions for water delivery and conservation. When villagers and community leaders work together, it facilitates innovation, because they may find unique solutions to overcoming infrastructure barriers that do not reach or are overlooked by larger, bureaucratic systems. Involvement of local communities in water management also raises their capacity to campaign for needed change at regional or national levels, ultimately leading to increased access to clean water by marginalized groups, including women and the elderly, who are typically disproportionately affected by inadequate water services (Yogesh et al., 2021). Economic implications of local management arrangements also point towards their advantages. Through the use of the local resources and human personnel, the communities are able to reduce water supply and distribution system costs. Cost-effectiveness is typically accommodated through the reduction of transport costs as water schemes are able to use community facilities already in existence, thereby realizing a more sustainable route to getting access to water. Also, when water management is under the control of a community, it is in its best position to develop financing requests with priorities based on its own requirements that will be able to obtain external financing and grants toward the expansion and upgradation of facilities. Local initiative not only adds to the economic and viability prospects of drinking water sources but also to the overall social and economic development goals of the community. Therefore, local administration stands as a vital variable in the pursuit of equitable access to safe drinking water (Yogesh et al., 2021) (Figure 6.4).

6.1.3. Case Studies of Successful Community Initiatives

The sophistication of locally-driven work usually reveals paths to sustainable solutions to long-standing water availability issues. A most dramatic example is that of farmers in sub-Saharan West Africa, who use traditional knowledge combined with scientific knowledge to devise effective water allocation practices. By syntheses of conventional and new farming research approaches, such communities have gained resilience against climatic change without undermining food security. At last, the programs that hold local knowledge to be important, as in Mali, Burkina Faso, and Benin, illustrate how involvement by the community empowers the people and promotes a community resource management policy. Thus, these case studies illustrate the value of community governance in addressing critical infrastructure questions on access to clean water, justifying the value of local methods in global efforts to provide drinking water and make it safe for all. Further, successful community programs are usually based on equitable access to resources, particularly where gender equality is incorporated into water management planning. The data provided by Galizzi & Herklotz. (2012) focuses on the interaction between gender inclusion in local administration and sustainable development across different areas, such as water supply networks. Women also carry the majority of the responsibilities of water collecting and safeguarding in most communities, and hence their inclusion in decision-making processes is essential to the success of water distribution schemes. By attaining gender equality, these programs not only bring women's status up but also support the general capacity of the community to survive. Just distribution of resources thus leads to a more just environment where all members of the community can define their needs and be part of the governing frameworks that oversee water accessibility so that long-term success and sustainability are attained. In addition, the commissioning of new water supply systems validates the value of cooperation between members of the community and the local authority. Grassroots interventions often use local material and resources for rollout, thus fostering sustainability and participant ownership. For example, efforts that mobilize community members to build and upkeep water supply systems demonstrate how cooperative efforts can contribute to effective solutions with infrastructure and accessibility benefits. These cooperative measures not only provide direct gains in the matter of water accessibility but also enhance social bonding at the grassroots level. The points by Nicolay & Fliessbach (2012) regarding agricultural research and localized cooperation also upholds the point that locally-led initiatives can contribute a significant percentage of access to clean drinking water, substantiating the role of community involvement in meeting long-term challenges concerning water supply system.

6.2. Challenges in Equitable Access to Clean Water

Multidimensional challenges in getting access to clean water proportionately mirror the complexities engaged in addressing global water crises. The poor, more so rural residents or low-income families, are likely to face insurmountable barriers that dampen access to clean drinking water.

Disparities arise from an array of causes such as socioeconomic status, geographical location, and lack of infrastructural facilities. For example, rural residents might not have effective distribution channels to provide clean water, hence they turn to contaminated sources. The ultimate outcome is that such disparities are observed expressed in health disparities that further increase public health challenges, and create a cycle of inequality and poverty.

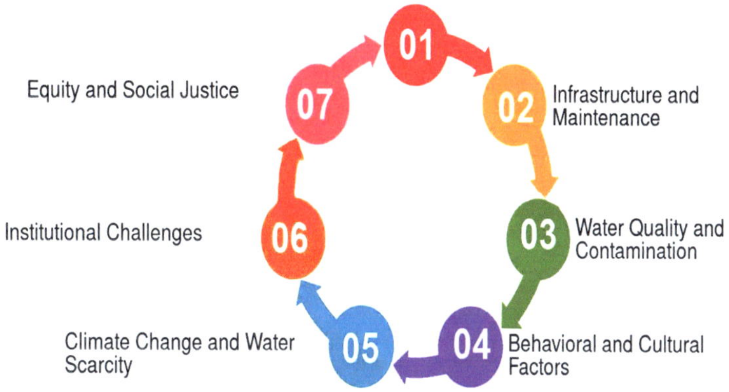

Figure 6.5. Challenges in access to clean water.

Source: FasterCapital. (n.d.). *Challenges in Access to Clean Water.*

The way out of these problems is an integrated approach to comprehending how infrastructure, governance, and socio-economic determinants are interconnected with respect to augmenting equitable access to needed resources such as safe drinking water. Institutional factors also have an important role in allocating who gets access to clean drinking water and to what extent. In most circumstances, institutions at the local level do not have either political will and sufficient resources required to invest in an enduring water supply system that supports existing inequalities. Mismanagement, corruption, and insufficient funding can also divert resources' attention from the most exposed and needy marginalized groups to other options. Additionally, traditional decision-making processes tend to exclude community members, particularly women and socially excluded groups, and in so doing, uphold inequalities in access to water. This exclusion serves to compound limitations to responses that can be effectively able to meet the specific needs of these groups. A transformation in patterns of governance with participatory involvement from the community is, therefore, necessary not merely to improve water access but also to enable citizens' sense of ownership, as expressed through enhanced maintenance and sustainability of water supply systems. With the urgency to address the contentious issues of water inequality, combining technology and novel strategies in community water supply systems is the order of the day. Technology innovations have the potential to facilitate enhanced monitoring and regulation of water resources with cost-effective interventions to the previously underfunded infrastructure. Decentralized water management systems, for example, can facilitate the management of communities' water supply needs while fostering stakeholder collaboration. Such systems can also be designed to incorporate marginalized groups by incorporating the specific issues of women and individuals with disabilities. Engaging communities in water system planning and management, for example, establishing fair tariff regimes and access levels, is also important in maximizing the sustainability and efficiency of these interventions. Lastly, adopting a holistic approach that prioritizes community involvement and innovative solutions is essential in overcoming existing impediments and ensuring equal access to clean water for all (Figure 6.5).

6.2.1. Socioeconomic Disparities Affecting Access

In thinking about the intricacies involved in having access to clean drinking water, one should keep in mind that infrastructure shortages disproportionately influence marginalized communities. Such communities also usually have numerous socioeconomic issues that interfere with adequate water supply distribution. For example, resource-poor communities may not have the resources to spend on necessary infrastructure development that enhances water quality and supply. This is supported by studies that show that steady funding to help with infrastructure growth is essential to ensure equal access to clean water.

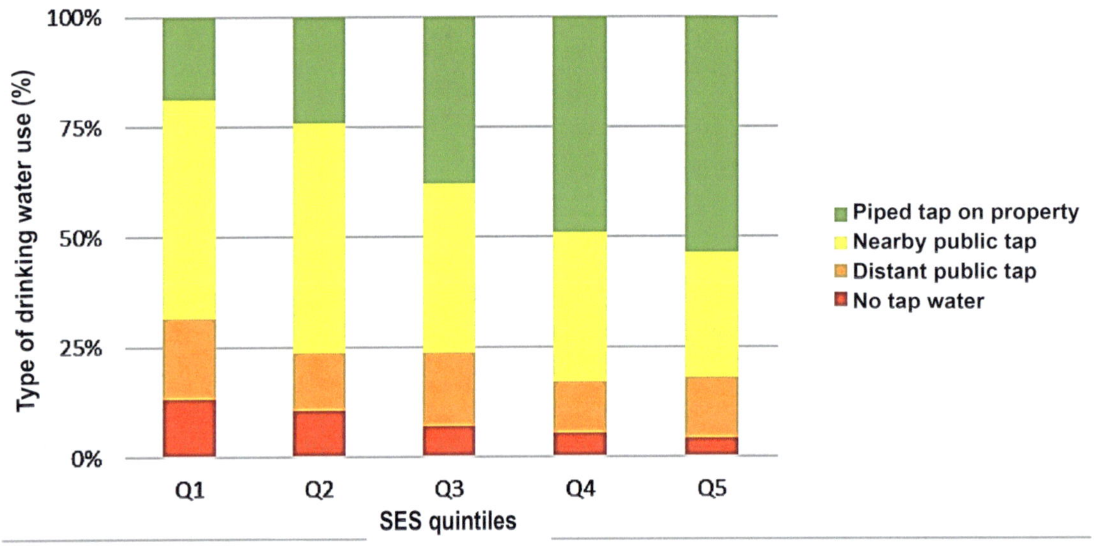

Figure 6.6. Type of drinking water use stratified by socio-economic status (SES) quintiles, where the first quintile (Q1) consists of the lowest SES households and the fifth quintile (Q5) the highest SES households.

Source: International Journal of Environmental Research and Public Health. (2021). *Type of Drinking Water Use Stratified by Socio-Economic Status (SES) Quintiles.*

As noted in research, functioning community participation strategies are key to functioning as a driver in providing redress for these gaps, enabling citizens to engage with local decision-making institutions and facilitate proper water usage in their communities (DeFries et al., 2024). In addition, the nexus between socioeconomic status and access to clean drinking water poses questions of basic policy equity and sustainability. More disadvantaged populations have greater exposure to contaminated water sources with concomitant negative health consequences. The intersection between socioeconomic inequality and municipal government may reflect these inequalities and necessitate increased emphasis on a comprehensive approach to water management. State policies favor the need for equitable distribution, promoting equitable billing practices to take the cost off poorer households (Birnbaum et al., 2011). Developing enabling policies that remove these systemic disincentives not only enhances water quality but also fosters a healthier community in general. Municipal government makes these issues easier because it is crucial that communities have a role to play in filling the infrastructure gap. Good governance frameworks are centered on openness and accountability in which citizens are actively involved in decision-making procedures involving their water supply. Community participation programs can ensure discussion about water management so that residents can voice out and collaborate in sustainable strategies tailored to their needs. The emphasis on inclusive governance in studies means that promoting such participation is essential to addressing socioeconomic disparities. Therefore, effective water distribution systems need to include mechanisms that empower communities and, at the same time, enhance fairness in accessing clean drinking water (DeFries et al., 2024) (Figure 6.6).

6.2.2. Geographic Barriers to Water Distribution

Geographical barriers mostly make efficient water distribution a big challenge, particularly where there are varied topographies and scattered populations. These barriers could take the form of mountain ranges, rivers, and even urbanization that isolates communities from water sources. Inadequate infrastructure also makes it harder as most of the rural communities lack the infrastructure like pipelines and water treatment plants that can ensure a clean water supply. As highlighted by the Integrated Regional Water Management (IRWM) policies and practices, the answer to solving water resource management (UN Water, 2017; The Local Government Commission, 2019) is through an integrated solution. However, the institutionally fragmented nature of governance will most likely discourage the application of comprehensive solutions. By ignoring the geographical facts, the policymakers will end up reinforcing the current inequalities, eventually shortening the time it takes to have equal access to clean drinking water. The existence of geographic barriers alongside socioeconomic facts creates a multifaceted environment for the provision of water. Population in distant or under-developed communities are likely to be burdened with extra cost and logistical issues to reach the water supplies, which may result in biased distribution. The Sustainable Development Goals (SDGs) demand seriousness in addressing such imbalances, basing their argument that the most vulnerable communities must be targeted to experience improvements in water service (Kullman et al., 2017). These objectives fuel the need for localized interventions that take local geographical contexts into account when designing distribution systems. Local community involvement becomes central, with approaches assuring that they are done specifically to their particular needs and circumstances. Allocation of resources should be evidence-based so that decision-makers can pinpoint and invest in solutions that address geographic obstacles pertinent to particular regions. Considering the role of local governance, it is apparent that effective water distribution largely relies on collaborative efforts that consider geographic conditions. Such coordination has the ability to facilitate the development of local solutions that touch upon the very particular needs of various communities. By combining policies that address land use as well as water management, for example, that of programs under SGMA, local governments can start breaking down obstacles that otherwise prevent fair access to water (UN Water, 2017; The Local Government Commission, 2019). But community meaningful participation in such systems of governance is still needed. When the residents themselves are involved directly in making decisions, they can bring worthwhile insight, thereby establishing more inclusive strategies that are specific to bridging geographic divides, thereby resulting in increased access to safe drinking water by all (Figure 6.7).

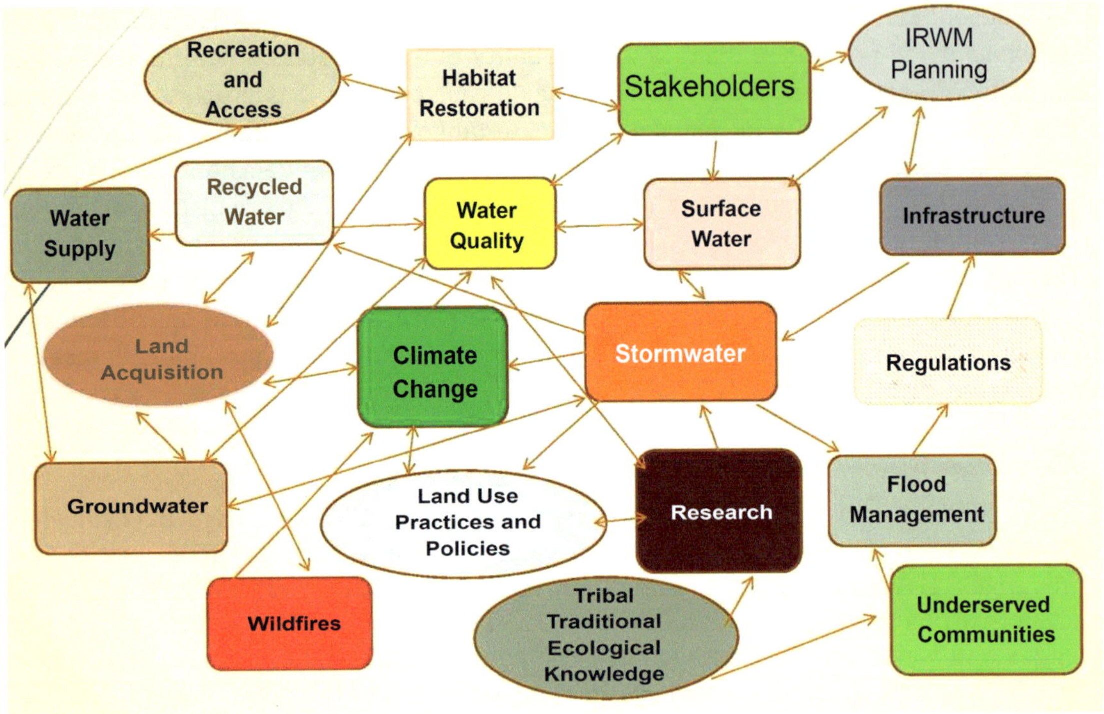

Figure 6.7. Integrated regional water management (IRWM).

Source: Maven's Notebook. (2021). *Integrated Regional Water Management.*

6.2.3. Impact of Climate Change on Water Availability

In analyzing the complexity of clean drinking water access, it is evident that increasing temperatures across the world and changed weather patterns exert serious pressure on water supply. These climatically induced alterations to precipitation regimes can cause interrupted precipitation cycles, influencing the quantity and quality of water sources. Gradual reduction in precipitation in specific areas can, in the long term, worsen water scarcity, leading to heightened competition for the resources and possible conflict between communities. The trends in these developing tendencies expose the challenges faced by local governments, particularly in cities where population density makes the provision of water a challenging exercise. By considering these factors, a more accurate picture of the weaknesses of existing water supply facilities can be built, which will assist in developing effective plans for the sustainable use of precious water resources. The condition is especially critical in susceptible areas, including the Rohingya refugee camps in Bangladesh, where climate change has exacerbated pre-existing water resource issues. Overpopulation in these camps leads to the over-extraction of groundwater, lowering the quality as well as quantity of water available to inhabitants. Seasonal fluctuations further aggravate this problem, contributing to peak crises with characteristics of contamination and scarcity. Climate change increases the occurrence of extreme weather events, and this renders current water infrastructures and others increasingly unreliable, as Ali & Shahreen (2024) argue. This development underscores the need for adaptive water management systems that are climate-resilient. With the application of community-centric strategies that prioritize local participation, stakeholders can not only make water resource systems sustainable but also equitable, thereby culminating in enhanced health outcomes for marginalized communities. Moreover, climate change effects on water availability extend beyond issues of access, having implications in broader urban health dynamics as evidenced by the recent World Health Organization's agenda. With increasing urbanization, the demand for safe water supplies increases, presenting stringent challenges to local governance institutions. The interdependency among water supply, environmental wellness, and population well-being becomes more pressing with growing disparities in access to clean water. In this regard, Roebbel et al. (2022) highlight the significance of multisectoral interventions to promote urban health outcomes through improved water management systems. Such strategies not only address the short-term requirements of city dwellers but also help build resilience against climate change, eventually contributing toward healthier communities that are capable of flourishing in the face of environmental uncertainties (Figure 6.8).

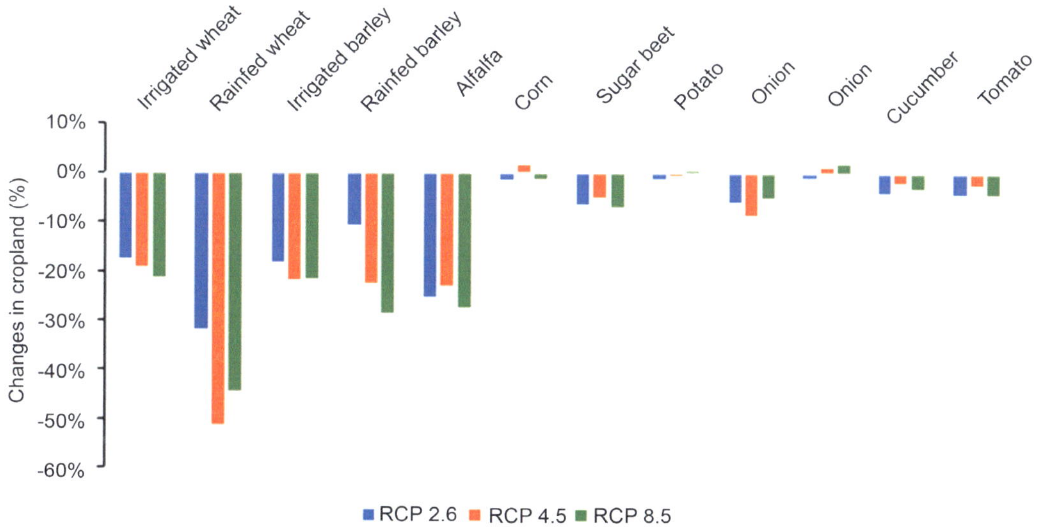

Figure 6.8. Impacts of climate change on water supply systems.

Source: Shayanmehr S, Porhajašová JI, Babošová M, Sabouhi Sabouni M, Mohammadi H, Rastegari Henneberry S, Shahnoushi Foroushani N. The Impacts of Climate Change on Water Resources and Crop Production in an Arid Region. *Agriculture*. 2022; 12(7):1056. https://doi.org/10.3390/agriculture12071056

6.3. Infrastructure Issues in Water Distribution

The issues behind effective delivery water systems are complex, with origins coming from the age of the system, lack of investment, and climate change impacts. Most existing systems fail to be effective in meeting needs due to the fact that they are not properly maintained and updated, and thus inefficiencies characterize drinking water quality and safety. Investigation reveals that there are a myriad of communities, particularly poor and rural communities, left behind by ineffective water supply systems that limit availability while, at the same time, placing the residents' health at potential risks. Secondly, as continued climate uncertainty ensures that it throws legitimate threats toward freshwater resources, the infrastructure finds itself under heightened pressure. Hence, investment in climate-resilient infrastructure that can withstand the shifting climatic patterns is of great significance in realizing fair access to safe water. The investment is essential not only for the purpose of efficiency but also in the establishment of trust and participation by the community in water management. Issues in infrastructure also converge with social injustices and therefore present additional challenges in achieving fair access to clean water. Marginalized people, either on the basis of socio-economic status (SES) or geography, typically face the greatest hurdles in enjoying sustainable water distribution systems. Inequities in infrastructure translate into unequal access, where more affluent communities might be enjoying renovated facilities while the poor are still dependent on outdated, unsafe systems. This disparity highlights the need for integrated planning that incorporates the voices of the marginalized groups, whose concerns are typically left out in policymaking. The function of local governances becomes essential in bridging these gaps by investing in the most needy areas first, making sure that every member of the community has access to clean drinking water. By actively involving marginalized groups in decision-making, the infrastructure can be designed to address the specific needs of multicultural communities. Furthermore, the function of community participation in planning and management of water distribution infrastructure cannot be overstated. Successful community-based processes facilitate locally based decision-making attuned to specific needs, allowing better ownership and accountability by the population. Direct involvement not only empowers people but also fosters ownership in keeping and securing water resources. Local government institutions can help make this a reality through forums of discussion that allow communities to vent their frustration and give input into enhancing water services. Collaborative efforts between government representatives, community members, and inhabitants lead to innovative solutions that address the existing infrastructure issues. These policies are becoming more and more realized as key to the achievement of SDG 6, aimed at universal safe access to water and sanitation, uncovering the importance of inclusive policies under local governance policies (Macura et al., 2021; Yogesh et al., 2021).

6.3.1. Aging Infrastructure and Its Consequences

The impact of aging infrastructure extends far beyond mere inconvenience; it poses significant public health risks and exacerbates existing inequities in water access. Leaking pipes and outdated treatment facilities are capable of polluting water, contributing to unsafe drinking water that is disproportionately impacting marginalized communities. These vulnerable groups are likely to experience compounded hardship, such as higher cases of waterborne disease as well as further financial hardship due to reliance on secondary, often more expensive, water sources. Involvement of the community in determining needs for infrastructure is important, as locals draw attention to particular issues that confront residents. For example, in Daly City, the analysis of community views regarding water affordability and quality identifies the need for localized approaches to meet these systemic challenges effectively (DeFries et al., 2024). Further, poor infrastructure may initiate a chain of socio-economic problems among affected communities, including lower educational achievements and higher food insecurity. In U.S. K-12 schools, to cite one case in point, availability of safe drinking water is closely linked to children's general health, academic achievement, and emotional well-being. When water supplies become polluted, schools are forced to turn to bottled water, a process that not only strains budgets but also erodes parents' and staff members' faith in water quality. This creates a context where children are deprived of necessary resources, which impacts their learning outcomes and development in a negative way (FitzGerald., 2024). Addressing such infrastructural deficiencies, therefore, becomes imperative for the establishment of equal access to clean water. The local government is at the forefront to mitigate the impacts of aging infrastructure. To effectively modernize water delivery systems requires successful planning and investment, yet these efforts again and again come short of their needs for long-term funding and public support. In order to reverse the spiraling costs associated with aging facilities, local governments must prioritize making decisions transparent and engaging communities in the decision-making process. Through cooperation between municipal governments and citizens, policies can be developed to address the unique needs of the community. In this way, decades of systemic disparities in the availability of water can be resolved, ultimately determining better health results and a more sustainable future for everybody (DeFries et al., 2024) (Figure 6.9).

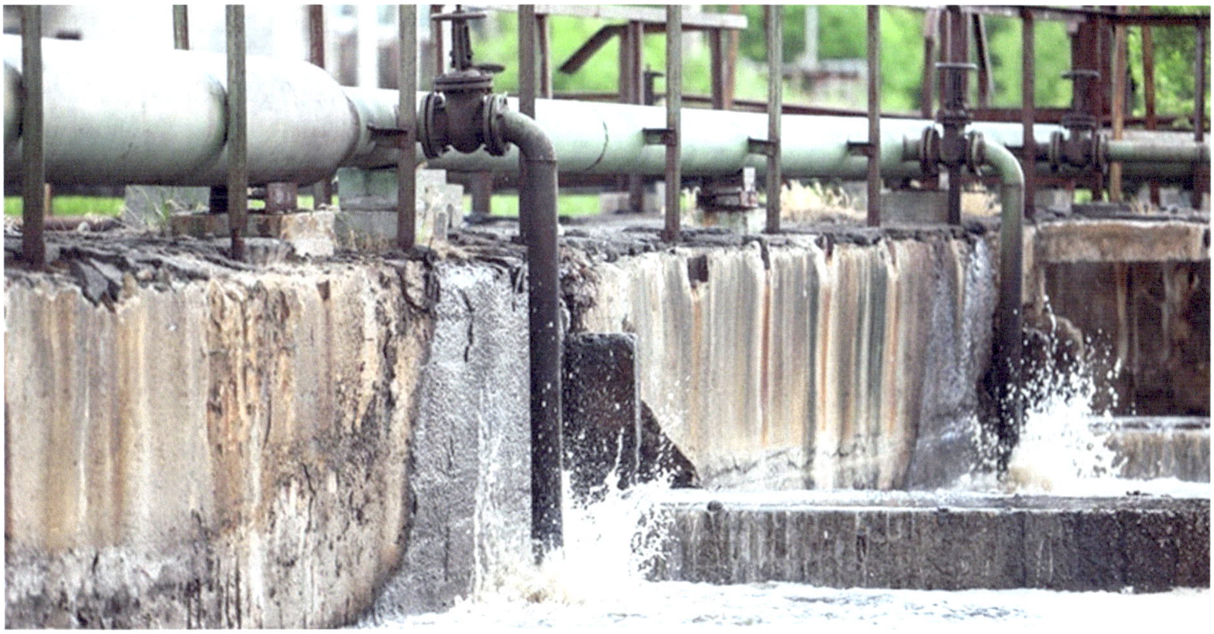

Figure 6.9. Aging and corroded infrastructure.

Source: https://urbanacres.in/wp-content/uploads/2024/10/Aging-Infrastructure-Cripples-Mumbais-Water-Supply.jpg.

6.3.2. Investment Needs for Modernization

The need to deal with the global shortage of water means that there must be a massive spend on upgrading water supply systems. Existing infrastructure is left behind as inferior and outdated, particularly in poorer areas, so it is even more difficult to deal with problems of access and quality. Hence, the money has to be spent on cutting-edge technologies for maximizing the performance and reliability of water supply systems. By investing in new and improved water treatment plants and piped distribution networks, the poor can minimize the risks of waterborne diseases that disproportionately affect the poor. Upgrading through investment can result in improved public health outcomes, thus breaking the cycle of poverty driven by poor-quality water supplies (UN Water, 2017; The Local Government Commission, 2019). In addition, financing such modernization efforts must account for both public and private expenses due to the intricacy of the issues involved. Governments also play critical roles in developing policy climates favorable to private sector participation, including investment incentives that aim to pursue water distribution priorities based on sustainability. The local authorities should be able to make decisions on priorities that represent the people's needs, where investments are not mere dictates of the upper echelons but inclusive processes engaging the local actors. The post-2015 Development Agenda emphasizes this requirement, calling for targeted policies that address unique regional water management challenges and in doing so promote equity and reciprocal accountability in the distribution of resources (UN Water, 2017; The Local Government Commission, 2019). Finally, community participation is a key factor in successfully modernizing water supply systems. Community participation makes sure that investment goes into local needs, enhancing ownership of the water resources. School and college programs and systems that raise the awareness of the people regarding water conservation and upkeep of infrastructure can make participating communities actively maintain their water systems. This model not only employs indigenous knowledge but also facilitates future resistance and resilience to systems and provokes involved stakeholders to be concerned about the sustainability of modern systems. Proper integration of investment, governance, and community participation can thus lead to a more just and sustainable access model to safe drinking water for both present and future needs (Figure 6.10).

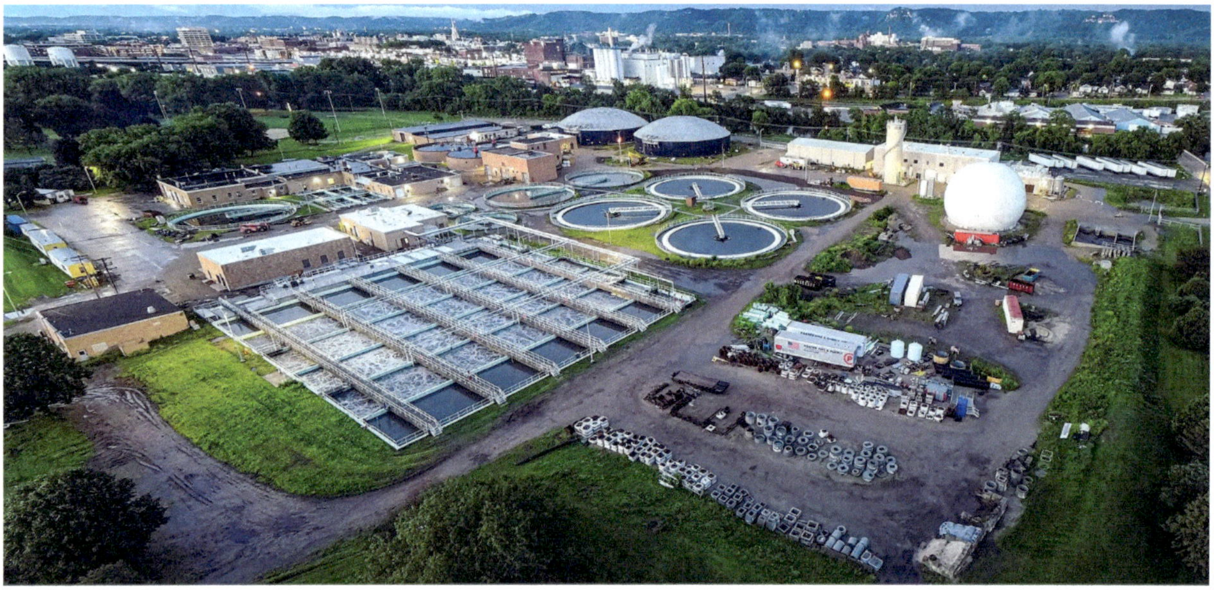

Figure 6.10. Modernization of water treatment plant.

Source: By Wikideas1 - Own work, CC0, https://commons.wikimedia.org/w/index.php?curid=150028072

6.3.3. Technological Innovations in Water Distribution

Water distribution technology innovation is the key to addressing the complex problems of equitable access to clean water. Modern systems allow easy monitoring and management of water supplies, particularly in under-served areas where traditional infrastructure does not exist. Technologies such as advanced metering infrastructure (AMI) and smart sensors allow real-time measurement of flow rates and water quality, allowing proactive maintenance and quick responses to leaks or contamination. This intersection of digital solutions is able to reduce water losses significantly and improve the reliability of services, which ultimately improves community trust in local governance systems. Through this integration of technologies, communities are capable of having greater insight into resource management such that water distribution is specialized according to the needs and preferences of their population. Prioritizing sustainability in water distribution networks requires a multi-faceted approach that involves community participation as well as good governance. Technological developments are not just for streamlining the process but for empowering citizens by making them included in the decision-making process regarding the management of water resources. Effective initiatives have a tendency to leverage social media and mobile apps in organizing community members in monitoring water usage and quality, rendering vital information more democratic in terms of access. Such participatory models guarantee that technology solutions are customized to fit local contexts, hence enhancing equity of access to safe drinking water. Local governance can also use such technologies to enable open communication with citizens, developing stronger partnerships that strengthen the role of the community in water stewardship. With the growing demand for clean drinking water amid urbanization and global warming, innovative and adaptive water distribution systems are needed that are resilient. Integrating smart grids and renewable energies into water infrastructure can greatly reduce the carbon footprint of water distribution while enhancing system reliability. Resilient technological infrastructure can facilitate the conservation of energy and maximize resource utilization, hence aligning with overall sustainability targets in global agendas (Yogesh et al., 2021; Kabeyi et al., 2022). With the implementation of these technologies and subjecting their application to current popular demands and environmental conditions, cities can meet current demands while also guaranteeing future water availability (Figure 6.11).

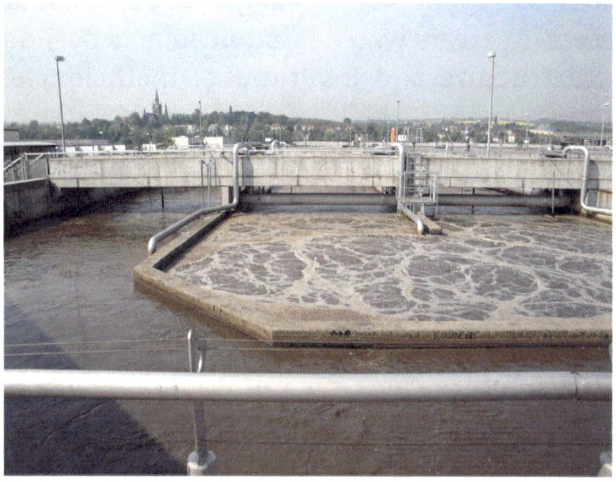

Figure 6.11. Advanced metering infrastructure allows water data to flow.

Source: By SuSanA Secretariat - https://www.flickr.com/photos/gtzecosan/12359229313/, CC BY 2.0, https://commons.wikimedia.org/w/index.php?curid=36440839

6.4. The Role of Local Governance

The coordination of community engagement and local authorities is central to the attainment of fair access to safe drinking water. Well-managed systems have the ability to facilitate CBWM systems in overcoming social, cultural, and economic obstacles that would otherwise hinder water access in poor environments. Studies have established that strong, well-executed governance systems at different levels of institutions would facilitate CBWM, enabling the operating and maintenance functions necessary for the sustainable water supply. The success of such models depends on the active participation of communities in decision-making. Where there is meaningful participation of communities in local government, they can better voice their needs and influence policies that directly affect their access to water and thus have a more guaranteed supply of clean drinking water, as supplied by Mugumya (2022). Unequal access to clean water is often joined by poor infrastructure and institutional inefficiencies. In most areas, including Uganda, safe water for drinking is significantly scarce, with fewer than 40% of the population having regular supplies of water. The local governments must deal with infrastructural shortages while providing highest priority to delivering water services to the poor. For instance, decentralized water infrastructure such as rainwater harvesting (RWH) can offer viable alternatives where conventional municipal supplies do not reach the most disadvantaged sections. Good local governance is important in mobilizing resources, implementing new water supply technologies, and building public confidence in such systems, thus ensuring increased acceptance and use. Without good governance, efforts to increase water access and supply can be in vain, leading to frustration both in service delivery and public trust in existing systems (Hanlon, 2021). Finally, that of the local government in running water distribution is not only that of control but rather one of building participatory institutions that give power to the people. Appreciate the different socioeconomic circumstances of places, local government can design strategies that integrate plural water security objectives, providing equitable access for all user groups to clean water. Through coordination between plural stakeholders such as NGOs, government agencies, and communities, governance can enable knowledge sharing and utilization of resources that foster sustainability and resilience in communities. This collaborative strategy is instrumental in resolving water distribution problems due to, apart from meeting immediate needs, the accumulation of shared ability for long-term water infrastructure maintenance and management necessary to improve the well-being of the populace and general health (Hanlon, 2021; Mugumya, 2022).

6.4.1. Policy Frameworks for Water Management

Efficient water management calls for a robust policy system that addresses diverse challenges, such as climate change, infrastructure gaps, and social inequalities. As outlined in recent studies, such systems must integrate scientific knowledge to forecast and prevent water scarcity and pollution risks. For instance, the Intergovernmental Panel on Climate Change (IPCC) report emphasizes the call for climate-resilient development that interlinks adaptation action and emission reductions under an integrated strategy of ensuring water resource protection (Intergovernmental Panel on Climate Change, 2023). This interconnection is fundamental to ensuring community-based water supply systems are not only sustainable but will also be able to ensure equal access to clean water for all socio-economic groups. Local government is essential in translating such policy arrangements into workable plans that are appropriate to specific community needs. Sound local governance guarantees that water management policies are based on and engage members of the community, thus encouraging ownership as well as accountability. This is particularly important where infrastructure is aging or badly maintained, contributing to issues of fair access to safe drinking water. Policies that grant the power to local authorities to interact with communities enable transparency within decision-making and assist in the implementation of context-specific and community-led solutions (Gatta, 2022). Participatory governance in this manner boosts the resilience of water supply systems as well as encourages sustainable infrastructure projects. Moreover, addressing water management infrastructure issues involves realizing that there are complex socio-economic dynamics at play within communities.

Inadequate investment in infrastructure not only expands access gaps but also poses a threat to public health and environmental sustainability. Therefore, policy systems need to accord priority to infrastructure development alongside local citizen participation programs to attain a harmonized approach toward water management. Lessons from adaptive practices to climate change can be tailored by policymakers in order to arrive at solutions that enhance not only the physical water supply system infrastructure but also the social network of the communities being served. The comprehensive approach ultimately results in a more equitable distribution of clean water and ensures long-term resource use sustainability (Intergovernmental Panel on Climate Change, 2023) (Figure 6.12).

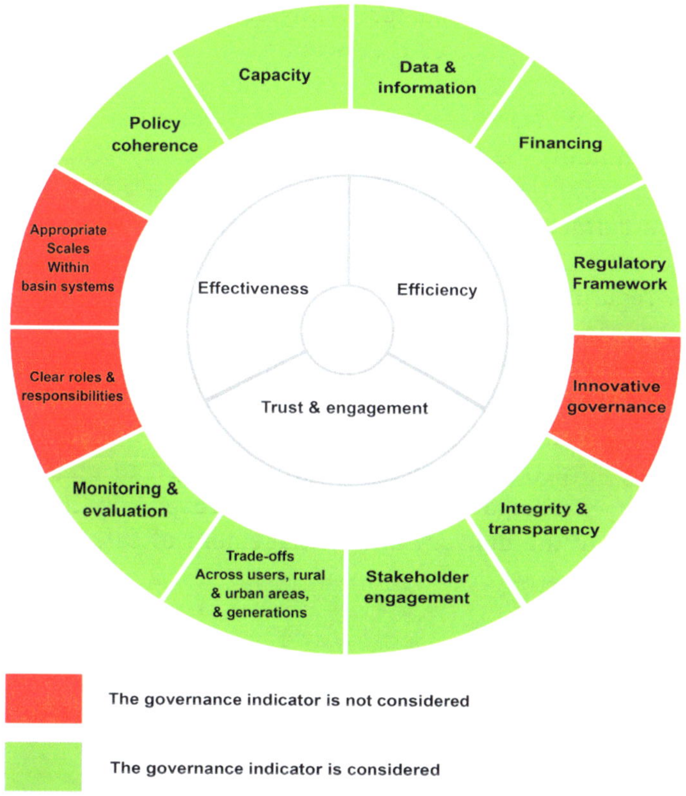

Figure 6.12. Jordan's water governance policy framework indicators.

Source: ResearchGate. (n.d.). *Jordan's Water Governance Policy Framework Indicators.*

6.4.2. Accountability and Transparency in Governance

The relationship between governance systems and investment in infrastructure has a major impact on the supply and quality of drinking water for people. Where institutions of governance place high value on transparency and accountability, they create a culture of trust that requires the involvement and participation of citizens. For example, it has been established through research that upgrading infrastructure has a corresponding relationship with better water quality, and open financial systems like equitable billing systems can help alleviate the fiscal tax burden on citizens dealing with rising costs (DeFries et al., 2024). This twofold practice not only makes water resources more sustainable but also allows for the empowerment of people's local governments. Effective engagement policies thus can facilitate the more equitable distribution of resources in a way that guarantees marginalized populations gain access to clean drinking water, thereby meeting past inequalities of access. There is also need for transparency of governance in successfully managing water resources, particularly in areas where water resource pressures continue to rise. River basin organizations (RBOs) are a case in point of a governing system that, if transparently well governed, can enhance accountability in various water management approaches. Research shows that adapting RBO roles and responsibilities highlights the necessity of adaptive governance practices emphasizing citizen engagement and transparent decision-making (Custodio et al., 2009). Through the presence of the mechanisms for giving feedback from the community and observation, RBOs can better make informed choices that account for local needs and circumstances. Not only does this enhance transparency regarding the efficiency of resource utilization, but it also results in improved maintenance of water infrastructure and compliance with conservation standards. Finally, organizing community participation in governance systems is essential in the name of responsibility in water supply systems. Whenever citizens are included in the local governance processes, it creates a culture of accountability that can be utilized to cultivate more sustainable methods of water governance. It has been observed that engaged communities exhibit increased rates of satisfaction regarding water quality and availability (DeFries et al., 2024). Through an understanding and appreciation of residents' experiences, local governments can create policies that target particular issues being confronted by given groups, ensuring there is more balanced access to clean water. In addition, the existence of mechanisms such as community monitoring committees can make institutions of governance function more effectively, in the sense that money is spent effectively and infrastructure projects are delivered to quality standards accepted. This interaction of community participation and governance responsibility serves as the foundation for sustainable development in the delivery and management of safe drinking water (Figure 6.13).

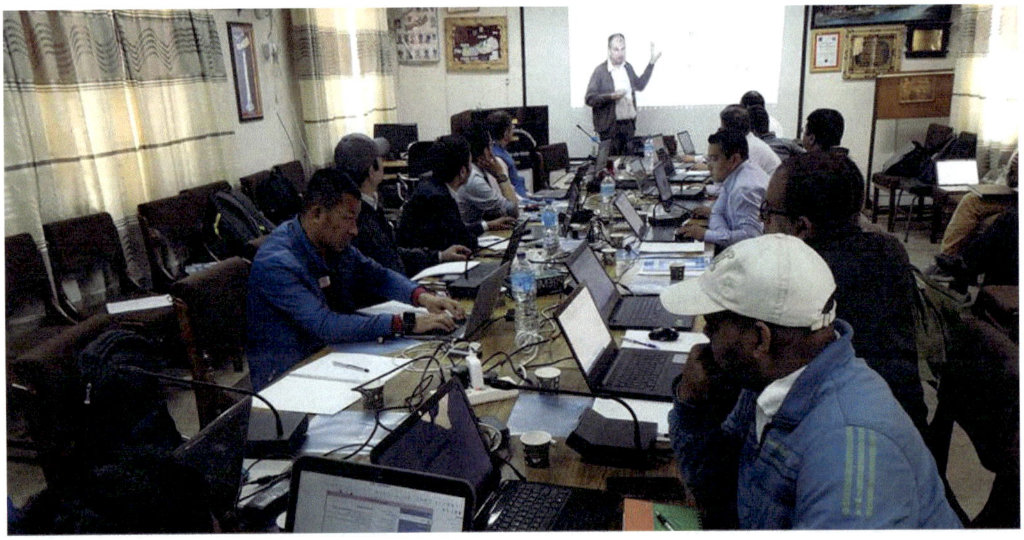

Figure 6.13. River basin organizations improve water security.

Source: Asian Development Bank. (n.d.). *River Basin Organizations Improve Water Security.*

6.4.3. Collaboration Between Local and National Authorities

The dynamics of access to clean drinking water typically depend on the quality of cooperation among national and local governments. This is particularly evident in regions where historically the distribution and administration of water have been overlooked. National policies, despite being very important, may not completely grasp the information that local governments have about the particular needs and challenges of their communities. Through the establishment of a two-way communication system, national decision-makers receive critical information and comments from national authorities. Such communication enhances decision-making that takes into consideration the most vulnerable members of society who have a propensity to fall between the cracks in the traditional system. As is evident in the GLAAS 2017 report, successful collaboration is not just about money but also about establishing plans and goals that relate to local realities (UN Water, 2017; The Local Government Commission, 2019). Lastly, efficient integration of national systems with local wisdom can significantly enhance the efficiency of overall water distribution systems. Moreover, the achievement of equitable access to safe drinking water also necessitates a brief specification of responsibility and authority limits between the national and local governments. Whereas national governments are usually focused on making broad policies, implementation and service provision are left to local administrations. This complementarity of approach is able to facilitate more targeted and responsive intervention at the local level. Local authorities, for example, can better identify infrastructural shortcomings, engage with locals, and adapt methodologies in line with feedback. Such resource imbalance and capabilities might make this partnership even more challenging as local authorities normally lack financial and technical capacities. Yet, mutual interaction can bridge these gaps to make sure that the local agencies are well-trained and funded by national authorities. The State of Health Equity Movement compendium of recommendations illustrates the importance of such collaborative platforms (Birnbaum et al., 2011), with the observation that consolidating the local government is at the heart of sustainable water management. Finally, effective collaboration among national and local government agencies depends not only on the structural setup but also on encouraging public participation. Engaging communities in the decision-making process of their water supply can enhance social cohesion and build mutual trust between citizens and authorities. Local governments, through engaging members of the community, can avail themselves of local knowledge and preferences and ascertain that water delivery systems are laid out in a manner that satisfies genuine needs. These participatory strategies are most important in order to perpetuate initiatives because collective ownership can make people proud to take care of and guard their water sources. In addition, as local governments promote stakeholder participation, they are able to more effectively lobby for national funding to respond to systemic issues regarding access to water. Therefore, cooperation that combines both local knowledge and community participation is needed to overcome the challenges in providing equitable access to clean water for everyone.

6.5. Community Participation in Water Distribution

For the achievement of the fair distribution of clean water, community involvement is a key element that can make water supply systems more effective and sustainable. Community involvement promotes ownership and responsibility, fostering initiatives addressing specific regional demands. In regions where the conventional systems of power have been unable to accommodate shifting demands, this kind of involvement becomes central. In addition, involving people's voices helps ensure that water supply plans are contextually appropriate and culturally acceptable. Research establishes that when people are engaged, they can better negotiate the nuances of water management at the local level, balancing their priorities with necessary infrastructure development and policy change. These collaborative systems not only empower individuals but also equate resources into a single common goal of better water availability and quality (Gael et al., 2025). Community-based solutions' impact is evidenced through instances where resident involvement and local governments intersect to bridge infrastructure gaps.

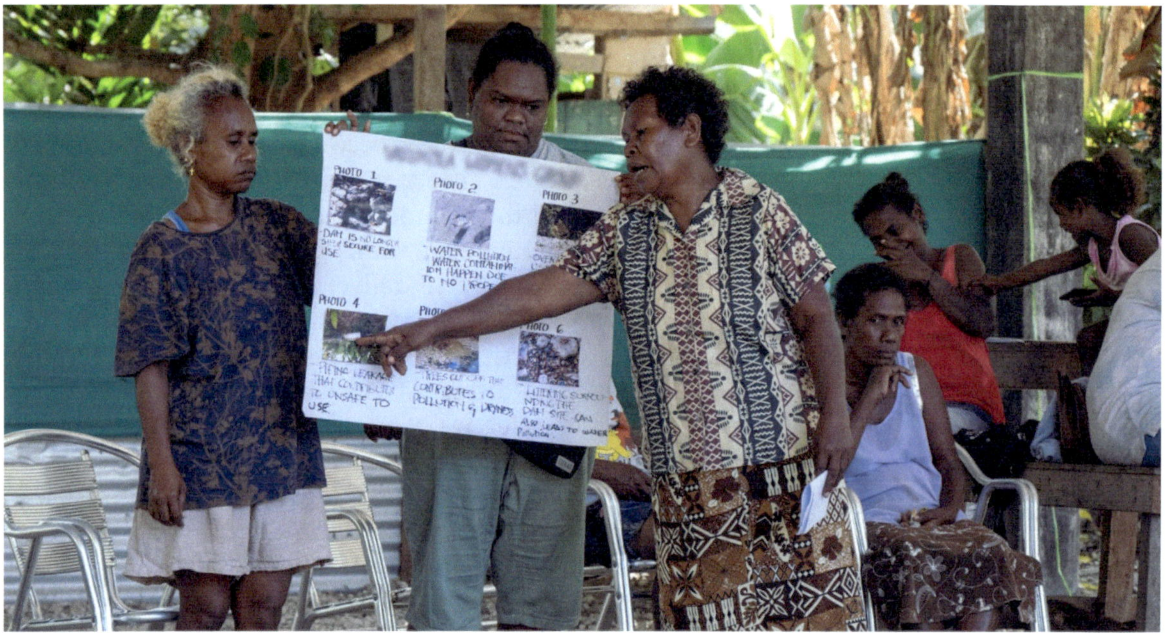

Figure 6.14. Women share their experience of water with fellow community members.

Source: Water for Women Fund. (n.d.). *A Group Discussion with Diverse Workshop Participants.*

In most cases, the absence of proper sanitation facilities contributes to the sophistication of water supply distribution, which calls for an holistic response that involves technical remedies and an appreciation of what people know works. For instance, grassroot efforts are likely to come up with creative solutions that improve water management, such as RWH and sustainable groundwater exploitation, tailored to local environmental conditions. In prioritizing people's involvement in decision-making, local governments can minimize corruption and discrimination that most commonly undermine fair access (Gael et al., 2025). Finally, the creation of opportunities for ongoing public dialogue advances the level of transparency and the level of public trust in the government, a vital factor in the creation of a water delivery system that is robust within the context of the wide-ranging infrastructure problems. Inequities with access to clean water continue to exist, but the vehicle of community engagement makes a point of entry in addressing these challenges systematically. The incorporation of local knowledge not only enhances policy recommendations but also provides advocacy avenues where communities can express their concerns and needs. Moreover, case studies have shown that collaboration between communities and local governments can yield transformative results, including enhanced water quality and service delivery. Such collaboration can bypass bureaucratic constraints and build innovation in water management practices, which makes the solution effective and sustainable. Through the focus on shared responsibility, societies are more able to organize governance systems and remain in charge of water distribution systems, thus enabling long-term improvement in access and equity (Bazaanah et al., 2024). Participatory system like this is needed for the implementation of human right to safe drinking water to everyone (Figure 6.14).

6.5.1. Importance of Community Engagement

Engaging communities within water supply schemes is pivotal to achieving sustainable access to clean drinking water. By including the population of the community within planning and implementation, stakeholders are able to assist in tailoring water delivery infrastructure to meet the unique needs of the community. This participatory approach enhances trust among people and local institutions while strengthening accountability as well as responsiveness to the needs of the population. Moreover, engaging residents in decision-making will enhance their sense of ownership of the local water resources, and hence there can be improved maintenance and utilization of the installed facilities. The attainment of such grassroots community projects to a large degree ensures equal access by eradicating flaws inherent with the traditional top-down approach to water management (Yürer et al., 2023).

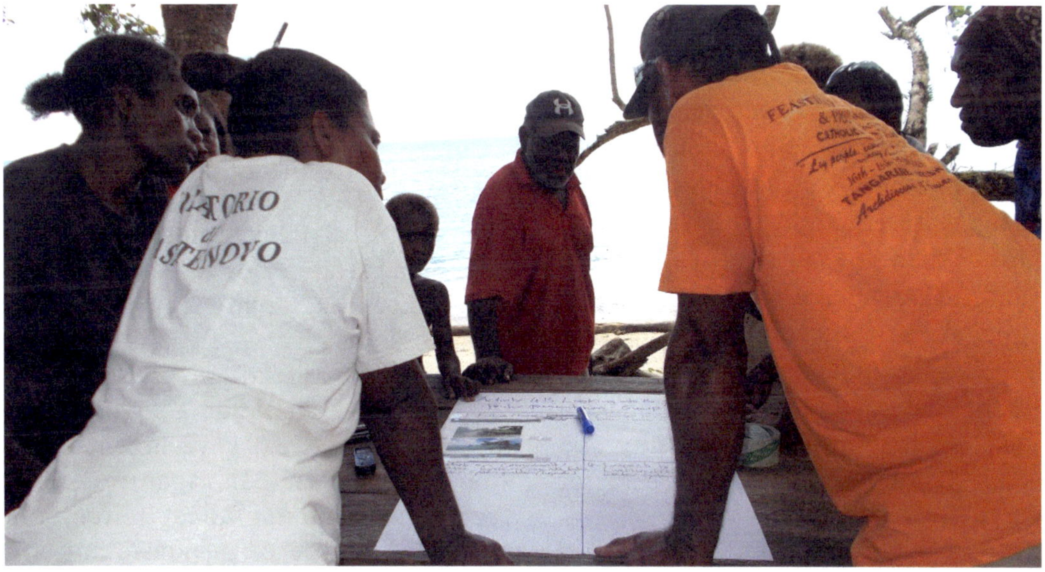

Figure 6.15. A group discussion with diverse workshop participants.

Source: Water for Women Fund. (n.d.). *A Group Discussion with Diverse Workshop Participants.*

For societies where unequal access to clean water continues to be an issue, community action is a driver for attainment and solving some problems. Local understanding of the communities enables them to recognize infrastructure issues that might otherwise remain unknown, such as ineffective distribution networks or socio-economic obstacles to access. Engaged communities have a high capacity for innovation, developing localized solutions to water quality and supply enhancement. The power of citizen engagement is not only in the recognition of the problem but also in the capacity for collective problem-solving between different stakeholders, such as the government, non-governmental organizations, and private sector organizations. The capacity to be their own advocate for their water rights through cooperative arrangements allows communities to compel reforms and investment in infrastructure that suits their unique conditions and desires (Abubakar et al., 2022). Finally, promoting community participation in water supply systems improves resilience to outside shocks that can interfere with access to safe drinking water. For example, local management greatly enhances the response rate to crises, such as droughts or contamination incidents, since members of the community are the first to respond. Such engagement not only guarantees faster mitigation measures but also helps in education and awareness at the community level and public sensitization regarding water conservation and sustainable utilization. Furthermore, engaging locals creates a stewardship culture that prompts individuals to take care of shared water supplies for their children and future generations. With climate change and other environmental factors progressively threatening the quality and supply of water, enhanced community involvement is vital in ensuring long-term sustainability and equity in the distribution of water (Yürer et al., 2023) (Figure 6.15).

6.5.2. Strategies for Effective Participation

Participation is most important in the provision of safe drinking water. Effective participation is in creating accessible channels where neighborhood residents have an opportunity to articulate their needs, concerns, and suggestions for water supply. This enables local people to claim ownership of their water resources, generating a sense of accountability required for sustainable management. Brokering such participation by local government is crucial. Involving citizens in cycles of implementation and planning, apart from promoting the trust of authorities and citizens with each other, also creates more locally tailored and more just solutions to clean water access. Such a model of inclusive government fits into broader commitments to righting systemic inequalities and is therefore core to determining obstacles and efficient elimination thereof. In addition, technological integration into mechanisms of participation will improve maximum community participation and sharing of information. Internet websites provide useful avenues for open communication and seeking the opinion of the inhabitants on water supply matters. Mobile applications or questionnaires online permit real-time data collection and enable communities to express their needs in an easy way. As has been noted earlier in modern climate action debates, technology utilization must also take into account ethical considerations so that data collection becomes equitable and equitable (Catherine et al., 2020). Additionally, sustainable digitalization ensures that e-waste and data privacy issues are minimized and thus guarantee that technology becomes an ally, not an adversary, when it is implemented in grassroots water initiatives. Through creating technology-driven but also morally upright systems, municipal government can enhance the efficiency of participatory action by the community to its fullest potential. Finally, having a culture of responsibility is required for ensuring that community involvement in water management can be sustained. This involves not only the municipal government but civil society organizations, civic organizations, and even private citizens collaborating to create a collective front in water management. Education efforts also raise public consciousness of the importance of access to clean water so communities can lobby on their own behalf. According to the wider data ethics context, the interests of marginalized groups need to be given precedence in order to balance the power imbalances in communities (Catherine et al., 2020). By placing the focus on inclusive approaches that amplify all voices, government agencies are able to shatter prevailing inequalities and thus unlock the gates to a more sustainable and equitable water distribution system. By these approaches, communities can be made strong active players in their water management, providing quick and lasting solutions to access issues.

6.5.3. Examples of Community-Led Water Projects

The complexity of water supply issues across the globe is usually relieved by innovative, community-driven schemes that focus on grassroots participation. There are a number of instances that confirm the effectiveness of grassroots water projects to provide sustainable access to clean drinking water. An example is providing RWH systems to rural villages, which has not only secured a consistent flow of water but also encouraged citizens to claim property in their assets.

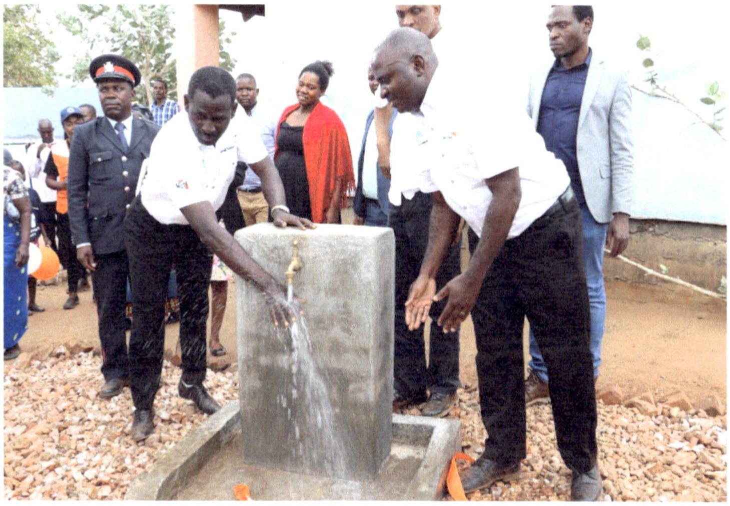

Figure 6.16. Community-led water projects in Zambia.

Source: World Vision. (n.d.). *Community-Led Water Projects in Zambia.*

These systems draw on natural rainfall, substantially reducing dependence on external water sources and enhancing resilience to climatic variability. Consequently, the integration of local knowledge with modern techniques supports the twin goals of supplementing water supply and the establishment of communal solidarity and, therefore, water resources sustainability. Apart from RWH, local borehole drilling operations reflect a commitment to meeting disparities in water supply. When communities finance the construction and maintenance of boreholes collectively, they can provide for the water supply to suit their specific needs and circumstances. This bottom-up approach allows for the creation of fair access to clean drinking water, especially in impoverished zones where government plans might fail. Through collective responsibility and community control, such plans also strengthen the social cohesion of these communities. The involvement of local communities in decision-making promotes more accountability, enhancing the lifespan of the infrastructure and building a culture of maintenance and preservation. Community-led development is an essential element of integrated strategies for providing universal access to safe drinking water. Programs such as the Community-Led Total Sanitation (CLTS) approach have been successful in changing community norms for sanitation and hygiene. By involving local stakeholders in determining problems and implementing solutions, these programs induce a sense of ownership and vested interest in public health solutions. Moreover, collective efforts toward water purification, filtration, and distribution not only minimize health hazards but also stimulate local economies. The long-term benefits of such community-led projects are in line with universal aspirations, emphasizing the requirement of adaptive responses that integrate local governance systems and embrace participative inclusion in water supply management, thereby enhancing community resilience against the variable pressures on access to water (Abubakar et al., 2022; Richard et al., 2022) (Figure 6.16).

SUMMARY

The search for safe access to drinking water is a problem more than technical in nature; it is a constellation of social, environmental, and governance problems that are interdependent and need an integrated solution. Good water supply systems need to address infrastructure building and community involvement in order to provide equitable access to clean water. Local government-community dialogue is key to developing strategies that are context-specific to the needs and conditions of every community. While the technology solutions are critical, they have to be implemented within environments that acknowledge social forces and local control of water assets. Through this, communities can actively engage in decision-making, enabling stewardship and maximizing the sustainability of water supply programs. A complete solution, as opposed to merely addressing the immediate case of water distribution, provides long-term resilience against the impending crises. Attaining the equal access to safe drinking water is closely associated with surmounting basic infrastructure challenges, usually compounded by inadequate investment and policy gaps. While countries attempt to meet SDGs, attention should be paid to how existing infrastructures could be upgraded and expanded to connect marginalized groups. Investment in both human capital and physical capital will be needed in order to put in place and maintain efficient water systems. Moreover, engaging communities in their planning and implementation can ensure that the communities' needs are being met in addition to the general efficiency in water distribution. Getting into an evidence-based practice, one with systematic monitoring instruments, allows policymakers to track improvement and identify areas that require further intervention so that community objectives are in sync with national goals for the access to clean water (Fanzo et al., 2021). The future of fair access to drinking water is not only based on short-term measures but on building systemic solutions to address profound inequities. Climate change introduces an extra layer of complication as unpredictable patterns of weather condition water availability and quality. Still, as it has been illustrated in many examples, an overall approach that carries technological innovation, community empowerment, and local administration can lead to transformational outcomes. For example, neighborhood-scale initiatives have been found to improve the availability and quality of water and also social coherence and resilience. They must become an example of increased use and are even able to have impact on international practices and policies. Ultimately, commitment to clean and equal access to water must be sustained through resilient adaptation systems that are efficient in responding to evolving challenges to ensure that the vision of global access to safe drinking water is a reality in the not-so-distant future (Yogesh et al., 2021).

Pure drinking water is being increasingly seen as a global human right, basic to public health and socio-economic development. Community water supply systems are an effective model for increasing coverage, especially where coverage is low. They depend on local participation in their planning, operation, and implementation, thereby ensuring that they are designed to suit the specific needs of the community. But just as much as possibilities for indigenous measures to enhance water supply access exist, there are also numerous challenges. Political instability, lack of funding, and poor infrastructure can all make it difficult to have a go at building sustainable sources of access to clean water. Such challenges call for joint efforts from the stakeholders such as community residents, local governments, and NGOs in order to set up an equitable and sustainable system for supplying water. Local governance application cannot be overemphasized while making consideration regarding the provision of safe drinking water. Strong governance systems allow communities to place water projects as a high agenda and allocate resources in a manner suitable to them. In addition, involving the people in decision-making enables greater ownership and accountability, which results in improved maintenance and sustainability of water infrastructure. Unfortunately, in most places, local government is beset by issues of corruption, lack of transparency, and limited resources, which reduce the efficacy of water management. Such governance challenges can also exacerbate existing inequalities, with disadvantaged groups having even less access to clean water. Governance structures have to be made firmer, and transparency and accountability promoted, to rectify such imbalances and provide equal access to water for all members of a community. Equitable access to water is deeply connected to other environmental and social concerns. As central as any argument regarding the environmental crisis, the relationship between accessibility to water and environmental integrity is fundamental. Areas experiencing environmental degradation tends to experience increased competition over water resources, and conflict as well as escalating vulnerabilities for groups already vulnerable are triggered. Besides, responding to these multi-faceted issues demands transformative strategies that integrate environmental regeneration as components of peace-building initiatives. The combined strategy is not only paramount in enhancing the access to water but also for sustaining the overall welfare of populations. By integrating the environment as a central part of water management, the stakeholders can implement a more secure and equitable socio-economic environment, which results in greater public health gains and community resilience (UN Water, 2017; The Local Government Commission, 2019; Richard et al., 2022).

KEY TERMS FROM THIS CHAPTER

- Safe drinking water systems
- Community participation
- Environmental sustainability
- Participatory governance
- Public health solutions
- River basin organizations (RBOs)
- Socio-economic status (SES)
- Unsafe resource management
- Water networks
- Water supply networks
- Water treatment plant
- Advanced metering infrastructure (AMI)
- Community-led total sanitation (CLTS) approach
- Local governments
- Policy-making process
- Rainwater harvesting (RWH)
- Seasonal fluctuations
- Supply distribution
- Water distribution systems
- Water resource management
- Water supply system
- World Health Organization

CLOSER LOOK

HUMAN RIGHTS TO WATER AND SANITATION

Water and sanitation access are also recognized by the United Nations as human rights – a right that underpins all individuals' health, dignity, and well-being. But billions of people lack access to safely managed water and sanitation.

Marginalized communities are often left behind, and at times discriminated against, when they seek access to the water and sanitation facilities they need. Governments must ensure a human rights-based approach (HRBA) to water and sanitation development, such that no one is left behind.

The Issue Explained

- The right to water makes everyone eligible for access to safe, sufficient, acceptable, physically accessible, and affordable water for domestic and personal use.
- The right to sanitation provides all people with the physical and affordable access to sanitation, in all aspects of life, that is safe, hygienic, secure, socially and culturally acceptable and that provides privacy and dignity.
- Physical presence is different from access. A water or sanitation service does not benefit the entire community if it is not affordable, not reliable, complex, dangerously placed, unsuitable for less able users or children, or unsegregated by gender, in the case of toilets and washing facilities.
- Toward all people water and sanitation must be provided equally without discrimination. Marginalized groups – women, children, refugees, indigenous peoples, disabled people and many others – are frequently forgotten by, and at times subjected to active discrimination from, those in power that plan and administer water and sanitation improvements and services, and other water and sanitation service users.

The Way Forward

- Governments must take on an HRBA for water and sanitation. Governments are duty-bearers of providing water and sanitation services to individuals, who are rights-holders. Rights-holders can claim their rights and duty-bearers must ensure the rights to water and sanitation equally and non-discriminatorily.
- Human rights law must have a 'pro poor' focus. Duty-bearers must focus on those most in need through their actions, and build the capacities of those people in order to fulfill their obligations. A HRBA also becomes a platform for rights-holders to interact, and hold duty-bearers accountable.
- All barriers to access to water and sanitation must be removed. Policy and law must accommodate all grounds of discrimination including sex, gender, ethnicity, religion, caste, disability, age, health status, and economic status. Other parameters influencing access to water and sanitation by marginalized groups like climate change, population growth, conflict, and migration must also be planned for.

References

1. Abubakar, I., Dalglish, S. L., Angell, B., Sanuade, O. A., Abímbọ́lá, Ṣ., Adamu, A. L., Adetifa, I., et al. (2022). The Lancet Nigeria Commission: Investing in health and the future of the nation. *The Lancet, 399*, 1155–1200. https://doi.org/10.1016/s0140-6736(21)02488-0.
2. Paolo Galizzi & Alena Herklotz, Missing in Action: Gender in International Environmental Law, in Powerful Synergies: Gender Equality, Economic Development and Environmental Sustainability (UNDP: 2012).(accessed on 14 May 2025).
3. Ali, M., & Shahreen, T. (2024). Climate-resilient water resource management for Rohingya refugee camps in Bangladesh. *International Journal of Science and Research Archive*. International Journal of Science and Research Archive, 2024, 12(01), 2661–2694.
4. Article DOI: 10.30574/ijsra.2024.12.1.1139(accessed on 14 May 2025).
5. Prosper Bazaanah, Smangele Johanna Buthelezi, Dina Afua Kobe Oppong; Qualitative study of drinking water, sanitation, and hygiene access: perspectives from the Central Gonja District, Ghana, and Mtubatuba Municipality, South Africa. *Journal of Water, Sanitation and Hygiene for Development* 1 November 2024; 14 (11): 1043–1065. doi: https://doi.org/10.2166/washdev.2024.021 (accessed on 14 May 2025).
6. Birnbaum, N., Masterson, E., & Schoomaker, H. (2011). *State of Health Equity Movement, 2011 Update Part C: Compendium of Recommendations (DRA Project Report No. 11-03)*. https://core.ac.uk/download/pdf/18491812.pdf (accessed on 14 May 2025).
7. Black, R. C., Busby, J. W., Dabelko, G. D., De Coning, C., Maalim, H., McAllister, C., Ndiloseh, M., et al. (2022). *Environment of Peace: Security in a New Era of Risk*. https://doi.org/10.55163/lcls7037.
8. D'Ignazio, C., & Klein, L. (2020). *Data Feminism*. MIT Press. https://doi.org/10.7551/mitpress/11805.001.0001.
9. DeFries, K. (2024). *Sustainable Management of Municipal Drinking Water Services: A Case Study of Daly City, CA*. https://core.ac.uk/download/622000605.pdf (accessed on 14 May 2025).
10. Dwivedi, Y. K., Hughes, L., Kar, A. K., Baabdullah, A. M., Grover, P., Abbas, R., Andreini, D., et al. (2021). Climate change and COP26: Are digital technologies and information management part of the problem or the solution? An editorial reflection and call to action. *International Journal of Information Management, 63*, Article 102456. https://doi.org/10.1016/j.ijinfomgt.2021.102456.
11. Fanzo, J., Haddad, L., Schneider, K., Béné, C., Covic, N., Guarín, A., Herforth, A., et al. (2021). Viewpoint: Rigorous monitoring is necessary to guide food system transformation in the countdown to the 2030 global goals. *Food Policy, 104*, 102163. https://doi.org/10.1016/j.foodpol.2021.102163.
12. FitzGerald, Shannon O'Donnell, "Water Insecurity in K-12 Schools in the U.S.: Understanding State Laws, Drinking Water Violations, and Lived Experiences" (2024). *Electronic Theses and Dissertations*. 2933. https://egrove.olemiss.edu/etd/2933(accessed on 14 May 2025).
13. Nicolay, Gian L. and Fliessbach, Andreas (2012) Production of Innovations within Farmer–Researcher Associations Applying Transdisciplinary Research Principles. In: *International Conference on Research for Development (ICRD 2012). Research for Global Transformation,*

Theme 4: Enabling Research in Global Transformation Session 26: Integrated Development Research Approach, NCCR North-South Dialogue, no. 44, p. 164.(accessed on 14 May 2025).

14. Gatta, P. P. (2022). *The State of World Fisheries and Aquaculture 2022*. FAO. https://doi.org/10.4060/cc0461en.
15. Gumbo, B., Indij, D., Coates, D., Lentini, E., Sewilam, H., Liebe, J., Bernaudat, L., et al. (2012). *Water in the Green Economy: Capacity Development Aspects*. UN-Water Decade Programme on Capacity Development (UNW-DPC) United Nations University UN Campus Hermann-Ehlers-Str. 10, 53113 Bonn, Microbeany. https://core.ac.uk/download/71360162.pdf (accessed on 14 May 2025).
16. Intergovernmental Panel on Climate Change. (2023). *Climate Change 2022–Impacts, Adaptation and Vulnerability*. https://doi.org/10.1017/9781009325844.
17. Kabeyi, M. J. B., & Olanrewaju, O. A. (2022). Sustainable energy transition for renewable and low carbon grid electricity generation and supply. *Frontiers in Energy Research, 9*. https://doi.org/10.3389/fenrg.2021.743114.
18. Kullman, C., Skoufias, E., Andres, L. A., & Srivastava, V. (2017). *Reducing Inequalities in Water Supply, Sanitation, and Hygiene in the Era of the Sustainable Development Goals*. https://core.ac.uk/download/141922872.pdf (accessed on 14 May 2025).
19. Macura, B., Del Duca, L., Espinoza Soto, A. E., Carrard, N., Gosling, L., Hannes, K., Thomas, J., et al. (2021). PROTOCOL: What is the impact of complex WASH interventions on gender and social equality outcomes in low- and middle-income countries? A mixed-method systematic review protocol. *Campbell Systematic Reviews, 17*, e1164. https://doi.org/10.1002/cl2.1164.
20. Mugumya, F. (2022). Governance dynamics disabling the sustainability of community-managed point-water facilities in rural Uganda. *Irish Studies in International Affairs, 24*, 165–177. https://www.semanticscholar.org/paper/c7cc6f8bf48ec56f7e1d6fb0e02f11d840283aa4 (accessed on 14 May 2025).
21. UN Water. (2017). *Financing Universal Water, Sanitation and Hygiene Under the Sustainable Development Goals: UN-Water Global Analysis and Assessment of Sanitation and Drinking-Water (GLAAS) 2017 Report*. UN-Water GLAAS 2017: Financing universal water, sanitation and hygiene under the Sustainable Development Goals. https://core.ac.uk/download/83111897.pdf (accessed on 14 May 2025).
22. The Local Government Commission. (2019). *Bringing Water and Land Use Together: Final Report to the Community Foundation Water Initiative on the Equitable Integration of Water and Land Use*. Final Report to the Community Foundation Water Initiative on the Equitable Integration of Water and Land Use. https://core.ac.uk/download/480184186.pdf (accessed on 14 May 2025).
23. Njouonang Djomo Harold Gael & Hamadou Bachirou Maazou, 2025. "Securing Land Rights for Young People and Their Role in a Win-Win Partnership Model for Agricultural Development: Issues and Perspectives for Northern Cameroon," International Journal of Research and Innovation in Social Science, International Journal of Research and Innovation in Social Science (IJRISS), vol. 9(3), pages 806-822, March.(accessed on 14 May 2025).
24. O'Hanlon, F. (2021). *Rainwater Harvesting and Community Water Security in South-West Uganda*. https://www.semanticscholar.org/paper/5b603cf613901ed2ed8fdc1ca1b1f46ecadc1b57 (accessed on 14 May 2025).

25. Roebbel, N., de Sá, T. H., Neira, M., & Krug, E. (2022). Global research priorities for urban health. *Bulletin of the World Health Organization, 100*, 750–750A. https://www.semanticscholar.org/paper/2ab193831e7d55d1b25b789e9819f943cfe55086 (accessed on 14 May 2025).

26. Rolnick, D., Donti, P. L., Kaack, L. H., Kochanski, K., Lacoste, A., Sankaran, K., Ross, A. S., et al. (2022). Tackling climate change with machine learning. *ACM Computing Surveys, 55*, 1–96. https://doi.org/10.1145/3485128.

27. Thürer, Y., Blanc, F., Ottimofiore, G., Castillo Morales, A., Amaral, M., Hernández, G., Karttunen, M. B., et al. (2023). *Better Regulation for the Green Transition* (Public governance policy papers). https://doi.org/10.1787/c91a04bc-en.

28. Bird, J., Arriens, W. & Von Custodio, D., (2009). *Water Rights and Water Allocation: Issues and Challenges for Asia*. Asian Development Bank. https://core.ac.uk/download/75783451.pdf (accessed on 14 May 2025).

Chapter 7

THE ROLE OF HYGIENE IN WATERBORNE DISEASE PREVENTION

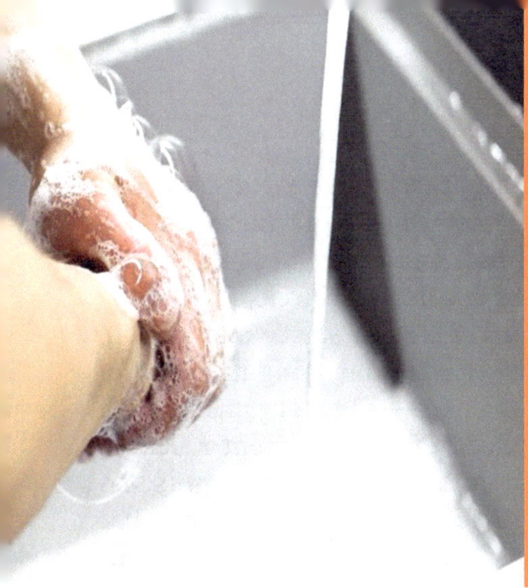

Contents

Introduction

Clean water and public health are two peas in a pod, particularly when it comes to maintaining waterborne diseases under control. Booming populations and yesterday's rapidly growing cities have turned water quality into an elusive problem; when simple cleanliness slumps, dangerous microbes gain a foothold very easily. WHO figures, for example, indicate that millions of people fall ill annually due to unsafe water and sanitation. It's not simply a matter of constructing new pipes or treatment facilities, however; maintaining keenness on daily cleanliness, at home and in public places, makes a significant difference in reducing these diseases. Considering the reuse of resources, a circular economy is perfectly part of this equation. In general, connecting these concepts with worldwide goals, such as SDG 6, which sets priorities for clean water and sanitation—unlocks intelligent approaches to resource management and waste reduction. Properly recycling wastewater isn't merely a tidy trick to alleviate water scarcity; it helps keep basic hygiene levels intact. For most instances, combining environmental responsibility with daily hygiene makes a virtuous circle, enhancing public health and balancing nature and society (Schroeder et al., 2018). Food safety also gets in on the act, even if it tends to receive less attention than water concerns. Challenging handling of food and water contamination share more than might appear at first glance—microorganisms such as *E. coli* and *Salmonella* quickly appear when conditions are not clean enough. Current research indicates that, overall, a risk-based approach (as opposed to solely emphasizing hazards) presents a smarter means to address the intricate web of interconnectedness between our food, water, and health (Bintsis, 2017). Ultimately, improved health occurs through spreading the news on full-scale hygiene—everything from the farm right to our plates, which emphasizes the necessity of an adaptive, multi-prong approach to truly overcome the spread of waterborne disease.

Importance of Hygiene in Disease Prevention

Hygiene and disease prevention are connected in a way that's difficult to overlook, particularly in the kind of areas where waterborne pathogens seem to be around every corner. Individuals washing their hands or keeping things clean can make a huge impact, particularly when clean water is scarce. The World Health Organization, for example, tends to emphasize that adhering to proper hygiene practices reduces the incidence of diseases, something that strikes even more forcefully in poor neighborhoods. Indeed, Schroeder et al. (2018) demonstrates that incorporating these practices is necessary for achieving Sustainable Development Goals (SDG) regarding clean water and sanitation. This type of ripple effect extends beyond health, but also boosts economic and social well-being. In some ways, it's not so much about what one does, but rather a community responsibility for ensuring communities are secure. Foodborne diseases further highlight why good hygiene is important where food and water intersect. When food or water spoils—tainted with microbes or lack of care, it often provokes outbreaks that can take a heavy cost in terms of disease and even fatalities. For instance, Kirk et al. (2015) posits that a considerable portion of foodborne disease originates from contaminated water, reminding us how much hygiene and food safety go hand in hand. Even a minor misstep, whether at harvest or preparation, can increase contamination risks. Populations that hold to strict hygiene protocols tend to enjoy improved public health outcomes, demonstrating that the fight against foodborne disease is one waged at every turn, not merely by individual behaviors but by community efforts. And then there's the influence education has on making habits stick. Informative campaigns—covering everything from handwashing to safe food handling, can shift attitudes about exactly how infections spread, leading to better habits over time. When folks learn how pathogens travel around, they often end up repeating those hygiene steps more consistently, even if it's not perfect every time. Several studies have shown that deeper knowledge of disease transmission equals more robust hygiene actions, particularly in areas hit hardest by waterborne diseases. By incorporating hygiene education into public health campaigns, communities are able to create healthier environments. Ultimately, dissemination of this information accomplishes more than merely preventing disease, it assists in creating sustained changes in overall well-being and fosters increased community involvement.

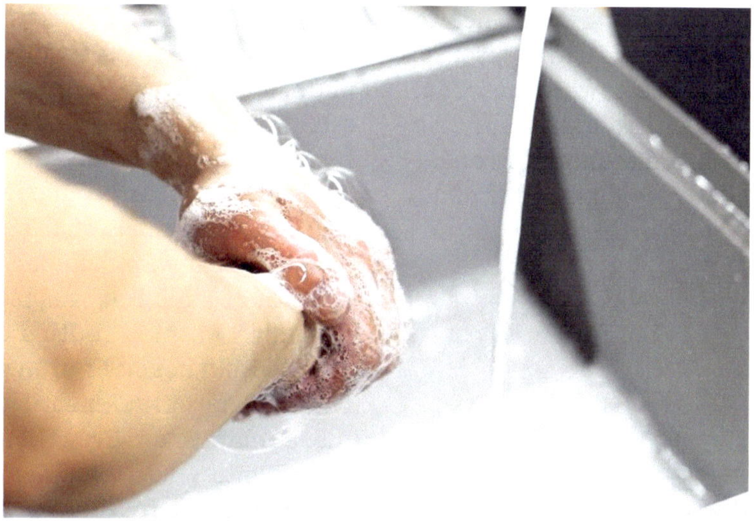

Source: https://d2jx2rerrg6sh3.cloudfront.net/images/Article_Images/ImageForArticle_22353_16497694860886539.jpg.

7.1. The Importance of Personal Hygiene

Water and wellness go hand-in-hand—bathing is truly the foundation of our protection from waterborne disease. Individuals who adhere to rudimentary but habitual cleansing routines typically don't catch anything, especially where water standards are low. Consider areas inundated with floods: when the quality of the water declines, disease spreads quicker. The Pakistan floods, for instance, demonstrate how quickly an absence of clean water can become a serious health emergency; and when the public's awareness is not where it should be, even proper hygiene measures break down. In the majority of instances, taking care of oneself is essential, since such habits serve to protect the entire community, especially the most vulnerable (Muhammad et al., 2023). Hygiene isn't merely an individual issue, it's an issue shared by the entire community. Washing your hands may sound simple, but it does more than safeguard you; it prevents microbes from spreading elsewhere. Community programs that take the time to instruct people on proper cleaning methods have been of great use, particularly where clean water is scarce. Recent experience tends to indicate that whereas a handful of easy repairs assist, far more mixed action involving education and improved infrastructure will be necessary to realistically address sanitation issues. , some new trials added that traditional methods such as WASH interventions sometimes fall short when implemented by themselves, and a broader strategy can truly turn the corner. Getting all parties involved on hygiene can ignite healthier settings and reduce disease in vulnerable populations (Cumming et al., 2019). If we look closer, improving personal hygiene also improves overall public health by causing individuals to notice how the little things they do make a huge difference. The more people learn why staying clean is so important, they automatically adopt preventive measures that reduce the risk of waterborne diseases. Health recommendations and vaccination campaigns are also more effective when individuals are aware of the actual value of hygiene—after all, everything is linked. On a certain level, personal hygiene and public health go together, compelling each individual to take an active role in preventing disease. By making cleanliness paramount, communities can create a more robust, more effective defense against health crises and reduce the overall burden of disease. Finally, taking a little effort toward personal hygiene not only protects individuals but also assists in making entire communities stronger against waterborne diseases (Muhammad et al., 2023) (Figure 7.1).

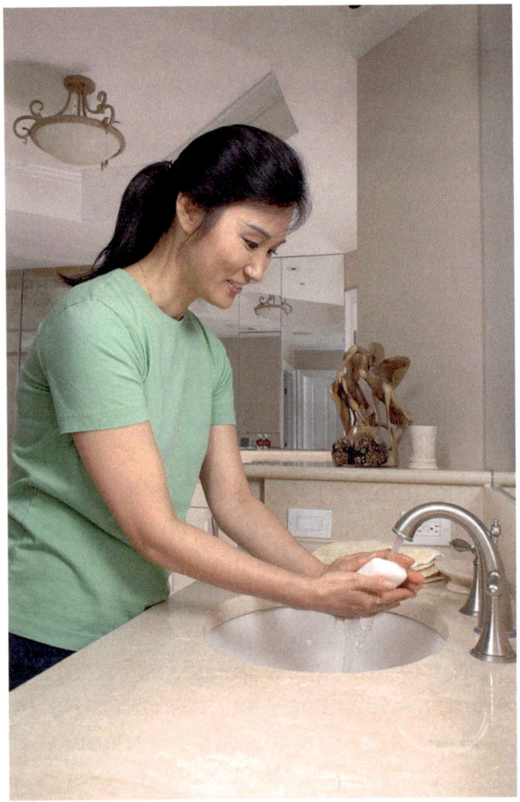

Figure 7.1. Importance of personal hygiene.

Source: By Bill Branson (Photographer) - This image was released by the National Cancer Institute, an agency part of the National Institutes of Health, with the ID 4396 (image) (next)., Public Domain, https://commons.wikimedia.org/w/index.php?curid=24030630

7.1.1. Handwashing Techniques and Their Effectiveness

Washing hands is just an ordinary day-to-day procedure that plays an important part in preventing waterborne insects' transmission. First, you rinse your hands in clean water, put soap into them, make lather from it (all about 20 seconds—take your time.), rinse off afterwards and dry in its entirety. Each step from the process repels dirt as well as microbes, even if it may possibly appear almost so normal. Health professionals, such as those of the Society for Healthcare Epidemiology (SHEA) (Glowicz et al., 2023), typically suggest that adherence to a regular washing routine can lower infection risks, within hospitals or in general life. In areas where waterborne infection is more prevalent, these routines are even more critical to making communities healthier. It's not only a matter of doing a set routine; what you use to do it also comes into play. For example, foamy soaps, sanitizers made of alcohol, or even specific antibacterial gels can add an extra kick to the cleanliness, minimizing the possibility of transference of icky microbes. In most scenarios, clean and flowing water plus a good grade soap assist in killing microbes such as *E. coli* and *Salmonella* (Ding et al., 2021). You may hear this repeated in several public health messages, stressing that both the method and the kind of materials are important. When a community knows these small but significant details, it tends to construct a stronger wall against waterborne diseases. Furthermore, the environment where you wash your hands should not be ignored. Having easy access to clean water and proper facilities is an important factor for making handwashing functional, and regions that lack these essentials are at risk for greater disease transmission. When sanitation does not exist, it requires more public health interventions that enable every day hygiene—sometimes with a bit of additional community education added. As soon as individuals recognize that a good handwashing routine is directly linked to improved health, they are likely to adhere to it even if the ritual is dull. At the end of the day, raising awareness and making resources accessible still is more than a central strategy for combating waterborne diseases and enhancing general community health (Figure 7.2).

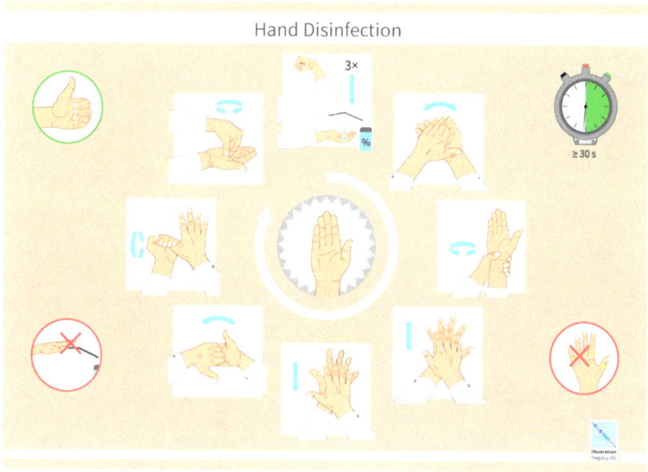

Figure 7.2. Hand washing steps.

Source: By Guido4 - Own work http://www.hegasy.de/, CC BY-SA 4.0, https://commons.wikimedia.org/w/index.php?curid=63765292

7.1.2. Role of Personal Hygiene in Disease Transmission

Keeping oneself clean is a simple habit that is important for community health, particularly in terms of waterborne diseases. So often, outbreaks are the result of oversights in daily hygiene—microbes hitching a ride on our hands or just sitting on surfaces. Where water isn't good and sanitation lags, these pathogens find a toehold. Health programs that prompt individuals to wash hands thoroughly and adhere to basic cleanliness can, in general, reduce disease transmission. The common understanding of good hygiene is a type of protector against infections that become exacerbated when water quality is poor. Even when targeting an individual's habits, more penetrative hygiene behaviors provide a greater foundation for public health. Animals can also bring extra challenges when it comes to keeping infections at bay. Nowadays, city living often means we're around animals more than before, which increases the chance of picking up microbes that come from them. Generally speaking, over 60% of microbes harming humans come from creatures, whether pets or wildlife. Climate change and rapidly expanding cities only fuel the fire further, creating more avenues through which these diseases can show up. When individuals engaging with animals go out of their way to maintain proper personal hygiene, it tends to shut down the passage of these infections. This unclean combination of sanitation and animal-borne disease truly points out how complex our public health tends to get (Rahman et al., 2020). And then there's the entire COVID-19 debacle, which reminded us that infections can creep in the most unsuspected manners. The pandemic taught us that in addition to coughing and sneezing, microbes could also live in, who knew, fecal matter—creating new worries about water contamination. Previous health guidelines were suddenly behind the times, and our habits needed to adapt to accommodate another type of risk. As we continue to learn more about these new threats, combining water safety with everyday cleanliness becomes increasingly important. New health guidelines that intertwine cleanliness advice with water quality testing may well reduce the likelihood of subsequent outbreaks of disease. Overall, maintaining pace with tidiness, updating our water quality standards, and keeping watch over how infections spread build improved resilience in everyday life (Amirian, 2020) (Figure 7.3).

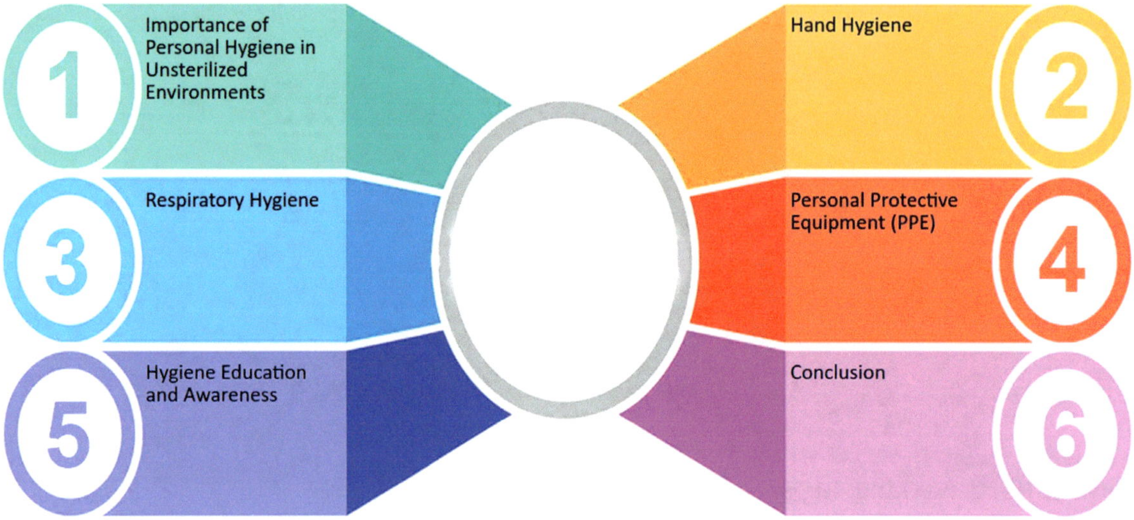

Figure 7.3. The-role of personal hygiene in preventing-pathogen spread in unsterilized environments.

Source: FasterCapital. (n.d.). *The Role of Personal Hygiene in Preventing Pathogen Spread in Unsterilized Environments*. FasterCapital.

7.1.3. Education and Awareness Programs on Personal Hygiene

Personal cleanliness is the best defense against waterborne disease, and education is a large—if occasionally apparently complex—part of making that defense effective. Projects tend to shake things up by staging community workshops, sprinkling informative tidbits into school curricula, and even providing brief tips on social media. These diverse methods encourage individuals to understand that microbes can be spread by contaminated water and poor cleanliness practices, encouraging them to make simple yet powerful measures for themselves. In most instances, where training speaks in the native language and makes references to cultural idiosyncrasies, the message regarding staying clean stays with the learner, silently echoing the same critical concepts without making it sound rote. Behavioral changes aren't so much about feeling better physically; they creep into the way groups think about hygiene in general. If people understand that bad hygiene can straightaway result in waterborne issues, they wash up more frequently, sometimes even making regular handwashing a societal standard. Local officials and familiar, culture-sensitive narratives—sometimes a little back and forth in how they are narrated—tend to generate increased interest and engagement. And, as identified in zoonotic disease management discussions (Rahman et al., 2020), learning how diseases leap from animals to humans can encourage individuals to become more proactive—all things considered, a minor adjustment that serves everyone well. Next is the encouragement of education regarding clean water, sanitation, and daily hygiene, collectively referred to as WASH programs. Studies indicate that when communities become enlightened about how safe drinking water, proper sanitation, and even proper hand hygiene are all interconnected, they're more likely to adopt measures that protect against frequent offenders such as *Giardia* and *Cryptosporidium* (Omarova et al., 2018). By publicizing these threats in a practical yet sometimes informal manner, these programs not only reduce the incidence of disease but also assist in the development of an elusive community resilience against future epidemics. Ultimately, such education sets the stage for healthier existence and improved overall quality even if the message must be repeated with minor setbacks along the way (Figure 7.4).

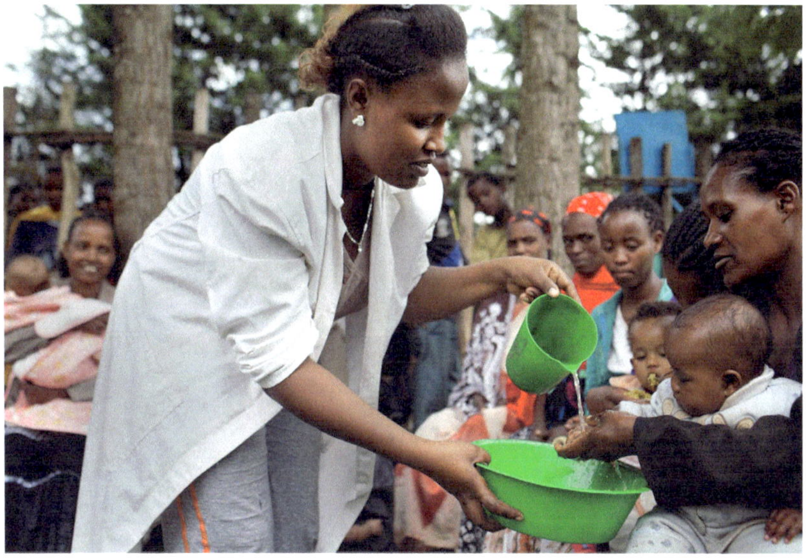

Figure 7.4. Hygiene promotion.

Source: International Medical Corps. (2017). *Hygiene Promotion.*

7.2. Community Hygiene Practices

Peoples usually confront the hygiene issues by relying on a combination of traditional knowledge and adaptable, occasionally improvised, methods. In times of crisis, such as disasters involving natural forces—individuals generally fall back on what they have been doing for generations instead of waiting for official assistance. Consider the tsunami in Aceh, 2004: residents promptly set to work by boiling water and even filtering it through fabric to ensure that they had clean drinking supplies. They also prioritized food safety and personal hygiene, a change that demonstrates real resilience and community action, something public health policy really cannot afford to overlook (Cipta et al., 2025). Research, in a number of instances, also indicates that Traditional Ecological Knowledge (TEK) has a large bearing on how communities maintain good health. This isn't intellectual mumbo-jumbo; it's about bringing indigenous eyes-on nature together with cultural wisdom to manage resources wisely. People tend to establish their own methods of keeping an eye on the environment and even utilize traditional remedies that sound, well, old-fashioned but really do the trick to reduce risky waterborne diseases. By doing so, they not only increase environmental sanitation but also weave a stronger social fabric, increasing trust and collective resilience (Suwono, 2024). As more individuals participate in daily hygiene habits, the entire community is likely to gain. People tend to adhere to health guidelines when they feel like active participants in the process, and knowing the importance of maintaining water sources and environments clean contributes to this attitude. Such participatory, community-wide mobilization has the promise, over a long-term horizon, of cleaning water and lowering the transmission of disease. Together with public health practitioners and local leadership, such campaigns can transform themselves into permanent behavior that can insulate communities against risk from waterborne diseases (Cipta et al., 2025; Suwono, 2024) (Figure 7.5).

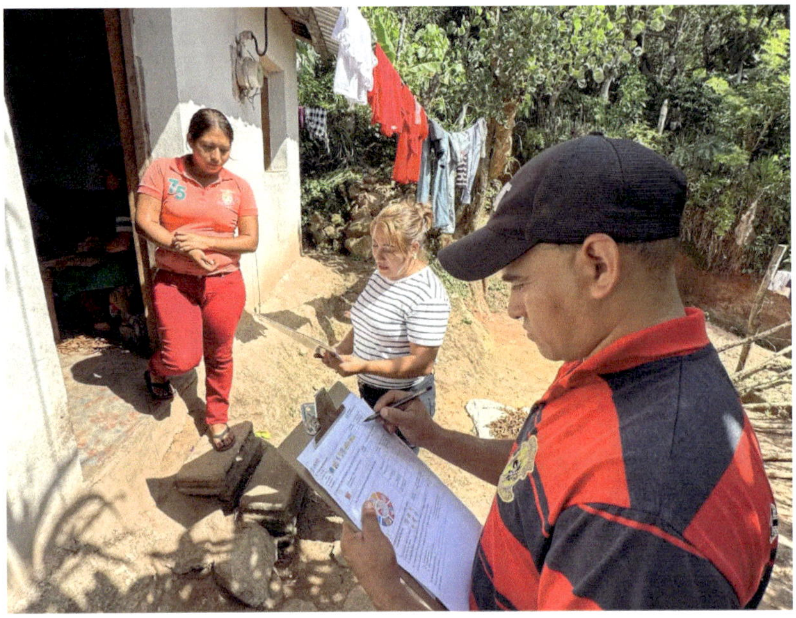

Figure 7.5. Hygiene promotion volunteers help make clean water count in communities.

Source: Water Mission. (2023). *Hygiene Promotion Volunteers Help Make Clean Water Count in Communities.*

7.2.1. Importance of Sanitation Facilities in Communities

Effective sanitation isn't a nicety, it's the key to keeping waterborne disease under control in communities. If clean facilities aren't provided, microbes are free to multiply, frequently igniting health problems on a massive scale. Installing effective waste disposal not only reduces disease but tends to raise the overall health of all those nearby. Most of the time, these arrangements provide a sanitary means of dealing with human waste, so water becomes less polluted. Without them, disease has simple routes to spread, and you can immediately appreciate how closely our daily cleanliness is connected to public health. Some studies, even some recent assessments of sanitation programs—indicate that improved facilities can push communities toward healthier practices in a more organic, nearly self-sustaining cycle. Sanitation is more than halting disease; it enhances the quality of life as well. Sanitary facilities preserve a person's dignity and privacy, particularly for vulnerable groups such as women and children who are most vulnerable. In the absence of sanitation, not only does physical health suffer but also community spirit, with people feeling and relating less positively. When communities rally their support behind good sanitation practices, they're not only battling disease, they're also creating a more equitable, more stable social fabric. Policymakers ought, in most instances, to integrate these facilities into community planning to address the wider social determinants of health. Otherwise, without such intelligent, customized solutions, the poverty cycle and poor health simply continue, highlighting the necessity of projects that suit each community's specific requirements (Rahman et al., 2020). Also, it's difficult to overlook the relationship between appropriate sanitation and the spread of diseases that leap from animals to humans. Experts note that more than 60% of the microbes that plague individuals regularly originate from animals; environmental circumstances have a lot to do with how these disease-causing agents are transmitted (Md. Rahman et al., 2020). Poor sanitation can exacerbate the interaction of individuals and animals, particularly in densely populated areas, inviting disease reservoirs to emerge. Solid sanitation strategies reduce these lethal contact points, providing a safeguard against transmission. A balanced strategy that combines sanitation with other public health interventions is essential to study the complex problems behind zoonotic disease. In the long term, investment in sanitation is not so much about short-term health solutions, it's about creating strong, resilient communities that can resist future outbreaks (Rahman et al., 2020).

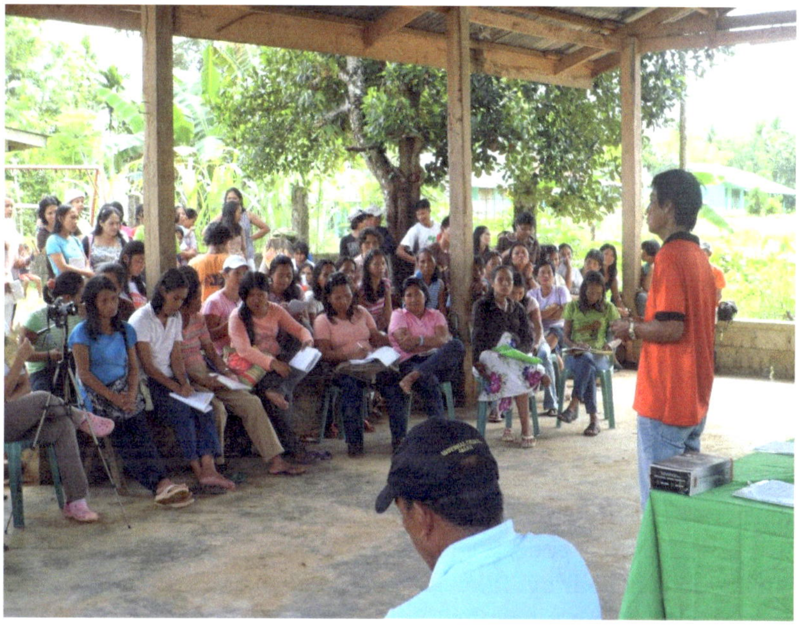

Source: https://blogger.googleusercontent.com/img/b/R29vZ2xl/AVvXsEgo-qf5a12U_QZhv7JWNSgKUnCzbxLX29FXdmWa1IakvImUQEuOvoKIZ8phrolYXdvPYlBE4XAN0Eg3jOozI6e5p44lWvt1JCFr3NQTQptmVuubmGOcN6txu4uJGfoA1UcA63vHfXcteUXL/s1600/Mr.+Albano,+Sanitary+Inspector+ talks+about+the+importance+of+sanitary+toilet+facilities+during+a+Family+Development+Seminar.jpg.

7.2.2. Waste Management and Its Impact on Water Quality

Waste disposal is a major factor in keeping our water clean and, by virtue of it, keeping everyone safe from diseases. Usually, when waste disposal is neglected, toxins from trash leach into surrounding waters, providing conditions where annoying pathogens can have a field day. This can be a particularly troublesome problem in areas with unreliable sanitation infrastructures. Poor waste habits not only drop harmful chemicals and poisons into leaves of water but also make warm nests for disease vectors, which subsequently raises the incidence of water-borne disease. More often than not, an effective plan that combines community education with actual policies that cut down on waste and promote recycling—appears totally indispensable. And with our constantly increasing food craving fueled by expanding populations, it's certain that farming practices, waste management, and their broader impacts on nature and health are all interlinked (Jason et al., 2019). Water quality, when it declines, straight increases the transmission of water-borne diseases, impacting small and large communities alike. Poor waste disposal is at the top of this list here, since the link between community health and environmental pressure is hardly a secret. Endless pollutants—from plastics to tiny microbes and miscellaneous chemicals—tend to find their way into our waterways, making it difficult to stay clean. As per the DPSIR framework, the interaction of all these forces (drivers, pressures, and effects on water bodies) heightens health issues, making focused action all the more necessary. Merging waste management with public health interventions may just relieve these pressures and improve overall results (Boelee et al., 2019). Even if it feels a little circuitous, these combined, practical measures really provide a means to combat the damaging impacts of contaminated water systems. Enhancing our strategy for waste management, quite honestly, could be the game-changer in preventing waterborne diseases. By cutting waste at its source and managing what they already have well, communities are able to limit the potential of water contamination enormously. New solutions, such as bioremediation or pretty sophisticated filtration processes—may transform the way we safeguard our water quality. Public health regulations supporting improved sanitation and hygiene on the other hand generally go along with cleaner water and less disease. It's really obvious that government agencies, nonprofit organizations, and communities themselves are going to have to work together to implement these strategies. Clean water and proper sanitation aren't so much about being clean; they're a genuine public health necessity. And with continuing population increase and intensive farming practices changing our world further, the reconsideration of waste management in terms of water quality appears more critical than ever before (Boelee et al., 2019; Jason et al., 2019).

7.2.3. Community-Led Initiatives for Improving Hygiene

Community-led initiatives have the power to ignite actual change in reducing waterborne diseases. Locals being involved in passing on good hygiene advice increases knowledge and even gives them a sense of ownership in keeping healthy. Take, for instance, local health workers holding workshops on sanitation, they demonstrate, in very explicit manners, that washing hands can prevent microbes from spreading. This is not only something that occurs in medical environments; the same concept easily applies to common neighborhoods. When people work in groups, they adhere to these routines, sort of validating that staying healthy isn't something one person does, it's something that all people share, which makes more resilient communities against waterborne issues (Glowicz et al., 2023). Sustaining sustainable hygiene routines truly relies on strategies that resonate with local culture and daily living. When hygiene messages are attuned to reflect local traditions, they resonate more naturally. Societies that have the opportunity to develop them usually sustain them because there are obvious gains—healthier families and cleaner environments, for example. By and large, concepts such as the One Health concept, which encourage us to remember that human, animal, and environmental health are intertwined, provide a bigger perspective. Mixing the insights and resources from various sections of the community will complete the gaps in knowledge and materials, establishing a solid groundwork for defense against waterborne diseases. All the same, ensuring these projects remain functional requires that they have continued support and space for expansion. Local committees or teams established to oversee hygiene habits keep everyone in line, even if the discussion gets slightly unbalanced at times. These small groups can identify a hygiene issue or two and quickly assemble the help required. Partnering with schools, local businesses, and health organizations also diffuses the message in a slightly off-the-cuff manner, creating a sort of day-to-day health savvy. Ultimately, this shared, imperfect effort not only reduces waterborne disease but also enables communities to become empowered to manage their own well-being on a day-to-day basis (Glowicz et al., 2023) (Figure 7.6).

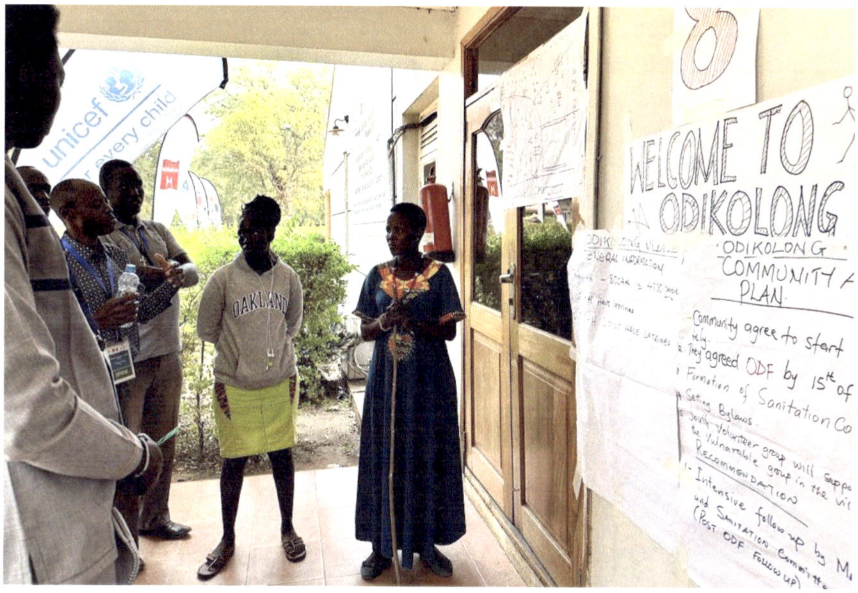

Figure 7.6. Community-led total sanitation archives.

Source: The MENTOR Initiative. (2023). *Community-Led Total Sanitation Archives.*

7.3. Water Treatment and Hygiene

We can't overstate how crucial clean water is for maintaining the health of people. Water from the outside or the ground tends to have stuff in it that isn't wanted, so ensuring it's okay to drink makes a big difference. Processes such as chlorinating, filtering, and allowing particles to settle remove the dirty things that make us sick. Consider chlorine, for instance – it tends to reduce bacteria such as *Campylobacter,* a prevalent food poisoning culprit in children and adults. Proper hygiene paired with these treatment measures reduces the chance of disease transmission within homes and community locations, and emphasizes that chemical solutions and physical solutions must be used together in order to provide everyone with access to safe water (Same & Tamma, 2018). Clean water is not just a matter of treatment procedures; it is also a matter of the way we behave toward it. Individuals should understand that maintaining cleanliness – from washing hands to keeping common areas clean – prevents harmful waste from ruining water quality. In a majority of situations, simple habits such as frequent washing and handling food correctly help prevent stomach worms and parasites that make you ill. Public health strategies should embrace these lessons, particularly for persons who may lack consistent access to adequate sanitation or learn all about the safe water habits. That repeated connection between intelligent hygiene and water treatment truly makes them central components of an effective system against disease (Daniel et al., 2018). Observe how water treatment and cleanliness practices appear near locations where individuals swim or congregate close to bodies of water. When water goes untreated, one can observe clearly the connection between forgoing correct hygiene and the opportunity for nasty microbes to breed – something that obviously increases the public health hazard. Outbreak stories related to untreated recreational water suggest that the whole spectrum of bugs gets its chance when we lower our guard. Individuals who disregard health notices or dive into fun even when they feel off not only risk becoming sicker themselves but may also transmit issues to others. Therefore, pools and beach areas within the local setting ought to have their focus on cleanliness, complement treatment schedules with hygiene advice, and enforce regulations to assist in keeping waterborne diseases at bay (Daniel et al., 2018; Same & Tamma, 2018).

7.3.1. Methods of Water Purification

Clean water is the pulse of public health – in the absence of it, communities are open to waterborne disease that can quickly spread. Individuals depend on all sorts of methods, ranging from simple physical filtration to more complex chemical solutions, each one keeping busy of ridding water of bothersome pathogens.

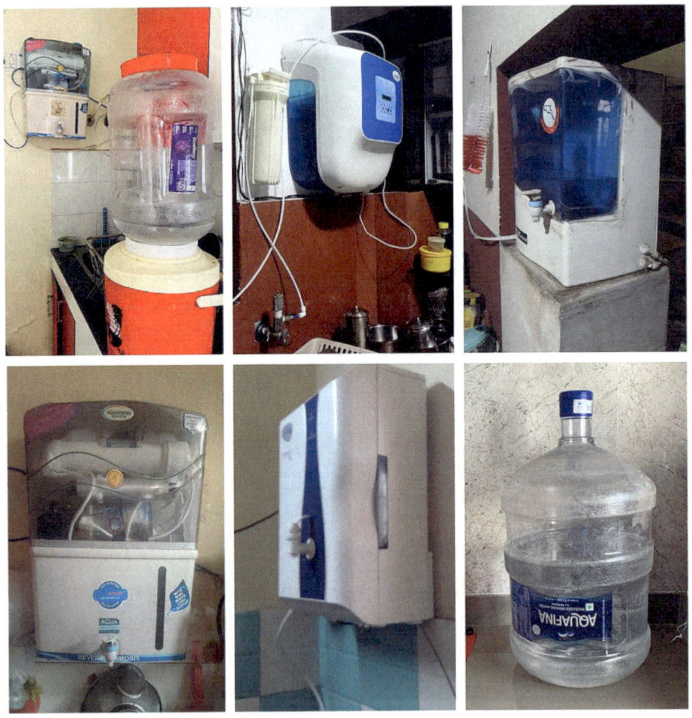

Figure 7.7. Water purification methods.

Source: https://en.wikipedia.org/wiki/File:Home_water_filters,_water_purifiers,_and_bottled_water_in_India.jpg

Consider, for instance, simple methods such as sand and activated carbon (AC) filters; such age-old favorites catch sediments and some pollutants with minute pores that allow the cleaner water to pass through. In most regions of the globe where state-of-the-art technology is not easily available, such basic solutions serve as effective alternatives for improving water safety. And occasionally, combining with ultraviolet (UV) light treatment, which disrupts the DNA of viruses and bacteria—gives that added oomph against disease threats. Chemical treatments continue to play a central role in water purification, with chlorination being a notable example. To summarize, chlorine is utilized to kill dangerous microorganisms to make water drinkable, although it gets problematic when undesirable byproducts are created; that is, monitoring chemical levels is essential. Nowadays, there has been a trend to combine ozonation with advanced oxidation processes (AOPs)—methods that complement each other in degrading organic materials. Ozone is quite cool because not only does it disinfect, but it also accelerates the breakdown of organic material, resolving issues of residual chemical residues. In most instances, the implementation of these chemical techniques is vital, particularly in regions fighting outbreaks of waterborne diseases, as evidenced by the worldwide effort toward improved sanitation against dangers such as giardiasis, which is commonly associated with contaminated water sources (Alexander et al., 2019). This multi-layered approach truly showcases how changing water treatment technologies ensure public health levels are maintained. New technologies are also rising to the challenge of transforming water purification. Membrane filtration systems, such as reverse osmosis (RO), are now favored because they have a talent for eliminating a wide range of contaminants, from disease-causing organisms to dissolved solids. Urban areas, which grapple with intricate water quality challenges, particularly find these systems helpful. And then there is nanotechnology; small, specially designed materials can now be used to remove a particular contaminant with specificity, providing a less invasive means of treatment. Increasing global need for clean water continues to escalate; these new approaches are becoming instrumental tools (Figure 7.7). Integration of these new methods with customary strategies reinforces joint action against waterborne disease and protection of community (OECD, 2020).

7.3.2. Role of Chlorination and Filtration in Disease Prevention

Clean drinking water is the foundation of public health and, to summarize, serves to keep waterborne problems from getting a foothold. Most communities make do with chlorination—a tried-and-true method—when it comes to addressing problematic organisms. Rather than frame it as a formal technical procedure, consider chlorination as a mechanism to disrupt the internal functioning of unwanted microbes such as bacteria, viruses, and protozoa, which otherwise, if left to themselves, can cause significant health issues. And chlorine isn't only effective for an instant; its residual action continues combating contamination even when water passes through distribution systems. This additional barrier of protection becomes particularly valuable where water systems are less dependable or more susceptible to contamination. Filtration, however, joins forces with chlorination in a beautifully synergistic manner. It removes from water particulates, disease agents, and other impurities by physical means. Sometimes this is accomplished with nothing more complicated than a sand filter; at others, more sophisticated membrane technologies enter the picture. These systems assist in minimizing the transmission of diseases brought about by recalcitrant organisms such as *Giardia* and *Cryptosporidium* that, in the majority of instances, don't recover with conventional treatments. By eliminating bits that could be hiding places for pathogens, filtration ensures not only that the water is chemically treated but also that it is freed of remaining debris. This method is especially crucial in much of the low- and middle-income world where access to safe drinking water and adequate sanitation is always a challenge. When you combine chlorination with filtration, you have a sort of tag-team effect that really emphasizes the concept of attacking water safety from every direction. There is an inherent synergy at play here that complements nicely with the concept of water, sanitation, and hygiene (WASH) all dovetailing together, an ecosystem in which all parts support each other. Improving both water quality and sanitation infrastructure often tends to increase the overall performance of these treatment methods. Even some research has it that addressing water management in increments may not be enough when it comes to disease prevention. Thus, building strong frameworks at both community and institutional levels is crucial for long-term success (Omarova et al., 2018; Shapiro et al., 2019). It seems clear that addressing all the connected components is key to reducing waterborne health risks effectively (Figure 7.8).

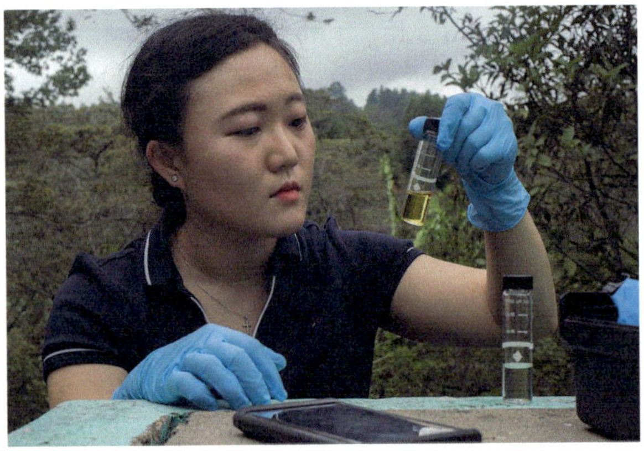

Figure 7.8. Checking chlorine level of the local water source.

Source: Wikimedia Commons. (n.d.). *Checking Chlorine Level of the Local Water Source.*

7.3.3. Importance of Regular Water Quality Testing

Water quality testing is important to safeguard our health and prevent waterborne diseases, particularly in areas where contamination is a serious concern. Routine tests provide valuable information regarding microbes, chemicals, and other uglies that intrude into our drinking water. We would usually find a correlation between compromised water quality and outbreaks of waterborne diseases such as cholera and typhoid – issues that, in the majority of instances, have a tendency to affect less dependable infrastructure-equipped places. Rapid monitoring and timely response such as Nichols et al. (2018) discusses can significantly trim down both rates of sickness and mortality attributed to contaminated water. Establishing a regular schedule for these tests isn't only about catching outbreaks in the moment, it's also going along with a longer game plan for health. Where there has been war or conflict or just where things are a little tough, having working water systems properly chlorinated has been known to reduce diseases spread through water significantly. Findings in Haar et al. (2023) indicate that communities with well-established water stations ultimately experience fewer severe diarrhea and other related cases. This type of checking extends beyond detecting contamination to also demanding having the proper treatment and distribution arrangements. When water testing that is simple combines with common sanitation practices, it brings us back to the realization that basic hygiene truly contributes to disease control. Ensuring that individuals are provided with water that is monitored and treated, even if the method becomes a little patchy at times, creates a layered public health defense, particularly where medical care is in short supply. Moreover, regular water testing isn't just about instant health victories, it sort of indicates a proactive attitude toward taking care of our planet, as well. The data collected can assist in informing plans to enhance water infrastructure and management, feeding into sustainable objectives, in general. By monitoring pollution and how climate change disrupts our water supplies, leaders can direct investments into improved purification techniques and improved sewage systems. These actions are quite crucial to reducing risks associated with anticipated climate changes as recorded in Nichols et al. (2018), which could even increase waterborne diseases. Overall, routine water quality monitoring goes far beyond checking compliance boxes; it sets a foundational stone for developing healthier communities and more resilient ecosystems (Figure 7.9).

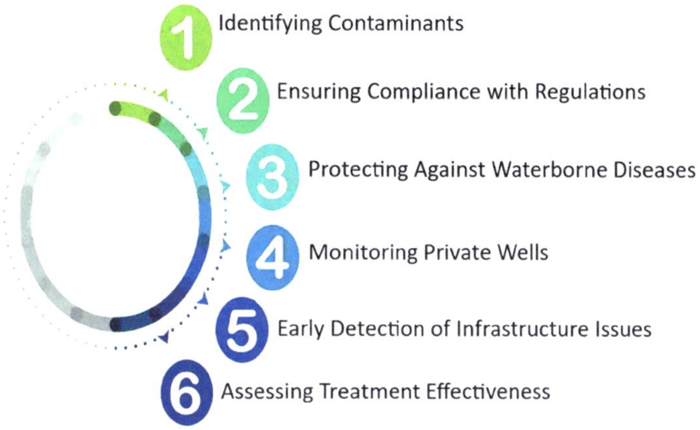

Figure 7.9. The-role of regular water testing in preventing diseases.

Source: FasterCapital. (n.d.). *The Role of Regular Water Testing in Preventing* Diseases.

7.4. Hygiene Education and Public Health Campaigns

Recently, however, public health campaigns appear to focus more on hygiene education, truly emphasizing the ways in which daily habits can combat waterborne diseases. They've discovered that sometimes simple tricks, such as hand washing or safe food preparation—reduce the chances of transmitting infection. Rather than sticking to a rigid schedule, campaign leaders shake things up by employing workshops, informal community collections, and other participatory methods to address various groups, sometimes repeating messages to make them stick. Research, in the majority of instances, indicates that when individuals become enlightened about the connection between cleanliness and health, there is a significant reduction in waterborne diseases (Todd, 2020). It's not all about individual habits, either. Hygiene classes merge into larger concepts that consider the overall picture, such as making sure clean water is accessible, good sanitation and even how the waste is managed, to improve public health. In a sense, putting these environmental perspectives with daily hygiene tips together explains why water quality is really important to health, particularly in communities that are under-served. Frequently, programs designed to reduce pathogen contact in water promptly remind us that being careful about our cleanliness can save a life. By encouraging an holistic understanding of what hygiene is, these strategies make environments safer, healthier spaces, even if, sometimes, the message comes full circle (Boelee et al., 2019). Cooperation, be it between government agencies or non-government organizations, is a key factor in making such campaigns linger. In general, when people put resources together, exchange know-how, and exchange best practices, the effect of public health initiatives gets a much-needed boost, even in regions where health services and facilities are, in a manner of speaking, behind schedule." Local perspectives assist in framing these campaigns such that the messaging feels appropriate for the community, so that efforts toward improved hygiene are not merely a matter of top-down imposition. When examining current investments in hygiene education, it is apparent that diligently organized, partner-facilitated initiatives can reduce waterborne diseases and improve overall global health (Boelee et al., 2019; Todd, 2020) (Figure 7.10).

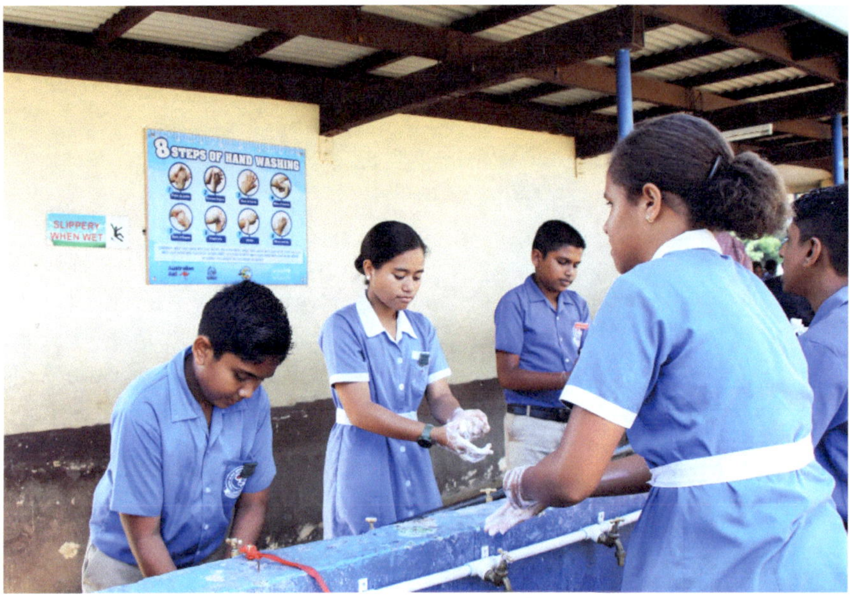

Figure 7.10. Promoting a culture of hygiene among children.

Source: UNICEF Pacific. (n.d.). *Promoting a Culture of Hygiene Among Children.*

7.4.1. Strategies for Effective Hygiene Education

Effective hygiene education begins with combining down-to-earth ideas that truly resonate with individuals from all walks of life. Simple programs emphasizing hand washing—with soap and water or even a good sanitizer, can significantly reduce how waterborne disease is transmitted. Occasionally, a brief campaign demonstrating just how easy washing your hands is does the trick, particularly when combined with images or hands-on sessions. It makes everything understandable, understandable enough that common people adhere to the habits. Periodic check-ups and some adjustments here and there keep the message new and helpful. Local leaders and health workers, for instance, tend to establish personal relationships that make it simpler for all to embrace these simple hygiene tips (Rao, 2024). Considering hygiene education from a wide angle involves understanding that communities are confronted with an entire array of issues. In most instances, it's necessary to understand that marginalized groups, particularly individuals with disabilities—tend to encounter actual obstacles when attempting to access WASH services. Bringing everyone along by modifying teaching approaches can assist in bridging those gaps, making individuals receive the information and assistance they require. Training facilitators to learn and work with special challenges contributes to a more inclusive atmosphere. And there's the dynamic climate, too; when changes in the environment disrupt water quality or availability, encouraging simple adaptive behaviors becomes increasingly important to forestall disease transmission. Ongoing conversations with vulnerable individuals assist in developing the resilience and adaptability needed as conditions change (Wilbur et al., 2024). Establishing real community ownership of hygiene habits is important as well. As individuals become engaged in shaping, implementing, and reviewing hygiene programs, they are much more likely to adopt the practice. Community initiatives such as establishing community hygiene committees can generate the natural sharing of ideas and resources, and group efforts become even more productive. Such grass-roots activity not only increases individual confidence but also creates a network that sustains good practice in the long term. In addition to that, with technology, even something as mundane as a cell phone app or social media post—word can really get out in unfamiliar ways. Ultimately, building an enduring culture of cleanliness requires work, consistent support, and a steadfast dedication to public health education (Rao, 2024) (Figure 7.11).

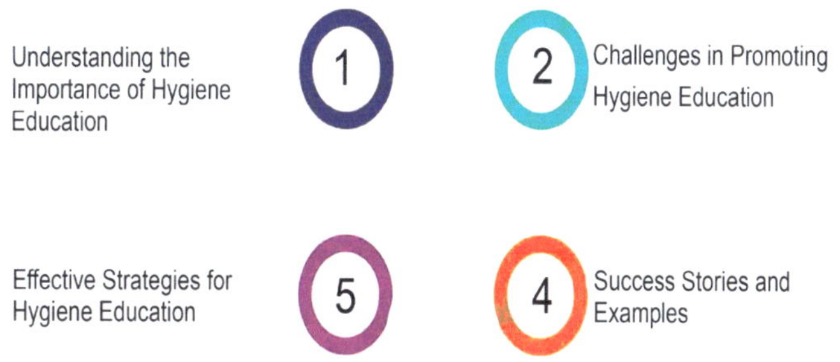

Figure 7.11. Empowering communities.

Source: FasterCapital. (n.d.). *Empowering Communities.*

7.4.2. Role of Government and NGOs in Promoting Hygiene

Encouraging cleanliness habits is a serious matter when battling water-borne diseases, and government organizations as well as NGOs get into the act here. Governments start by laying down regulations and fundamental directives that maintain day-to-day sanitation under control; they don't only make these directives—their large-scale publicity campaigns about them also target areas of neighborhoods where water problems appear more frequently. They maintain public health by overseeing waste systems and water sources, attempting to nip would-be contamination in the bud. It's remarkable how much we rely on groundwater, a fact that barely receives the attention it should (Gr Jönwall et al., 2020). NGOs, meanwhile, jump headfirst into community work, collaborating with locals to disseminate practical know-how regarding hygiene. They also combine training sessions with sharing of resources so that easy, enduring practices can truly take hold at the grassroots level. They have a special focus on groups who may otherwise fall through the cracks, such as women and children, to spread the hygiene message. By organizing informal health discussions and assisting in obtaining clean water, NGOs not only inform but also empower individuals to be responsible for their own health, which reduces waterborne disease—sometimes with a few bumps along the way (Nzung, 2018). When governments and NGOs collude, things work far better when they do it together than apart. Governments can contribute money and even put down some heavy infrastructure, while NGOs provide local knowledge and on-the-ground networks that are less formal but do the trick. It is this combination of top-down assistance and grassroots expertise that weaves together a multi-layered response to waterborne issues. In the majority of instances, such an alliance, as imperfect as some of its execution, demonstrates a co-responsibility among official institutions and social groups working toward safer water and improved sanitation in the locations that most require them (Gr Jönwall et al., 2020) (Figure 7.12).

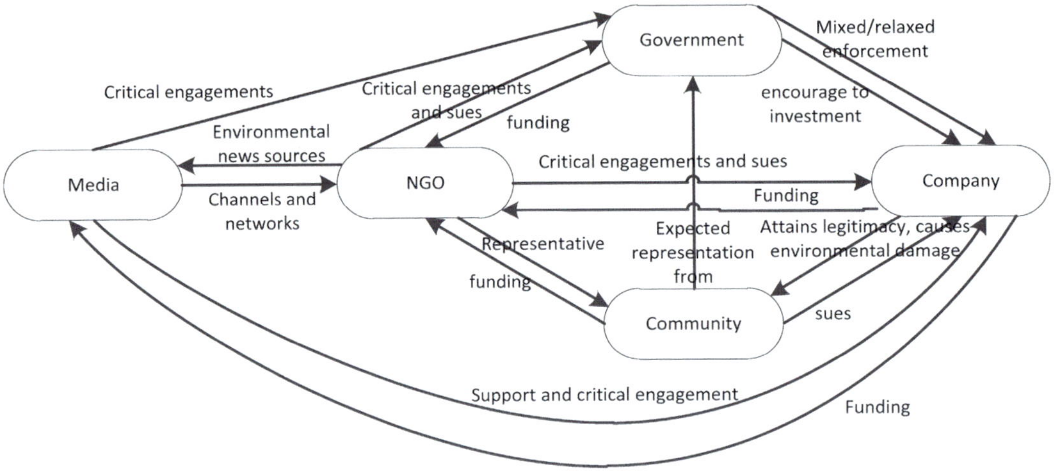

Figure 7.12. Sanitation sector actors and roles played by NGOs – opportunities for engagement.

Source: Wichianrak J, Khan T, Teh D, Dellaportas S. Critical Perspectives of NGOs on Voluntary Corporate Environmental Reporting: Thai Public Listed Companies. *Sustainability*. 2023; 15(7):6195. https://doi.org/10.3390/su15076195

7.4.3. Case Studies of Successful Hygiene Campaigns

Hygiene initiatives that have been implemented in the recent past are truly making their impact felt in how waterborne disease is addressed. In countries such as Haiti and Mozambique, where cholera erupted, officials began monitoring diseases more closely and pulled out all the stops for water, sanitation, and hygiene (WASH) services, throwing in oral vaccination campaigns to boot. The figures dropped significantly, which tends to indicate that combining various strategies can prove to be magical in crisis-ridden environments (Mercogliano et al., 2025). In Nigeria, it is more of a community-based atmosphere. Locals have come forward by enhancing hygiene and operating hands-on educational sessions regarding day-to-day hygiene. Certain case studies support that these measures not only reduce short-term problems such as cholera and typhoid but also establish a sustainable resistance to water pollution. Engaging citizens in policy reform and offering on-the-ground training appears to lay a strong foundation for keeping water clean, ultimately reducing the risk of diseases (Vosa et al., 2025). It also seems that such hygiene campaigns work best when tailored to local practices and environments. Consider, for instance, the Kumbh Mela festival in India—swift surveillance and rapid action were able to catch potential outbreaks in their infancy. This type of outcome tends to highlight the value of adapting hygiene promotion to cultural events to gain true community acceptance. Combining known public health messages with the local culture, in the majority of instances, enhances the success of these campaigns, illustrating that a sensitive, context-informed strategy is able to confront public health issues successfully (Mercogliano et al., 2025).

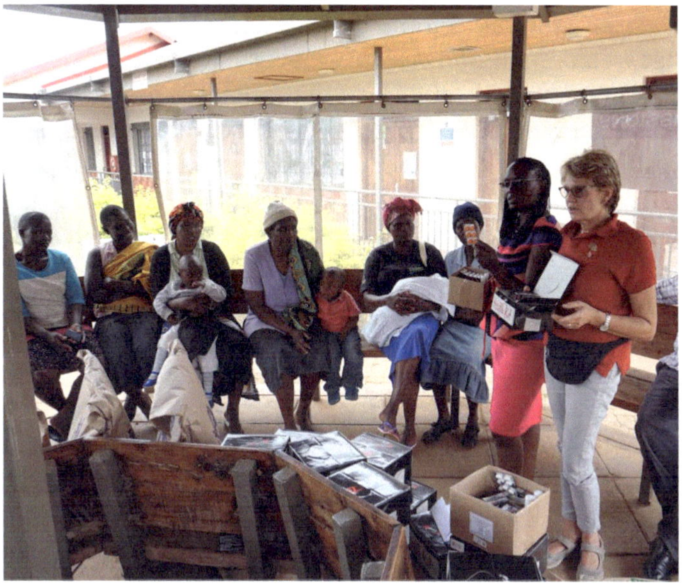

Source: https://familycare.or.ke/wp-content/uploads/health-and-hygiene/Talk-on-Hygiene-for-Support-groups.jpg.

7.5. Challenges in Implementing Hygiene Practices

Often, encouraging good hygiene ends up getting derailed by a combination of system issues and daily routines, particularly in areas where waterborne disease is prevalent. Clean water, for example, is a large obstacle; public health initiatives can become derailed if the region doesn't have good sanitation or good water treatment. When we are talking about the Global South, we usually consider that it doesn't have a sufficient amount of clean water. And therefore, the ground is set for the development of dangerous microbes. When you think about it, not meeting these minimum requirements for hygiene means any attempt to reduce disease may not quite find its target (Jamie et al., 2024). And in addition, the perception that people have of cleanliness can additionally slow things down, and this illustrates just why community education and outreach are necessary. Socio-economic status also heavily influences whether communities and individuals are able to implement suggested hygiene routines. In a lot of under-served places, even accessing basic things like soap or sanitizer is a challenge, and in doing so, this usually results in substitute practices that inadvertently increase disease risk. Public health officials, in most instances, must operate within these economic constraints—some studies even cite that many diseases are attributed to both shared and individual water systems that lack the care they require since funds are limited (Jasen et al., 2024). Thus, knowing these economic factors in depth is paramount if interventions are to prove effective while also being sustainable, leading overall community health to rise. And then there's the matter of rules and regulations, which adds another spanner to the works. In many parts of the world, particularly where waterborne disease is rampant, the regulations on hygiene and water treatment either don't exist or aren't being enforced adequately. Without effective legislation, checking on water quality and sanitation tends to be inadequate, allowing pathogens space to thrive. Rising numbers of outbreaks linked to inadequately regulated water systems remind us, rather graphically, that weak regulations can have dreadful consequences (Jasen et al., 2024). All things apart, establishing and implementing effective hygiene regulations is essential in preventing the spread of waterborne diseases, an achievement best attained by combining regulation with intimate collaboration between governments, local communities, and other organizations.

7.5.1. Socioeconomic Factors Affecting Hygiene

Clean water and a good spot to wash usually depend on how much money people have. In most low-income communities, not much cash means people generally can't get enough clean water or consistent sanitation, and this deficiency not only prevents regular handwashing but also increases the likelihood of contracting waterborne diseases. Households that just can't get hold of clean water, for instance, end up experiencing more episodes of diarrheal diseases – issues that particularly affect children. With not enough basic health tips available, most individuals simply don't realize the real significance of being clean; so it's not only a matter of money but also of having the know-how. All of this is made even more difficult in regions that are addressing issues such as climate changes and rapid urban sprawl (Stenberg et al., 2017). Unstable employment and low wages also disrupt the way people live from day to day, making hygiene issues even more difficult. In areas with high unemployment, you tend to see overcrowded housing combined with patchy waste management, which makes fairly unsanitary conditions. These living conditions not only make it more difficult for personal hygiene routines to take hold but also appear to permit waterborne pathogens to flourish. Where a person lives may trap them in a vicious cycle of poverty and disease—imagine housing that exposes residents to the extra vulnerability of standing water carrying cloudy, contaminant-laden water into buildings during severe weather storms. This combination of economic hardship and ecological blunders most often requires steps in public policy to resolve these problems and enhance hygiene in general (Jonathan et al., 2014). Lastly, whether people or entire communities can remain committed to plain hygiene habits all comes down largely to how well they are educated and have access to medical care. Low education in most regions may mean individuals won't necessarily have an appreciation of how important a matter it is to practice daily hand washing or proper food handling in staying at bay from waterborne diseases. This lack of knowledge generally serves to promote not even minimum sanitation measures being observed, and with good health treatment generally also coinciding with more income, impoverished groups will mostly find additional difficulties when in need of medical consult or care regarding hygiene issues. Therefore, these populations not only are exposed to a greater spread of waterborne diseases but also receive poorer overall health outcomes, making it all the more necessary to dismantle these educational and economic barriers for improved hygiene and health outcomes (Stenberg et al., 2017).

7.5.2. Cultural Beliefs and Practices Related to Hygiene

Cultural practices determine the way people get clean in ways that may not be immediately clear. Many groups combine ancient custom with concepts regarding health, such that practices like washing one's hands before a meal—something that feels all but automatic in so many communities—becomes a way in which people tie themselves to the people around them in a bond of cleanliness. In most societies, this has little to do with individual health. It's also a means by which communities can sign their history and religious origins, even when those traditions may not exactly fit with current guidelines. Sometimes, if health messages bypass these long-established practices, the outcomes can be, well, not as effective, illustrating that campaigns must communicate in a manner that honors people's cultural seasoning but still urges safer, newer practices. Around the world, conflicting perceptions of hygiene produce highly divergent health outcomes. In some places, traditional thoughts about water , and about the way it must be treated – can cause people to be shy about experimenting with new sanitation solutions, even though the science is on their side. Much of the time, this type of hesitation arises because of a combination of misinformation and experience that is remembered, and, quite frankly, sometimes just a little old-fashioned community gossip. You may observe a town with restricted exposure to fresh water depending on word-of-mouth customs, which by extension can sometimes nourish additional concern over waterborne diseases. Being able to speak freely with local authorities and locals, in general, is how trust is established and how health measures that seem authentic and knowledgeable regarding local values are implemented. Religion and spirituality complicate, and occasionally assist—this entire hygiene scenario. Most religions do have practices that emphasize cleanliness as part of maintaining spiritual purity, which can support attempts to encourage good hygiene. On the other hand, how these practices are interpreted can differ significantly, sometimes conflicting with contemporary health regulations. For instance, some long-standing religious washing rituals, although rich in cultural significance, may not meet all the requirements of contemporary health codes. Closing that gap involves offering education that, while it honors ancient traditions, also clearly demonstrates the advantages of employing evidence-based practices. This balancing act is not one for the faint of heart; it takes a little bit of negotiating, some surprising halts, and in certain situations, even a little bit of typo here and there—reminding us that marrying tradition and modernity is as much art as it is science.

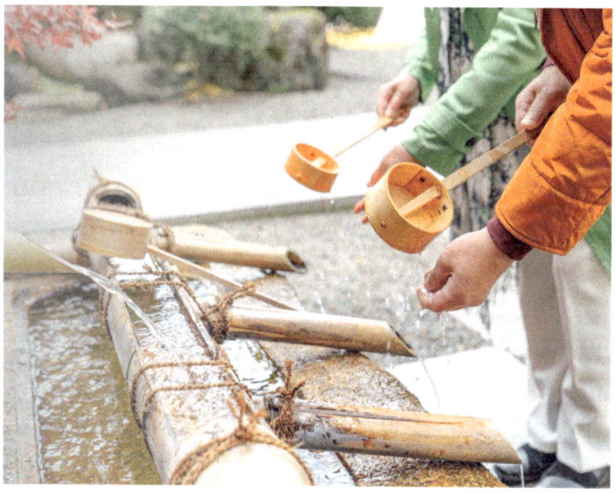

Source: Sterillium. (n.d.). *Hygiene Customs Around the World.*

7.5.3. Barriers to Access to Clean Water and Sanitation

Accessing clean water and proper sanitation is a true challenge in most areas, where meager finances and few resources are in the way. Weaker communities experience a double blow—too little money both delays government initiatives and inhibits local efforts to improve water, sanitation, and hygiene infrastructure. In areas where even basic infrastructure is lacking, health hazards rise up, triggering increased instances of waterborne diseases. It's not only a matter of busted pipes and limited facilities; lots of people lack sufficient information on appropriate hygiene, too, and that keeps the vicious cycle going. Studies for the most part find that if local officials, NGOs, and government agencies sit down together, sharing resources and creating daily awareness about improved sanitation, things begin to change. These types of collaborations, while perhaps not perfect, have the effect of easing funding problems and rolling out answers that really make sense for the local environment and keep disease surges at bay. Geography gets in on the act too of making clean water inaccessible. Rural or remote locations mean sheer distances where many individuals simply can't have a steady supply of secure water. Too often, the poor condition of local transport infrastructure and systems only exacerbates the issue—water delivery sometimes fails even before it leaves the source. On top of that, changes in the environment, such as those caused by climate change, can tighten water supplies even further, further complicating matters. In most instances, communities that invest in education about water conservation and simple sanitation fare a little better. Small, grassroots projects that encourage sustainable methods and involve everyone in the equation can gradually chip away at these obstacles, making it progressively simpler over time to reduce disease spread through polluted water. Added on top of physical obstacles are cultural and social elements that complicate access further. Local tradition, customary beliefs, and even ingrained gender roles can influence why and how water and sanitation facilities are utilized. For example, it's often women, and sometimes even girls—who shoulder the heavy burden of collecting water, a task that can cut into their schooling and chances at work. In many cases, you'll see girls missing class to fetch water, which not only drags down their academic performance but also leaves them more exposed to health risks. Community-based programs that engage individuals in decision-making can assist in infusing a sense of ownership and applicability into water and hygiene initiatives. When programs explain simple hygiene in a manner that is appropriate to local customs, the outcomes can take hold. By repairing these social deficits, stakeholders can create a more inclusive setting that improves health as a whole and gradually reduces the incidence of waterborne diseases.

SUMMARY

Inadequate water hygiene can trigger a massive outbreak of waterborne diseases. If sanitation is not stringent enough, things get out of hand fast—microbes ride free and disease escalates. Some of the newer indicators, such as those strange microbiological signatures, indicate that we seriously need to tidy up our ways. There was this research in the Russian Federation which cited that as much as 70% of acute intestinal infections are not of known causes (Trukhina et al., 2022); this type of fact really cries out for stronger pathogen control in water bodies. Monitoring these markers more closely will help to limit the risk and protect people who are particularly at risk. It's difficult to exaggerate how extensively water quality, hygiene, and public health are intertwined. Proper sanitation not only appears pleasing on chapter; it reduces the likelihood of transmission of unpleasant pathogens that play havoc with our digestive tracts. Consider the function of entities such as *Escherichia coli* and enterococci—those indicators mark fecal pollution and serve to eliminate possible infections. When everyone abides by concrete rules, the chances of large outbreaks decrease significantly, demonstrating that simple hygiene habits seriously keep public health dangers at bay. Even recent studies suggest that by maintaining clean water systems, communities can anticipate and avoid future outbreaks (Nigro & Muselli, 2023). Overall, having a good understanding of how hygiene prevents waterborne diseases is essential to long-term public health. Sound hygiene habits don't only break short-term threats; they also lay the groundwork for healthier futures. There's wide agreement among experts that water safety regulations are in need of some drastic renovations, so investing more in hygiene education and improved infrastructure is a well-played gamble. Ultimately, this multi-faceted strategy can stem the infection cycle and make a significant impact on community health. And, in addition, specialized study programs, particularly in clinical practice—again show just how vital proper hygiene is in preventing infections (Trukhina et al., 2022; Nigro & Muselli, 2023).

When you consider hygiene and how it prevents waterborne diseases, a good picture emerges. Keeping everything clean simply reduces the microbes that tend to find their way into water supplies, resulting in fewer cases of diseases such as cholera and dysentery. In most instances, communities with inadequate water treatment depend on rigorous cleanliness regimens to provide a safer environment. Educating individuals on how to wash their hands and how to get rid of waste is not only a temporary solution, it creates the type of long-term health gains that specialists have been advocating for. In general terms, these sorts of information campaigns and community engagement on a long-term basis combine to create a wide, solid protect against sickness. Taking it further, there's another aspect of this topic that connects how cleanliness is handled with social and economic factors. Poverty-stricken areas are more likely to be affected by water-related disease, which indicates that hygiene is not necessarily about clean water, it's connected to education, local resources, and local decision-making. In this instance, César et al. (2024) explains that education programs tailored to the local community can make a huge difference in people's understanding of the need to be clean in order to keep disease away. Additionally, good local leadership tends to facilitate easier roll-out of these cleanliness practices and establish a sort of informal structure wherein communities would be more likely to maintain their sanitary practices. The trickle-down effects of enhanced hygiene go far and wide. In addition to preventing disease outbreaks, improved sanitation can help create a healthier community and even spur economic growth. Sanz-Fernández et al. (2023) is one case in point; it explores practical solutions to monitor cleanliness in agricultural settings, suggesting that similar solutions may have application to larger health initiatives as well. Many of these steps toward preventing diseases also reduce healthcare costs because there are fewer individuals who require treatment for issues that could otherwise be prevented. Short answer: when healthy habits are integrated into daily life, they don't just guard our well-being, they also help set the stage for economic stability over the long term and an improved ability to deal with health issues that lie ahead (Dhaliwal et al., 2010).

KEY TERMS FROM THIS CHAPTER

Community education
Contaminated water sources
Disease prevention
Disease-causing agents
Environmental pressure
Hands-on educational sessions
Health recommendations
Hygiene practices
Public health education,
Reverse osmosis (RO)
Solid sanitation strategies
WASH interventions
Community-based atmosphere
Contemporary health codes
Disease vectors
Economic constraints
Food handling
Health guidelines
Hygiene advice
Personal cleanliness
Public health interventions
Society for Healthcare Epidemiology (SHEA)
Treatment facilities

CLOSER LOOK

HYGIENE IN PREVENTING WATERBORNE DISEASES

Hygiene is important in the prevention of waterborne diseases because it helps curb the transmission of pathogens through fecal-oral route and polluted water supplies. Proper handwashing, safe food preparation, and proper access to clean water and sanitation amenities are important aspects to reducing the risk of these infections.

Key hygiene practices for waterborne disease prevention:

1. Safe Water Practices:

   i. **Boiling or Purifying Water:** Boiling water for a minimum of one minute (longer at altitudes above sea level) or using a filter or purifier kills harmful pathogens.

   ii. **Proper Water Storage:** Keep water in clean, covered containers to avoid contamination by insects, soil, or other contaminants.

   iii. **Avoidance of Contaminated Water:** Do not swallow water during swimming in pools, hot tubs, or natural water bodies and do not drink tap water or water from natural water bodies in high-risk zones.

2. Hand Hygiene:

   i. **Regular Hand Washing:** Wash hands with soap and clean water before meals, after using the toilet, and after touching animals or excreta.

   ii. **Handwashing Facilities:** Think about providing “tippy taps” or using other inventive techniques to promote and make handwashing possible, particularly in situations with low availability of clean water.

3. Safe Food Handling:

   i. **Avoid Eating Raw or Undercooked Food:** Raw and undercooked food can carry pathogens that can cause waterborne diseases.

   ii. **Proper Food Storage:** Cover food and keep it in the refrigerator to prevent contamination.

   iii. **Avoid Street Food:** Street food is often prepared with unhygienic practices and may be contaminated.

4. Sanitation and Waste Disposal:

   I. **Use Sanitary Facilities:** Properly dispose of human waste using toilets and sewage systems to prevent water contamination.

   Ii. **Avoid Open Defecation:** Open defecation can contaminate water sources and spread pathogens.

5. Personal Cleanliness:

   I. **Regular Bathing:** Bathing regularly helps prevent skin infections and other health problems.

- **Ii. Clean Teeth and Hair:** Regular oral hygiene and hair washing are important for overall health and hygiene.

6. Community Engagement:

- **i. Educate Communities:** Encourage the practice of hygiene measures and proper water use to limit waterborne disease spread.
- **ii. Community-Level Interventions:** Institute community-level programs such as water purification, proper waste management, and health education to reduce the transmission of these diseases.

By giving these hygiene habits a high priority, people and communities can greatly lower the risk of getting and spreading waterborne diseases, enhancing general public health and well-being.

References

1. Haar, R., Abdelrahman, S., Muzzall, E., Aladhan, I., Shobak, K., Kawas, M. R., Aksh, A., Blair, A. H., Reingold, A., & AlMhawish, N. (2023). Water and war: The effect of functioning chlorinated water stations in reducing waterborne diseases during conflict in northwest Syria, 2017-2021. *PLOS global public health*, *3*(12), e0002696. https://doi.org/10.1371/journal.pgph.0002696 (accessed on 14 May 2025).
2. Amirian, E. S. (2020). Potential fecal transmission of SARS-CoV-2: Current evidence and implications for public health. *International Journal of Infectious Diseases, 95*, 363–370. https://doi.org/10.1016/j.ijid.2020.04.057.
3. Anushya, S., & Subramaniyan, D. J. (2024). Role of NGOs and Civil Society Organizations in Enhancing WASH Facilities in Government Schools: Lessons from Kallakurichi District, Tamil Nadu. *South Eastern European Journal of Public Health*, 1034–1046. https://doi.org/10.70135/seejph.vi.3167 (accessed on 14 May 2025).
4. Dhaliwal, W., Shawa, T., Khanam, M., Jagatiya, P., Simuyandi, M., Ndulo, N., Bevins, C. L., Sanderson, I. R., & Kelly, P. (2010). Intestinal antimicrobial gene expression: impact of micronutrients in malnourished adults during a randomized trial. *The Journal of infectious diseases*, *202*(6), 971–978. https://doi.org/10.1086/655903 (accessed on 14 May 2025).
5. Bintsis, T. (2017). Foodborne pathogens. *AIMS Microbiology, 3*, 529–563. https://doi.org/10.3934/microbiol.2017.3.529.
6. Boelee, E., Geerling, G., van der Zaan, B., Blauw, A., & Vethaak, A. D. (2019). Water and health: From environmental pressures to integrated responses. *Acta Tropica, 193*, 217–226. https://doi.org/10.1016/j.actatropica.2019.03.011.
7. César Neto, J. B., Dos Reis, I. N. R., Lazarin, R. O., Naenni, N., Villar, C. C., & Pannuti, C. M. (2024). Ten-year follow-up after peri-implantitis treatment using resective surgery: A case report. *Clinical advances in periodontics*, 10.1002/cap.10310. Advance online publication. https://doi.org/10.1002/cap.10310(accessed on 14 May 2025).
8. Hendra Cipta, Muslim, Rahmad Julianto, Rosnidawati, Teuku Maulana, Ambia Nurdin, Harri Santoso, & Aisy Al-Khansa. (2025). COMMUNITY-DRIVEN HEALTH STRATEGIES FOR PREVENTING DISEASE OUTBREAKS AFTER THE 2004 ACEH TSUNAMI. *Jurnal Penelitian Progresif*, *4*(1), 16-31. https://doi.org/10.61992/jpp.v4i1.204 (accessed on 14 May 2025).
9. Cumming, O., Arnold, B. F., Ban, R., Clasen, T., Esteves Mills, J., Freeman, M. C., Gordon, B., et al. (2019). The implications of three major new trials for the effect of water, sanitation and hygiene on childhood diarrhea and stunting: A consensus statement. *BMC Medicine, 17*. https://doi.org/10.1186/s12916-019-1410-x.
10. Department of Health. (2023). Health Smart City toward improving public health and citizen engagement. *The European Journal of Public Health, 33*. https://www.semanticscholar.org/paper/addae99d4d4ce09ea58b4e5561389e64f399de06 (accessed on 14 May 2025).
11. Ding, S., Du, Y., Lü, H., Wang, W., Cheng, H., Chen, S. Y., Chen, M., et al. (2021). Chinese consensus report on family-based *Helicobacter pylori* infection control and management (2021 edition). *Gut, 71*, 238–253. https://doi.org/10.1136/gutjnl-2021-325630.
12. Garrido-Cantero, G., Longo, F., Hernández-González, J., Pueyo, A., Fernández-Aparicio, T., Dorado, J. F., Angulo, J., et al. (2023). Impact of the COVID-19 pandemic on cancer diagnosis

in Madrid (Spain) based on the RTMAD tumor registry (2019–2021). *Cancers, 15*. https://www.semanticscholar.org/paper/e200788add4b50591f4c40f9a7ea69d025c869bc (accessed on 14 May 2025).

13. Glowicz, J., Landon, E., Sickbert-Bennett, E., Aiello, A. E., deKay, K., Hoffmann, K. K., Maragakis, L. L., et al. (2023). SHEA/IDSA/APIC practice recommendation: Strategies to prevent healthcare-associated infections through hand hygiene: 2022 update. *Infection Control and Hospital Epidemiology, 44*, 355–376. https://doi.org/10.1017/ice.2022.304.
14. Graciaa, D. S., Cope, J. R., Roberts, V. A., Cikesh, B. L., Kahler, A. M., Vigar, M., Hilborn, E. D., et al. (2018). Outbreaks associated with untreated recreational water–United States, 2000–2014. *American Journal of Transplantation, 18*, 2083–2087. https://doi.org/10.1111/ajt.15002.
15. Grönwall, J., & Danert, K. (2020). Regarding groundwater and drinking water access through a human rights lens: Self-supply as a norm. *Water, 12*, 419. https://doi.org/10.3390/w12020419.
16. Nichols G, Lake I, Heaviside C. Climate Change and Water-Related Infectious Diseases. *Atmosphere*. 2018; 9(10):385. https://doi.org/10.3390/atmos9100385(accessed on 14 May 2025).
17. Jaffee, S., Henson, S., Unnevehr, L. J., Grace, D., & Cassou, E. (2018). *The Safe Food Imperative: Accelerating Progress in Low- and Middle-Income Countries*. Washington, DC: World Bank eBooks. https://doi.org/10.1596/978-1-4648-1345-0.
18. Kirk, M., Pires, S. M., Black, R. E., Caipo, M., Crump, J. A., Devleesschauwer, B., Döpfer, D., et al. (2015). World Health Organization estimates of the global and regional disease burden of 22 foodborne bacterial, protozoal, and viral diseases, 2010: A data synthesis. *PLoS Medicine, 12*, e1001921. https://doi.org/10.1371/journal.pmed.1001921.
19. Kunz, J. M., Lawinger, H., Miko, S., Gerdes, M., Thuneibat, M., Hannapel, E. J., & Roberts, V. A. (2024). Surveillance of waterborne disease outbreaks associated with drinking water–United States, 2015–2020. *MMWR Surveillance Summaries, 73*, 1–23. https://www.semanticscholar.org/paper/d1319df1c02a528ae6987479287150b6f7e1e67d (accessed on 14 May 2025).
20. Leung, A. K. C., Leung, A. A. M., Wong, A. H. C., Sergi, C., & Kam, J. (2019). Giardiasis: An overview. *Recent Patents on Inflammation & Allergy Drug Discovery, 13*, 134–143. https://doi.org/10.2174/1872213x13666190618124901.
21. Luyckx, V. A., Tonelli, M., & Stanifer, J. W. (2018). The global burden of kidney disease and the Sustainable Development Goals. *Bulletin of the World Health Organization, 96*, 414–422D. https://doi.org/10.2471/blt.17.206441.
22. Mercogliano, M., Spatari, G., Noviello, C., Di Serafino, F., Mormile, M. E., Granvillano, G., Iagnemma, A., et al. (2025). Building evidences in public health emergency preparedness ("BePHEP" project)—A systematic review. *International Journal for Equity in Health, 24*. https://www.semanticscholar.org/paper/0bfd654b7eb15706b237951668c74f90d5a5de23 (accessed on 14 May 2025).
23. Moon, S. J., & Ku, I. Y. (2012). Research on cognition of infection control by dental hygienics students in some areas. *The Journal of the Korea Contents Association, 12*, 313–320. https://www.semanticscholar.org/paper/6cb12e09e06c4080071be1f6cb8b4ffd923d8f75 (accessed on 14 May 2025).
24. Muhammad, A., & Noor, S. (2023). Climate change, COVID-19, and flood disasters in Pakistan. *Journal of the Pakistan Medical Association, 73*, 1754. https://doi.org/10.47391/jpma.9231.

25. Nigro, G., Muselli, M., & On Behalf Of The Congenital Cytomegalic Disease Collaborating Group (2023). Prevention of Congenital Cytomegalovirus Infection: Review and Case Series of Valaciclovir versus Hyperimmune Globulin Therapy. *Viruses, 15*(6), 1376. https://doi.org/10.3390/v15061376(accessed on 14 May 2025).

26. OECD. (2020). *Environmental Health and Strengthening Resilience to Pandemics.* OECD Policy Responses to Coronavirus (COVID-19). https://doi.org/10.1787/73784e04-en.

27. Omarova, A. O., Tussupova, K., Berndtsson, R., Калишев, М. Г., & Sharapatova, K. (2018). Protozoan parasites in drinking water: A system approach for improved water, sanitation and hygiene in developing countries. *International Journal of Environmental Research and Public Health, 15*, Article 495. https://doi.org/10.3390/ijerph15030495.

28. Patz, J. A., Frumkin, H., Holloway, T., Vimont, D. J., & Haines, A. (2014). Climate change. *JAMA, 312*, 1565. https://doi.org/10.1001/jama.2014.13186.

29. Rahman, M. T., Sobur, M. A., Islam, M. S., Ievy, S., Hossain, M. J., El Zowalaty, M. E., Rahman, A. T., et al. (2020). Zoonotic diseases: Etiology, impact, and control. *Microorganisms, 8*, 1405. https://doi.org/10.3390/microorganisms8091405.

30. Rao, V. (2024). The effectiveness of hand hygiene in preventing zoonotic diseases among zoo workers: A critical evaluation and strategic recommendations. *EPRA International Journal of Multidisciplinary Research (IJMR).* https://www.semanticscholar.org/paper/93b12838d7eca2cde5e91d30fe4fb642239fdd44 (accessed on 14 May 2025).

31. Same, R. G., & Tamma, P. D. (2018). *Campylobacter* Infections in Children. *Pediatrics in review, 39*(11), 533–541. https://doi.org/10.1542/pir.2017-0285

32. Jamie M. Reedy, Dana Pousty, Beldeen W. Waliaula, Josephat Maniga, Hadas Mamane, Richard M. Mariita. Enhancing quality of life, public health, and economic development in the Global South through waterborne disease prevention with ultraviolet C light-emitting diode technology. *Global Health Economics and Sustainability* 2024, 2(1), 1984. https://doi.org/10.36922/ghes.1984 (accessed on 14 May 2025).

33. Rohr, J. R., Barrett, C. B., Civitello, D. J., Craft, M. E., Delius, B. K., De Leo, G. A., Hudson, P. J., et al. (2019). Emerging human infectious diseases and the links to global food production. *Nature Sustainability, 2*, 445–456. https://doi.org/10.1038/s41893-019-0293-3.

34. Sanz-Fernández, S., Díaz-Gaona, C., Borge, C., Quintanilla, R., & Rodríguez-Estévez, V. (2023). Multi-criteria evaluation model of management for weaned piglets and its relations with farm performance and veterinary medicine consumption. *Animals, 13.* https://www.semanticscholar.org/paper/259cfafa6441cd744a7951aff99f96759271f126 (accessed on 14 May 2025).

35. Schroeder, P., Anggraeni, K., & Weber, U. (2018). The relevance of circular economy practices to the Sustainable Development Goals. *Journal of Industrial Ecology, 23*, 77–95. https://doi.org/10.1111/jiec.12732.

36. Shapiro, K., Bahia-Oliveira, L., Dixon, B. R., Dumètre, A., de Wit, L. A., VanWormer, E., & Villena, I. (2019). Environmental transmission of *Toxoplasma gondii*: Oocysts in water, soil and food. *Food and Waterborne Parasitology, 15*, e00049. https://doi.org/10.1016/j.fawpar.2019.e00049.

37. Sila, O. N. (2018). Physico-chemical and bacteriological quality of water sources in rural settings: A case study of Kenya, Africa. *Scientific African, 2*, e00018. https://doi.org/10.1016/j.sciaf.2018.e00018.

38. Stenberg, K., Hanssen, O., Tan-Torres Edejer, T., Bertram, M., Brindley, C., Meshreky, A., Rosen, J. E., et al. (2017). Financing transformative health systems towards achievement of the health Sustainable Development Goals: A model for projected resource needs in 67 low-income and middle-income countries. *The Lancet Global Health, 5*, e875–e887. https://doi.org/10.1016/s2214-109x(17)30263-2.

39. Suwono, I. (2024). Community behavior based on traditional ecological knowledge (PET) toward environmental health and disease prevention. *Global International Journal of Innovative Research*. 2(9):2305-2316. https://www.semanticscholar.org/paper/6702921b04bb2c1cf011219d53d13289c09ecaf2 (accessed on 14 May 2025).

40. Todd, E. C. D. (2020). Food-borne disease prevention and risk assessment. *International Journal of Environmental Research and Public Health, 17*, Article 5129. https://doi.org/10.3390/ijerph17145129.

41. Trukhina, G. M., Iaroslavtseva, M. A., & Dmitrieva, N. (2022). Current trends in sanitary microbiology within implementation of sanitary and epidemiological surveillance of safety of water bodies. *ЗДОРОВЬЕ НАСЕЛЕНИЯ И СРЕДА ОБИТАНИЯ–ЗНиСО / Public Health and Life Environment*. https://www.semanticscholar.org/paper/9d4a41ec4c1b2330215aadf57da0cac1ad0a454e (accessed on 14 May 2025).

42. Vosa , O., Salibi, G., & Tzenios, N. (2025). Water pollution and its impact on human health in Nigeria. *Special Journal of the Medical Academy and Other Life Sciences., 3*(2). https://doi.org/10.58676/sjmas.v3i2.110(accessed on 14 May 2025).

43. Wee, S. Y., & Aris, A. Z. (2019). Occurrence and public-perceived risk of endocrine disrupting compounds in drinking water. *npj Clean Water, 2*. https://doi.org/10.1038/s41545-018-0029-3.

44. Wilbur, J., Ruuska, D., Nawaz, S., & Natukunda, J. (2024). Climate risks to water, sanitation and hygiene services and evidence of inclusive and effective interventions in low and middle-income countries: A scoping review. medRxiv 2024.08.21.24312122; doi: https://doi.org/10.1101/2024.08.21.24312122 (accessed on 14 May 2025).

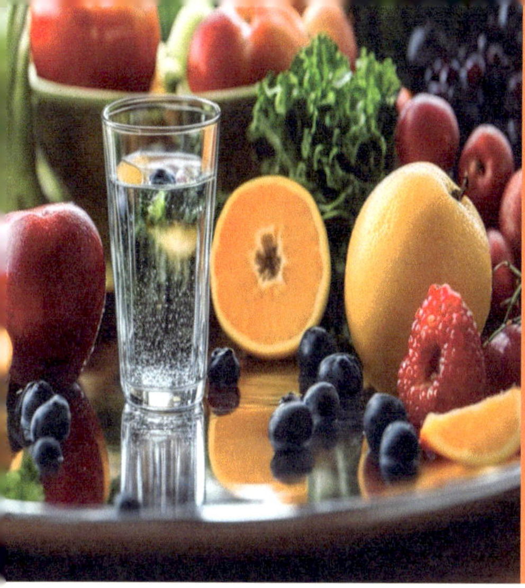

Chapter 8

THE LINK BETWEEN WATER, NUTRITION, AND HEALTH

Contents

Introduction

Clean water is essential for solid health. It does more than just satisfy thirst; it actively works to help your body get the best out of nutrients (Figure 8.1). Taking a closer look, water assists in breaking down food and transporting major vitamins and minerals, ensuring that your body receives what it truly needs. Poor water quality, even slightly off, can cause waterborne diseases that throw the entire system into chaos. When water runs low, the issue isn't solely drying up; it disrupts food security, balanced diet, and public health initiatives intended to address such concerns as malnutrition and diseases more often. When it's a matter of eating correctly, water stays with you like an old companion. Not having sufficient throws your metabolism off and leads to nutrient deficiencies, particularly for those already vulnerable. We tend to speak about big and little nutrients, but hydration humbly underpins all of that. In general, regions that don't have access to clean water lose some of the crucial things like iron and vitamin A, which then affect both physical wellbeing and mental acuity. Some research even suggests these deficits can damage not only overall health but also workplace or school performance—potentially impacting broader community well-being. Global health truly exemplifies the effect of water and nutrition as a combined effort. Areas having trouble accessing clean water typically have increased malnutrition levels as well as other accompanying health problems—a cycle that is difficult to overcome. Studies, such as the Global Burden of Diseases study, tend to indicate that with longer lives, insufficient clean water and adequate nutrition cause more deaths and even more years of living with disabilities. This twin burden puts enormous pressures on health systems in poorer countries. Creative, community-oriented initiatives and global partnerships are more increasingly essential, as an across-the-board, one-size-fits-all strategy to water and nutrition appears the best hope for making sustained gains in health.

Definition of Water and Its Role in the Human Body

Water is the unheralded hero within our bodies, it's what makes it all go. It regulates temperature when we perspire and transports nutrients through our bloodstream. It breaks down minerals, vitamins, and other necessities so that our cells can utilize them, ensuring our metabolism converts energy and eliminates waste. Even the slightest dehydration can disrupt our attention or mood, demonstrating that water is not merely another nutrient but a vital contributor to maintaining us healthy. Breastfeeding, for example, exemplifies the role water plays to aid nutrition from birth. This natural process is commonly recognized as the healthiest means of nourishing infants, as it gives essential nutrients along with antibodies that assist in developing an infant's immune system. Recently, however, the increasing adoption of commercial milk formulas (CMF) makes it more complicated—taking 1 kg of CMF uses approximately 699 liters of water, which is really mind-boggling (Baker et al., 2021).

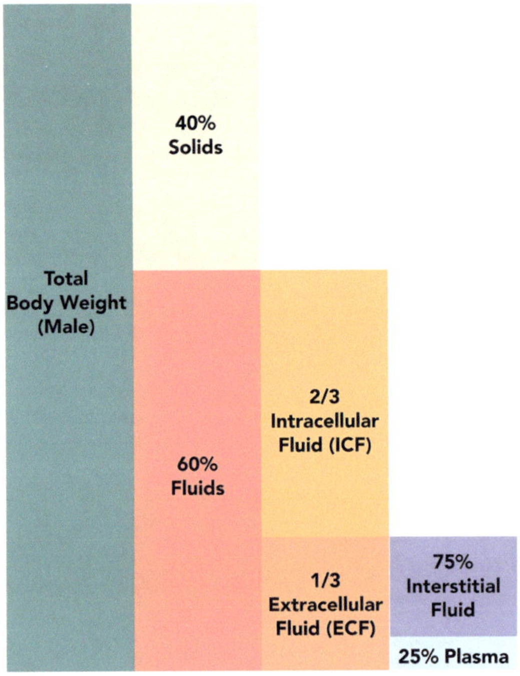

Figure 8.1. Water in the human body.

Source: By Alan Sved and David Walsh - Own work, CC BY-SA 4.0, https://commons.wikimedia.org/w/index.php?curid=81541888

It makes one reflect and think about how our activities in terms of nourishment come with environmental expenses, prompting us to prefer activities like breastfeeding and local food cultivation where we can. And then there is the social aspect of water availability, which frequently impacts women in particular ways. In most locations, women balance water responsibilities for agriculture and domestic use—a combination that links water security to nutritional status directly. When water is limited or polluted, it's not merely a matter of having a beverage; it can result in worse sanitation and lower food security. A collection of studies indicates that improved access to water can enhance physical health and even mental well-being in women who regularly deal with these issues (Mitra et al., 2019). Overall, ensuring everyone has safe, dependable water isn't only an issue of supply, it's an integral component of building healthier, more resilient communities.

Overview of Nutrition and Its Components

The connection between the food we eat and how well we do isn't quite so black-and-white as one might imagine; our diet consists of a multitude of important components that interact in unforeseen methods. Carbohydrates, proteins, fats, they don't merely energize us but keep our bodies functioning day after day. And then, of course, there are the smaller players such as vitamins and minerals that do their work unseen to keep our metabolism ticking and at bay pesky health troubles. Water, also, has its contribution to make by making nutrient absorption go smoothly throughout our system. And in most instances, it's balancing these pieces that keeps our internal state constant, reminding us that a balanced plate is indeed the foundation of good health. Combining a big variety of nutrients truly gets the machinery of the body running in ways you may not immediately notice upon a cursory glance. Consider carbohydrates, for example; they fuel everything from brain activity to cellular function in a very literal sense. Proteins, which consist of a collection of amino acids, assist in repairing tissues and fortifying our defenses, while fats, much maligned, store energy and assist in making hormones and absorbing nutrients. And indeed, hydration is no small note; it aids in digestion and keeps everything moving along at an appropriate rate. For the most part, when you look at how all of these pieces work together, it is apparent that selecting nutrient-dense foods is an important approach to maintaining health problems at bay. Adding a range of foods to the plate not only increases your nutrient level but also creates a more natural connection between your diet and your overall well-being. Both animal and plant sources bring their own spin, such as fruits and vegetables packed with vitamins, antioxidants, and fiber, which may help ward off issues like obesity or heart disease; whole grains and lean proteins add more to your metabolism's benefits. Water, despite usually flying under the radar in nutrition conversation, is a big part of staying hydrated and making every nutrient perform. Overall, the interworking of these ingredients brings a vision of nutrition as an intricate, sometimes complex, but in the end, rewarding endeavor to feel your best.

Importance of the Relationship Between Water, Nutrition, and Health

Water, nutrition and health are inextricably linked – they constitute the foundation of our general health. Clean water is not just something to consume; it sets the ball rolling for cooking food that does us good. Without safe water, nutritional issues often develop, as waterborne diseases can cause malnutrition, particularly among children. The World Health Organization, for instance, commonly points out that daily determinants such as hygiene and sanitation have a major influence on how children develop, broadly stated, which means that improved health around them tends to prevent stunting. Investing in improved water quality, sanitation, and simple hygiene, therefore, is not merely a matter of addressing immediate needs; it lays the groundwork for long-term gains through supporting nutrient uptake and development (Shatriadi et al., 2024). Pure water also influences the way we consume food and the diets we choose. Numerous caregivers incorrectly assume that sweetened beverages are healthy for children, thus they give out those sugary drinks too frequently. Studies indicate that this behavior can water down the advantages of having sufficient clean water - water that our bodies require for maintaining metabolism in check and transporting nutrients to the correct locations. One investigation revealed that many caregivers continually provide sugary beverages, generally because they misinterpret wellness labels on the label; this practice not only encourages children away from healthy hydration but can also trigger issues such as obesity and gastrointestinal issues. Confronting such misconceptions with public health education is, in most instances, the most important factor in promoting better hydration patterns for families (Yoon et al., 2022).

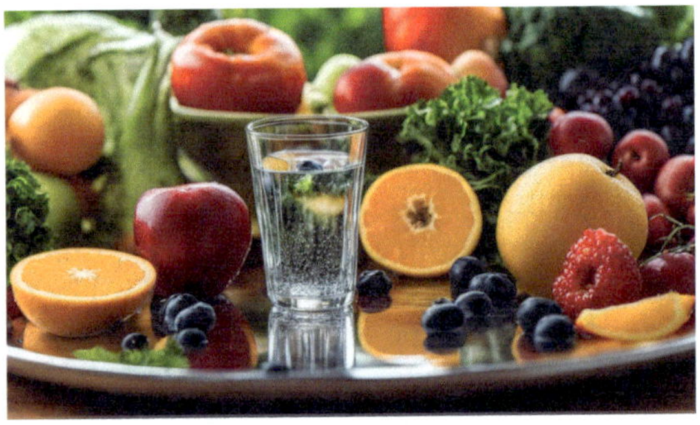

Source: Water Diet (2024). *The Role of Water in a Balanced Diet: Essential Tips.*

Source: https://www.waterdiet.com/wp-content/uploads/2024/06/The-Role-of-Water-in-a-Balanced-Diet-Essential-Tips.jpg.

It's also necessary to consider how water, nutrition, and health are interconnected when developing public health initiatives. A combined strategy - one that enhances water access, enhances nutritional training, and fosters healthier eating habits - can have surprisingly robust positive effects on populations. For example, the availability of safe drinking water immediately reduces foodborne disease, and by doing so, it assists our bodies in utilizing the nutrients we intake to the fullest. Studies commonly identify that cleaner water correlates with decreased stunting; when both water and nutrition are treated as one problem, the public health gains can be substantial and permanent. It is thus important to recognize this interdependent association to design holistic interventions with a focus on supporting long-term health and nutritional benefits for diverse populations (Shatriadi et al., 2024).

8.1. The Role of Water in the Body

Water is at the center of our daily bodily processes, maintaining our system in balance in ways we tend to take for granted. It constitutes about 60% of an adult's body weight, a fact that translates to it always being hard at work cooling us down, transporting nutrients, and removing waste (Figure 8.2). All of the cells are reliant on water to initiate the chemical processes to generate energy and absorb nutrients; when you fail to get a sufficient amount, those functions are quick to shut down, in some cases leading to disease. For the most part, hydrating isn't so much about preventing thirst as it is to keep everything humming along. Connecting water to our food has a story of its own. Lots of fruits and vegetables contain lots of water in addition to vitamins and minerals, showing they are capable of adding to hydration without you realizing it. For instance, certain species of macroalgae have a water content of as much as 93.5485% (Tuaputty et al., 2024). This being the case, in all but a few instances, means that adding water-rich foods to your diet is a healthy decision for overall wellness—foods that not only quench but also provide necessary nutrients for cell activity and energy control. Whether obtained from a beverage or a bite of fruit, a balanced hydration strategy can pay big dividends. Water is also responsible for an enormous role when it comes to recovery and exercise. Sportspeople, and even busy people, usually notice that even the slightest decrease in water consumption can drain energy, endurance, and overall performance. Proper hydration regulates body temperature during exercise and, as an added bonus, delivers nutrients to your cells while sweeping away waste – accelerating recovery after a tough workout. A few researchers even comment that intelligent hydration practices can impact not just short-term recovery but overall long-term physical well-being (Pelc et al., 2024). Simply put, recognizing the numerous functions of water—everything from helping us stay upright to powering workouts, is essential to increasing both daily well-being and sports performance.

8.1.1. Functions of Water in Physiological Processes

Water does a great deal for our bodies, although it may not appear so at first glance. It transports important things such as nutrients, hormones, and waste throughout us, sort of playing a universal dissolver's role. Because it disassembles ions and molecules, most of our chemical processes required for energy and work in the cells can take place; think of it as the quiet assistant behind a well-running engine. It even keeps us cool when we are working hard—sweat and additional breaths assist in losing heat. A lack of water can decelerate all these processes, sometimes creating health problems. In most instances, knowing how water assists in our daily processes is central when we are talking about nutrition and overall health. When metabolism is examined, water is absolutely critical. It's essential for enzyme reactions that process food and initiate energy production. Several metabolic pathways rely on water to divide big molecules into tiny pieces accessible to the body — a process that impacts both calorie consumption and energy expenditure. Frequently, if someone doesn't remain hydrated, they may not be able to take in nutrients as they might otherwise, which subsequently leaves them with less energy. Intriguingly, studies indicate that dehydration can even play havoc with mental functions, which can possibly influence academic performance in children and adults (Woodhouse et al., 2012). So, maintaining hydration is not only important for body health; it also contributes to how we operate mentally and academically. Another huge job for water is maintaining our internal equilibriumor homeostasis. It supports the body's capacity to maintain pH levels, electrolytes, and temperature in balance, keeping cells functioning at their optimal level. If the water balance is off — whether you're underhydrated or even overdoing it — these sensitive systems can fail. Even other studies indicate observable changes in the way our bodies process nutrients and dispose of energy (Zou et al., 2007), suggesting that our water consumption plays a role in the way food is metabolized. Overall, being adequately hydrated is important to the metabolic functions linking nutrition back to our health.

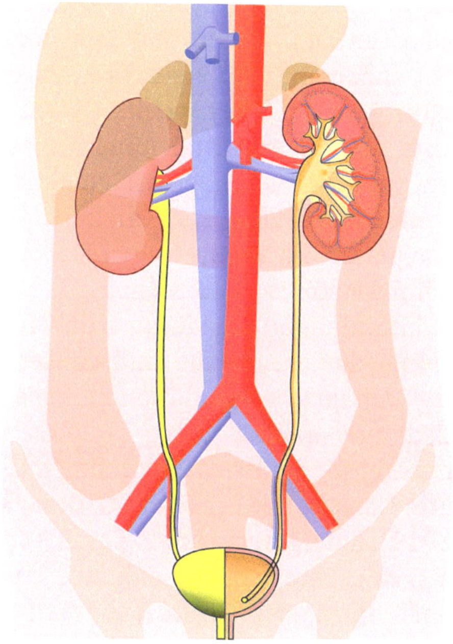

Figure 8.2. Function of water in the body.

Source: By Andrewmeyerson - Own work, CC BY-SA 3.0, https://commons.wikimedia.org/w/index.php?curid=49411619

8.1.2. Water as a Medium for Nutrient Transport

Water is not simply present to satisfy our thirst, it's the very vehicle that transports the nutrients our bodies require. When you consume food, food dissolves in water, and that water absorbs both the large macronutrients and the small micronutrients to disperse them throughout. Cells receive what they require for metabolism due to this natural process, and without sufficient water, that delivery system breaks down, at times resulting in nutrient deficiencies that can impact your health. It's almost like a dance: hydration assists in moving nutrients, and if the steps are incorrect, everything suffers. In general, this relationship between water as a dissolver and transporter is vital to maintaining our bodily functions in balance and in good order. The significance of water extends beyond our individual bodies, it's a foundation for farming and food sustainability, as well. In agriculture, water allows soils to dissolve essential nutrients and transport them to plants, enhancing crop yields in ways we tend to take for granted. When plants absorb water, they also take in essential minerals such as nitrogen, phosphorus, and potassium that power development and ultimately make their way onto our plates. Naturally, things may become altered if the water is polluted; heavy metals and other contaminants can disrupt this nutrient path, doing damage to soil and consequently affecting crop quality. Resolution of these issues is critical for making water effective in its function, thereby inextricably binding improved agriculture and better human nutrition (Kumar et al., 2019). Emerging technologies are opening up surprising avenues to enhance nutrient transport in agriculture. Nanotechnology, for instance, has smart solutions—small nanofertilizers can ensure that nutrients are delivered effectively while addressing water quality as well. The method, which in most instances increases yields and reduces waste through fertilizing, also addresses larger problems such as environmental runoff. It's a win-win: by optimizing how water transports nutrients, we can move toward a system that is not only more productive but more sustainable as well. Innovations such as these secure the crucial nexus of water, nutrition, and overall health, providing a more robust foundation for global food systems (Prasad et al., 2017).

8.1.3. Impact of Hydration on Bodily Functions

Hydration is not all about quenching thirst – it's one of the main ingredients in how our bodies operate day to day (Figure 8.3). Water maintains our inner equilibrium, regulates our temperature, and transports nutrients around our body. When you have adequate hydration, you may observe more acute focus and clearer memory; when you don't, decision-making and mental stamina can decline significantly. It's not just about downing water, either; what you're eating throws its own weight into the equation. Everyday variables—exercise, surroundings, and even diet—factor into how much water you require, so determining your body's needs isn't quite so simple as it seems at first glance. Recent research has recently brought to light the fact that all water is not created equal. Take alkaline reduced water (ARW), for example – its antioxidant-like properties may help ease the oxidative stress that can flare up when you're underhydrated. Generally speaking, when your body isn't well supplied with water, oxidative stress may worsen and stir up problems linked to metabolic conditions. ARW might have a role in calming this internal chaos, even offering potential benefits for issues like obesity or diabetes mellitus. In general, knowing what type of water is best for you can be as crucial as eating the right foods, combining hydration and health in a somewhat surprising manner. When we have large-scale global health crises, like what happened during COVID-19, hydration becomes even more critical. Our immune system is dependent on being sufficiently watered – not having enough water can easily disrupt your body's natural defenses and leave you more susceptible to infections like SARS-CoV-2. It's a bit startling to realize that the choices made day in and day out, all the way down to remembering to take a glass of water, have a ripple effect on long-term health. Even during colossal health emergencies, staying hydrated isn't solely an issue of personal health; it becomes part of the grand narrative of public health, highlighting an elaborate web of relationships between water, diet, and overall well-being.

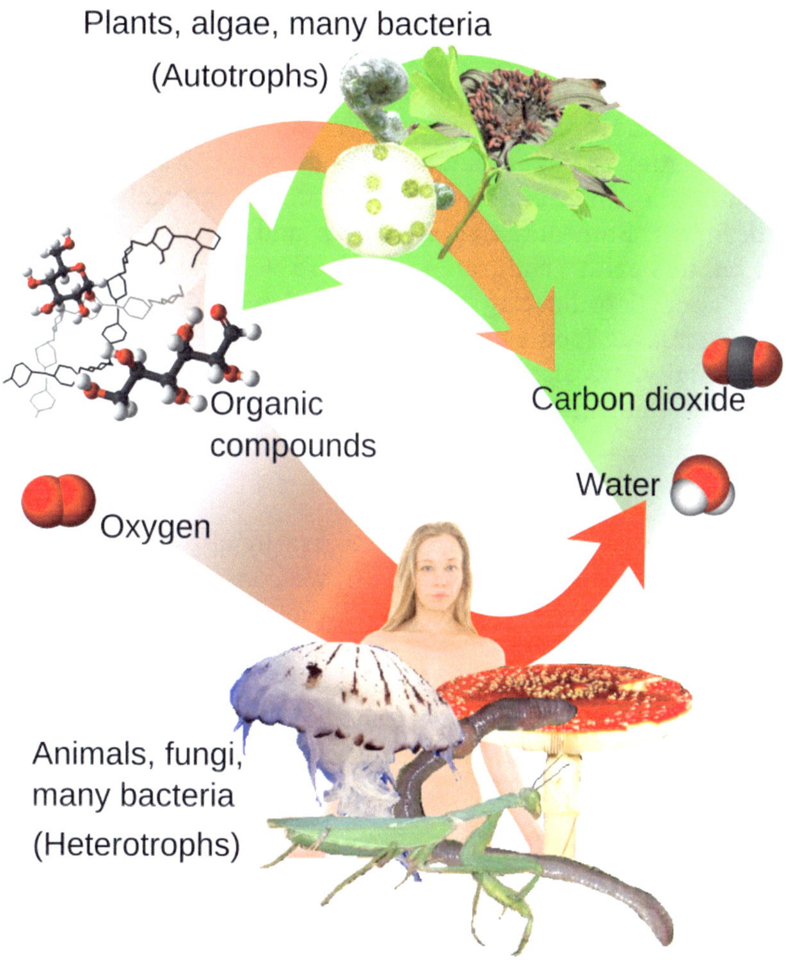

Figure 8.3. Body functions and hydration.

Source: By Mikael Häggström - Images used:GlucoseAnimalsCarbon dioxideGlucose (open form) OxygenPlantsFungiStarchWaterHuman, CC BY-SA 3.0, https://commons.wikimedia.org/w/index.php?curid=6602428

8.2. Nutritional Components Essential for Health

Remaining well-hydrated is the key to unlocking your body's nutritional advantages. Water enables food to break down and cause nutrients to move around – it serves as the platform where proteins, vitamins, and minerals function. If you don't stay hydrated, the vital components like electrolytes and small micronutrients may become sidelined, throwing off how your body functions. Glancing over, it's evident that intelligent meal planning works hand in hand with keeping your water levels topped up and that improved water quality and constant hydration can contribute substantially toward overall health (Mahmud & Mbuya, 2016). Water also has a connection with the actual ingredients of vegetables and fruits in our diets. Carbohydrates, proteins, and fats all require water to process them efficiently, for instance, protein digestion forms urea which has to be eliminated lest it become toxic. Carbs are metabolized into glucose for energy, and fats break apart so they can be absorbed. Even vitamins and minerals will use water to effectively pass through your system. And, to boot, areas with improved water sanitation tend to have less undernutrition, which suggests that combining nutritional education with water improvement will pay off (Habicht et al., 2025). Nutritional literacy is a matter of understanding how diets and water are paired together. Clean water usually accompanies healthier eating, something that's especially true where malnutrition's worst effects have been felt. Both nutrition education and water quality programs can lead to enormous strides in public health , children, in fact, are vulnerable to the deleterious effects of dehydration and poor diet. Coordinating water, sanitation, and nutrition activities appears to unlock streets toward increased food security, reduced child stunting, and overall better health. Integrating the varied local views also assists in scaling these activities to respond to the actual needs of each community (Habicht et al., 2025).

8.2.1. Macronutrients: Carbohydrates, Proteins, and Fats

Nutrition and health intersect in ways that aren't necessarily apparent at first glance, and a large part of that is the result of the three macronutrients we consume—carbohydrates, proteins, and fats (Figure 8.4). Carbs, for instance, get our energy going by being metabolized into glucose, which our brains and muscles require to stay in motion. Studies in most cases show that our carbohydrate intake can sway things like cholesterol and triglyceride levels as well as influence our weight management (Thom & Lean, 2017). In places where food choices are narrower, like in parts of Kenya, finding that proper balance of carbs becomes a must to help fight malnutrition and boost overall community wellness (Pierre et al., 2019).

Proteins, conversely, do not merely serve as fuel. They're the building blocks that enable growth, repair, and even our immune systems—constructed from amino acids that drive a lot of our body's critical processes. In many cases, consuming adequate protein not only repairs tissues that require repair but also keeps you feeling fuller for longer, which is a welcome bonus when it comes to controlling your weight. Further, as some new research suggests, high-protein diets could even result in gains in body composition and metabolic health, providing additional benefits such as benefits to cardiovascular function, particularly in those remaining active or experiencing food insecurity (Thom & Lean, 2017). It's evident that protein somehow supports both energy balance and general health outcomes across a wide range of circumstances (Pierre et al., 2019). Fats don't get as much credit, but they're important in their own right, too, they contribute to hormone synthesis and aid the absorption of the fat-soluble vitamins A, D, E, and K. They deliver a strong energy wallop in a very small serving. Of course, what fat you consume is important; unsaturated fats from nuts or olive oil typically improve heart health, while trans fats in processed food could potentially destroy it. You may find that disparities in fat intake reflect greater concerns, as they do in such places as Kenya where malnutrition remains an overwhelming issue (Pierre et al., 2019). Finally, having the proper balance of fats, and with them, the other macronutrients, is not only important for individual health, but also for informing public health policy to decrease malnutrition and encourage improved dietary patterns (Thom & Lean, 2017).

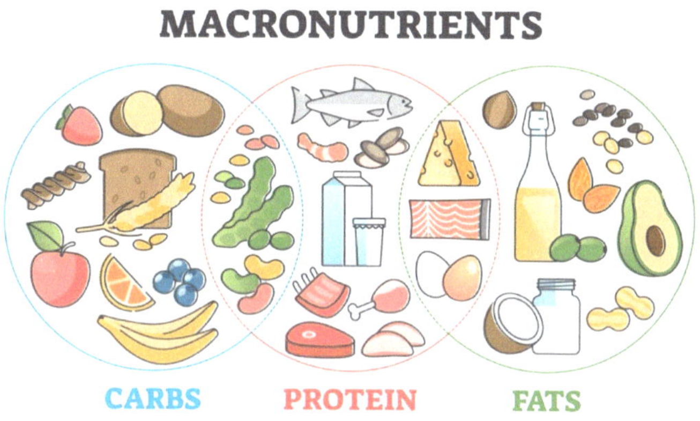

Figure 8.4. Macronutrients.

Source: Cedars-Sinai (2022). *What Are Macronutrients?*

8.2.2. Micronutrients: Vitamins and Minerals

Micronutrients have a surprisingly large impact on our day-to-day health, although they tend to go under the radar (Figure 8.5). Vitamins and minerals—the small but mighty helpers, one might say, are crucial for simple things such as burning energy, maintaining defenses, and even maintaining sharp thinking. Some studies hint that even a brief stint with multivitamin supplements can give our minds and moods a boost, especially when we're pushed hard mentally or physically. One recent piece of research, for example, noted that after some extra micronutrients, males tended to burn more energy and break down carbohydrates faster during brain-heavy tasks (Dodd et al., 2020). It also happens that when individuals have no access to clean water or proper food, not having adequate amounts of these necessary nutrients really initiates a cascade of diseases. In environments where food is scarce, catching sufficient vitamins and minerals is an important issue, frequently exacerbating the typical problems. That deficit can cause challenges such as hindered mental development and a compromised immune system, holding communities in a tough loop of worsening health (Webb & Thorne-Lyman, 2006). Closing these gaps in nutrients appears to be essential not only for personal health but also for building more robust, more resilient communities. More people are paying attention today to the significance of these micronutrients, and that's triggering a whole array of new health initiatives. Fortifying common foods and advocating for adequate supplements, particularly among risk groups—has become a top priority. Overall, improved vitamin and mineral consumption is associated with less incidence of mental exhaustion and enhanced physical function, so the call for educational efforts and resource dissemination is rather pressing (Dodd et al., 2020). There's also the developing buzz in the world of research that men and women may not react to these supplements exactly identically, a reminder that more specific approaches to diet can be the key to successful public health initiatives.

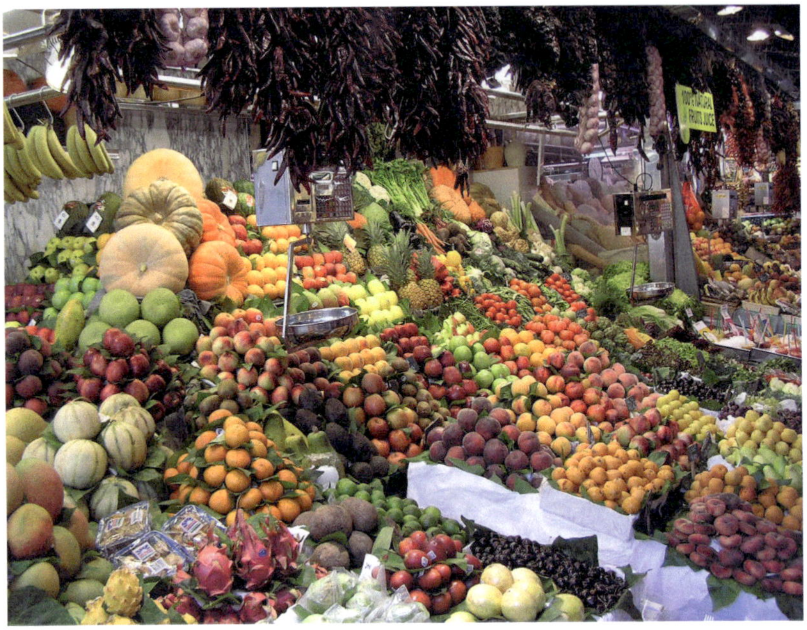

Figure 8.5. Micronutrients.

Source: By Dungodung - Own work, Public Domain, https://commons.wikimedia.org/w/index.php?curid=227289

8.2.3. The Role of Fiber in Nutrition and Digestion

Fiber is not a single thing – it presents in various forms that operate in unexpectedly different ways within our gut. Insoluble fiber, which you more often than not obtain from whole grains, nuts, and many vegetables, makes your stool bulkier and generally keeps everything going smoothly. This function is critical to overall health of the gut, more often than not preventing problems such as constipation and even diverticulitis. Simultaneously, soluble fiber , present in oats, beans, and fruit , combines with water to create a gel-like substance that, in the majority of instances, helps to regulate blood sugar levels and reduce cholesterol. You could argue this combination of effects indicates that fiber is not just about making digestion easier, but it also has something to do with systemic metabolic health. The natural equilibrium between these types of fiber strongly points toward why so many professionals currently suggest a high-fiber diet for enhancing one's overall health. The effect of fiber extends beyond digestion; it also affects the gut community of microbes. More recent studies (Högberg et al., 2003) have shown that an increase in fiber intake can shift the environment of the intestine, which leads to a more populous population of bacteria. In most cases, soluble fiber functions almost as a prebiotic, feeding beneficial bacteria and encouraging them to grow. This shift is not entirely about enhanced digestion – a balanced gut community can assist in strengthening the immune system and may decrease inflammation disorder risk. Apart from its function in maintaining blood sugar levels stable by gut fermentation, fiber also appears to provide a good solution for controlling chronic conditions like diabetes. Overall, this close relationship between fiber consumption, a varied microbiome, and well-being implies that increasing one's fiber might really pay off. Water is also a key to how fiber functions, and without sufficient fluid, even the finest high-fiber foods can be a problem. When fiber is consumed without its watery companion, it may at times cause discomfort or even exacerbate constipation instead of preventing it. Conversely, water and fiber in combination have a tendency to make the passage of food through the digestive system smoother, so that nutrients are absorbed in the process. It is curious to observe that the normal hydration retains the integrity of fiber during its passage through the gut, thereby enhancing its beneficial effects on health. Identifying this intimate connection between fiber and fluid use highlights the point that a healthy diet requires an abundance of both water and fiber in order to maintain overall digestive health (Barnes Hospital Bulletin, 1975; Welsh Network of Healthy School Schemes, 2007).

8.3. The Interdependence of Water and Nutrition

Water and food always had something to do with each other in ways that are difficult to study, and these days concerns like climate change and urban sprawl only make this connection more apparent. While cities continue to expand, the demand for both water and food increases, and our existing supplies tend to be stretched too far. Handling these sectors together isn't merely wise, it's crucial if we ever hope for decent food security and good lives. Garrett et al. (2000) noted that when cities expand and redefine our communities, it becomes a serious challenge to keep up with how resources circulate. Meanwhile, not having sufficient water disrupts agriculture and even reduces the small but significant minerals in our food, which consequently results in more instances of malnutrition. This endless cycle truly demands a bird's-eye perspective, combining water management with agricultural methods to increase the overall nutritional content of what we put on our plates, particularly in high-activity urban areas. Water quality, furthermore, has its voice in what we consume and how we remain healthy. If the water is contaminated, it can cause diseases that mess with the body's ability to absorb nutrients—making the malnutrition problem even worse for people who are already vulnerable. Families stuck with unsafe water often end up choosing meal options that are high in calories but low in nutrients, which only deepens the deficiency issue. There's an intense back-and-forth relationship here, in which diseases that are carried by water and nutrition issues interact with one another; for example, improved hygiene combined with education on nutrition can truly be beneficial. Therefore, projects aimed at achieving safe water should also involve attempts at educating people on the need to consume a balanced diet.

Research even points out that when communities become engaged in health and nutrition education, it ignites actual, long-term change for individuals struggling with these intersecting issues. Attempting to study the water–nutrition relationship isn't a single-group effort, it requires teamwork among the health, agriculture, and education communities (and perhaps more). Leaders must recognize that you can't effectively increase food security if you don't address water resource management. Effective strategies that include cover water conservation efforts, more intelligent irrigation systems, and community-based nutrition programs can really make people healthier. By implementing policies that emphasize the close connection among these resources, communities may develop some much-needed immunity to health panics along with better general nutrition. And with continuing education and skill acquisition (whoops, a couple typos there, but that's life.), individuals can begin to make better decisions regarding both water and food, generating a kind of give-and-take that elevates general well-being. When concepts across disciplines cross-fertilize, they lead us down new avenues to a secure future, a future that more closely mirrors how water and nutrition challenges are all wound together.

8.3.1. How Water Affects Nutrient Absorption

Water's crucial function in enabling our bodies to utilize nutrients can scarcely be exaggerated. Our body depends on water to break up vitamins, minerals, and other treats so that they can pass easily through cell membranes. Within the gut, water springs into action to initiate hydrolysis—the enzyme-catalyzed breaking up of large molecules—streamlining digestion. Under- consumption of water sees enzymes functioning less effectively and nutrient uptake suffering. Dehydration can even make the goo in your bowels thicker, so it takes longer to move through, which over time can really mess with how well you digest what you eat, particularly in older individuals who frequently struggle with less effective gut function (Rémond et al., 2015). Now consider food. Sometimes the combination of what we consume plays with water's role in our body. Eat a high-fiber diet: as wonderful as it is for making things move along, with not enough water, that fiber can bind together and become constipating, reducing the nutrients your body so badly needs. Proteins and fats don't miss out either—proteins require water to break down into amino acids, and fats rely on bile acids, which are largely water, to get digested. Even some vitamins such as vitamin C or those B vitamins possess their own little idiosyncrasies in how they dissolve. Most of the time, balancing what water you drink with the type of food that you're eating is a good idea for maintaining nutrient absorption on track (Högberg et al., 2003). It isn't merely a matter of personal health, either; it cascades out into larger public health concerns as well. In places where clean water is hard to come by, many people face higher risks of malnutrition and other health issues. As people age, natural drops in gut function combined with shifting hydration needs can ramp up these dangers. Research tends to indicate that as we age, shifts in gut function and motion can influence how well our bodies are able to capture nutrients—underscoring why dietary recommendations should really consider hydration. And when you add the gut's overall ecosystem—water, fiber, and those teeny microbial assistants—the picture becomes even more complicated. Overall, having a clear understanding of the numerous roles of water is important in developing effective nutritional strategies that benefit everyone (Rémond et al., 2015).

8.3.2. The Role of Hydration in Metabolic Processes

Water is at the center of how our body functions—a reality that is frequently unheralded. It isn't merely something you consume when you are thirsty; it silently facilitates the transport of nutrients and removal of waste. When our body metabolizes macronutrients such as carbohydrates, fats, and proteins to obtain energy, water is present, facilitating enzyme reactions (particularly in processes such as aerobic respiration). In the majority of instances, when the body lacks sufficient water, enzyme activity is slowed, resulting in inefficient energy production and paving the way for some metabolic problems. Not having enough water doesn't just impact metabolism; it disrupts the way the body stays cool as well. A body that's dehydrated can't maintain its temperature, which can lead to a rise in heart rate, decreased volume of blood, and even heat stress or exercise difficulties at times. In general terms, it is for these reasons that scientific research identifies hydration as a vital component of diets such as the Mediterranean and DASH diets—those that blend plenty of vegetable foods with adequate amounts of water. It turns out that adequate hydration isn't merely a fallback; it's an essential component of healthy living. Water also marries well with the body's natural harmony and the signals guiding millions of biochemical processes. There's proof that even a little bit of mild dehydration can cause hormonal changes that affect our hunger and the way energy's utilized, which sometimes makes it difficult to adhere to a diet. And, besides, if hydration dips, the balance of electrolytes can falter, affecting muscle function and even mental acuteness. So, it's obvious that water isn't just about replenishing fluids but calibrating our entire nutritional approach to forestall disease. As nutritionists persist in exploring the ups and downs of diet and hydration, combining these factors into larger wellness plans will probably be a foundation for improving public well-being (Berg et al., 2020; Cena et al., 2020).

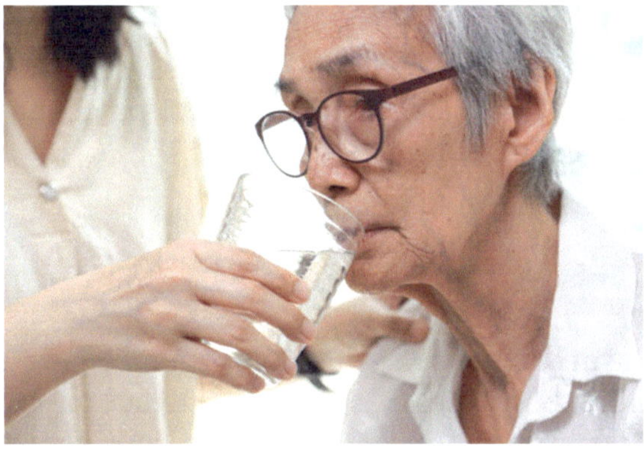

Source: https://t4.ftcdn.net/jpg/04/95/38/53/360_F_495385366_Yh5sWoCay8c6ncFfQz2CN3BnNTNnf84r.jpg.

8.3.3. Consequences of Inadequate Water Intake on Nutrition

Not getting enough water can really mess with the way our bodies use nutrients. When hydration is low, the digestive system may not work as well as it should, which in turn makes it hard to break down food and let vital vitamins and minerals in. Even under a well-balanced diet, in most instances, if water is limited—because the body is effectively shuffling water around, slowing down major enzymes critical to digestion—this can be a problem. This problem is particularly critical in aged care settings, where residents tend to have multiple health issues (Agarwal et al., 2016). Chronic low water intake also has a tendency to disrupt appetite messages and food consumption. Hydration levels have a direct impact on hormones like ghrelin and leptin, the ones that generally tell us when we're hungry or full. Sometimes, a lack of water makes people mistake thirst for hunger, prompting unnecessary eating that doesn't fix the real hydration deficit. This can lead to weight gain and further mess up nutritional balances. Also, individuals who are not consuming sufficient amounts of water may experience their energy levels and mental acuity decreasing, so that even a simple process like cooking dinner becomes challenging. Such associations of water with hunger highlight the importance of assisting individuals in being aware of their thirst signals, particularly for those whose diseases or hectic lifestyle may lead them to overlook these cues (Cohen et al., 2008). Apart from influencing personal health, inadequate water consumption has a ripple effect, influencing public health and increasing the cost of healthcare. Dehydration-related malnutrition can make individuals more vulnerable to infections and contribute to increased hospital stays—both of which contribute to additional burden on the healthcare system. For instance, in aged care facilities it's documented that close to half the residents exhibit signs of malnutrition, and hydration tends to be an afterthought when nutritional assessments are made (Agarwal et al., 2016). Broadly speaking, these trends serve to illustrate the value of examining water and nutrition as a combined entity. Optimal strategies must involve educating individuals regarding the significance of hydration, monitoring fluid consumption regularly, and developing customized plans to increase water intake among high-risk populations. With an understanding of the complex relationship between proper nutrition and good hydration, healthcare systems can more effectively contribute to preventing malnutrition and its attendant complications (Cohen et al., 2008).

8.4. Health Implications of Water and Nutrition Deficiencies

Water and food are intertwined in ways that usually go unnoticed, and this connection can have tremendous health implications throughout the world. Dehydration isn't merely a small nuisance, it can disrupt digestion and interfere with nutrient absorption. For most people, inadequate fluids result in a reduced efficiency of the enzymes that assist in the breakdown of foods, so our bodies have less access to those vital vitamins and minerals. Strangely, individuals who are malnourished might not even feel thirst so strongly, trapping them into a vicious cycle of both water loss and nutritional decline simultaneously. This convergence of concerns occasionally appears as gastrointestinal issues, a compromised immune system, or other challenges that make it all the more difficult to obtain and utilize the proper nutrition and water, which is why having knowledge of the connection between hydration and nutrition is so important (Intergovernmental Panel on Climate Change, 2023). Pregnant women and children, for instance, have particular challenges in finding a balance of their nutritional and hydration requirements. Iron-deficiency anemia—most often the product of a bad diet combined with insufficient amounts of water—may strike both maternal and fetal well-being fairly significantly. Studies typically reveal that pregnant women with low levels of iron are disproportionately fatigued, a fatigue that frequently carries over into their day-to-day lives throughout and beyond pregnancy. Such fatigue can even influence infants in later life, possibly inhibiting their mental and physical development. Additionally, lack of adequate water consumption can increase the risks associated with nutritional deficiencies, at times contributing to conditions such as gestational diabetes or even preterm deliveries. Obviously, maintaining care over food and hydration is paramount in maternal health interventions to prevent these risks (Pavord et al., 2019). Community-based efforts targeting both proper nutrition and adequate hydration have also proven to be a true game changer. Local initiatives that combine education about why water is important with concepts for consuming better have been found to alter public health figures in a positive direction. For instance, initiatives that educate individuals on the advantages of iron content foods alongside sufficient hydration have reduced anemia cases among pregnant women and children. This combined emphasis on food and water not only assists people in making more intelligent decisions but also promotes a more general consciousness of health that accumulates community resilience to different health problems, both acute and chronic (Intergovernmental Panel on Climate Change, 2023).

8.4.1. Dehydration and Its Health Effects

Dehydration is something most people tend to ignore, but it has a significant impact on how our bodies work. If you don't drink enough water, it disrupts the body's natural balance, with symptoms that can set in in unpredictable ways (Figure 8.6). Occasionally, if you lose more water than you ingest, your blood volume could decrease and—broadly speaking—this deficiency can make it harder for your blood to transport oxygen where it is required. You could quite easily feel drained or notice that your focus isn't precisely optimum. Even moderate dehydration could initiate a headache or make it difficult to concentrate, which can in turn affect your daily energy and mental acuity. In the majority of situations, staying ahead of your fluids keeps your body and brain communicating more effectively, something that's fairly significant in today's round-the-clock world. Failing to drink water over an extended period of time really raises the stakes, especially for your organs.

Your kidneys, for instance, are really sensitive; without proper fluid levels, they wedded to issues such as kidney stones or even urinary tract infections become probable. The body's fight to eliminate toxins due to low fluid levels can develop into an accumulation that's no laughing matter. And if you already have an disease such as diabetes or heart disease, low chronic hydration can just make it all the more difficult to manage those conditions. It's particularly problematic for older adults or individuals with underlying health issues because they sometimes miss the cues that signal it's time to hydrate. There's also a powerful connection between water consumption, nutrition, and overall health that isn't always given the attention it deserves. Dehydration isn't merely inconvenient, it's tied to a host of problems like weaker immunity and a higher risk of falling ill. On the flip side, when you're well-hydrated, your body can better absorb nutrients, which in turn can boost your metabolism and energy levels. During times of disease, such as bouts of diarrhea or fever, your need for fluids really goes up to ward off any extra complications. Overall, attempting to maintain a constant supply of water within your system, in addition to a healthy diet, works wonders when it comes to how efficiently your body operates on a daily basis. Public health initiatives more and more lead back to the concept that incorporating water intake as a habitual activity is as important as anything else in healthy maintenance.

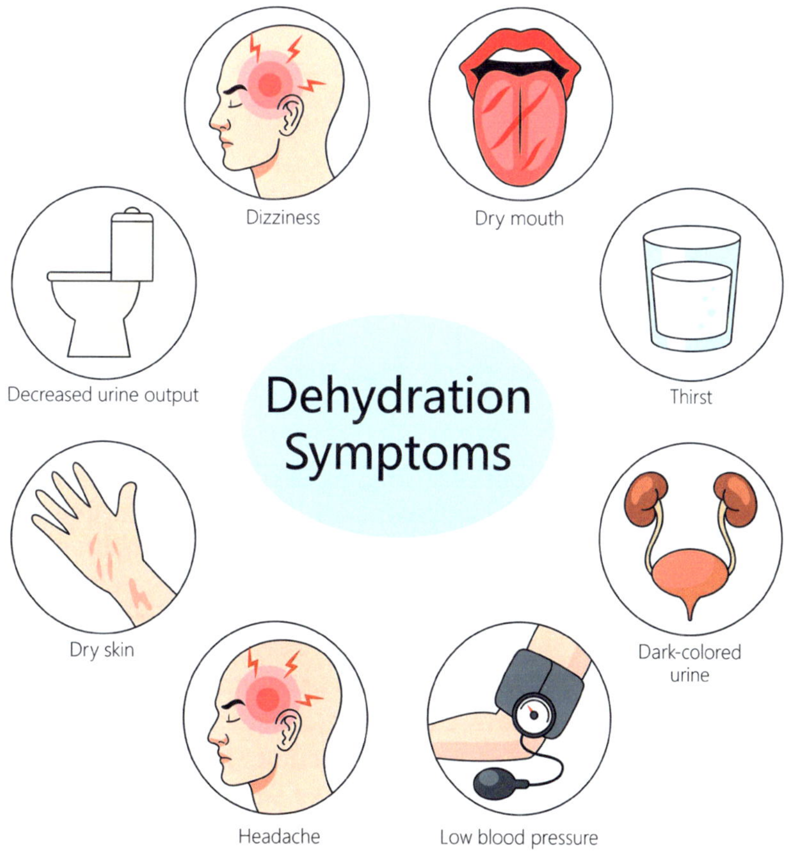

Figure 8.6. Dehydration symptoms.

Source: Pokusai, O (n.d.). *Common Symptoms of Dehydration Including Dizziness, Dry Mouth, and Thirst Diagram Hand Drawn Schematic Vector Illustration*. Dreamstime.

8.4.2. Malnutrition and Its Impact on Overall Health

Global sustainability challenges are intertwined with problems of water, nutrition and health. Increased undernourishment in combination with increased rates of obesity describe a double burden that most populations experience in the modern era. Where clean and sufficient water simply is not an option, poor nutrition has a tendency to set off a combination of problems of health. There is a significant correlation between water scarcity and food concerns that makes it apparent we can no longer address one without considering the other. Fresh thinking that locks in food and advances more intelligent use of water is necessary. When resources are not managed properly, not only do individual health opportunities get hurt, but larger public health initiatives to combat malnutrition get derailed, illustrating just how interconnected these issues are (Committee UNSS on Nutrition, 2020). Taking a slightly closer look, malnutrition goes on to have a whole host of detrimental effects on the body and the mind. Children are particularly vulnerable; many have stunted growth and appear to be more susceptible to infection. In most instances, the immediate issue is just half of the picture – in the longer term, malnutrition's persistent effect can keep communities trapped in poverty and uneven health prospects, especially where communities are already challenged with poor water and sanitation.

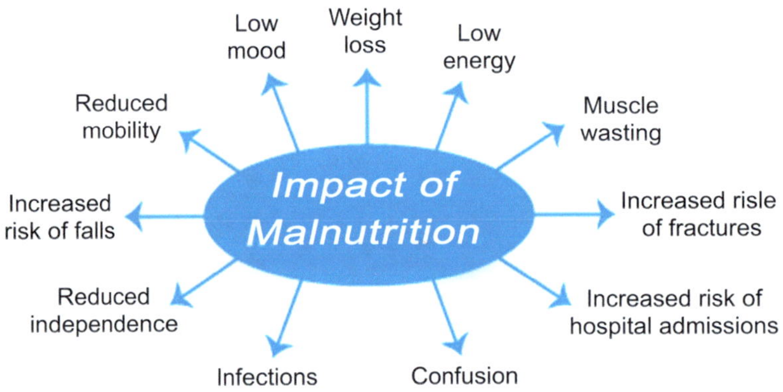

Figure 8.7. Impact of malnutrition.

Source: https://blogger.googleusercontent.com/img/b/R29vZ2xl/AVvXsEgq7JMcRCKFQGCkpeYjeAUd8FEV1qO4-N5o-nqqQn7ekF-e487pZnbKvPLxWjohw40Umxx53sZoYxDC4F-a6EwG-H_7Lc2JphnG_8TYuzBnNEYZC32W0MMt5m-pOtpX3lEbz2e6LH6103c/s1600/malnutrition-diagram.gif.

Lacking sufficient clean water only widens these nutritional deficiencies, such as missing out on critical micronutrients, and this can put a person's health at risk throughout their lifetime (Menon et al., 2018). When you pull all these threads together, it is apparent that any strategy to improve public health must operate across various sectors, combining efforts and resources in a wide, integrated manner (Menon et al., 2018). Correcting malnutrition is not simply a matter of isolated measures of health; it requires a concerted effort from disciplines such as agriculture, water management and healthcare. It is generally the case that recognizing the way food problems tie back to water security is crucial, as prioritizing one aspect could unwittingly hinder the other. The continuing debate on global sustainability reminds us that we need a combination of expertise, particularly with climate change making these connections even more complex. It is important to bring together clusters that specialize in nutrition, water and food safety in order to construct something that would truly address the far-reaching impacts of malnutrition (Figure 8.7). It is only with such integrated, flawed but authentic strategies that our society can strive to enhance overall well-being and leave future generations the tools they must need to flourish (Committee UNSS on Nutrition, 2020).

8.4.3. The Combined Effects of Water and Nutrient Deficiencies

Clean water is essential—without it, the body withholds from nutrient deficiencies in a way that erodes overall well-being. When water isn't present in adequate amounts, dehydration creeps in and disrupts the way vitamins and minerals are absorbed, putting many critical processes out of whack. Water is not merely a fundamental necessity; it supports many of our most critical bodily processes, so in shortage, the body is unable to utilize nutrients effectively, and when attempting to correct one problem in the absence of the other, most often just falls short. In a majority of situations, an expanded effort that brings food and health policies together, coupled with a re-engineered strategy in agricultural research and investment, could truly make an impact (Pinstrup-Andersen et al., 2025).

Inadequate availability of nutrient-dense foods places an additional layer of burden, particularly on those who are already vulnerable. Usually, water scarcity results in reduced crop yields, which subsequently decreases the local availability of vitamin-rich alternatives; local populations are left with fewer options that contain the nutrients required to maintain the immune system strong. Vitamins A, C and B12, for instance, are crucial in ensuring health, and their absence can lead to serious conditions such as scurvy or anemia (Yu et al., 2015) (Figure 8.8). In regions where water scarcity or drought have become the norm, traditional agriculture at times just is not sufficient anymore, and this further heightens the need for nutrient-dense crops. Thus, addressing the problem of water needs to go hand in hand with encouraging more diversified agriculture if people are to remain resilient. If you consider the combined impact of water and nutritional deficiencies, the public health issues truly accumulate.

People residing in areas where clean water or wholesome sustenance is difficult to access are exposed to threats that add up over the long term; ongoing water scarcity can trap populations in a malnutrition cycle that only aggravates health and further restricts access to survival necessities.

Public health interventions usually have to be able to observe this interaction in some way—otherwise, there's a chance of allocating resources in the wrong direction or winding up with useless measures. A more holistic, integrated strategy incorporating education, infrastructure development and community participation could in the end assist in ending this cycle and improving overall health and stability (Pinstrup-Andersen et al., 2025).

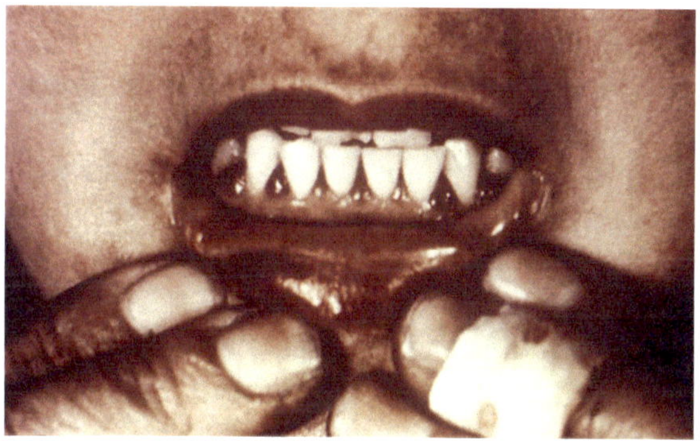

Figure 8.8. Scorbutic gums due to a vitamin C deficiency, a symptom of scurvy.

Source: Scorbutic gums (n.d.). *Wikimedia Commons*. https://upload.wikimedia.org/wikipedia/commons/thumb/8/88/Scorbutic_gums.jpg/1024px-Scorbutic_gums.jpg.

8.5. The Importance of Hydration in Different Life Stages

Water is important from the beginning. Babies and toddlers contain much more water than grown-ups, so even a small amount of dehydration can result in serious problems. Their kidneys, which are still learning how to handle fluids, make it even more challenging, they absolutely need frequent drinks from both liquids and foods. Not enough water? That's a recipe for things like cloudy thinking and developmental delays. Other research, for instance, indicates that when mothers are able to keep themselves hydrated during pregnancy, it will provide the infant with a healthier beginning in life at birth. In the majority of situations, a continuous supply of water early in life sets the stage for robust development and improved general health. Once children enter adolescence, hydration needs take on a different set of challenges. Growth spurts strike quickly, and with a whole lot more physical activity, sports, outdoor play, and all that, they're losing fluids faster than ever before. Sometimes they just aren't attuned to how much water they require, which could disrupt energy levels, sports performance, or even mood. There are apps that attempt a little bit of additional coaching on drinking sufficient water, and studies tend to indicate that adolescents who keep on top of their water intake also tend to concentrate better at school. Water, it appears, isn't just about keeping the body in gear but about keeping the head in gear too. Down the line later in life, hydration becomes increasingly critical. As we get older, our feeling of thirst disappears, and retaining water doesn't function the same. Older people—already struggling with chronic disease and even certain medications such as diuretics—run additional risks when they're not adequately hydrated. This can cause problems like mental slowing or an increased risk of infection, which really takes its toll on quality of life. Habits are simple, such as keeping water in arm's reach and taking care to drink periodically, and can make a difference in these issues. Generally, viewing hydration as an essential component of nutrition has benefits both for body and brain throughout the later years (Berg et al., 2020; Livingston et al., 2020).

8.5.1. Hydration Needs During Childhood and Adolescence

Children, particularly when they are young or teenagers, badly need to consume lots of water. Their bodies undergo significant changes during these years, which forces them to require additional fluids so that everything functions properly. You see, children naturally contain more water in their bodies than adults do, so they're slightly more at risk of dehydration if they don't get enough water. Things such as how much they're moving around, the weather, and even the type of snack they have can tip their water balance. Failing to drink enough water can disrupt the way they think and play, and even in some instances, harm their overall well-being later on. That is why it's really important that both parents and children understand why drinking water often is important. Overall, each child's hydration requirements can literally change with their daily life and environment. For instance, a sporty child or a child who is continually active will require more water to replenish the loss of water that occurs when they sweat. And, considering that obesity is increasingly prevalent in children, having extra weight may even alter the way effectively a body regulates its water – certain research suggests that excess body fat has the potential to modify how water balance is maintained. In most scenarios, monitoring water consumption becomes a simple component of guidance on eating healthily and exercising regularly, particularly when energy is high. It almost sounds like proper hydration is one of those easy steps that will keep a lot of health problems at bay later in life. Then there's the entire effect of external factors , such as commercials and what everyone around them is consuming – that can completely alter a child's behaviors as well. Quite frequently, though, sweet drinks come on the scene and take over from plain water, creating a sort of confusion about what true hydration really is. Caregivers and parents must lead the charge here, demonstrating by example that water will be the drink of choice above soda or other sweet drinks. Also, ensuring that water is readily available to grab at school or home can also go a long way in directing children toward improved decisions. Ultimately, once all is said and done and children are establishing their own habits of eating and drinking, maintaining good hydration is important for reaching those health goals. And within the larger context of how water fits into general nutrition and health, keeping hydration in mind is a pillar of assisting youths in leading healthier lives (Figure 8.9).

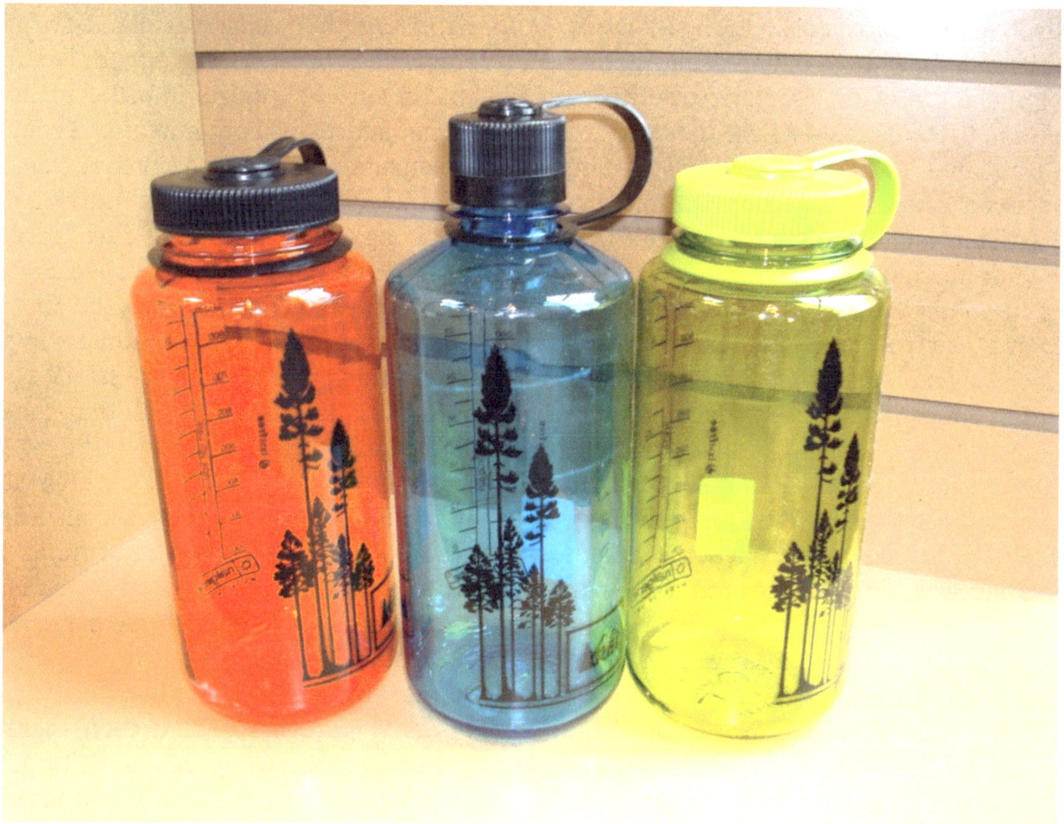

Figure 8.9. A young soccer team drinking from water bottles.

Source: By Amraepowell - Own work, CC BY-SA 3.0, https://commons.wikimedia.org/w/index.php?curid=19133754

8.5.2. The Role of Water in Adult Health

Water is the secret to staying healthy, particularly for adults. Drinking sufficient water initiates some seriously important body processes. It levels out your temperature, powers your metabolism, and even transports nutrients from place to place like a mini delivery system. If you don't meet the proper water intake, you may start to feel remarkably tired, foggy-headed, or just not really functioning physically. This works against athletic individuals more because they lose more water as they perspire. And, frankly, if the water is not in top condition, things only get worse. All this demonstrates an evident correlation between good hydration and maintaining both work and personal demands. Water is not merely for thirst, though. It has a tremendous influence on how your body breaks down food and absorbs nutrients. When you're short on water, your gut can slow down—often resulting in constipation and a drop in nutrient absorption. In many cases, not drinking enough only makes existing dietary imbalances worse, such as obesity or malnutrition. Urban areas—where these issues often spring up—really show how water and nutrition need to work together. Uniting the two can assist in establishing interventions that enhance your nutrition and increase hydration, resulting in enhanced overall health outcomes (Nogaski et al., 2010). Taking the larger picture, worldwide problems such as water shortage and malnutrition appear to be intertwined. Climate change, for instance, is driving more individuals into water shortage, which then disrupts food production and our general nutritional security. The United Nations has noted that achievement on targets such as zero hunger and access to clean water tends to be sluggish, revealing a lag between water, food, and nutritional efforts. That entails implementing serious initiatives that not only provide clean water but also increase the nutritional value. Lacking close focus on how nutrition and water do intersect, attempts at correction for undernutrition can have the unintentional effect of increasing water shortages, and conversely (Committee UNSS on Nutrition, 2020).

8.5.3. Special Considerations for the Elderly

As one ages, new issues usually appear that affect overall health, so it is necessary to find means to maintain healthy nutrition and sufficient fluids. Daily routines and normal body changes sometimes blend together in surprising ways and create obstacles that are not always visible. For instance, a reduced feeling of thirst could lead an individual to not consume enough water, which can subtly push up the risk for dehydration, and that, in turn, could exacerbate chronic conditions many older adults already struggle with. Proper hydration is not solely about general health but also has a significant role in keeping the mind active and the body moving. Oftentimes, meeting these needs involves piecing together such variables as personal preferences, pre-existing health issues, and available social supports in order to develop a plan that addresses both nutritional content and fluid consumption. It's also key to remember that special health issues arise as individuals grow older. Long-term conditions such as diabetes and high blood pressure need special attention when it comes to what is consumed and, equally importantly, how much is consumed. In general, research, such as some on COVID-19 outcomes (Choi et al., 2023)—indicates that those with chronic health conditions may be at greater risk of severe complications, which suggests that food and drink balance is an important aspect of managing these conditions. Adding foods that are high in nutritional density and also hydrate can fulfill the dual requirement of necessary nutrients and adequate fluids, ultimately improving quality of life for elderly patients (Figure 8.10). And then there is the social component, which cannot be forgotten. At times, loneliness or reduced social interactions can quietly alter the quantity and quality of food and fluids that older persons consume. Research on workers over 60 shows that casual, supportive interactions can really make a difference in daily health outcomes. Encouraging community programs or even just more family time can lead to better eating habits and more regular fluid consumption—small steps that pile up over time. Overall, if we bring together both the bodily needs and the human touch aspect of things, we can aid in alleviating some of the health issues that come with age and encourage sustained wellness among our seniors (Choi et al., 2023).

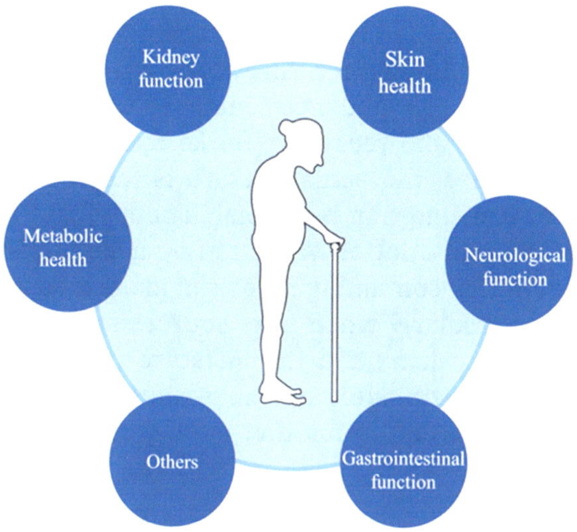

Figure 8.10. Hydration and major health outcomes in older people.

Source: Li S, Xiao X, Zhang X. Hydration Status in Older Adults: Current Knowledge and Future Challenges. Nutrients. 2023; 15(11):2609. https://doi.org/10.3390/nu15112609

8.6. Strategies for Maintaining Proper Hydration and Nutrition

In our hectic world, it's simple to overlook something as straightforward as drinking water and healthy eating. It's easy to forget that hydration is an important part of feeling good, so the simplest trick is simply to have a water bottle handy and sip throughout the day. Every now and then it's a good idea to add a serving of water-dense fruits or vegetables to your meal, they're not just great for hydration, but also are filled with vitamins. Having a random alarm or utilizing a hydration-monitoring app will remind you to take a glance at your water consumption—this small push really makes a significant impact. Getting proactive about staying hydrated appears to keep the not-so-fun symptoms of dehydration at bay, and adapting your water routine to your own daily living schedule increases both physical and mental energy. Having a good understanding of nutrition complements staying hydrated. In general, incorporating nutrient-dense foods into your diet assists your body in getting the most out of the water you consume. Balanced meals that contain carbs, proteins, and fats, and, of course, the smaller micronutrients—also appear to enable your system to utilize water better. For instance, combining a healthy dose of carbs with some protein in some cases may improve hydration while exercising. It may seem redundant, but being familiar with portion control as well as knowing what's in what you eat can give you more control over making smarter decisions. In the majority of instances, programs aimed at combating childhood obesity emphasize the importance of balanced meals accompanied by adequate hydration (Brown, 2011), demonstrating that a full-circle approach truly counts when it comes to long-term health. Today, technology is coming in as a convenient assistant for hydration and nutrition objectives. New programs such as FitPot blend intelligent technology with daily routines, reminding you to monitor water, watch nutrition, and adhere to better habits. Devices and programs that provide instant feedback can encourage you to drink up and even provide suggestions on how to make your habits better—consumer interest in these devices is definitely on the increase (Podder et al., 2023). When fitness influencers begin to discuss their own regimens, that added hype does count, inspiring more people to make hydration and healthy food a normal way of life. Ultimately, the combination of intelligent tech, social buzz, and individual commitment does appear to lead the way to improved overall health results.

8.6.1. Recommended Daily Water Intake Guidelines

Hydration is most important for body and mind. Our functioning, in fact, tends to be dependent on the availability of water, and our requirement varies a little from one individual to another. Age, activity level, weather, and general health contribute to individualized water requirements. Consider sports people—many need to make alterations in their liquid intake in terms of the training they undertake and the ambient conditions. In general, sports nutrition guidance reinforces this notion, citing that adequate hydration is important for performance and recovery (Burke & Cox, 2020). So, even if typical recommendations provide a general sense, the actual picture is much more individualized. It's also important to mention that water consumption isn't solely about what you drink. Consuming fruits and vegetables, which already contain a lot of water, can be a significant contribution to meeting your daily quota. At times, these water-containing foods can make it easier to manage the stress of having to drink a lot of water, particularly when pure sources are scarce or at the height of activities. Observing both the liquids you drink and the moisture trapped in your foods can open up the door to a more effortless and sustainable drinking routine. Several nutritionists recommend incorporating these hydrating foods into your diet as a great plan to maintain your fluid equilibrium.

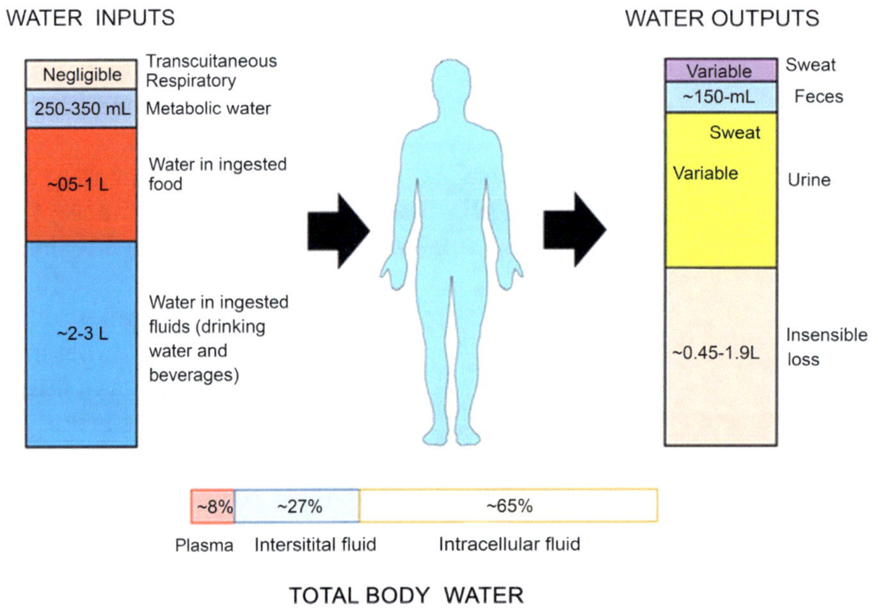

Figure 8.11. Recommended daily water intake.

Source: Li S, Xiao X, Zhang X. Hydration Status in Older Adults: Current Knowledge and Future Challenges. Nutrients. 2023; 15(11):2609. https://doi.org/10.3390/nu15112609*8.6.2. Nutritional Strategies for Balanced Diets*

Even with the various daily guidelines out there, having something in place for being hydrated is critical to both your physical energy and mental acuity. Health officials often remind us that women need to target some 2.7 liters a day while men may require up to 3.7 liters, encompassing everything from drinks to water-dense foods (Figure 8.11). This minimum provides a rough guide to good practice. In addition, with our diet getting more processed nowadays, there is an increased necessity for reconsideration in how we consider drinking water, particularly for older adults who could use some adjustments in their diets (Lumbis et al., 2018). In general, connecting hydration to nutrition and health appears to be a wise, proactive step that benefits improved well-being across populations.

Nutrition and wellness isn't solely about adhering to a tight set of rules; it's really about observing all the individual pieces that make up our day-to-day foods. Individuals can thrive when they consume a variety of fruits, vegetables, whole grains, lean proteins, and healthy fats, albeit at times, a long list does sound. A diverse diet ensures you receive the vitamins, minerals, and other fundamental nutrients your body needs. Plain, unprocessed foods tend to reduce the risk of chronic issues related to nutrition, and even a splash of water now and then helps significantly in enabling your body to absorb everything it needs to continue functioning properly. Diet is not just what ends up on your plate; it also what you're born into and what's local. Cultural patterns, how convenient it is to obtain various foods, even economics – all that's in the equation. Consider Vietnam: recent reports tend to show that a movement toward more Western food has resulted in imbalances of nutrients and a steep increase in obesity. Local efforts, in turn, that address food environments and community education can bridge the gaps left behind by these transformations. Most of the time, integrating traditional measures with new measures leaves space for healthier options while still supporting local agriculture measures. Public health policies also contribute significantly to determining to what extent our diets promote our well-being. Recent studies indicate that as food systems evolve so quickly, there are requirements for definite yet adjustable rules to meet emerging dietary issues. The governments and other stakeholders need to work together (yes, it's true—sometimes it's not perfect) to implement food safety measures, improve food literacy, and promote local food production. Subsidies for healthy food and nutrition education programs, for instance, can smooth out nutritional deficiencies for those most vulnerable. As these policies integrate with good dietary recommendations, they construct an architecture that not only enhances individual nutrition but also raises public health as a whole (Wellesley et al., 2015; Raneri et al., 2020).

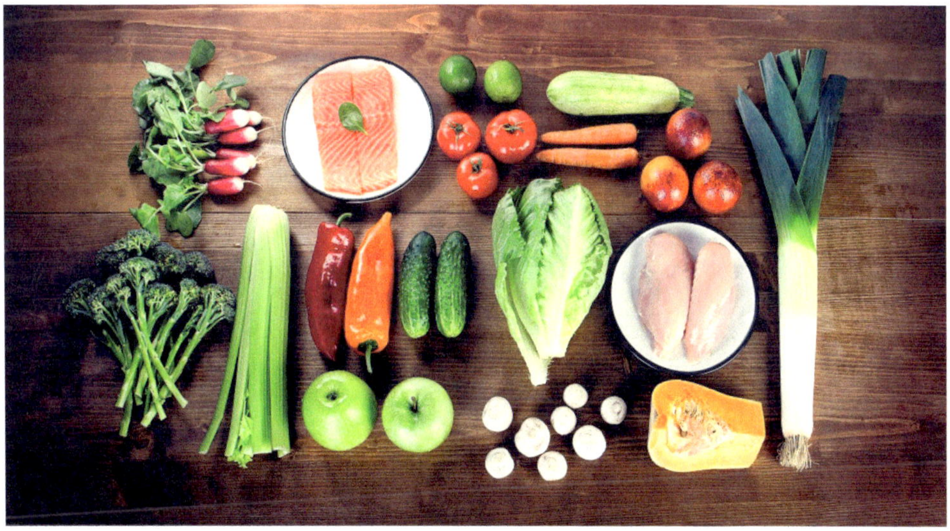

Source: Analyzing Media (2023). *Balanced Diet Feature.*

8.6.2. The Role of Education in Promoting Healthy Habits

Schools these days appear to combine nutrition and health in a manner that is new and surprising. Recently, a change has been seen as many programs, consider StarBites, for instance, combine art with health education, evoking real interest in food (Figure 8.12). Drama, dance, poetry, and music appear in surprising ways, capturing student interest and reinforcing their understanding of what healthy eating is. This imaginative approach is not merely recalling facts; it encourages children to think about better meals on a daily basis. In the majority of instances, when learning is presented in interactive, diverse ways, it really influences children's eating habits and prepares them for long-term health (Perry & May, 2006). There's also something to be said for when schools take a broad definition of health education, which can result in food and fitness policies that ring with credibility in the local community. Most schools, in their own rushed but determined manner, are trying to integrate physical activity, nutrition, and overall health lessons into a single cohesive approach. Even smaller schools tend to gain from a single, unified policy that simplifies action toward improved living. This combined and sometimes rather haphazard process—tended by parents and community groups alike—reminds everyone that good food and proper exercise count, reinforcing a collective sense of responsibility for health. In general, these concerted actions create awareness and contribute to a culture of wellness that far transcends school grounds (Barnes Hospital Bulletin, 1975; Welsh Network of Healthy School Schemes, 2007). Learning isn't limited to classroom pages or school books; it overflows into daily decisions that influence a child's existence. Schools often become the stage for illustrating the reasons behind keeping water and healthy food balanced. Teachers, informally yet efficiently, unveil the fact that proper hydration is crucial for digestion, mental sharpness, and the functioning of the body. And when hydration lessons become integrated into physical education and health class, kids end up considering their own behaviors—sometimes even twice. Setting these concepts early on creates a generation that, with its own flawed but sincere efforts, appreciates both water intake and healthy eating, eventually leading to healthier habits and better public health results.

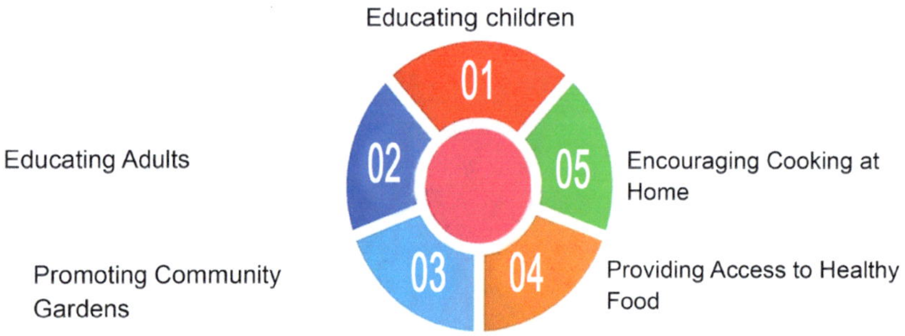

Figure 8.12. The importance of education in promoting healthy eating habits.

Source: FasterCapital. (n.d.). *Healthy World: Disinvesting from Fast Food for Well-Being—The Importance of Education in Promoting Healthy Eating Habits.*

SUMMARY

Water, nutrition, and health combine in ways that define our day-to-day well-being. Proper hydration is a big deal—when you're drinking enough, your body absorbs nutrients and operates its metabolism more efficiently. On the flip side, not getting enough water can mess with the body's ability to use all the good stuff you eat, even if your diet seems just fine, and that can lead to shortages over time. In general, drinking enough water and eating well go hand in hand when it comes to keeping you healthy. Studying, for example, typically demonstrates that adequate hydration not only energizes your metabolism but also keeps plenty of other health issues at bay, particularly for children, the elderly, and others who do more poorly when dehydration sets in. Knowing how water consumption relates to various aspects of nutrition is crucial, too, it may even direct local health schemes into new avenues. Consider that: if individuals understand that water is so important, even in all those difficult feeding regimens for preterm infants, it creates a new arena that requires attention and clear guidance. The connection between nutritional outcomes and hydration in these populations is still surprisingly under researched (you hardly ever hear much about how preterm babies grow when their feeding involves smart hydration), and that sort of research is still just beginning. Efforts to pin down firm guidelines should take into account the specific issues that these individuals encounter, ensuring that water and food strategies both have their full measure of attention (Liotto et al., 2020). Overall, the interaction between water, nutrition, and health requires a wide, general perspective on diet and well-being. When various studies highlight the significance of water in assisting nutrients in their job, it is evident that stand-alone tips simply won't cut it. What we require is a strategy that combines frequent consumption of water with healthy, well-balanced meals to ward off diseases. We need ongoing studies that continue to poke at these specifics, examining how variation in drinking and eating patterns impacts individuals of all backgrounds; this could ultimately result in public health recommendations and legislation that really strike the right note (Mazidi et al., 2021).

Pure water stands at the center of our daily good health, it's so much more than a drink to quench our thirst. Occasionally, not drinking sufficient water won't just cause dehydration; it can play havoc with the way that our bodies process food and transport vitamins and minerals. Once dehydration takes hold, the delivery of these important nutrients slows considerably, and that deceleration can cascade through our metabolic systems, sometimes even pushing us toward chronic disease. In most instances, a lack of water simply compounds nutrient problems, illustrating why any good health plan must consider hydration and nutrition as one, bundled package. Children experience the effects of water purity in a variety of ways, particularly when it comes to receiving adequate nutrition. Contaminated water, for example, can cause gastrointestinal distress that contributes to a child's inability to process essential nutrients, which can stifle growth and influence development. A UNICEF research, for instance, demonstrates that when societies prioritize clean water and improved sanitation habits, nutritional health improves significantly, especially for the most vulnerable. Initiatives in areas such as maternal and child care, and combating tropical diseases—often have tie-ins with these water, sanitation, and hygiene (WASH) interventions. Combine all these elements, and it's obvious that addressing access to water with nutritional education can reduce malnutrition rates, increase school attendance, and even help end the cycle of poverty. It's now widely accepted that proper nutrition and adequate hydration are the primary factors in preventing a variety of diseases, even certain cancers. Consider it: the nutritional quality of what we consume and drink directly determines our risk profile. Solid evidence indicates that by enhancing diets and providing regular access to clean drinking water, we can reduce the risk of developing a range of health ailments, including cancer. On this basis, most experts recommend public health interventions combining nutrition advice with provision of good hydration. When policy makers and community leaders value how water quality combines with eating habits, they are able to make actual strides in ending preventable disease. Ultimately, a well-crafted plan that addresses both nutrition and hydration not only improves personal health but also creates stronger, healthier communities.

KEY TERMS FROM THIS CHAPTER

- Alkaline reduced water (ARW)
- Commercial milk formulas (CMF)
- Dehydration
- Food security
- Global food systems
- Human nutrition
- Hydrolysis
- Iron-deficiency anemia
- Multivitamin supplements
- Nutrient-dense crops
- Nutritional security
- Sensitive systems
- Sugary beverages
- Balanced diet
- DASH diets
- Food literacy
- General health
- Global sustainability challenges
- Hydration-monitoring app
- Intelligent hydration practices
- Mental acuity
- Nutrient deficiencies
- Nutrition education,
- Nutritional value
- Small nanofertilizers
- Water consumption

CLOSER LOOK

ORAL REHYDRATION THERAPY

Oral rehydration therapy (ORT) is a method of fluid therapy administered for the treatment and prevention of dehydration, particularly that caused by diarrhea. ORT entails taking water in small quantities accompanied by some sugar and salts, such as sodium and potassium. It may also be administered through a nasogastric tube. Therapy may involve the administration of zinc supplements to decrease diarrhea duration in children and infants under 5 years old. Utilization of ORT has been estimated to reduce the risk of diarrhea-related death by up to 93%.

Side effects could be vomiting, elevated blood sodium, or elevated blood potassium. If vomiting, use should be stopped for 10 minutes and then restarted slowly. The preferred formulation is sodium chloride, sodium citrate, potassium chloride, and glucose. Glucose can be substituted with sucrose and sodium citrate can be substituted with sodium bicarbonate, if available, though the resulting solution is not shelf stable in humid environments. It functions as glucose increases the absorption of sodium and consequently water by the intestines, and the potassium chloride and sodium citrate prevent hypokalemia and acidosis, respectively, which are both frequent side effects of diarrhea. Several other preparations are also found such as formulations that can be prepared at home. Yet, the use of home preparations is not well documented.

ORT was introduced in the 1940s based on electrolyte solutions with or without glucose empirically for mild or convalescent patients but did not become widely used for rehydration and maintenance therapy until following the discovery that glucose stimulates sodium and water uptake in cholera in the 1960s. It is included in the World Health Organization's List of Essential Medicines. Globally, up to 2015, ORT is employed in 41% of children who have diarrhea. Its employment has been instrumental in lowering child mortality under the age of five years.

References

1. Cohen, M. J., Aberman, N. L., et al. (2008). *Impact of Climate Change and Bioenergy on Nutrition*. International Food Policy Research Institute (IFPRI)

2. Preece, J. (2011) Nurturing lifelong learning in communities through the National University of Lesotho: prospects and challenges. International Journal of Lifelong Education . ISSN 0260-1370(accessed on 14 May 2025).

3. Agarwal, E., Marshall, S., Miller, M., & Isenring, E. (2016). Optimising nutrition in residential aged care: A narrative review. *Maturitas, 92*, 70-78. https://doi.org/10.1016/j.maturitas.2016.06.013 (accessed on 14 May 2025).

4. Tuaputty, H., Papilaya, P., Tuapattinaya, P., Parry, C., & Alimudi, S. (2024). Macroalgae As a Source of Food And Health For Coastal Communities in Moluccas Province. *BIOEDUPAT: Pattimura Journal of Biology and Learning*, *4*(1), 153-164. https://doi.org/10.30598/bioedupat.v4.i1.pp153-164 (accessed on 14 May 2025).

5. Marmot, M; Atinmo, T; Byers, T; Chen, J; Hirohata, T; Jackson, A; James, W; + view all (2007) Food, Nutrition, Physical Activity, and the Prevention of Cancer: a Global Perspective. (WCRF/AICR Expert Report). World Cancer Research Fund / American Institute for Cancer Research: Washington DC, US. (accessed on 14 May 2025).

6. Baker, P., Karlsson, J., McCoy, D., Pope, D., et al. (2021). Examining the environmental impacts of the dairy and baby food industries: Are first-food systems a crucial missing part of the healthy and sustainable food systems agenda now underway? https://core.ac.uk/download/491343308.pdf (accessed on 14 May 2025).

7. Pelc, Z., Sędłak, K., Mlak, R., Chawrylak, K., Mielniczek, K., Leśniewska, M., Skórzewska, M., Kwietniewska, M., Paśnik, I., Gęca, K., van der Sluis, P., Banasiewicz, T., Pędziwiatr, M., Polkowski, W. P., Pawlik, T. M., Małecka-Massalska, T., & Rawicz-Pruszyński, K. (2024). MalnutritiOn assessment with biOelectrical impedaNce analysis in gastRic cancer patIentS undergoing multimodaltrEatment (MOONRISE)-Study protocol for a single-arm multicenter cross-sectional longitudinal study. *PloS one*, *19*(2), e0297583. https://doi.org/10.1371/journal.pone.0297583 (accessed on 14 May 2025).

8. Berg, G., Rybakova, D., Fischer, D., Cernava, T., Champomier Vergès, M. C., Charles, T. C., Chen, X., et al. (2020). Microbiome definition re-visited: Old concepts and new challenges. *Microbiome, 8*, Article 103. https://doi.org/10.1186/s40168-020-00875-0.

9. Menon K, Puthussery S , Ravalia A, Panchal P, Rana R, Mistry S, Tseng P, Bhandol J, Mavalankar D (2018), Effectiveness of nutrition interventions in low and middle income countries: An evidence summary. London: EPPI-Centre, Social Science Research Unit, UCL Institute of Education, University College London (accessed on 14 May 2025).

10. Rémond, D., Shahar, D. R., Gille, D., Pinto, P., Kachal, J., Peyron, M. A., Dos Santos, C. N., Walther, B., Bordoni, A., Dupont, D., Tomás-Cobos, L., & Vergères, G. (2015). Understanding the gastrointestinal tract of the elderly to develop dietary solutions that prevent malnutrition. *Oncotarget*, *6*(16), 13858–13898. https://doi.org/10.18632/oncotarget.4030 (accessed on 14 May 2025).

11. Sofia Jimenez. Assessing Market Incentive Policies in Kenya with a Food Security and Nutrition Perspective: a Macro-Microsimulation Approach. 2020.Bray, F., Ferlay, J., Soerjomataram,

I., Siegel, R. L., Torre, L. A., & Jemal, A. (2018). Global cancer statistics 2018: GLOBOCAN estimates of incidence and mortality worldwide for 36 cancers in 185 countries. *CA: A Cancer Journal for Clinicians, 68*(6), 394–424. https://doi.org/10.3322/caac.21492.

12. Brown, S. (2011). Using a Social-Ecological Model to Examine Obesity Interventions Susan Lee Brown. http://lib.dr.iastate.edu/etdCarmichael, J. C., Keller, D. S., Baldini, G., Bordeianou, L., Weiss, E. G., Lee, L., Boutros, M., et al. (2017). Clinical practice guidelines for enhanced recovery after colon and rectal surgery from the American Society of Colon and Rectal Surgeons and Society of American Gastrointestinal and Endoscopic Surgeons. *Diseases of the Colon & Rectum, 60*, 761–784. https://doi.org/10.1097/dcr.0000000000000883.

13. Cena, H., & Calder, P. C. (2020). Defining a healthy diet: Evidence for the role of contemporary dietary patterns in health and disease. *Nutrients, 12*(2), 334. https://doi.org/10.3390/nu12020334.

14. Choi, T., Chan, B., Grech, L., Kwok, A., Webber, K., Wong, J., Nguyen, M., et al. (2023). Factors influencing COVID-19 vaccine hesitancy among patients with serious chronic illnesses during the initial Australian vaccine rollout: A multi-center qualitative analysis using the health belief model. *Vaccines, 11.* https://www.semanticscholar.org/paper/e2c9992ab160a8b7f25c447cb9cdbfaeb4a5619b (accessed on 14 May 2025).

15. Choi, Y. Y., Jensen, M., Fleming-Milici, F., & Harris, J. L. (2022). Caregivers' provision of sweetened fruit-flavored drinks to young children: Importance of perceived product attributes and differences by socio-demographic and behavioral characteristics. *Public Health Nutrition, 25*, 2308–2316. https://www.semanticscholar.org/paper/41e4fc0e6e91faafb1164bdfa6bfe4ca0d1fff37 (accessed on 14 May 2025).

16. Delos Reyes, F. S. L. G., Mamaril, A. C. C., Matias, T. J. P., Tronco, M. K. V., Samson, G. R., Javier, N. D., Fadriquela, A., et al. (2021). The search for the elixir of life: On the therapeutic potential of alkaline reduced water in metabolic syndromes. *Processes, 9*, 1876. https://doi.org/10.3390/pr9111876.

17. Raneri; J.E.; Kennedy, G.; Nguyen, T.; Wertheim-Heck, S.; Do, H.; Nguyen, P.H. (2019) Determining key research areas for healthier diets and sustainable food systems in Viet Nam. IFPRI Discussion Paper 1872. Washington, DC: International Food Policy Research Institute (IFPRI). 127 p. https://doi.org/10.2499/p15738coll2.133433 (accessed on 14 May 2025).

18. Dodd, F. L., Kennedy, D. O., Stevenson, E. J., Veasey, R. C., Walker, K., Reed, S., Jackson, P. A., & Haskell-Ramsay, C. F. (2020). Acute and chronic effects of multivitamin/mineral supplementation on objective and subjective energy measures. *Nutrition & metabolism, 17*, 16. https://doi.org/10.1186/s12986-020-00435-1(accessed on 14 May 2025).

19. Esteves Mills, J., & Cumming, O. (2016). *The Impact of Water, Sanitation, and Hygiene on Key Health and Social Outcomes: Review of Evidence*. https://core.ac.uk/download/75761114.pdf (accessed on 14 May 2025).

20. Laura Wellesley, Catherine Happer, Antony Froggatt (2015). *Changing Climate, Changing Diets: Pathways to Lower Meat Consumption*. Publisher Royal Institute of International Affairs, Chatham House, 2015. ISBN 1784130559, 9781784130558. https://core.ac.uk/download/42367153.pdf (accessed on 14 May 2025).

21. Garrett, James & L, James & ed, & Ruel, Marie & T, Marie. (2000). Achieving urban food and

nutrition security in the developing world:. International Food Policy Research Institute (IFPRI), 2020 vision focus. (accessed on 14 May 2025).

22. Habicht, J. P., Kim, S. S., Menon, P., Stoltzfus, R., et al. (2025). *How do Programs Work to Improve Child Nutrition? Program Impact Pathways of Three Nongovernmental Organization Intervention Projects in the Peruvian Highlands.* https://core.ac.uk/download/pdf/6254914.pdf (accessed on 14 May 2025).

23. Hijdra, T., Health Science, D. of, Department of Sociology and Social, University, et al. (2023). Work participation of elderly construction workers: A systematic review and qualitative analysis. *The European Journal of Public Health, 33.* https://www.semanticscholar.org/paper/7bdf53db6ec6dd402384561640a135c7d32fed84 (accessed on 14 May 2025).

24. Högberg, A. (2003). *Cereal Non-Starch Polysaccharides in Pig Diets.* https://core.ac.uk/download/11694626.pdf (accessed on 14 May 2025).

25. Intergovernmental Panel on Climate Change. (2023). *Climate Change 2022–Impacts, Adaptation and Vulnerability.* https://doi.org/10.1017/9781009325844.

26. Kumar, P., Lee, S. S., Zhang, M., Tsang, Y. F., & Kim, K. H. (2019). Heavy metals in food crops: Health risks, fate, mechanisms, and management. *Environment International, 125*, 365–385. https://doi.org/10.1016/j.envint.2019.01.067.

27. Woodhouse, Allison and Lamport, Ph.D., Mark A. (2012) "The Relationship of Food and Academic Performance: A Preliminary Examination of the Factors of Nutritional Neuroscience, Malnutrition, and Diet Adequacy," *Christian Perspectives in Education*, 5(1). Available at: https://digitalcommons.liberty.edu/cpe/vol5/iss1/1 (accessed on 14 May 2025).

28. Thom, G., & Lean, M. (2017). Is There an Optimal Diet for Weight Management and Metabolic Health?. *Gastroenterology, 152*(7), 1739–1751. https://doi.org/10.1053/j.gastro.2017.01.056 (accessed on 14 May 2025).

29. LeBoff, M. S., Greenspan, S. L., Insogna, K., Lewiecki, E. M., Saag, K. G., Singer, A., & Siris, E. S. (2022). The clinician's guide to prevention and treatment of osteoporosis. *Osteoporosis International, 33*, 2049–2102. https://doi.org/10.1007/s00198-021-05900-y.

30. Liotto, N., Cresi, F., Beghetti, I., Roggero, P., Menis, C., Corvaglia, L., Mosca, F., et al. (2020). Complementary feeding in preterm infants: A systematic review. *Nutrients, 12.* https://www.semanticscholar.org/paper/1094fe85c1f7239b08c6bc24aac7f534a33950d6 (accessed on 14 May 2025).

31. Livingston, G., Huntley, J., Sommerlad, A., Ames, D., Ballard, C., Banerjee, S., Brayne, C., et al. (2020). Dementia prevention, intervention, and care: 2020 report of the Lancet Commission. *The Lancet, 396*(10248), 413–446. https://doi.org/10.1016/s0140-6736(20)30367-6.

32. Lumbis, R. H. (2018). *Nourishing Dogs and Cats Through Their Twilight Years.* https://core.ac.uk/download/154422917.pdf (accessed on 14 May 2025).

33. Mahmud, Iffat, 1982- author.; Mbuya, Nkosinathi, author.; World Bank, issuing body.

34. Washington, DC : International Bank for Reconstruction and Development/The World Bank; 2016

35. Library Catalog ; MMS ID 9916637343406676; ISBN 9781464806988 (paper); NLM Unique ID 101663734 (accessed on 14 May 2025).

36. Perry, C., & May, S. ((2006). *Increasing Awareness of Healthy Eating Through the Use of*

Performing Arts: An Evaluation of the StarBites Project. Chester: Centre for Public Health Research, University of Chester, 2006. https://core.ac.uk/download/363942.pdf (accessed on 14 May 2025).

37. Mazidi, M., Dehghan, A., Mikhailidis, D., Jozwiak, J., Covic, A., Sattar, N., Banach, M., et al. (2021). The association between coffee and caffeine consumption and renal function: Insight from individual-level data, Mendelian randomization, and meta-analysis. *Archives of Medical Science: AMS, 18*, 900–911. https://www.semanticscholar.org/paper/8e477e6b4f2a5c204b6fa3e010c91058720dc448 (accessed on 14 May 2025).
38. Mitra, A., & Rao, N. (2019). *Gender, Water, and Nutrition in India: An Intersectional Perspective*. https://core.ac.uk/download/196593849.pdf (accessed on 14 May 2025).
39. Murray, C. J. L., Ikuta, K. S., Sharara, F., Swetschinski, L. R., Robles Aguilar, G., Gray, A. P., Han, C., et al. (2022). Global burden of bacterial antimicrobial resistance in 2019: A systematic analysis. *The Lancet, 399*(10325), 629–655. https://doi.org/10.1016/s0140-6736(21)02724-0.
40. Barnes Hospital Bulletin, June 1975. Bernard Becker Medical Library Archives. Washington University School of Medicine.(accessed on 14 May 2025).
41. Welsh Network of Healthy School Schemes. (2007). *Developing a Whole School Food and Fitness Policy*. https://core.ac.uk/download/4158108.pdf (accessed on 14 May 2025).
42. Burke, L. M., & Cox, G. R. (2020). Nutrition Strategies for Triathlon. In S. Migliorini (Ed.), Triathlon Medicine (pp. 261-287). Springer. https://doi.org/10.1007%2F978-3-030-22357-1_17 (accessed on 14 May 2025).
43. Nogaski, A., Rynell, A., Terpstra, A., Roberts, A., & Carrow, L. (2010). *Running on Empty: Nutritional Access for Children in Cook County, Illinois*. https://core.ac.uk/download/71345397.pdf (accessed on 14 May 2025).
44. Nogueira-de-Almeida, C. A., Del Ciampo, L. A., Ferraz, I. S., Del Ciampo, I. R. L., Contini, A. A., & Ued, F. V. (2020). COVID-19 and obesity in childhood and adolescence: A clinical review. *Jornal de Pediatric, 96*, 546–558. https://doi.org/10.1016/j.jped.2020.07.001.
45. Pavord, S., Daru, J., Prasannan, N., Robinson, S., Stanworth, S., & Girling, J. (2019). UK guidelines on the management of iron deficiency in pregnancy. *British Journal of Hematology, 188*(6), 819–830. https://doi.org/10.1111/bjh.16221.
46. Pinstrup-Andersen, P. (2025). *Agricultural Research and Policy for Better Health and Nutrition in Developing Countries: A Food Systems Approach*. https://core.ac.uk/download/pdf/7055873.pdf (accessed on 14 May 2025).
47. Podder, C., & Sritharan, K. (2023). *Early Market Entry Strategies for Commercialization of Digital Innovation in the Welfare Sector: A Case of Smart Nutritional Bottle "FitPot."* https://core.ac.uk/download/588315645.pdf (accessed on 14 May 2025).
48. Prasad, R., Bhattacharyya, A., & Nguyen, Q. D. (2017). Nanotechnology in sustainable agriculture: Recent developments, challenges, and perspectives. *Frontiers in Microbiology, 8*, Article 1014. https://doi.org/10.3389/fmicb.2017.01014.
49. Yu, Christina and Sarkar, Indra Neil, "A Computational Approach for Identifying Plant-Based Foods for Addressing Vitamin Deficiency Diseases" (2015). *UVM Patrick Leahy Honors College Senior Theses*. 212. https://scholarworks.uvm.edu/hcoltheses/212(accessed on 14 May 2025).

50. Shatriadi, H., Putra, C., Mohd. Said, F., & Abd Rashid, N. (2024). Healthy environment for optimal growth and development: Preventing stunting early. JIKA (ProceedingsThe 2 nd INHOSTEC (Institut Ilmu Kesehatan dan Teknologi Muhammadiyah Palembang) (accessed on 14 May 2025).

51. Singhal, T. (2020). A review of coronavirus disease-2019 (COVID-19). *The Indian Journal of Pediatrics, 87*, 281–286. https://doi.org/10.1007/s12098-020-03263-6.

52. Webb, P. , Thorne-Lyman, A. (2006) Entitlement Failure from a Food Quality Perspective: The Life and Death Role of Vitamins and Minerals in Humanitarian Crises. Research Paper 2006/140. Helsinki: UNU-WIDER. (accessed on 14 May 2025).

53. United Nations System Standing Committee on Nutrition. (2020). *Water and Nutrition: Harmonizing Actions for the United Nations Decade of Action on Nutrition and the United Nations Water Action Decade*. https://core.ac.uk/download/288633623.pdf (accessed on 14 May 2025).

54. Vos, T., Abajobir, A. A., Abate, K. H., Abbafati, C., Abbas, K., Abd-Allah, F., Abdulkader, R. S., et al. (2017). Global, regional, and national incidence, prevalence, and years lived with disability for 328 diseases and injuries for 195 countries, 1990–2016: A systematic analysis for the Global Burden of Disease Study 2016. *The Lancet, 390*(10100), 1211–1259. https://doi.org/10.1016/s0140-6736(17)32154-2.

55. Wei, P. F. (2020). Diagnosis and treatment protocol for novel coronavirus pneumonia (Trial version 7). *Chinese Medical Journal, 133*, 1087–1095. https://doi.org/10.1097/cm9.0000000000000819.

56. Zou, M. L. (2007). *Variation in the Apparent Fecal Digestibility of Macronutrients and Urinary Energy Excretion for Three Diets Varying in Fat and Fiber Content—Assessment of the Atwater Factors and Related Energy Conversion Factors* (Master's thesis, Massey University, Palmerston North, New Zealand). https://core.ac.uk/download/162617248.pdf (accessed on 14 May 2025).

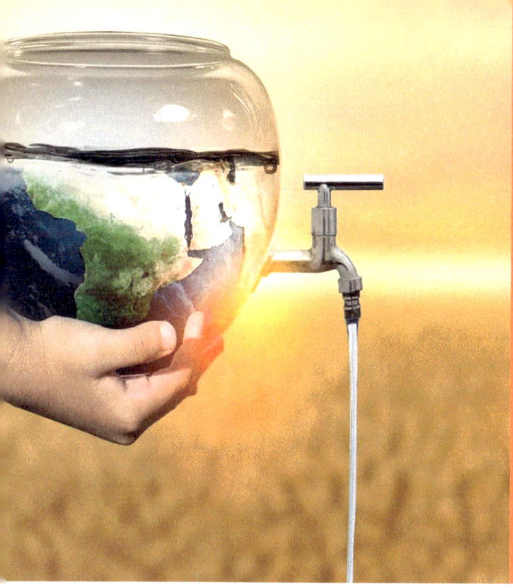

Chapter 9

CLIMATE CHANGE AND WATER HEALTH

Contents

Introduction

Climate change and water health have been much in the news recently, water infrastructure takes the hit as temperatures rise and weather acts erratically. Increased heat and changing weather patterns push both freshwater availability and quality into uncharted territory. Changes in rainfall combined with warmer days don't simply translate to less water in total; they can also threaten water purity, igniting problems for public health and natural ecosystems. Really, knowing these complex details is key if we're going to come up with fixes that help both people and ecosystems. Extreme weather events pile on the pressure too, such as floods, droughts, even hurricanes—that often upset water supplies in unexpected ways. A heavy downpour might contaminate tap water one moment, while rising sea levels can allow saltwater to creep into once-reliable aquifers, making them suspect. Such disruptions compel communities to find new, innovative approaches, ones that combine technical work with larger social support to maintain water systems strong even when nature throws a curve. Policy is no less crucial here. Sound policies that connect local needs to global challenges are, by and large, the foundation of good water management. In most instances, diligent planning and explicit examples from various parts of the world indicate that when climate realities are integrated into water policies, the outcomes are stronger. Finally, the combination of environmental changes, water quality concerns, and governance choices makes this subject a rich soil for continued investigation, and for taking timely, needed action.

Definition of Climate Change

Climate hasn't been writing a straightforward script for many years now, it's influenced by the natural rhythms of nature intertwined with what we do. Greenhouse gas emissions, rising day by day, have triggered a domino effect that goes far beyond a few degrees extra on the thermometer. You begin to notice peculiar shifts not only in the average temperatures but also in phenomena such as weather fluctuations, rising sea levels, and even the way the air itself moves. When we say climate change, we're referring to those gradual, long-term modifications and the steep, abrupt variations in the weather. This confusion lands particularly hard in fields such as agriculture and water supplies, where recognizing these changes is necessary to understand how water's availability and quality can decline over the long term (Mukherjee, 2021). It's not just a matter of getting cozy; climate change introduces extreme occurrences into the discussion as well. Consider droughts, floods, and rain that just don't play by the book. Higher heat tends to increase evaporation, which then diminishes the quantity of freshwater we can rely on. All these influencing factors ultimately mess with water's quality and availability in both unexpected and concerning ways. Aquatic ecosystems and biodiversity suffer, and globally we could end up with significant water distribution gaps—adding to the burden on regions already tight on water. In most instances, communities are left to scramble for adaptation plans, trying to find ways of managing these quickly changing conditions (Mukherjee, 2021). Being confronted by these urgent issues implies that strong policy interventions are downright necessary in order to assist in keeping our water systems in balance. Policymakers have to delve into scientific data and climate projections, mixing knowledge from environmental science, economics, and even social considerations. This type of interdisciplinary combination is usually the sole method to design flexible solutions that can withstand upcoming uncertainties. Effective policies may cross the divide between today's challenges and tomorrow's demands, making water accessible and safe for all. When we truly understand all the turns and twists of climate change, we lay the groundwork for strategies that not only safeguard water health but also ensure equitable access to this life-giving resource (Denisow et al., 2016).

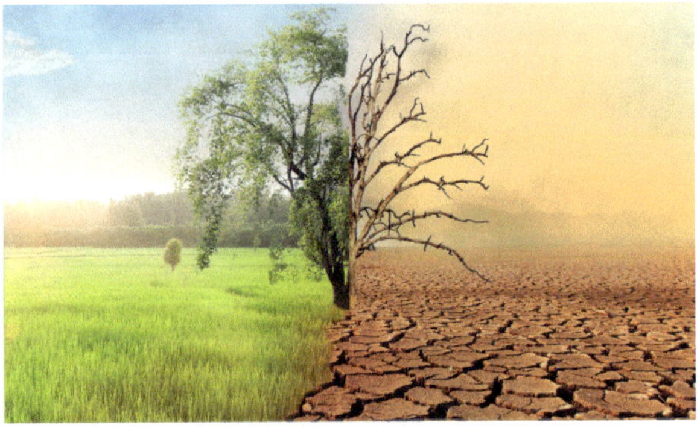

Source: Shopequo (2023). *What is Climate Change: Causes, Impact on Humans and Animals.*

Importance of Water Health

Climate change and water health are connected in ways that disturb both nature and our everyday lives. Increasing heat and erratic rain disrupt the regular flow, leaving water sources—both in terms of quality and quantity—to bear the brunt. The IPCC looked into these twists and turns, and its Synthesis Report tells us that getting a grip on these complex associations is key if we're going to form smart water policies. Clean water isn't just about human well-being; it's also the backbone of vibrant aquatic habitats that a host of species call home. And when water slips up, the ripple effects reach food supplies and even local economies—with effects that spin outwards (Calvin et al., 2023). Wild weather is making things yet more unpredictable. Floods can spill pollutants directly into our freshwater locations while droughts make everyone vie for what little water is around. The IPCC Working Group II explored these many effects, and they revealed to us that these extreme weather conditions cause both short-term crises and enduring vulnerabilities. On average, investing in sustainable construction projects may absorb the impact of heavy rain or extended dry periods. In the majority of instances, even minor repairs or enhancements can assist in maintaining clean water on hand, but implementing those changes isn't always simple or routine (Intergovernmental Panel on Climate Change, 2023). Acting now is still our best bet at maintaining water health in the face of a changing climate. Strong policies, based on science, are necessary to combat declining quality and scarcity without becoming mired in bureaucracy. Governments, local businesses, and ordinary communities must cooperate—often in unorthodox partnerships—to create plans that address today's bumps while protecting tomorrow's priorities. The truth is that water challenges don't abide by boundaries or budgets; they propagate everywhere. With a little more insight and some real collaboration, there's a promise that today's and tomorrow's generations will not have to fight over a fundamental, life-sustaining commodity (Calvin et al., 2023).

9.1. Effects on Water Availability

Climate change is turning things upside down, particularly when you consider how it scrambles our water cycles. We're experiencing more extreme weather—big fluctuations such as longer dry spells and precipitous rains—that really get to the bottom of how much fresh water we can rely on (Figure 9.1). Certain places that were once flowing with water are now under surprise stress, with groundwater and surface water supplies shrinking. This decline not only exacerbates water scarcity but also appears to be correlated with additional instances of waterborne disease from contaminated supplies. It's quite apparent that grasping how climate changes and water supplies interact is central to determining our next move (Zhang et al., 2023). Exploration a bit further into water quality shows a quite complex picture. Increased temperatures and bizarre, unpredictable rain patterns are stimulating poisonous algal blooms, which in turn disrupt surface and subsurface water systems. When torrential rains occur, they tend to wash just about any kind of pollutant into these water bodies. This unexpected runoff reveals vulnerabilities in our water treatment facilities, which may threaten public health. Addressing these problems involves not only concentrating on water cycles, but also taking into account the socio-economic aspects involved in the availability of water and its purity. More often than not, investing in more infrastructure and in smarter, more sustainable approaches is an imperative (Intergovernmental Panel on Climate Change, 2023). On top of everything, our policies must keep pace with these multifaceted challenges. Today's leaders have the daunting task of combining new scientific insights with pragmatic water management while also encouraging long-term, sustainable utilization of resources. This may include supporting green infrastructure, such as wetlands and permeable surfaces—so that nature can do its work with water capture and filtration. Creating balanced laws based on current climate data can inform communities on how to conserve water and avoid some of the most adverse outcomes of extreme weather. Short, the key is combining intelligent policy, robust science, and authentic community effort for coping with the daunting intersection of water health and climate change (Zhang et al., 2023).

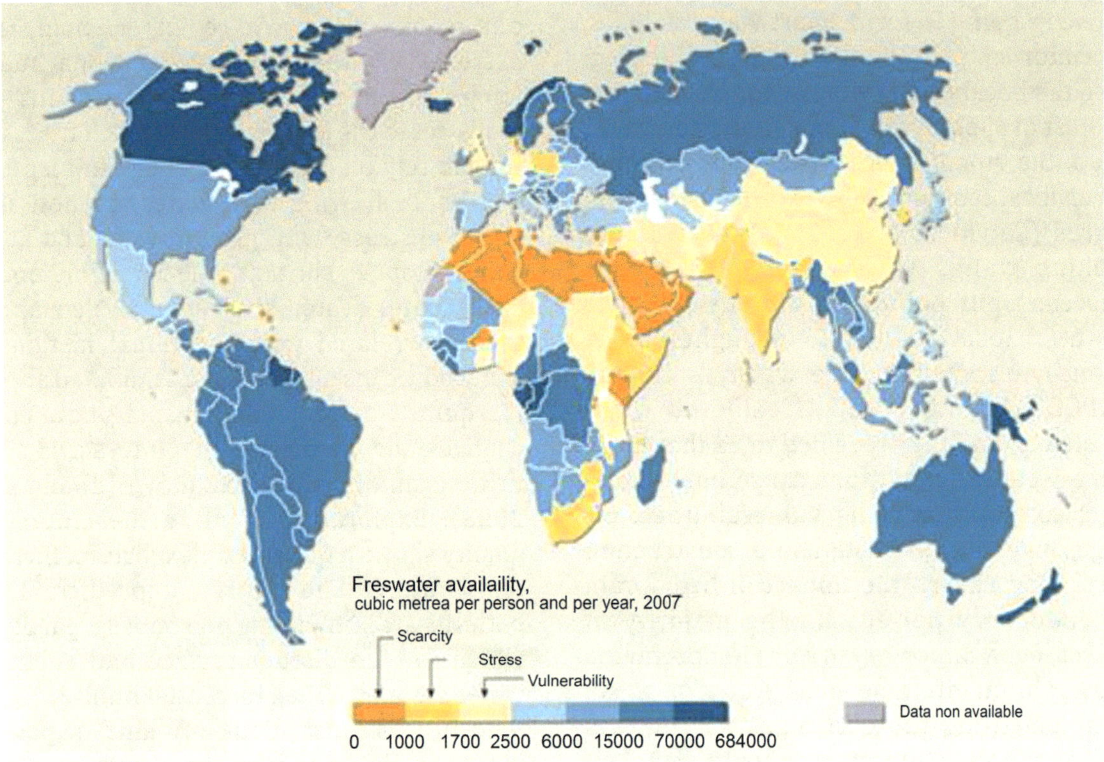

Figure 9.1. Fresh water availability and country classification.

Source: Gebrechorkos, S. H (2014). *Fresh Water Availability and Country Classification.* In *The Role of Information and Communication Technology (ICT) in Water Resource Management.*

9.1.1. Changes in Precipitation Patterns

Climate change is not simply about warmer days, it plays havoc with our weather in strange ways. You know, it's not only increasing temperatures but also distorting the normal rainfall patterns. Heavy rains bang down on some areas out of the blue while others become dry, affecting water availability and quality. The IPCC broadly asserts that such uneven changes result in flooding intensifies here and dries out there, adding on water scarcity where we least anticipate. Strangely, some areas receive excess rain while others receive hardly any, and this topsy-turvy trend disrupts the hydrologic cycle, necessitating adaptive strategies and intelligent policies (Intergovernmental Panel on Climate Change). Attempting to define what's going on with all this wild-and-woolly rain requires sly new tools. Consider the CHIRPS dataset—short for Climate Hazards Group Infrared Precipitation with Stations, it slyly sews together satellite images and ground station measurements to provide us with a high-resolution view of rainfall patterns over time. This combination of satellite snapshots and neighborhood data reveals information and subtleties in the manner in which precipitation wanes or increases, particularly in regions such as the Greater Horn of Africa. In most instances, these dense analyses, although somewhat unsightly at times, assist decision-makers as they map out adaptive measures to confront the changes head-on (Funk et al., 2015). Water management nowadays must contend with wild fluctuations—floods one place, droughts somewhere else, and what that means is science and policy need to talk. As threats from excess rain to protracted dryness accumulate, crafting a resilient water infrastructure (gosh, even professionals trip on this term now and then) becomes a necessity. Policymakers are commonly advised to invest in projects that fortify our water systems for both deluges and deficits. Frequently, conclusions from panels such as the IPCC push us toward more adaptable, in-the-field solutions. Finally, securing water safety for people and the environment requires a collective, sometimes makeshift effort that blends scientific sophistication with practical solutions (Intergovernmental Panel on Climate Change, 2023).

9.1.2. Increased Evaporation Rates

Our heating planet isn't all about increased temperature, it's also altering the way water acts. As temperatures rise, water evaporates more quickly from rivers and lakes, and that translates to our water cycle becoming out of balance. When water evaporates more rapidly, levels fall and toxins become more concentrated. This isn't just a numbers problem, it's already an issue of tight water supplies in many areas, and quicker evaporation just means that shortage becomes even more acute. Clean water gets less plentiful, public health suffers, and agriculture hurts as well. In most instances, it appears that knowing these accelerating rates of evaporation is the key to developing workable methods to address climate-driven water issues. Consider Senegal, for instance—there, heightened evaporation collides with other social and economic problems already present. Rainwater-dependent farmers discover that as more water evaporation occurs, their crops begin to diminish. Where rainwater is not sufficient, they're driven toward the use of groundwater; yet, excessive usage there only worsens the lack and contributes to environmental strain. In a nation already struggling with severe poverty, these additional climate stresses really make matters worse. It becomes clear that any solution has to integrate water management with environmental stewardship and agricultural requirements, understanding that climate, water, and economic issues are heavily interconnected.

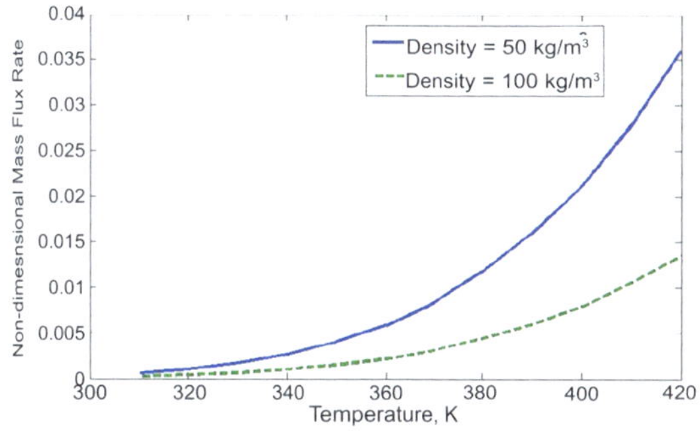

Figure 9.2. Non-dimensional water evaporation rate as a function of temperature for two different effective density parameter values.

Source: Gokoglu, S., et al. (2014). *Non-Dimensional Water Evaporation Rate as a Function of Temperature for Two Different Effective Density Parameter Values.* In *Analysis of Water Extraction from Lunar Regolith*. NASA Glenn Research Center.

Policy-makers, however, have a substantial undertaking before them if they're going to contain such challenges. They must invest in good research and get good data on evaporation patterns, not only to address the problems of today but also to prepare for a more opaque future. More monitoring is required so that, when conditions change, policies may be tweaked on the fly. Most importantly, cooperation between the sectors of agriculture, water resource management, and the environment is critical. As different places have demonstrated, when scientists collaborate with communities, they can design adaptive strategies that not only minimize the negative impacts of enhanced evaporation but also make water resources equitable and safe for all (Figure 9.2).

9.1.3. Groundwater Depletion

Climate change is stretching our water resources to their limits, and it's affecting groundwater in all sorts of unforeseen ways. Excessive withdrawal of water—driven by strange changes in rainfall and increased evaporation—has led to underground storage decreasing significantly. As levels decrease, it's not only that there's less water; the water quality also diminishes because lower levels allow more salt and even surface contaminations to enter. Wild weather, whether protracted droughts or unseasonal rain, only ratchets up the stakes, causing those levels to fluctuate erratically. All that sort of chaos serves to illustrate that we require water management strategies which function immediately and in the future as well, integrating with larger schemes to maintain our water sustainable (Calvin et al., 2023). There is no single silver bullet to solve groundwater depletion; we must blend a combination of adaptive measures that consider both environmental and socio-economic perspectives (Figure 9.3). In the majority of situations, tightening water conservation and management is essential, particularly in areas where aquifers are heavily depended upon for agriculture and domestic purposes. Regulations that encourage more responsible water draws and incentivize water-saving technology can help soothe the nasty impacts of climate change. And community education and outreach have a large role to play in fostering a culture of conservation, encouraging people and businesses to use water more conservatively. Once all the science is combined, it becomes clear that working together between policymakers, scientists, and local communities is essential to truly understanding and addressing groundwater issues in our changing world (Intergovernmental Panel on Climate Change, 2023). It is difficult to overemphasize how critical policy is when addressing our increasingly strained groundwater resources. As a general rule, sound government—to bring together all elements of water management, is needed to address both the short-term consequences of depletion and the long-term issues of shifting weather patterns. In a lot of instances, policy must promote investments in infrastructure that assists with groundwater recharge and safeguards aquifer systems. And because a lot of aquifers extend across national frontiers, global coordination is all but obligatory. With increasing populations and changing water behaviors driving demand upwards, proactive groundwater-sustaining policies are going to be central to keeping our water safe in the future for generations to come (Calvin et al., 2023; Intergovernmental Panel on Climate Change, 2023).

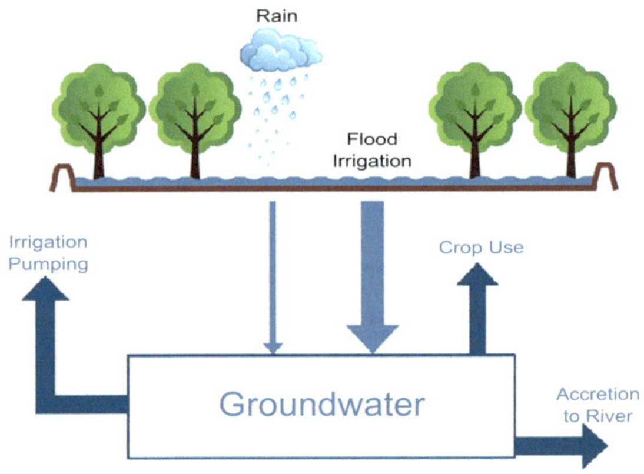

Figure 9.3. Groundwater depletion.

Source: World Green Bridge. (n.d.). *Climate Change: The Magnitude of the Problem.* https://www.worldgreenbridge.org/wpimages/wpbd56d200_06.png.

9.2. Effects on Water Quality

Ecosystems are being compelled to adjust as our weather changes, and water quality is struggling more than ever before. Dissolved oxygen—a crucial indicator of water health, can float up and down with higher temperatures and choppy fluctuations in water levels. Warmer water, for the most part, just can't contain as much oxygen, occasionally leading to low-oxygen areas that threaten aquatic life. Simultaneously, more intense rains will cause greater runoff, which tends to carry along a combination of fertilizers, sediments, and other contaminants into rivers and lakes. This added load of nutrients can trigger those very toxic algal blooms that disrupt water quality and ultimately harmed our health as well as the local ecosystem. All of these factors, combined, ensure that it is evident that the comprehension of such complex dynamics is imperative in ensuring that water resources are well managed in a shifting climate (Calvin et al., 2023). Extreme weather occurrences provide a new dimension to the issue, one that goes beyond the typical impact of warmer days and erratic rains. Heavy rains and flooding can overburden sewage and wastewater systems, even cause them to overflow, while urban pollutants leak out in unanticipated fashions. That situation tends to increase the concentration of pathogens and chemicals in surface waters, with severe public health implications. Drought gets in on the action by reducing water bodies and further concentrating pollutants. In general, all these diverse events scream out the necessity for continued, cautious water monitoring so policymakers can make adjustments to frameworks in order to assist populations in preparing for abrupt environmental shocks (Intergovernmental Panel on Climate Change, 2023). Combining adaptive approaches into water management is quite important if we're going to mitigate climate change's ugly punch on water quality. Smart policy can unlock the door to green infrastructure that leverages nature's own mechanisms to filter water and slow down runoff. Methods such as reforestation, restoration of wetlands and sustainable agriculture not only improve water quality but also provide a cushion against stormy weather. In addition, when local residents and educational programs take hold, they serve to encourage responsible use of water and ongoing surveillance, even if that involves a little bit of experimentation in the process. As voices at the local level become more concerned with maintaining their water systems, the collaborative effort to maintain clean water gains speed. Finally, collaborative efforts between governments, scientists, and ordinary people are essential for creating a sustainable arrangement that caters to the well-being of our aquatic habitats as well as the health of our communities (Calvin et al., 2023).

9.2.1. Contamination from Runoff

Urban expansion and changing land use, coupled with climate change, slammed our water infrastructure. Increased heat and altered rain patterns result in storms growing more ferocious, and with them, runoff spikes more erratically. This runoff is not simply water, it takes along a complex cocktail of city and farm runoff. Fertilizers, some pesticides, heavy metals, even small pathogens all catch a ride into our rivers and lakes. In most places where solid water management just isn't there, it becomes a perpetual loop where bad stuff just keeps accumulating, seriously straining on water quality and supply—as several studies have pointed out (Jöm et al., 2023). Clever policy is more important than ever, since climate change and runoff contamination intersect in ways that require rapid, adaptable action. Increasing numbers of people in decision-making positions are realizing that reducing pollution while managing sweeping climate changes is a delicate, yet inevitable, dance. Concepts such as rain gardens and permeable pavements—a type of green Band-Aid, can cut down on runoff and trap contaminants before water bodies get hit. And when severe weather makes its appearance, these problems just intensify, pushing the levels of contamination even greater during heavy rain periods. Overall, we need strategic policies that blend environmental concern with the power of communities (Birnbaum et al., 2021). It is also true that education and community action cannot be overlooked in addressing concerns of runoff. Sharing some elementary information about where pollution originates and what it does to our water equips individuals to get into action and defend local resources. Practices that deconstruct land stewardship, such as monitoring pesticide application or maintaining natural cover where water runs, can truly make inroads on the pollutant burden. Even engaging locals in periodic inspections can kindle feelings of responsibility and ownership. Where policy, technology, and grassroots activism come together in most instances, you have a stronger strategy for warding off water quality issues fueled by global warming (Jöm et al., 2023).

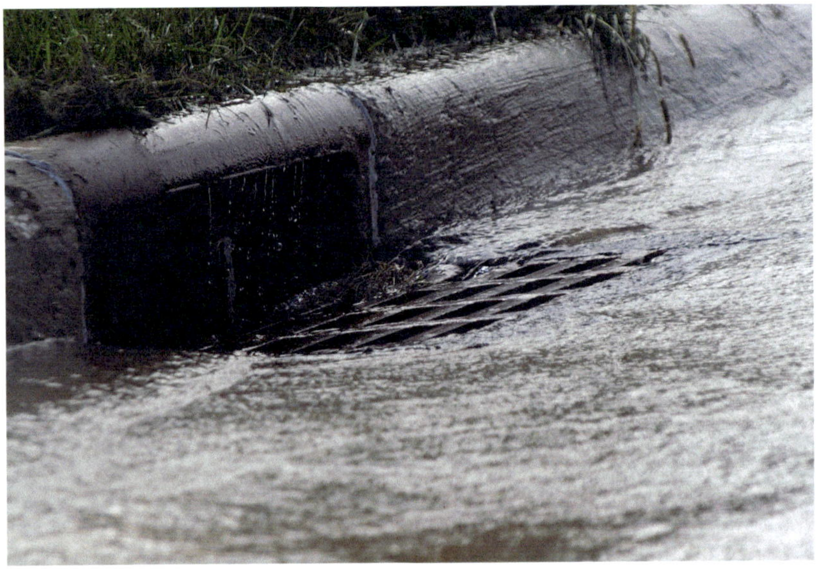

Source: By Robert Lawton - Own work, CC BY-SA 2.5, https://commons.wikimedia.org/w/index.php?curid=1243835

9.2.2. Altered Water Temperature

Climate change and increasing water temperatures have been disrupting aquatic ecosystems in unpredictable manners. The warm weather disrupts long-standing biological routines—both water-dwelling organisms and the water quality itself left in pretty unstable positions. At times, when water heats up, dissolved oxygen concentrations decrease, which many organisms rely on. Furthermore, the added warmth can induce toxic algal blooms that ultimately release noxious compounds and possibly pollute drinking water. Detailed descriptions by the Intergovernmental Panel on Climate Change (IPCC) describe how these interlinked changes play out (Figure 9.4) (Calvin et al., 2023). Changed water temperatures don't only disturb biodiversity, they also pose serious threats to human health and water supplies. Severe weather, when combined with increasing heat, tends to amplify droughts and floods and render water sources far less dependable. When the surface heats up, evaporation kicks in, leading to lower water levels that can really mess with agricultural irrigation. It isn't only about having less water immediately available; the water's quality often takes a hit too, forcing costly filtration and treatment processes. In many cases, this degradation piles extra strain on water management systems, so understanding these multifaceted effects is essential if we're to develop workable adaptation strategies. Overall, the IPCC identifies climate-resilient development as part of the solution (Intergovernmental Panel on Climate Change, 2023). Managing these changes in water temperature requires strong policy responses at the local, national, and even international levels.

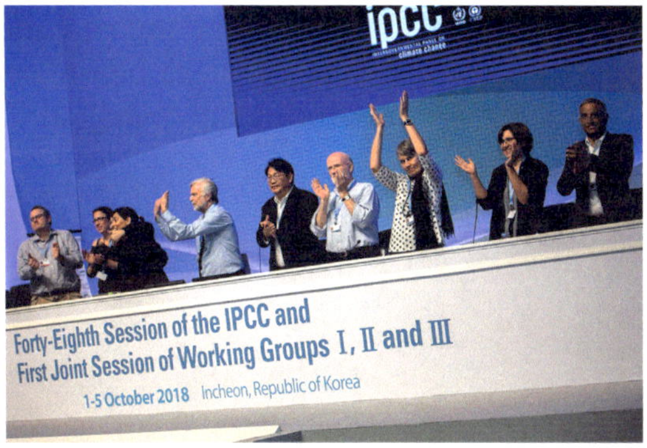

Figure 9.4. Adoption of the Summary for Policymakers of the IPCC Special Report on Global Warming of 1.5°C in 2018*Source:* By User:Sean Wu, International Institute for Sustainable Development - Photo by IISD/ENB, Sean Wu (Attribution Requirements for online use: visible Text: Photo by IISD/ENB Sean Wu (https://enb.iisd.org/attribution-guidelines)), CC BY 4.0, https://commons.wikimedia.org/w/index.php?curid=126405791

Decision-makers must incorporate climate data into water management strategies in an effort to more effectively address these dynamic thermal conditions (Figure 9.5). Actions may include installing monitoring systems for water temperature, investing in green infrastructure that increases water retention and quality, and even cross-sector collaboration to promote sustainable use. Engaging communities, and making the public aware of these changes in water, can catalyze the type of collective action that underpins ecosystem resilience. Finally, effective policies convert scientific understanding into effective practical strategies for conserving water resources, as argued by the IPCC (Calvin et al., 2023).

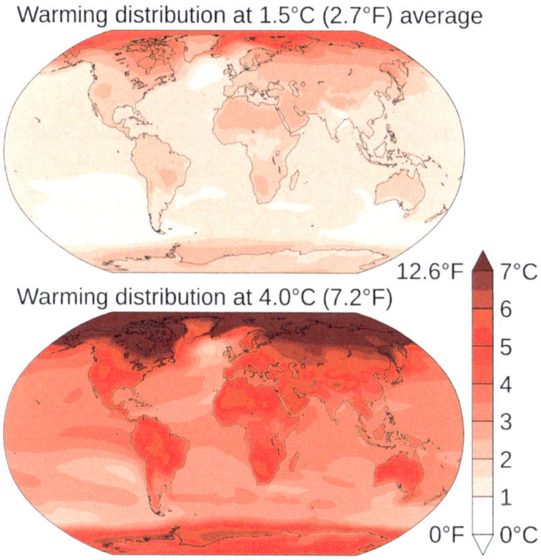

Figure 9.5. Water temperature.

Source: By Efbrazil - Own work, CC BY-SA 4.0, https://commons.wikimedia.org/w/index.php?curid=87862027

9.2.3. Increased Algal Blooms

Warming temperatures combined with additional nutrients from agricultural runoff are bubbling up more than talk about our water. Warming waters allow toxic algae to thrive (Figure 9.6), and these blooms pull oxygen out of lakes and rivers, which forces aquatic life to struggle to survive. Large storms and heavy rains tend to pour even more nutrients into our waters, exacerbating the situation. For the most part, when water quality declines, toxins from these algae migrate into seafood, threatening those who rely on these resources for sustenance and livelihood (Philip et al., 2020). Already delicate ecosystems find themselves displaying just how stressed they become when harmful algal blooms establish themselves. Most communities rely on water recreation and tourism for local revenues, and when those blooms spread, they can quite literally throw a spanner in the works. Frankly, a lot of local governments haven't got the right regulations in place to deal with these uninvited water quality issues, issues that accompany climate change. It does appear obvious that stricter controls on nutrient runoff, combined with outreach, could pay dividends. And, furthermore, when scientists and policymakers, in collaboration with voices on the ground (albeit sometimes things get complex), engage, they are able to design strategies that catch up to an evolving climate scenario (Fawzy et al., 2020). Climate change, degraded water quality and the rapid proliferation of algal blooms are all enmeshed among themselves; they require a multi-pronged strategy to our water management. Small, sustainable steps, such as converting to cover cropping or more precise use of fertilizers—could reduce the nutrient surplus pouring into water bodies. Restoring lost wetlands can even perform like a built-in filter, catching up on pollutants before reaching lakes and streams. Continued investigation into climate's influence on water networks remains essential to informing wise, responsive policy. Overall, as investment in water health increases and pollution-targeted rule-making is tightened, policymakers are able to slow the pace of these blooms and protect both our aquatic environments and public health in an age of continually rising climate changes (Philip et al., 2020).

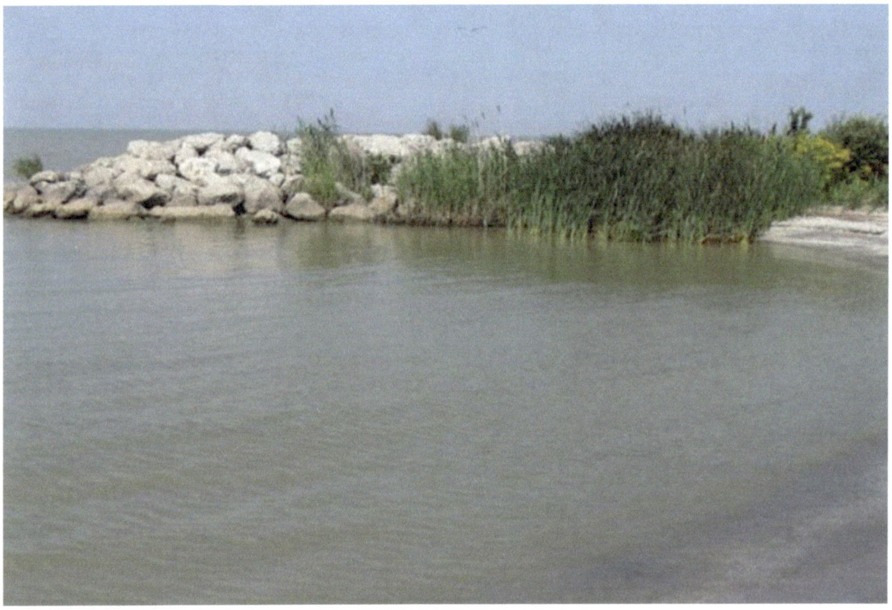

Figure 9.6. Harmful algal blooms.

Source: Wikipedia Contributors. (n.d.). *Nonvisible Cyanobacteria Harmful Algal Bloom (HAB).* Wikimedia Commons. https://upload.wikimedia.org/wikipedia/commons/a/ae/Nonvisible_cyanobacteria_HAB.png.

9.3. Impact of Extreme Weather Events

Severe weather strikes us harder and more frequently nowadays—a pretty good indication that climate change is playing havoc with our water resources. Endless droughts combine with sudden, intense floods to disrupt freshwater systems and reduce water quality. Severe droughts reduce water supplies, which then disrupt farms and drinking supplies, while intense rainstorms tend to wash contaminants and pathogens into our water sources. The Lancet Countdown 2023 report even highlights that when wild weather and health consequences meet, it indicates, in the majority of instances, a pressing need for climate action that is focused on people's wellbeing (Zhang et al., 2023). Without speedy solutions and adjustments in how we do things, communities, particularly those at highest risk, are increasingly threatened by the health of their water. Policy, not surprisingly, has much to do with all this. Effective water management regulations can enhance resilience against the unpredictable fluctuations of climate-driven water crises. Most present configurations are a little fuzzy with regard to health effects, even though public health and clean water are closely connected. IPCC's Sixth Assessment Report tends to point out how beneficial it is to incorporate adaptation strategies within overall environmental strategies in an attempt to build a model of development that assists those most exposed (Intergovernmental Panel on Climate Change, 2023). Overall, policies must address these complex challenges from all sides, making sure water is managed sustainably and community health remains protected. This frequently requires bringing health professionals, farmers, environmentalists, and even ordinary citizens—together against climate-driven water problems. Molding to these changes requires strategies that are as varied as the threats we confront. Local residents becoming involved is not only a good decision but an essential one to counter the idiosyncrasies and dangers of climate change. More advanced early warning systems, for instance, can more effectively predict floods or droughts, alerting individuals in advance to prepare in whatever manner possible. Investing in more environmentally friendly infrastructure, such as restoring wetlands or even installing a few rain gardens—allows nature to purify water and repel flood-caused contamination. All this, of course, requires a concerted action from local administrations, civic organizations, and health organizations. As these adaptation measures merge into broader public health policies, they establish a system that not only saves water resources but also supports community health, particularly as increasing extreme weather occurrences continue to intensify (Zhang et al., 2023).

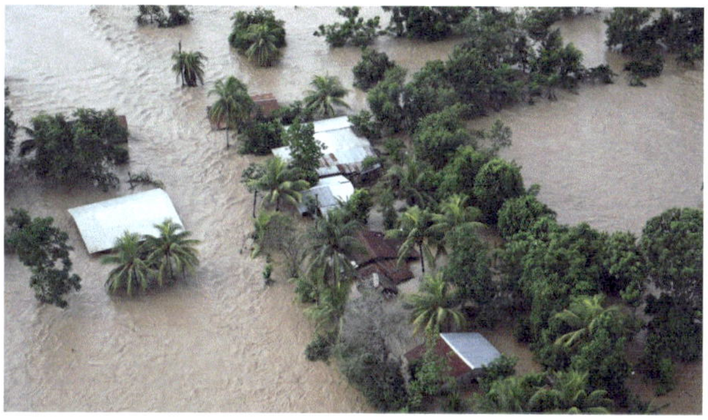

Figure: Editorial Team (2025). *Extreme Weather Events*. Carbon Impacts.

Source https://carbonimpacts.info/uploads/2025/03-March/19-Wed/Extreme-weather-events_67dacc617ff21.jpg.

9.3.1. Flooding and Its Effects on Water Resources

Climate change and flooding are entwined in ways that impact our water supplies severely—both in terms of quantity and quality. Global warming appears to churn up our weather until floods become more common and more powerful, frequently overwhelming what our water infrastructure is able to take. These unexpected deluges drench regions directly, but they also trigger longer-term troubles such as soil eroding and nutrients being washed out. Floodwaters get in the way of both surface puddles and deeper wells by combining with pollutants and altered sediments, which subsequently contribute to making our drinking water less clean (Figure 9.7). Urban areas, especially, flaunt their vulnerable places when floods occur, which necessitates immediate policy remedies. In most instances, correcting these issues requires a plan that brings various ideas together, similar to the strategy presented within the IPCC's Sixth Assessment Report (Calvin et al., 2023). Flooding not only spoils the sanctity of our water; it disturbs nature as well. When heavy water sweeps in, it has the tendency to force plant life and animals out of their typical hotspots.

This displacement is enough to change the entire balance of nature, impacting the natural services offered by an ecosystem. The destruction of such in-built water filters makes other environmental problems even more complicated. As observed in the Working Group II section of the IPCC report (Intergovernmental Panel on Climate Change, 2023), these variations tend to need adaptive and flexible responses because water systems under climatic pressure don't have a script to follow. Initiatives such as restoration and conservation activities can enable nature to recover, balancing human requirements and wildlife concerns. Considering policy, it's obvious that wise interventions are essential for controlling the various aspects of flooding's effect on water. Good governance can enable communities to be more prepared for severe weather by combining science insights with practical plans. Steps could vary from constructing additional green buffers and adjusting zoning regulations to prevent development in flood zones, to providing our stormwater infrastructure with the upgrade it so desperately needs. Local voices count as well; when community members are able to contribute their on-the-ground knowledge, it gives real substance to any plan. Policymakers need to lean into forward-looking steps bridging today's gaps while being prepared for tomorrow's shocks, mirroring the climate-resilience concepts articulated in recent IPCC reports (Intergovernmental Panel on Climate Change, 2023).

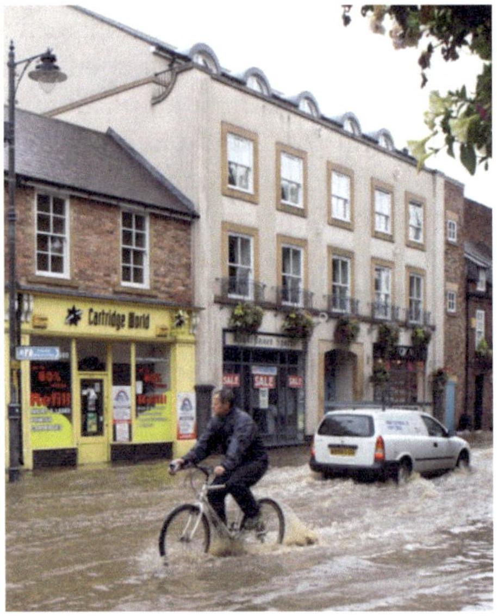

Figure 9.7. Surface water flooding.

Source: By johndal - https://www.flickr.com/photos/johndal/2835286257/in/photolist-5jxzPP-GMYPh-dxZ6YV-99EMz9-dgJGFN-dxSC3t-2jsbwH-5jBTQ5-5jxB8X-gF2qp-GMYQf-5jBUBC-5jxBgX-99ENnh-dgJP17-dgJMcb-9id1Bv-7XTr9i-7PFpsk-5jxz1x-7XWG8j-ampKGU-ampJwY-dgJE6G-5jBSSY-9N5KiH-9ig5N1-dgJQK1-5puhdW-ampMuj-dgJN3h-qXd4uv-4YfCmX-rQv3W4-dy5AQm-7PFpAT-9c7vP2-7cwNtp-5jxARv-9BAN4A-8ChMYf-7-PFptx-99P3vb-6zszRC-k7x8Dw-7PJAVs-9bWQFh-Ure6Cq-iYJaX4-aHKMLg/, CC BY-SA 2.0, https://commons.wikimedia.org/w/index.php?curid=62293788

9.3.2. Drought Conditions and Water Scarcity

Drought has been popping up in so many areas recently, and global warming is making it worse (Figure 9.8). Weather that once followed reliable patterns now catches us off guard—with ridiculously long stretches of dryness and spurts of rain that occur at random and leave water supplies scrambling. Temperatures continue to rise, so even the established patterns just seem to disappear, leaving communities with strained local water systems. The United Nations indicates that, in the majority of situations, close to half of the world's population may be facing water shortages soon (Zimmermann et al., 2025). This does not just translate to less potable water; it also translates to a greater likelihood of water-borne diseases since unsafe sources move in. Obviously, if we are to manage water responsibly, we must consider nature and what is required on the ground. Drought isn't only an ecological problem, it disrupts local life, as well. Farmers, who depend on consistent water flows, are affected by reduced crop yields and increasing food insecurity, which then propagates shockwaves throughout entire local economies. In much of the world, agriculture is the cornerstone of daily life, so when water weakens, communities are deeply affected. At the 2023 United Nations Water Conference, it was pointed out that water shortages can even trigger social tensions and conflicts related to access (Zimmermann et al., 2025). With these long-term socio-economic consequences in mind, decision-makers must become creative with cooperative measures, arranging a fair distribution of water even if it involves stretching the normal rules a little (Figure 9.9). Communities recovering from drought rely on strong policies and new, sometimes surprising, strategies. It's not merely a matter of following rain or doing math; it's about knowing genuine needs in the present and what may arrive in the future. We require drought plans that consider present vulnerabilities while also looking into the future possibilities. When local leaders, experts, and community members are able to come together, usually in impromptu conversations, it can catalyze creative policies in support of sustainable use of water and equitable access. Giving people the right tools and aid can take a dismal problem and turn it into a moment of authentic resilience, even when the process is a bit complex along the way. Ultimately, maintaining our healthy water in a variable climate requires combining robust research, common sense, and creative policy-making into a mixed, sometimes flawed, but real attempt.

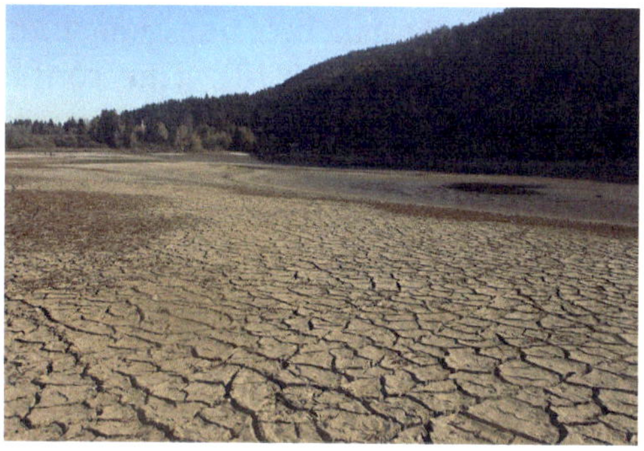

Figure 9.8. Limited water and parched soil as evidences of drought condition.

Source: By Pmau - Own work, CC BY-SA 4.0, https://commons.wikimedia.org/w/index.php?curid=73958040

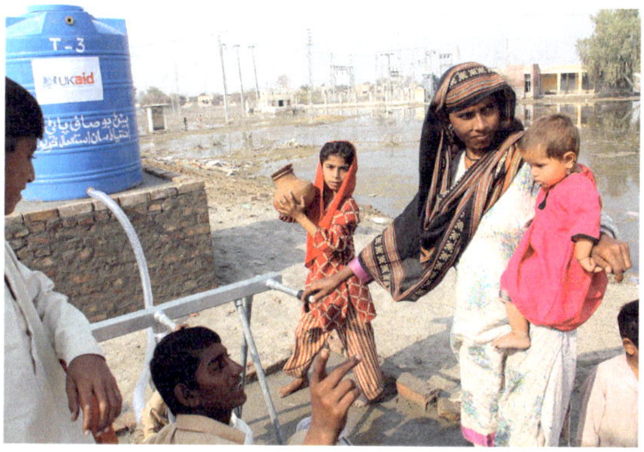

Figure 9.9. People collect clean drinking water from a tap stand.

Source: Department for International Development (DFID) (2010). *Collecting Clean Water with the Help of UKaid*. Wikimedia Commons.

9.3.3. Storm Surges and Water Contamination

Climate change's influence on storm surges is getting increasingly difficult to deny – with sea levels inching up and extreme weather events disrupting our water systems. Coastal communities, for instance, already contend with antiquated infrastructure that can't handle it, and when surges arrive, saltwater seeps into aquifers while contaminants ride along into our drinking water (Figure 9.10). This confusion not only lowers water quality but also incites public health concerns, compelling authorities to move quickly. In most instances, you find yourself in a situation where you need short-term fixes as well as longer-term infrastructure improvements in order to truly deal with these issues (Birnbaum et al., 2021).

Apart from the initial burst of storm surges, the impact on freshwater systems is quite disturbing. Agricultural runoff, sewage, and even factory discharges peak along with wild weather, occasionally producing low-oxygen patches and reducing biodiversity. Coastal wetlands – those natural barriers we rely on – take the worst of it, their capacity for filtering out pollution really suffers when water flows and sediments shift abruptly. In essence, when these wetlands fail, the quality and supply of water in surrounding communities suffer, which adds urgency to the mission to protect and restore them (Newton et al., 2020).

As storm surges become more frequent and strong due to climate change, it's evident we require a strong policy approach. This strategy should typically involve increasing disaster preparedness, investing in more sustainable infrastructure, and, yes, strengthening action against polluters before they reach our waterways. Integrating the ideas of local people, researchers, and policymakers can assist in identifying risk hotspots and fitting solutions to local needs. Additionally, integrating new technology into real-time water monitoring has a tendency to hone our policy reactions. Overall, a forward-looking, adaptive strategy may be our best bet at protecting water quality from threats posed by climate change (Birnbaum et al., 2021).

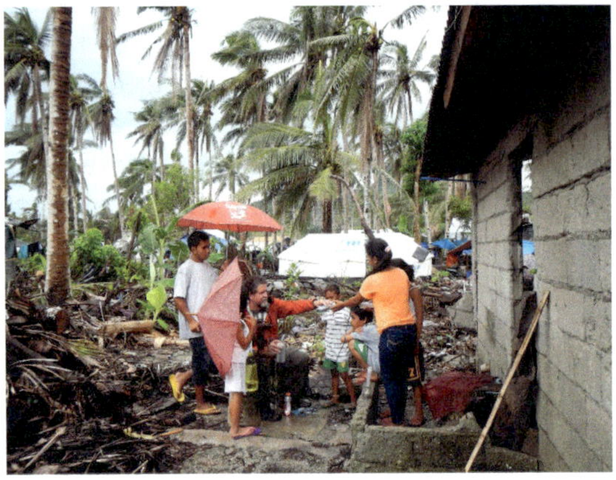

Figure 9.10. Testing water wells in the rural village after Typhoon.

Source: Jackson School of Geosciences (n.d.). *Testing Water Wells in the Rural Village After Typhoon.* https://www.jsg.utexas.edu/news/files/DSCN2333.jpg.

9.4. Adaptation Strategies

When it comes to water health and climate change, acting isn't something nice to do, it's quite literally a necessity. It isn't all about avoiding short-term water disasters; in the majority of instances, it's also about establishing protection for what could be coming down the pipeline. One solution that always comes to mind is to improve water management infrastructure so that water consumption and supply become a bit wiser, which matters in countries hit hard by unanticipated weather fluctuations. Consider China, for instance—countries like those are beginning to integrate health issues directly into the heart of their climate agendas, demonstrating that a health-led approach can be a game changer. Merging local health information with weather forecasts (as identified by the Lancet Countdowns (Zhang et al., 2023) provides policymakers an edge in ensuring individuals most vulnerable receive assistance when water quality or availability suffers. Incorporating natural, green solutions into our plan plays its own critical role in responding to these challenges, particularly in our cities. Urban areas thrive when green areas come in to screen out pollutants and retain water for a while longer, making it easier to alleviate flooding, purify the air, and increase overall public health. It's not even necessarily about cities, though; regenerating farm practices can have a significant impact as well. Methods such as harvesting rain and planting crops that dismiss drought (which, all things considered, assist in holding water resources and protecting food security) are going to have to be on our list, even if the circumstances aren't ideal. All of these steps do rely on maintaining firm, if slightly yielding, policies that keep nature and community health on the same page, consistent with our increasing faith in whole-scale solutions for climate resilience (Calvin et al., 2023). Engaging people and sharing information gets a lot of people moving and helps to build readiness at the community level as well. When people get wind of how changing weather conditions can upset water quality, they, and even local officials—begin taking actions that may at first appear modest but collectively amount to something quite substantial. Occasionally, community initiatives in water management breed innovative solutions that are custom-suited to local peculiarities; otherwise, equipping local governments with the appropriate tools and expertise is the key to achieving effective outcomes. This chaotic, but pragmatic, strategy not only makes society more resilient in the face of climate surprises, but it also aligns with global action plans, demonstrating that a little collaboration between sectors is just what the doctor ordered (Zhang et al., 2023).

9.4.1. Water Conservation Techniques

Conserving water is more and more important as our climate becomes more challenging (Figure 9.11). Farmers today attempt a combination of innovative techniques – consider contour bunds and terracing – which not only prevent soil from washing away but also retain water in fields in ways that sometimes surprise you. As these techniques are applied properly, water will penetrate into the earth more easily and runoff is minimized, enhancing natural recharge to aquifers. Vegetative barriers, for example, not only stabilize slopes but also function essentially like natural filters for contaminants, enhancing water quality overall. Then there are percolation pits and surprise small infiltration trenches that operate unobtrusively to recharge underground water storage. In most instances, the preservation of such sustainable strategies is essential to food security and environmental resilience at large – concepts that usually align with climate adaptation measures policymakers are increasingly being asked to support (Rithika et al., 2025). Climate change has also affected livestock and crop yields fairly severely, and it is evident that water-saving strategies must adapt to certain agricultural environments. The majority of studies indicate that increased temperatures and erratic weather conditions reduce water supplies to livestock, which thereby disrupts farmers' yields and financial security. In regions such as the Siavonga district, smallholder farmers have begun experimenting with different strategies; from applying heat-resistant breeds on crops as well as animals – which naturally reduces water use – to installing rainwater tanks and precision-controlled irrigation. These measures, while at times a little mixed and ad-hoc, not only facilitate reduced water scarcity but also more sustainable agriculture systems. Most would acknowledge that policies that focus on informing farmers about such methods further add to our response to the negative impacts of climate change (Likomba & & Chibomba, 2025). Ultimately, the actual success of these conservation techniques lies in how well they integrate into larger, climate-resilient policies. It requires collaboration—from researchers to policymakers and local communities—to disseminate these methods and get them implemented. Funding and capacity-building programs, for example, can provide the momentum needed for communities to implement practices that are tailored to their own environmental idiosyncrasies. Sometimes, combining local, indigenous wisdom with modern scientific ideas even sparks innovative solutions that might not have emerged otherwise. Establishing networks for sharing knowledge, and even reworking current policies in light of growing climate challenges—appears essential if we're to boost our adaptive capabilities. As the relationship between water health and climate change becomes increasingly complex, moving toward strong, sustainable water management practices is simply essential in order to preserve agricultural productivity and water quality for generations to come (Rithika et al., 2025).

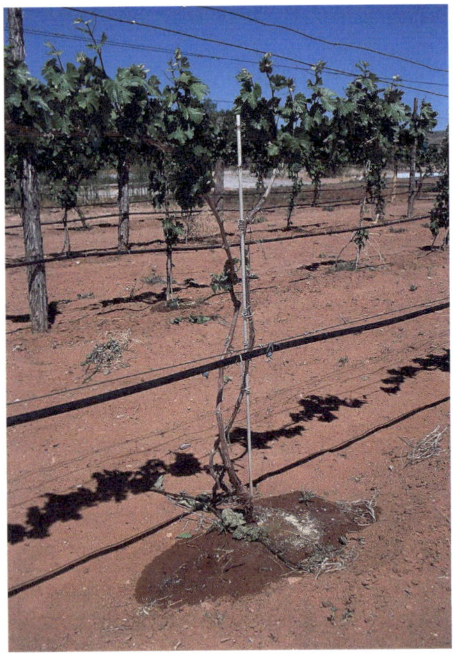

Figure 9.11. Illustration of water conservation.

Source: By Jeff Vanuga, USDA Natural Resources Conservation Service - http://photogallery.nrcs.usda.gov/Index.asp, Public Domain, https://commons.wikimedia.org/w/index.php?curid=688757

9.4.2. Infrastructure Improvements

Water infrastructure improvements appear more important than ever as our climate extremes intensify. The improvement of water treatment plants, redesigning distribution systems, and even increased storage can assist systems in coping with unpredictable weather, such as floods and droughts, that are becoming all too frequent these days. Certain cities are even experimenting with concepts such as combining green elements with sustainable drainage that not only reduces stormwater more effectively but also gives a new breath of life to the urban environment. It all interconnects—a functional necessity for clean water and a gesture toward larger climatic and health concerns, as certain reports have highlighted (Zhang et al., 2023). Constructing these enhancements is not something one segment can accomplish independently. Government agencies, private investors, and community folk are all in the mix. Policy makers may opt to invest in things such as flood walls or water recycling facilities so that everybody still gets clean water when disaster hits. Engaging the community often identifies local idiosyncrasies and requirements that could otherwise be pushed apart, resulting in investments that suit each region's climate issues and health hazards. Additionally, adding measures such as real-time monitoring and predictive information sometimes can catch problems early before they become entrenched—something that has been subtly suggested by public health professionals for some time now (Calvin et al., 2023). Spending money on more sustainable, more durable water equipment addresses short-term concerns and lays the groundwork for sustainability in the future. Implement wetlands restoration or rain garden installation: these actions support water filtering and uptake while providing a boost to native biodiversity and community green spaces. They also reduce stress on city drainage during intense rains and reduce runoff contaminants. Combining nature-inspired concepts with conventional solutions tends to be less costly in the end. Overall, this type of balanced approach illustrates just how closely ecological health and public health are intertwined. Policies in the years ahead will probably integrate climate-resilient infrastructure more intensively into the blend, as the moment is clearly at hand to address health and climate concerns together (Zhang et al., 2023).

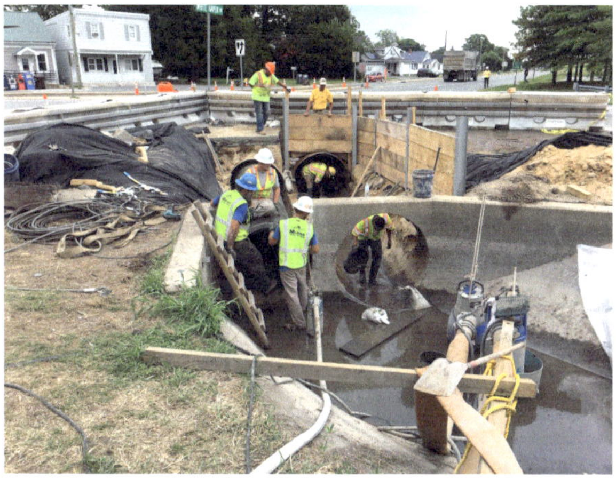

Source: A. Morton Thomas and Associates, Inc. (AMT) (2020). *Slip Lining Installation at MD 16 Drainage Improvements Project.*

9.4.3. Community Engagement and Education

Local participation is essential when it comes to addressing how climate change disrupts water health. Neighbors, officials, and scientists combine their thoughts in innovative ways, creating a sort of collective knowledge that—well, it works in developing means to adapt. Occasionally workshops, community meetings, and those in-person conversations end up making individuals understand just how crucial it is to manage water wisely. When people begin discussing these matters, they get more enthusiastic about supporting changes that can, in the majority of instances, make local water systems harder and more attuned to the region's idiosyncrasies. Sometimes school-like programs that delve into the economics aspect of climate topics also contribute to this enthusiasm. In general terms, the more that individuals witness how water woes impact their pockets or even their well-being, the more likely they are to demand changes within local government. Such a push not only creates more water-conscious citizens, but puts real pressure on decision-makers to make sustainable decisions. Teachers, by demonstrating how water health, climate, and community life are all intertwined, can occasionally span that pesky gap between dull theory and practical action. Overall, combining community conversations with useful schooling has the potential to inspire better policy and even new, homegrown ideas. And then, of course, there's technology, which seems to have a rather cool function in all of this. With digital resources such as webinars and mobile applications, just about anyone can get involved, sharing information in ways that sometimes are a little more grounded.

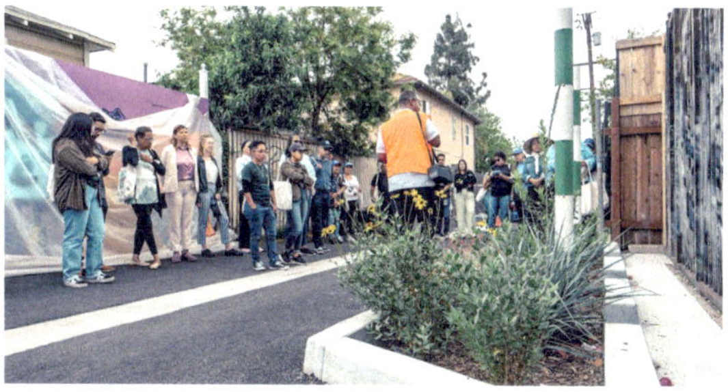

Figure 9.12. Engaging community.

Source: Safe Clean Water LA (2024). https://safecleanwaterla.org/content/uploads/2024/06/200-53012036165_3167e06b88_k-e1717523627143.jpg.

These platforms are able to dissect complex problems into bite-sized information, allowing communities to observe their water quality and even collect data on the go (Figure 9.12). Organizations that experiment with these technology tools may even direct local research, so that residents actively assist in studies that inform water policies. Not only does this provide policymakers with valuable information, but it also creates a sense of ownership and concern for local water spots, making communities more resilient. In short, combining tech with community outreach is fairly crucial to building flexible, informed communities prepared to meet a changing climate.

9.5. Role of Policy in Water Management

Climate change is disrupting our strategy for managing water. It's not only about fretting over short-term issues such as water quality or shortages; there is also the long-term effect of wild, out-of-the-ordinary weather occurrences that we can't possibly turn a blind eye to. Policymakers now realize that these water issues are complex up with economic growth and environmental health. Governments can become better equipped to deal with unpredictable water supplies when they combine water strategy with larger climate adaptation strategies. Overall, as the Sixth Assessment Report of the IPCC recommends (Intergovernmental Panel on Climate Change, 2023), neglecting these interlinked approaches only escalates threats to both ecosystems and societies. Apart from that, examining water in terms of its overall "footprint" is increasingly becoming significant. This perspective isn't just about monitoring how much water is consumed—from agriculture to industry—but also monitoring the pollution that comes along with it. In a sense, these measurements are useful guidelines, pushing stakeholders toward more sustainable practices while establishing goals for effective water use. In most instances, applying the water footprint concept can guide policies that halt over-extraction and pollution, ensuring that our use of water mirrors environmental conditions (Rick, 2020). A definite necessity is to incorporate a range of voices into discussion of water policies (Figure 9.13). Combining various inputs from government, business, and local community organizations tends to generate solutions that feel both reasonable and equitable. When water is in short supply, leaving out any group can even create social inequality or strife. Gradually, encouraging frank discussion appears to assist in shaping policies that weigh human requirements against protecting ecosystems. As water problems intensify across the world, sharing responsibility isn't merely a pleasant notion, it's nearly a necessity for securing our future (Intergovernmental Panel on Climate Change, 2023).

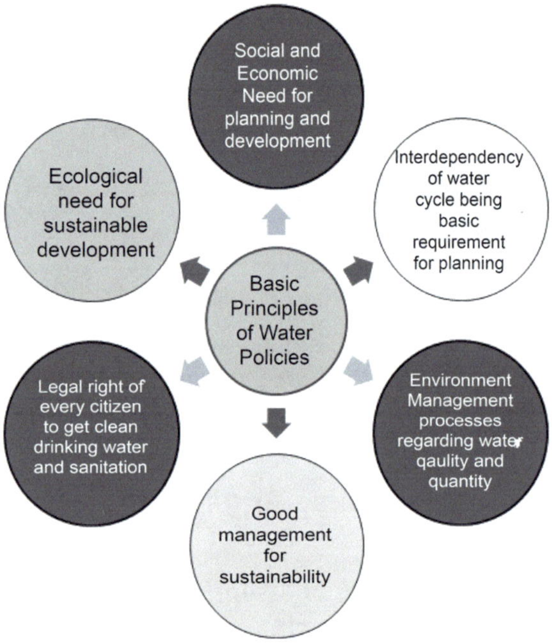

Figure 9.13. Basic principles of water policies.

Source: India Water Portal (2024). *Water Policies in India.*

9.5.1. Regulatory Frameworks for Water Quality

Oversight of water quality can't be treated lightly anymore with climate change seemingly refusing to ever hit the brakes. Increased temperatures disrupt our normal patterns of rain and cause more severe weather, which then puts both the quantity of water that we have and its cleanliness at risk. Officials are typically left to implement wide-ranging safety regulations that are intended to keep contaminants away and our sources of water sustainable. In most cases, these changing circumstances compel us to experiment with adaptive management strategies – a genuine necessity, especially in areas badly affected by floods or drought. Combining sound scientific evidence with policy formulation has enabled us to study the complex interconnections between climate fluctuations and water well-being, as the Synthesis Report of the IPCC (Calvin et al., 2023) reminds us with a quiet nuance. Water regulations also need to contend with a whole heap of issues stemming from industrial expansion and urban sprawl, problems that only exacerbate water pollution. Greenhouse gas emissions – primarily the result of fossil fuel combustion – increase climate change as much as they contaminate water bodies through runoff and infrastructure failure during extreme weather occurrences. That's why our systems of regulation must rapidly add prevention and bounce-back measures. Coordination across local, state, and federal levels is essential to patching together rules that truly work while spending resources more efficiently. And when local stakeholders and communities become part of the action, it assures that policies reflect the actual needs of people on the ground (Chen et al., 2022). While existing water standards provide a starting place, they tend to gloss over the nuance that is required to address the entirely new issues that climate change presents us. Our regulatory structures need to move toward more flexible strategies that allow us to adjust standards quickly whenever new information or unanticipated climate effects come along. Policies should encourage innovation in water technology—imagine new filtration systems or even local, small-scale treatment alternatives—that can mitigate threats from climate-linked contaminants. And closing the economic and social disparities in access to water simply has to be a top agenda item. By advocating for more equitable policies that truly encompass vulnerable populations, regulators can make the transitions needed for water health and climate resilience Just and inclusive, ultimately clearing the way for resource management that can withstand our increasingly dynamic world.

9.5.2. International Agreements on Water Resources

Confronted with mounting climate concerns, nations now realize that water management treaties are more important than ever before. Nations come together in treaties, albeit at times through treaties such as the United Nations Watercourses Convention—to address both the quality and the supply of water. Severe weather patterns, such as severe droughts and abrupt floods, accelerate this cooperation further, demonstrating that river and lake management across borders is critical for shared environments. These agreements blend short-term solutions with longer-term agendas, allowing countries to react to a changing climate while enhancing regional water resilience. Water management is not easy, and these global systems rely so much on science and data. You may see that new techniques and technology for mapping water in high resolution enable countries to collaborate in new ways and make policy adjustments on the fly. For instance, input from institutions like the IPCC , with their meticulous excursions into the ways water cycles respond to shifting climates — provides policy-making with a solid injection. Collaborating gets the process of conserving water, reducing pollution, and improving infrastructure for wacky weather done faster, and overall, combining scientific wisdom into policy-making just makes these agreements stronger. Also, these treaties do more than establish principles, they influence economic decisions and push sustainable development. With water shortages usually following economic inequalities, there's an evident call to address social equity as well as resource management. International agreements can trigger financial actions, such as investment in low-carbon technologies and renewable energy, which are determinative for countries facing water issues amidst climate fluctuations. Linking economic incentives to approaches emphasizing healthy water practices sometimes can unlock opportunities for improved agriculture and more effective use of water. Ultimately, cooperative international collaboration with the flexibility to adapt to changing water challenges under these agreements remains the solution to managing the complex effects of climate change on water, providing safe water for all.

9.5.3. Local Government Initiatives

Local authorities have emerged as lead actors in addressing water issues fueled by climate change. Too often, what happens is that the communities themselves hatch their own innovative solutions—a combination of green infrastructure, rainwater harvesting, and stormwater adjustments—that really resonate with their specific requirements. Most of the time, these solutions are what arise organically when individuals observe nearby water quality problems and scarcity. Policies today encourage such things as permeable pavement, which reduces the risk of flooding while providing a recharge for groundwater. In most cases, this down-to-earth, locally based strategy demonstrates that when you know the local climate effects, you end up with solutions that work, however unorthodox. Combining in climate adaptation is not a one-size-fits-all solution; local governments are frequently the first point of contact. Community discussions, such as spontaneous workshops and even town halls—invite in inherited knowledge as well as innovative perspectives to inform these policies. Public forums (and occasional impromptu neighborhood gatherings) enable all to have a say about the use of water in ways that are relevant to their own culture and environment. It's not uncommon for local groups to collaborate with state or federal agencies, and by doing so, they share both resources and experiences and take on the threat of adverse weather occurrences (Calvin et al., 2023; Intergovernmental Panel on Climate Change, 2023). For the most part, these partnerships prepare places not only for short-term issues but also for the uncertainties of the future. Local leaders also guide policies that emphasize sustainable water management on multiple fronts. They establish rules that restrict pollutants and close loopholes in land use, ensuring important water sources are properly maintained. Occasionally, they even retrofit items such as wastewater treatment centers so such plants can cope with heavier rainstorms—a very forward-thinking step. Meanwhile, strategies such as providing low-interest loans or subsidies for water-saving devices in homes and workplaces encourage mass-scale sustainable habits. Collectively, these initiatives not only maintain healthy water resources but also enhance overall climate resilience, so that both our communities and natural ecosystems can weather future adversity.

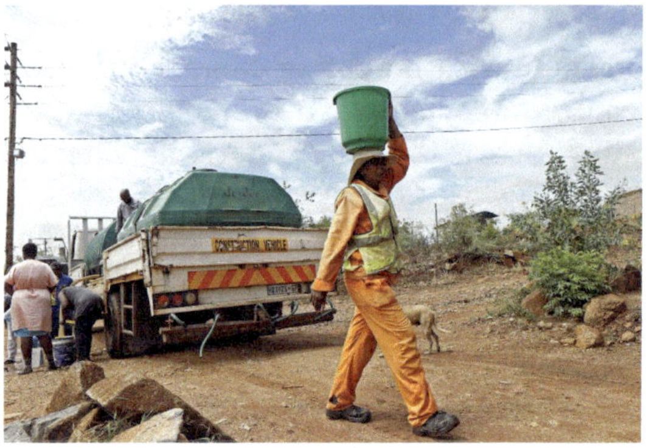

Source: https://assets.bwbx.io/images/users/iqjWHBFdfxIU/iDceq4qjDvXY/v1/-1x-1.jpg.

SUMMARY

Climate change and water health are complex together in such a way as to truly make us consider the here-and-now and the long term for our ecosystems and society. Global warming—much of it due to our own doing—has thrust rainfall and severe weather into new, uncertain patterns, which in turn disrupt how much water we have and its quality. You may have observed that studies like the IPCC continue to persist that these changes also play havoc with our health and biodiversity; in essence, we require intelligent, adaptive approaches to keep our water and the world of nature in balance (Intergovernmental Panel on Climate Change, 2023). Unless we combine good science with practical policy, communities are likely to face more difficult water management problems as the climate changes. It's fairly evident from what's going on that climate effects on our water resources aren't an issue for the future, they're standing at our doorsteps today. Floods, droughts, and even hurricanes not only slice into the quantity and purity of our freshwater supply, but they also place public health, agriculture, and the economy under severe pressure. Numerous studies, and disaster evaluations especially, indicate that massive populations of individuals worldwide are already experiencing the squeeze from these water issues, triggering calls for policy solutions (Fawzy et al., 2020). When governments, NGOs, and community people come together, there is a chance of creating a structure that allows everybody to address water problems more agility as situations continue to shift. Policy has an enormous role in this; genuinely, you cannot overemphasize it. We require legislations that step in promptly in addition to creating long-term assistance systems to weather climate fluctuations. For example, the Paris Agreement is a type of shared commitment to maintaining global temperatures under control and safeguarding vulnerable assets such as water (Fawzy et al., 2020). Most times, combining new scientific information with strong policies may be the very turning point that not only protects our water sources but also stocks up on our future resilience—no matter how many curveballs the climate continues to hurl in our direction.

Weather health and climate change blend in so many unforeseen ways—you receive changes in the amount of water we do have, alterations in its purity, and even those weather extremes we typically take for granted. Warming temperatures puts the water cycle into overdrive, so rain patterns deviate from script and evaporation increases more quickly than ever before. Such changes can instigate long droughts or sharp, heavy rainfall, each posing its own challenges. For the most part, the IPCC reminds us that the understanding of these changes is imperative, requiring that any plan of adjustment must integrate concepts regarding climate, nature, and human existence into one (Intergovernmental Panel on Climate Change, 2023). It's worth remembering that extreme weather not only interferes with our freshwater sources but also gets in the way of the quality of water, a thing to consider when trying to determine the solution. Climate changes don't only influence the quantity of water around us, they come at water quality quite heavily as well. When floods arrive, agricultural runoff, factory refuse, and urban remnants usually get swept into the water, threatening public health and our environment. Temperature spikes also accelerate the development of nuisance algal blooms and dangerous microorganisms, complicating water treatment further. The Food and Agriculture Organization, for example, has noted that infusing a bit of adaptive management into the mix is vital to maintaining water safe and plentiful, particularly in areas already under stress (Gatta, 2022). With such challenges continuously unfolding, it then becomes evident that communities and decision-makers truly require the appropriate instruments and expertise to handle our fine water balance. Addressing climate change-related water challenges requires an assortment of approaches—clever policies and everyday adaptation practices alike. All people, including grassroots leaders and individuals, must contribute to creating approaches that are not only sustainable but also resilient and prepared for shocks. In general, the IPCC has long preferred integrating strong scientific findings into policy-making, observing that climate-resilient development occurs when various groups collaborate across sectors (Intergovernmental Panel on Climate Change, 2023). Simple solutions, such as rainwater collection or improved irrigation, can work wonders in strengthening our water resilience. In the end, the challenge is not merely about solving today's issues; it's about arranging proactive policies that foretell future climate turns, providing a stable and sustainable future for water wellness and general well-being.

KEY TERMS FROM THIS CHAPTER

- Aquatic habitats
- CHIRPS dataset
- Climate action
- Climate fluctuations
- Climate resilience
- Climate-resilient policies
- Coastal communities
- Diligent planning
- Droughts
- Ecosystems
- Flood zones
- Freshwater supply
- Global warming
- Greenhouse gas emissions
- Groundwater-sustaining policies
- Health implications
- Local authorities
- Precision-controlled irrigation
- Rainwater harvesting
- Resource management
- Uncharted territory
- Urban expansion
- Wild weather

CLOSER LOOK

CLIMATE CHANGE IMPACT ON WATER QUALITY

Climate change greatly affects water quality, directly influencing community health by raising the risk of waterborne diseases and widening preexisting health inequalities. Variations in precipitation patterns, temperature, and the number of intense weather events interfere with water sources, resulting in both water shortages and pollution, ultimately weakening public health.

How Climate Change Impacts Water Quality:

- **Water Scarcity:** Increased temperatures and altered rainfall patterns lead to reduced water availability, straining existing water sources and potentially forcing communities to rely on contaminated water sources.
- **Contamination:** Extreme weather events like floods and droughts can contaminate water sources with pollutants, including fecal matter, industrial waste, and agricultural runoff.
- **Waterborne Diseases:** Changes in water quality, coupled with inadequate sanitation and hygiene practices, can increase the prevalence of waterborne diseases like cholera, typhoid, and dysentery.
- **Vector-borne Diseases:** Climate change also influences the spread of vector-borne diseases like malaria and dengue fever, which are linked to water availability and stagnant water conditions.

Impacts on Community Health:

- **Increased Risk of Disease:** Waterborne diseases pose a significant threat to community health, particularly among vulnerable populations like children and the elderly.
- **Exacerbation of Health Disparities:** Climate change disproportionately affects marginalized communities, leading to wider health inequalities and increased vulnerability to health risks.
- **Mental Health Impacts:** Climate change and its related impacts, such as displacement and food insecurity, can also negatively affect mental health.
- **Strain on Healthcare Systems:** The increased burden of water-related diseases and other health consequences of climate change can strain already limited healthcare resources.

Addressing the Challenge:

- **Climate Adaptation and Mitigation:** Implementing strategies to adapt to and mitigate climate change, such as reducing greenhouse gas emissions and improving water management practices, is crucial for protecting water quality and public health.
- **Improved Sanitation and Hygiene:** Strengthening water, sanitation, and hygiene

(WASH) infrastructure, promoting good hygiene practices, and ensuring access to safe drinking water are essential for preventing waterborne diseases.

- **Community Engagement:** Engaging communities in climate adaptation and mitigation efforts, as well as promoting awareness about the link between climate change and health, can empower them to take action and protect their health.
- **Research and Monitoring:** Conducting research on the impacts of climate change on water quality and health, and monitoring water quality parameters, is essential for understanding the risks and developing effective strategies. (Abera, 2025)

References

1. Abera, M. (2025). Response of dairy cattle to thermal stress: Implications for designing animal breeding strategies for sustainable productivity under changing climate. Applied Veterinary Research, 3(4), 2024011. https://doi.org/10.31893/avr.2024011 (accessed on 14 May 2025).
2. Calvin, K., Dasgupta, D., Krinner, G., Mukherji, A., Thorne, P., Trisos, C. H., Romero, J., et al. (2023). *Climate change 2023: Synthesis report. Contribution of Working Groups I, II and III to the Sixth Assessment Report of the Intergovernmental Panel on Climate Change* (H. Lee & J. Romero, Eds.). IPCC. https://doi.org/10.59327/ipcc/ar6-9789291691647.
3. Chen, L., Msigwa, G., Yang, M., Osman, A. I., Fawzy, S., Rooney, D. W., & Yap, P. S. (2022). Strategies to achieve a carbon neutral society: A review. *Environmental Chemistry Letters, 20*, 2277–2310. https://doi.org/10.1007/s10311-022-01435-8.
4. Denisow, B., & Malinowski, D. (2016). Climate change and the future of our world–Implications for plant phenology, physiology, plant communities, and crop management. *69*. DOI: https://doi.org/10.5586/aa.1683 (accessed on 14 May 2025).
5. Dwivedi, Y. K., Hughes, L., Kar, A. K., Baabdullah, A. M., Grover, P., Abbas, R., Andreini, D., et al. (2021). Climate change and COP26: Are digital technologies and information management part of the problem or the solution? An editorial reflection and call to action. *International Journal of Information Management, 63*, Article 102456. https://doi.org/10.1016/j.ijinfomgt.2021.102456.
6. Fawzy, S., Osman, A. I., Doran, J., & Rooney, D. W. (2020). Strategies for mitigation of climate change: A review. *Environmental Chemistry Letters, 18*, 2069–2094. https://doi.org/10.1007/s10311-020-01059-w.
7. Faye, A., Dieye, M., Diakhaté, P. B., Beye, A., Sall, M., & Diop, M. (2021). *Senegal–Land, Climate, Energy, Agriculture and Development: A Study in The Sudano-Sahel Initiative for Regional Development, Jobs, And Food Security*. Agricultural Economics eJournal. https://www.semanticscholar.org/paper/cdcae054e6e72a5d9cf5bc7170cdb69fc9cac398 (accessed on 14 May 2025).
8. Funk, C., Peterson, P., Landsfeld, M. F., Pedreros, D., Verdin, J. P., Shukla, S., Husak, G. J., et al. (2015). The climate hazards infrared precipitation with stations—a new environmental record for monitoring extremes. *Scientific Data, 2*, Article 150066. https://doi.org/10.1038/sdata.2015.66.
9. Gatta, P. P. (2022). *The State of World Fisheries and Aquaculture 2022*. FAO eBooks. https://doi.org/10.4060/cc0461en.
10. Hogeboom, R. J. (2020). The water footprint concept and water's grand environmental challenges. *One Earth, 2*, 218–222. https://doi.org/10.1016/j.oneear.2020.02.010.
11. Intergovernmental Panel on Climate Change. (2023). *Climate Change 2022–Impacts, Adaptation and Vulnerability*. https://doi.org/10.1017/9781009325844.
12. Korkmaz, M. (2024). Impacts of climate change: Examining precipitation, temperature anomalies, and effects on water resources in Turkey. *Journal of Anatolian Environmental and Animal Sciences*. https://www.semanticscholar.org/paper/9304110e74f55621da860ab05fa88948e489e5bd (accessed on 14 May 2025).

13. Landrigan, P. J., Stegeman, J. J., Fleming, L. E., Allemand, D., Anderson, D. M., Backer, L. C., Brücker-Davis, F., et al. (2020). Human health and ocean pollution. *Annals of Global Health, 86*, 151. https://doi.org/10.5334/aogh.2831.

14. Likomba, I., & Chibomba, D. (2025). To analyze climate change on agricultural productivity and livestock productivity: Case study of Siavonga District. *International Journal of Advanced Multidisciplinary Research and Studies.* DOI: https://doi.org/10.62225/2583049X.2025.5.2.3849 (accessed on 14 May 2025).

15. Lindner A, Stamm J. Integrating Climate Change Adaptation and Water Resource Management: A Critical Overview. *Standards.* 2025; 5(1):4. https://doi.org/10.3390/standards5010004 (accessed on 14 May 2025).

16. Mukherjee, D. (2021). Food security under the era of climate change threat. *Journal of Advanced Agriculture & Horticulture Research.* DOI: 10.55124/jahr.v1i1.78. https://www.semanticscholar.org/paper/bbb1f043da9b76a44b8238bbbd61d0e927a4b2a2 (accessed on 14 May 2025).

17. Newton, A., Icely, J., Cristina, S., Perillo, G. M. E., Turner, R. E., Ashan, D., Cragg, S. M., et al. (2020). Anthropogenic, direct pressures on coastal wetlands. *Frontiers in Ecology and Evolution, 8*, Article 144. https://doi.org/10.3389/fevo.2020.00144.

18. Ríos-Núñez, S. (2025). Smart Wines 4.0 inclusive: Climate change adaptation strategies in Northern Patagonia, Chile. *Brazilian Journal of Animal and Environmental Research.* https://www.semanticscholar.org/paper/a02f2bb80cfe6c7120d1d9630a95cded79ebd223 (accessed on 14 May 2025).

19. Rithika S, Malaisamy A, Raswanthkrishna M, Parimalarangan R, Balaji R, Prabakaran K. Review of assessing the impact of climate change on tank irrigation: vulnerabilities and adaptation strategies. Plant Sci. Today [Internet]. 2025 Mar. 7 [cited 2025 Jun. 17];12(1). Available from: https://horizonepublishing.com/journals/index.php/PST/article/view/6100 (accessed on 14 May 2025).

20. Rockström, J., Gupta, J., Qin, D., Lade, S. J., Abrams, J. F., Andersen, L. S., Armstrong McKay, D. I., et al. (2023). Safe and just Earth system boundaries. *Nature, 619*, 102–111. https://doi.org/10.1038/s41586-023-06083-8.

21. Zhang, S., Zhang, C., Cai, W., Bai, Y., Callaghan, M., Chang, N., **Чэн, Б.**, et al. (2023). The 2023 China report of the Lancet Countdown on health and climate change: Taking stock for a thriving future. *The Lancet Public Health, 8*, e978–e995. https://doi.org/10.1016/s2468-2667(23)00245-1.

22. Zimmermann, K., Abadi, A. M., Brauman, K. A., Maestu, J., Oude Essink, G., Schuster-Wallace, C., Smith, R., Madani, K., Adeel, Z., & Gribble, M. O. (2025). Addressing water scarcity to support climate resilience and human health. *Integrated environmental assessment and management, 21*(2), 291–300. https://doi.org/10.1093/inteam/vjaf001 (accessed on 14 May 2025).

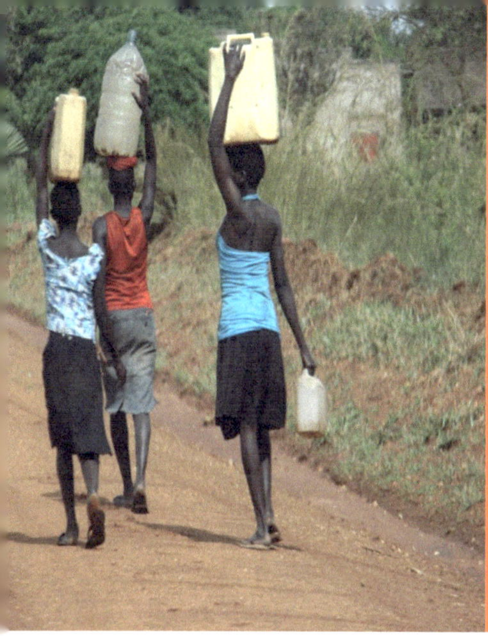

Chapter 9

WATER AND GENDER: ROLES, HEALTH RISKS, INEQUALITIES, AND COMMUNITY SOLUTIONS IN WATER MANAGEMENT

Contents

Introduction

Water management and gender roles are inextricably linked in such a way as to influence day-to-day life, sometimes in unexpected ways. In most areas, the responsibility of water fetching falls predominantly to women and girls—a chore that can result in actual health hazards and even damage their prospects at school. This task is not new but has been wedded to customary cultural routines and established economic routines that are prone to perpetuating gender imbalances. As populations expand and climate change erodes water resources, these problems are likely to get uglier, so we have to see the whole picture. Studies from bodies such as the IPCC (Intergovernmental Panel on Climate Change, 2023) caution us, as is often the case, that our health, economy, and ecosystem are intimately blended.

If water is not managed properly, it has a habit of hitting those who can least afford it hardest. Women, who are usually tasked with fetching water, are left to use dirty sources exposing them to a range of waterborne diseases. These health complications derail them from school and work, and the impacts trickle down to families, halting progress in communities. Studies even suggest that poor water quality is responsible for increasing antibiotic resistance (Intergovernmental Panel on Climate Change). It's a trend that reveals how gender and health cross paths in ways that are not predictable when it comes to water. Getting everyone equitable access to water requires that communities, governments, and NGOs all contribute. Bringing women into the water decision-making process not only raises their social status but can also introduce innovative, out-of-the-box thinking that might otherwise be overlooked. Their own experiences tend to create new perspectives, and neighborhood education on clean water can generate backing for improved infrastructure and policy. Ultimately, equitable water management can result in healthier communities, enhanced economic prospects, and a more equitable society. By borrowing from solutions that emanate from the people themselves, there's a likelihood of us being able to forge through the complicated connections between water and gender and create resilience for the future ahead.

Overview of Water as a Critical Resource

From much of the globe, the fight to have access to safe, reliable water continues. Women, in especially, tend to bear the responsibility of water carrying—a burden that encompasses not just numerous health threats but also restrictions on learning time or working time. In a lot of societies, you can observe how this daily task perpetuates gender disparities and, consequently, hinders the progress of communities. Water is at the center of everyday life, providing a lens into how gender roles intersect with access to such a fundamental commodity. For the most part, this circumstance demands intelligent, well-focused measures that guarantee all members of a community have fair access, without regard to gender or societal position. Regulating water resources directly intersects with bigger concepts regarding governance, economic security, and social equity. While climate change intensifies water scarcity, communities reveal dramatically differing responses to it. Many times, these groups with inferior leadership are having a harder time maintaining water resources as sustainable. The specifics, formed by history, culture, and even politics, can truly distort the way a community addresses water shortage and its accompanying health threats. Poor people, for example, will end up carrying much of the impact of such environmental hazards. Considering it all, one realizes easily that ingrained disparities shape water management, and locally led solutions become key to achieving resilience against climate-driven issues (Thomas et al., 2018). Not having access to clean water isn't a mere individual nuisance, it resonates across communities and knocks public health off balance. Where sanitation is inadequate and clean water is limited, waterborne diseases tend to erupt, usually among vulnerable populations such as children and the elderly. The combination of scarce water, deeply rooted gender roles, and severe health issues truly highlights the necessity of public health strategies that do not leave anything behind. In most instances, concentrating on the dual challenge women experience as caregivers and water gatherers proves to be central. Local responses, based on cooperative community, can mitigate these risks by enhancing water quality and increasing access. As communities begin to see water as a human right in a broader context of gender equality, they're more likely to develop sustained, inclusive strategies that address both health concerns and empower people (Dwivedi et al., 2022).

Importance of Gender in Water Management

Women and water management are now a burning issue, linking social justice to ecological health. In most developing societies, women do a lot, even if what they do tends to go unnoticed, and they're on the ground in terms of managing water resources. Research typically reveals that when women are included in making decisions about water, our systems really end up functioning better and serving communities more effectively. Tripathi et al. (2012) even highlight how many women smallholders, with practical knowledge of their own, devise innovative, locally adapted solutions that enable communities to cope with climate ups and downs. Poor water management also entails dire health consequences, and women typically bear the brunt. Most often assigned to fetch water or maintain household sanitation, they often get water-borne diseases. An absence of clean water harms not only daily life but also erodes their capacity to work and take care of family, triggering cycles of poverty and inequality. Statistics in most instances link poor water quality with increased disease among women and children. In order to truly address these risks, policies must address the specific challenges women encounter regarding water, as noted in (UNDP, 2016)—this intersection between gender equity and climate action is fairly central to overall, sustainable development. Involving women's perspectives in water management does more than correct inequities, it makes stronger communities as well. As women's practical knowledge and new perspectives blend into water management, communities end up having surprisingly adaptive approaches to climate change and scarcity. Local projects championed by women not only boost biodiversity but help strengthen the social fabric of the community itself. Once gender champions, grassroots organizations, and policymakers get together (or sometimes get involved in unlikely alignments), it brings down old dividing lines that separated women from real participation. Ultimately, providing more prominence to women in these schemes isn't all about fairness-it makes societies more resilient and better equipped for the challenges yet to come.

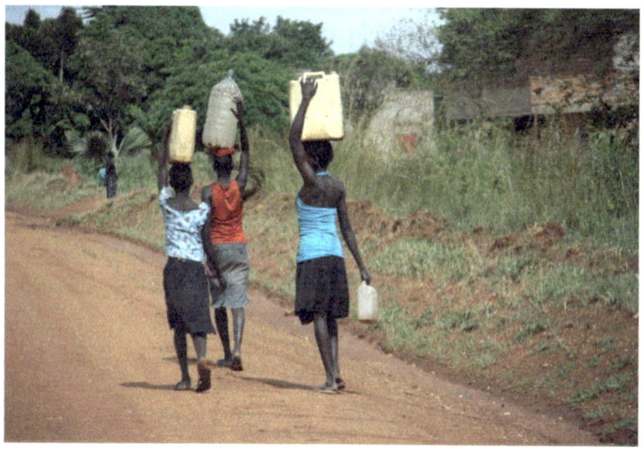

Source: https://iucn.org/sites/default/files/water-3936378_1280_s._zappi_from_pixabay.jpg.

10.1. Historical Context of Water Management

Water management has a complex, circuitous history that entwines throughout various ages. Early societies learned resourceful methods of collecting, distributing, and storing water not just for farming and performing routine tasks but also for early types of industry. Consider the areas of Mesopotamia and the Indus Valley, canals were constructed and irrigation systems established that increased agriculture and, in a very real way, laid the groundwork for power struggles. Control over water frequently became control over society, with groups like women, who typically were tasked with drawing water, having to endure the bruteness of scarcity directly. Contemporary research, for instance, indicates that the combination of water resource problems and climate change still sets communities out of kilter, compelling all of us to glance back to the past while creating new initiatives (Intergovernmental Panel on Climate

Change, 2023). When you step back and consider the way societies dealt with water through history, you will see it tends to replicate the general social landscape shaped by cultural idiosyncrasies and economic dynamics. In most conventional societies, women were the pillars of water management, making their homes never run dry, even though their role was hardly ever brought to the limelight in official discourse. This has, in most instances, conserved ancient inequities, curtailing the roles of those who had so much to play in decision-making. A closer examination of such patterns highlights necessity in combining gender-sensitive understanding into planning for water, demonstrating that history continues to speak solutions to today's woes (Dwivedi et al., 2022). There's another side of the story wherein water history comes up against issues of the environment. As civilization grew, its growing need for water occasionally contributed to activities detrimental to the environment—a definite collision between addressing urgent needs and keeping long-term environmental health in sight. Next was industrial age, and cities came to tap out enormous supplies of water in practices that frequently served to make country areas worse off. As climate anxiety increases, new strategies emphasize building resilience and viewing traditional approaches differently. Numerous leading scientific voices of today's generation contend that past mistakes must be learned from, and that even overlooked contributions of those who were otherwise marginalized must not be ignored—for us to create a water management regime that is not only just, but effective enough for today's complex world (Panel I on Change C, 2023).

10.1.1. Traditional Roles of Men and Women in Water Collection

Water collecting in most locations flaunts some of the ancient, obstinate notions about what people do. For centuries, women have been regarded as the fetchers of water, even in rural locations where water is distant and frequently unreliable, which is to say they do not only the long treks to obtain water but a whole host of tasks that are part of daily life such as cooking and cleaning (Figure 10.1). Men, however, typically do things such as taking care of storage facilities or controlling irrigation on farms. This division tends to maintain men in the public eye in terms of decisions while women are left with household chores, a matter that obviously denies women the opportunity to achieve equality (Intergovernmental Panel on Climate Change, 2023). These old roles don't only determine who gets hard work done, they also play with health and economic well-being. Most often, women and girls with long hours doing these tasks tend to suffer from physical stress, ranging from muscle pains to perpetual tiredness. Hours spent fetching water sometimes translate into less time going to school, which also impacts their futures. And when there's no clean, safe water, communities have larger health risks, with waterborne diseases affecting women and their households especially (Dwivedi et al., 2022). Several communities are beginning to wake up to these imbalances and experimenting with fresh concepts. There is an increasing feeling that addressing water challenges requires both men and women to be part of the conversation. In most instances, even miniature projects that educate women in water management become not only empowering for them but also promote more diverse and cooperative methods of managing their needs for water. Having these responsibilities shared can simplify the burden for women and, in the majority of instances, enhance their status in communal life. By including both sexes in the conversation about access to and management of water, people are able to collaborate toward practices that enhance health, create economic opportunities, and drive gender equity forward (Intergovernmental Panel on Climate Change, 2023).

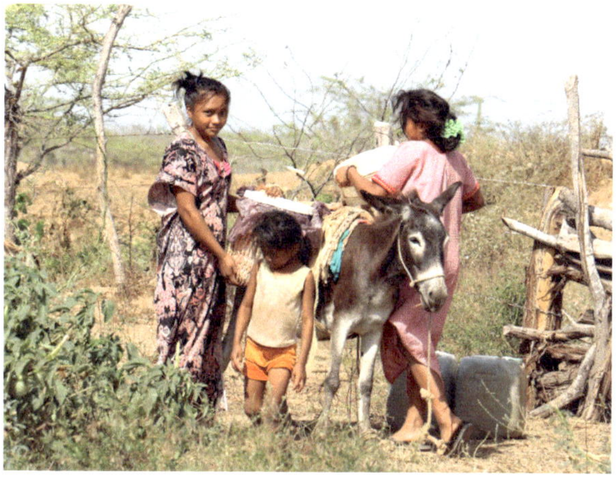

Figure 10.1. Colombia women collecting water.

Source: World Business Council for Sustainable Development (WBCSD). (n.d.). *Women Collecting Water in Colombia*.

https://s7d1.scene7.com/is/image/wbcolla/b/colombia-women-collecting-water?qlt=90&fmt=webp&resMode=sharp2.

10.1.2. Evolution of Water Management Practices

Water management's history goes back a long way, combining culture, technology, and nature in ways that are not always tidy. People long ago, consider the Mesopotamians, for example, established irrigation systems essentially to extract more from their fields, demonstrating an early ability to associate water with both survival and economic power. In a few locations, neighborhoods used gravity-fed channels, but in other areas, people dug into elaborate canal systems that defied easy description. Eventually, who received water and who did not begin to reflect social roles, and women tended to do the water collecting—a responsibility that, apart from reaffirming gender roles, occasionally accompanied health consequences when water was inadequate or poor quality. In the majority of cases, you notice that controlling water has always been involved with local tradition, influencing community health and way of life in untidy, volatile manners. Nowadays, discussions about water elicit many age-old gender disparities that are difficult to ignore. Women's efforts in providing, managing, and even inspecting the quality of water for families and entire communities usually go unnoticed. Throw in the rising imperatives of climate change – which essentially ratchets up the stakes for water quantity and quality , and things can become even more complicated.

The Sixth Assessment Report of the Intergovernmental Panel on Climate Change (IPCC), for instance, tends to emphasize how our climate and community existence are closely interrelated (Intergovernmental Panel on Climate Change, 2023). This type of understanding calls for solutions that are community-led, where the voices and experiences of women come forward to influence policies addressing both health risks and underlying social imbalances. In recent times, measures to increase water practices are shifting toward community-driven solutions that blend in gender perceptions and an ability to participate. Projects increasingly bring together diverse people, particularly the marginalized such as women, to construct water management that is both equitable and feasible. Occasionally, such community projects even incorporate informal schooling on the dangers of polluted water, which further empowers women as central actors in public health and sustainability. While local communities struggle with the dilemmas of climate change, integrating local expertise with true social equity appears nearly essential. Overall, when local knowledge is combined with authentic knowledge of gender dynamics, it winds up honing water plans that are directed toward improved health and sustainability in the long term, making the connection between the way we manage water and the way we strive for gender equity (Dwivedi et al., 2022).

10.1.3. Impact of Colonialism on Gender Roles in Water Access

Colonial power imprinted itself on society in ways that still resonate to this day, particularly regarding water. Pre-existing water management practices, ones that had been keeping communities alive for ages—were suddenly discarded as colonial authorities imposed their agendas. Established practices, which had been rich in balance and complexity, were junked in favor of expediency. Women, long responsible for getting and distributing water, had their tried-and-true expertise politicized and even erased; in most instances, it not only intensified gender disparities but also made it more difficult for those communities to gain access to something as fundamental as water—a commodity crucial to survival as well as to community health. In much of the region, the new colonial facilities weren't about equality at all. Quite straightforwardly, water systems were established to serve colonial ventures instead of serving everyone in an equal manner. That left old disparities far worse. Women, with the burden of managing everyday water necessities, became more and more relegated, with their contributions minimized to that of dependents instead of strong contributors. In general, this imbalance of power also meant that they participated less in decision-making regarding water control. Contemporary ideas of progress consistently benefited male leadership; consequently, the disparity of who was allowed to speak out regarding water concerns only increased, leaving scars on the mannerisms of how communities currently handle resources. Even in post-colonial times, the fight for equitable access to water still persists. Several countries have attempted to incorporate gender insights into water policy, but those same long-standing divisions seem to creep in again. Women still struggle with poor supplies of clean water—those in turn affecting their health, education, and general quality of life, and particularly when you consider obstacles like climate change and economic uncertainty (Figure 10.2). Typically, these complications are part of a complex web of issues, as described in discussions around sustainable development goals (SDGs), specifically SDG 5 (Gender Equality) and SDG 6 (Clean Water and Sanitation). Ultimately, it is evident that we have to resort to community-centric strategies that effectively enhance women's participation and value their long-standing efforts in managing water (Newell et al., 2021; Shulla et al., 2021).

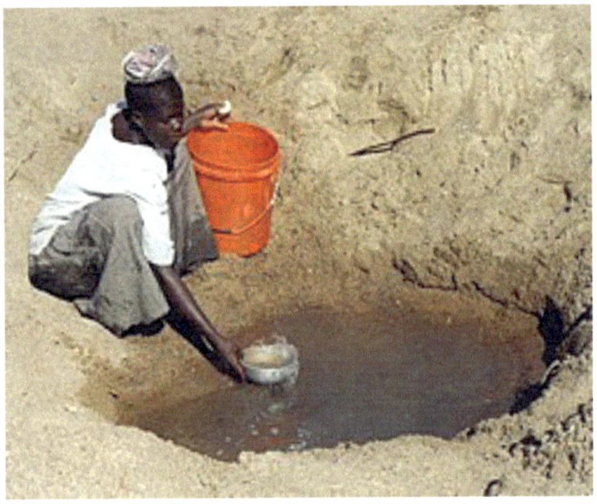

Figure 10.2. School student collects drinking water from a makeshift filtration arrangement at a nearby stream at Nyamphota Village, Chikwawa District, Malaw.

Source: https://en.wikipedia.org/wiki/Water_scarcity_in_Africa#/media/File:Mwamongu_water_source.jpg

10.2. Gender Roles in Water Access and Usage

Water access isn't merely a matter of who comes to fetch it, it's caught up with long-standing notions of gender. Women are largely responsible for the work of fetching water in many settings, an activity that saps time and energy and eats into school or work opportunities. Frequently, society portrays doing housework as a woman's role, which has a way of perpetuating economic inequalities and reinforcing past inequities. When women spend hours carrying water, their ability to contribute at home or in the community suffers. And not having safe water readily available tends to add additional health concerns, particularly when conditions like menstruation or pregnancy enter the picture, illustrating just how closely gender and public health are connected when it comes to water resource management and policy-making. At times, when water and sanitation services are not meeting the mark, the cost to women is all too evident.

Left out of the room, women's needs and everyday difficulties are easily overlooked, and decisions often result in services that fall short of safety and wellbeing. Consider, for example, spaces where latrines are not planned for privacy or safety; here, women can be at higher risk of harassment or even assault. When water management incorporates women's voices—yes, hearing what they have to say, it creates the opportunity for infrastructure upgrades that improve not only water quality but also women's empowerment. In general terms, factoring in their ideas helps communities create solutions that solve both for safety and equity. And of course, rediscussing gender roles in water management is the way to long-term community solutions. Getting not just women, but men and young boys as well involved in the discussion can start to break down long-held stereotypes and share the burden more equitably. Education efforts that, in the majority of cases, focus on water as a shared resource for all can initiate changes in traditional cultural perspectives. When programs engage families in working together—whether it is fetching water, maintaining sanitation, or making choices, it close people and makes communities stronger. Ultimately, prioritizing gender equity in water strategies gives everyone an even chance of being able to contribute and benefit from better systems, resulting in healthier outcomes and a more equitable division of labor.

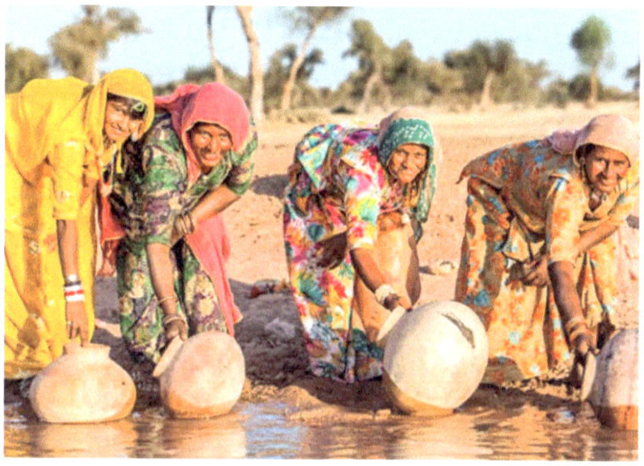

Source: https://www.orfonline.org/public/uploads/posts/image/652bc854d7d8e.png.

10.2.1. Division of Labor in Water Collection

Most communities have an unusual division in the matter of fetching water—a tendency more influenced by social convention than by functional demand among them. In many places, economic pressure and social conventions send men to tackle large jobs such as installing meters or manning major irrigation, while women tend to find themselves doing the day-to-day task of bringing water to the household. This arrangement, which initially may appear to be natural, really reflects deeply ingrained gender roles and ultimately perpetuates inequalities. Frequently, the numerous hours women spend collecting water crowd out opportunities for education or wage work, locking them into a cycle that prevents them from fully participating in community life. In practice, this practice not only freezes in time traditional roles but is also wedded to fundamental ideas that exclude opportunities for greater advancement. The impact is pervasive, extending into community health and even school attendance. Women often have to make long journeys for water, excursions that fatigue them and even sometimes put them at risk for physical strain or even harm due to violence. Children are also attracted to such work at home, and more often than not, this results in a routine of absence from school. Wherever you combine gendered work with issues of health and poor academic performance, you have severe impediments to equitable development. On the whole, if we are to break this cycle, we must examine closely the outdated norms that determine what people do and make way for new, more egalitarian thoughts. Viewing possible solutions, various local experiences suggest the ways through which these imbalances can be tempered. Various local governments now recognize the necessity to integrate gender into water policies—sometimes by initiating community-based initiatives that relieve the burden on women and, in the process, increase their voice in decisions. Such a strategy, which weaves together ordinary issues with social and environmental objectives, has genuine potential for more equitable results. Just look at cities such as Barcelona, where collective action on the part of a diverse set of community voices has generated grassroots movements that address these historically entrenched divisions (Amorim et al., 2021; Radics et al., 2023). Oftentimes, such innovative solutions may be just the thing to open the door for sustainable and equitable water management practices.

10.2.2. Gendered Patterns of Water Usage in Households

Home water management unleashes underlying gender dynamics. Women tend to end up doing most of the water-related work—from fetching and organizing supplies to portioning them out for cooking, cleaning and even hygiene purposes. In most instances, particularly where water is limited or has to be carried over long distances, these tasks can become a daunting physical and mental burden; recent research suggests such burdens build up unobtrusively in such environments. This disproportionate allocation of duties not only underscores entrenched disparities in health, well-being and economic condition but also indicates the necessity of water practices that can empower entire communities (Calvin et al., 2023).

Another facet is how water use and gender entwine with health hazards, especially where sanitation and hygiene are lacking. Women, typically carrying the bulk of home water tasks, are exposed to greater risks from conditions such as waterborne disease—a truth rendered all the more distressing in areas without strong infrastructure. The challenge of finding clean water for consumption and sanitation simply further exacerbates health inequities already present, typically also impacting local productivity in the process. In the majority of instances, efficient water management must consider such gender disparities to balance how resources are distributed. Strategies involving education and community initiatives have been promising in empowering women while alleviating overall health burdens (Gamage et al., 2023). Developing solutions that really take into account how water tasks divide along gender lines requires a collective effort of all members of the household and society. Often, merely involving men in the discussion of daily water chores can go a long way in reducing the disproportionate burden. Local efforts—whether through training programs or water systems managed collectively by groups, can bring about a more participatory approach to accessing and controlling water resources. Such projects not just enhance water security but also recognize the critical inputs made by women, and improve gender equality. As communities gravitate toward such equitable approaches, the beneficial outcomes for public health, environmental conservation and social equity become obviously manifested, presenting strong evidence for gender-sensitive water policy (Calvin et al., 2023).

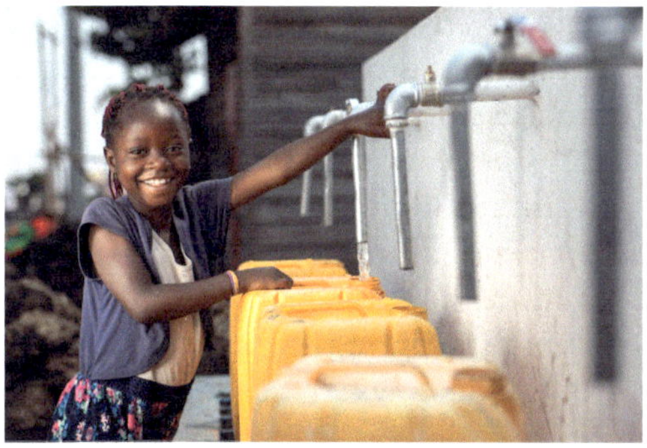

Source: https://www.unwater.org/sites/default/files/styles/d12/public/2022-08/un0549961.jpg?itok=ZqFVJ58F.

10.2.3. Cultural Perceptions of Water-Related Responsibilities

Everyday water work blends with cultural beliefs in unexpected ways, showing definite differences in the way genders manage water. Everywhere, it's taken for granted that women are responsible for fetching and managing water at home—placing them smack in the middle of the water shortage battle. This position influences not just their day-to-day activities but also, in the majority of instances, their health; the physical labor of transporting water occasionally precipitates long-term diseases. Examining these perspectives allows us an opportunity to get at how gender affects water access and the consequent health issues, connecting cultural concepts with the everyday practices of water work within communities. These same cultural concepts also influence decisions regarding who receives what regarding water resources. The positions of men more frequently than not receive additional attention in community leadership and decision-making, with women's experiences often going unconsidered. This lopsided view can hinder progress toward more effective water management because women are likely to possess valuable local expertise on water use and conservation. Omitting their wisdom not only widens long-held gaps, but also overlooks pragmatic thoughts that might drive community solutions. For the most part, it is important to challenge these long-held perceptions in order to develop equitable water management plans that combine what all bring to the table. We must also understand that these cultural lessons are accompanied by a larger context of social and political conditions. For instance, when indigenous customs blend with the effects of climate change, the outcome can be even more acute gender inequalities. As highlighted in the IPCC's comprehensive reports, climate change disproportionately affects women because they are primarily responsible for water and domestic work (Intergovernmental Panel on Climate Change, 2023). This intersection reveals that to address water management isn't solely a matter of technology, it's just as much a social and cultural challenge. So, embracing community-based approaches that respect and incorporate local traditions (all their flaws and all) feels practically necessary for the creation of water systems that are sustainable, equitable, and capable of alleviating health hazards while enhancing community resilience.

10.3. Health Risks Associated with Water Inequality

Everyone should have access to safe drinking water, but it's not available to all in equal proportions. Several communities, particularly the marginalized, are at serious risk of health due to water shortages. In most cases, households use untreated sources—a decision due to water scarcity, and end up contracting diseases such as cholera or dysentery. Hospitals get clogged, and the poorer sections suffer the hardest. Girls and children, traditionally responsible for collecting water, become more vulnerable, linking water management to gender equity (UNDP, 2016). Overall, repairing this water deficit is central to enhancing community health and daily living conditions. Water disparity extends far beyond physical health; it pervades mental health, as well. In general terms, the long hours of water fetching—largely by women—elicit stress and anxiety, both from the physical impact and the ongoing concern with whether the water is safe or even accessible. In most instances, all that time might be devoted to school or work, only perpetuating poverty cycles. Research indicates that when water infrastructure is planned with gender in mind, the advantages transfer over to wider community empowerment, having a tangible impact on health and social justice (Fisher & Mohun, 2015). It's a reminder that issues of water are as much concerned with human dignity as they are with managing resources. Climate change just makes the challenges more difficult. Severe weather such as floods and droughts can deplete valuable water resources or pollute what's present, exacerbating local health emergencies. In most cases, these environmental shocks not only perpetuate the spread of diseases but also precipitate conflict over scarce resources, affecting mental health and social bonds. Here, there needs to be a gender-sensitive solution to addressing climate effects, one that focuses on how water is handled closely. Engaging local people in designing such solutions can strengthen resilience and promote useful, sustainable habits. Clearly, embracing inclusive policies to overcome water inequality is vital if we're going to weather these unpredictable changes (UNDP, 2016).

10.3.1. Waterborne Diseases and Their Impact on Women and Children

Waterborne diseases strike communities severely, and they are connected to an entire combination of social and gender concerns (Figure 10.3). In much of the world, clean water and good sanitation simply aren't evenly distributed—further exacerbating the health issues already in the mix.

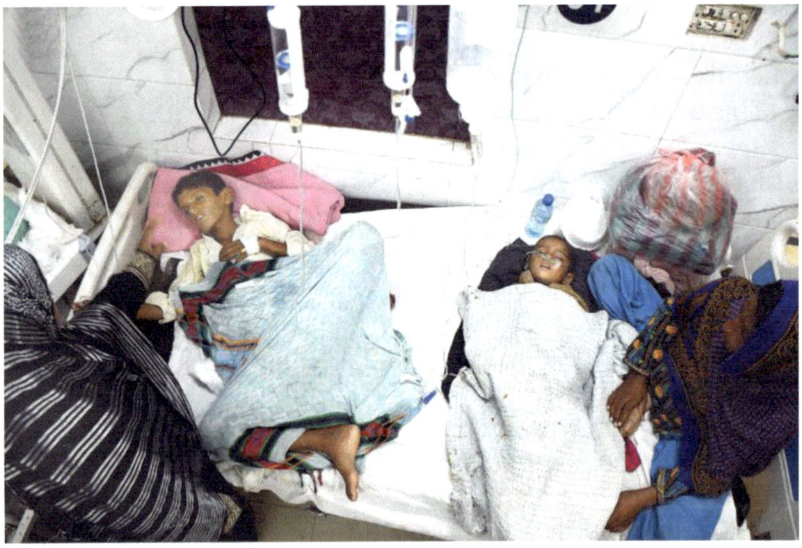

Figure 10.3. Waterborne diseases spread among children.

Source: The Nation (2022). *Waterborne Diseases Spread Among Children, Women as Floods Death Toll Surpasses 1500.*

Children, particularly children under the age of five, frequently endure such conditions as diarrhea or even cholera when water systems are lacking, and women who typically bear the responsibility for water collection are left to encounter hazardous, unsanitary situations that increase their risk of contact with contaminants. These health conditions don't just end at disease; they radiate out to disturb the social and economic life of the community. Usually, when family members get sick, it's the women—who already have a lot on their plates—losing out on time and resources, sometimes entering into a poverty trap. The pressure to find household water can also interfere with school and participation in community life, so economic prospects and education suffer for women and children. Solving these issues involves examining them from all sides. Developing improved water, sanitation, and hygiene (WASH) facilities can reduce disease incidence while alleviating the everyday hassles many experience. Education programs on safe water handling can in most instances educate women and children with the skills to minimize hazards. And, when societies own water management, it invites women to become more involved in decision-making—no matter how imperfect things become. All of this, with the support of strategic investments, not only increases public health but also moves society a little toward equality, as recent research and (Hans-Otto Pörtner et al., 2023) show.

10.3.2. Mental Health Implications of Water Scarcity

Natural resources and our brains are closely linked together—water isn't only an issue of bodily survival; it's an important component of how we experience things on a day-to-day basis. In much of the world where water starts to get tight, folks all of a sudden have irregular supplies that induce a combination of tension, worry, and even episodes of depression. Clean water, therefore, is not just a basic want; it's the subtle underpinning that prevents our mental health from collapsing. In a majority of situations, individuals who have to live with erratic water supplies experience this burden again and again, and the worst part is that the downtrodden sections, particularly women and children, who usually bear the water-fetching burden—bear the brunt. It's also important to mention that water shortage neatly falls within the larger environmental justice debate. In general, when groups of people aren't provided with sufficient water, it isn't just a physical shortcoming; it's a question of social and emotional balance. Individuals in these conditions tend to experience both shortages of resources and the stress that accompanies feeling neglected.

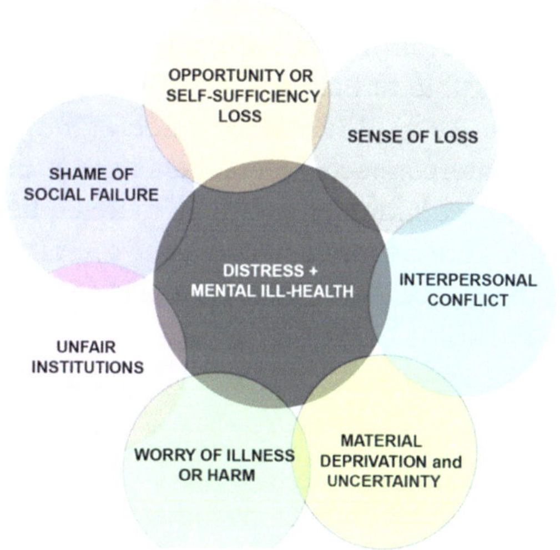

Figure 10.4. Possible mechanisms connecting water insecurity to distress and mental ill-health.

Source: Wiley. (n.d.). *Possible Mechanisms Connecting Water Insecurity to Distress and Mental Ill-Health.*

https://wires.onlinelibrary.wiley.com/cms/asset/cd0275cd-2a77-4bed-a586-f8349dce2093/wat21461-toc-0001-m.jpg.

Local programs that provide educational resources and mechanisms for generating local support can truly help lighten this load, providing people with additional resilience to ride out the fluctuations of water shortages. On top of that, reinforcing community bonds tends to work behind the scenes but effectively to promote mental well-being, and in many respects, this is an important component of a sustainable water plan. Culture and daily social roles complicate the picture further, as customary practices at times put most of the water collection work on women, causing additional physical burden and psychological stress. This unequal division of labor can destabilize not just individual mental well-being but also family and community dynamics in the long run; at times, the burden even radiates out, slightly unraveling the social fabric. By inserting a gender-informed vision into water management and mental health projects, even if it is a seemingly minor shift, it is possible to heal some of those distortions (Figure 10.4). Ultimately, understanding all these interconnected elements is necessary for creating community solutions that see beyond simple access to water, addressing overall health and resilience in a way that is whole and organic.

10.3.3. Physical Health Risks Linked to Water Collection Burdens

It is not an easy job to collect water. In most areas, it largely becomes the responsibility of women and girls, who walk long distances carrying heavy loads at a great personal expense. They end up with muscle strain, joint pains, and persistent fatigue that weakens them day after day, even when it looks like mere routine work. This imbalance in burden not only leads to profound health issues but also makes everyday life more difficult, fueling a cycle where the physical weight continues to grow. The issue is beyond mere pains and aches. In poorer or rural settings, the journey for water can lead individuals into really dangerous situations—settings where harassment or violence could be precipitated at any moment. The backbreaking labor involved in carrying water leaves insufficient time for simple self-preservation, such as eating adequately or sleeping well. As (Intergovernmental Panel on Climate Change, 2023) posits, cultural pressures tend to restrict women's mobility, leaving them even more vulnerable to these threats. An end to this situation, in most instances, would involve a combination of practical community education, enhanced local facilities, and enlightened policy action. Climate change is further complicating the entire picture. With weather patterns becoming more unpredictable, water sources tend to be farther away or of poorer quality, so longer journeys and higher risks of dehydration and waterborne disease. The lack of clean water has profound implications for families, particularly mothers and children, as dehydration and poor sanitation can cause risky conditions such as sepsis, as defined in (Intergovernmental Panel on Climate Change, 2023). Ultimately, combining gender inequality with health and climate issues demonstrates just how crucial effective WASH programs are. If societies are able to lighten the burden of water collection and address these interrelated threats, there is hope to create a just and sustainable future.

10.4. Socioeconomic Inequalities in Water Management

Clean water is a fundamental right that all people ought to enjoy—but if you examine it, disparities in wealth and opportunity tend to alter the way water is controlled between communities (Figure 10.5). In most poor communities, individuals encounter all sorts of barriers (consider crumbling infrastructure, minimal investment in water infrastructure, and poor government support) that prevent them from accessing safe water. Studies, in the majority of instances, indicate that those who are left behind, particularly women and children—lose out more, and this is detrimental to their health and restricts opportunities for an improved life. Different studies suggest that when economic disparities increase, the struggle for clean water becomes even more challenging, and there is a critical need to work toward more equitable solutions (Intergovernmental Panel on Climate Change, 2023). Now, if you add the issue of gender in terms of economic status, it only gets more complex. In many developing areas, women tend to take on most of the water collection responsibilities—a time-consuming daily chore that can consume a great deal of their day. This backbreaking labor chops off school time and employment opportunities and even, sometimes, jeopardizes their own physical health as they expose themselves to risks along the way. In most cases, some research writes that if women are provided with a firmer voice in controlling water, the benefits cascade throughout the community, enhancing overall well-being. Identifying these special challenges allows policymakers to devise innovative solutions that tackle gender concerns and financial issues in water access (Yoshikawa et al., 2020).

In addition, numerous local, community-based initiatives are proving to be effective in addressing these very same disparities. Rather than trusting solely in top-down edicts, local groups that listen to people who are typically overlooked help ensure water gets shared more equitably. Participatory methods sometimes result in more efficient use of resources and improve trust in water service providers—albeit if, on occasion, the coordination is a tad uneven. And, in addition, collaborative efforts among government agencies, nongovernmental organizations, and community groups have been able to mobilize additional resources and disseminate useful knowhow on water conservation and hygiene. Ultimately, as communities come together to confront poverty and gender disparities, they not only enhance short-term water management but also create a sort of resilience that benefits all in the long term (Intergovernmental Panel on Climate Change, 2023).

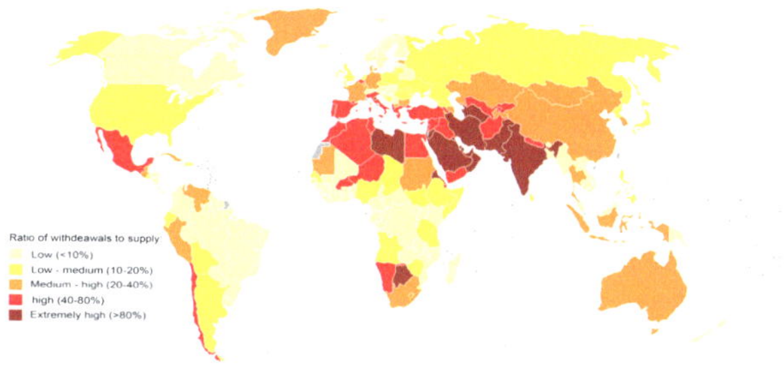

Figure 10.5. Water inequity.

Source: https://en.wikipedia.org/wiki/File:Water_stress_2019_WRI.png

10.4.1. Access to Clean Water and Its Correlation with Poverty

Clean water isn't merely about making people healthy, it's a lifeline that directly connects to the way our society operates, particularly in communities where poverty is severe. Without a constant source of water, many communities are locked into a never-ending cycle of survival. Too often, fetching water is left to the most resource-poor members of society, typically children and women, and this time drain seriously curtails opportunities for school or employment. When communities have to live on unclean, dirty water, diseases spread rapidly and further burden already strained resources. A few attempts at being more water-efficient have begun to yield benefits, yet most concur that if the core of the disparity is not fixed, the cycle will simply continue (UNDP, 2016). Poorer neighborhoods truly illustrate how access to water and gender inequality go hand in hand. Women—who are usually responsible for water collection—may spend their entire day on the task, robbing them of opportunities for education or work. When water is more equitably distributed, new opportunities arise, opening the door for women to play larger roles in society and in economies. Research typically indicates that more convenient access to clean water not only improves family health but also results in more girls being able to remain in school rather than missing school days to gather water. This change, in a majority of instances, trickles out to improve entire communities, demonstrating that equitable water management is an integral component of gender disparities reduction (Galizzi & Herklotz, 2012). Dealing with the complex problems of water scarcity and poverty indeed demands a joined-up effort from local communities, governments, and global agencies (Figure 10.6). Water conservation programs, sustainable living, and equitable distribution are essential in enabling vulnerable populations to weather the harder knocks of climate change. Local, community-based projects, such as organizing neighborhood water committees, can have a significant impact both in terms of how water is handled and in creating a sense of ownership. And when there are education programs that teach people the health hazards of contaminated water, they can create wider efforts toward sanitation and hygiene improvements. By linking water management with poverty reduction, communities are able to experience not only improved well-being and health but also more long-term sustainable development (UNDP, 2016).

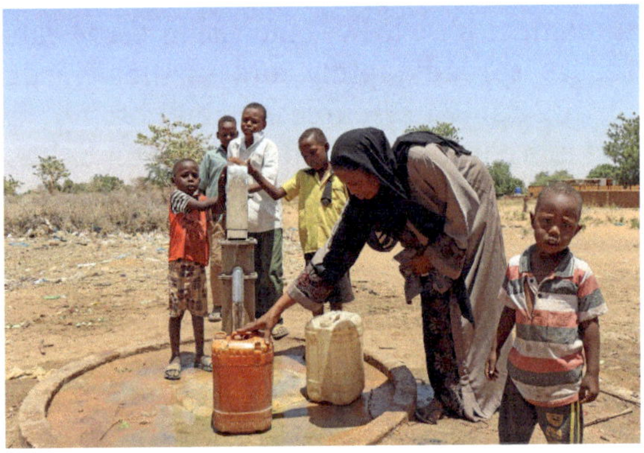

Figure 10.6. Access to water linked to poverty.

Source: Islamic Relief South Africa. (2021). *Access to Water is Linked to Poverty.*

https://www.islamic-relief.org.za/access-to-water-is-linked-to-poverty.

10.4.2. Gender Disparities in Decision-Making Roles

Traditional historical gender roles have always had a great role to play in determining who gets to make the decisions in water management. Men have long been in the driver's seat, usually silencing women's perspectives—despite locations where water plays a direct role in food security and health, fields where women typically have much to contribute. For the most part, infrastructure projects really don't even factor in what women require, and decisions get made without taking that crucial input; after all, when structures aren't created with everyone in mind, it could even endanger women's safety. Obviously, giving space for additional female voices in these conversations is essential to equal outcomes and increased community bonding (OECD, 2021). The effects of these gender disparities extend far, far beyond individual experience, it is spilling over into the health of communities as a whole. Women tend to approach water issues in a distinctive, practical manner, and this is particularly important when you add in issues such as climate change and scarce resources. The COVID-19 pandemic, for instance, has illustrated that social inequality and environmental issues go hand in hand. Very often, local women have a near-instinctive understanding of their environments; their observations, married at times to conventional expertise, can inform genuinely adaptive approaches to challenging situations. Overall, removing the obstacles preventing women from exercising decision-making capacity opens the door to more equitable and sustainable water habits (Folke et al., 2021). Changing this ancient pattern will not occur by itself. We require clear, deliberate action to increase women's participation in water management. This may involve constructing structures that promote women's leadership through training workshops, mentorship, and other capacity-building activities that bridge the gender gap. Creating coalitions to lobby for gender-sensitive policies shakes up the old narratives we have used for water governance. Finally, the expansion of women's participation isn't solely an exercise in checking a social justice box, it also gets at a wider set of ideas and solutions that are desperately needed for navigating an age of expanding environmental uncertainty (OECD, 2021).

10.4.3. Economic Implications of Inadequate Water Access for Women

Women in most communities are locked in a daily battle for water, and the battle seeps deep into their opportunities for reliable income and improved living. Passing hours collecting water, usually from places that do not have the adequate infrastructure, takes away valuable hours for work and self-improvement (Figure 10.7). Loss of time trickles down to exacerbate age-old inequalities, making it increasingly difficult for them to be economically independent. Bad water facilities, for instance, appear to trap them in a vicious cycle where economic prospects fade, leaving women's potential and roles repeatedly eroded (OECD, 2021). Lack of access to dependable water also creates a chain reaction of health issues and financial difficulties. Women end up depending on contaminated water sources, which exposes them to waterborne diseases; when they fall ill, lost work and increasing healthcare costs add to the burden. Sickness upsets their routine daily lives and pervades home life, reaching families and even communities. Whereas in most situations, the repeated shortage of healthy water and related poor health implies that women increasingly find it difficult to sustain their households, this again explains how the problem repeatedly couples setbacks in health and the economy (Eriksen et al., 2021). Addressing these concerns requires integrating women's voices into every stage of planning for water management. Engaging women in local water infrastructure decisions isn't just a desire for equality, it's a pragmatic move that can unlock improved resource management and increase economic benefits. Frequently, when women offer their advice at the table, outcomes speak for themselves: enhanced community well-being and economic opportunity more within reach. Even some studies indicate that when women are excluded, vulnerabilities expand (Eriksen et al., 2021). In short, establishing a dialogue in which ordinary women assist in guiding water policies could very well be the secret to transforming a health problem into an actual opportunity for economic gain.

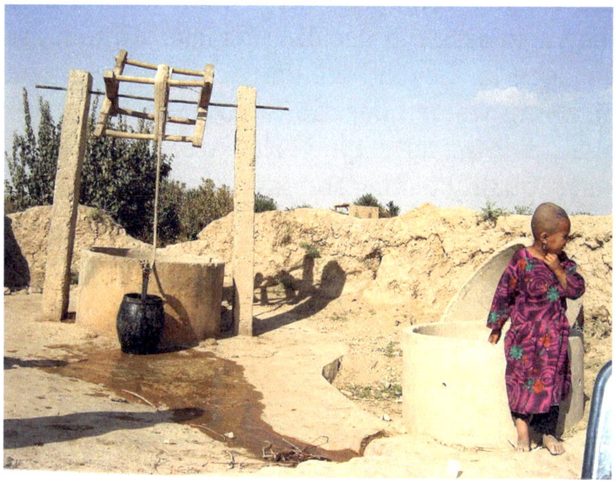

Figure 10.7. Women at a village well.

Source: https://en.wikipedia.org/wiki/File:Faryab-_village_dug_well.JPG

10.5. Community Solutions to Water Management Issues

Communities may find that addressing water management issues requires new, local solutions instead of the typical top-down regulations. People on the ground understand their own territory in ways that outsiders typically do not, so they often meet together, sometimes serendipitously, to decide how to best conserve and share water. In such small-scale projects, individuals make use of ordinary experience and practical planning, and this blend can result in plans that suit special local conditions. Women, who are most often responsible for most of the water collection, are an important part of these initiatives, with the result being that systems developed work both fairly and effectively. More often than not, as the IPCC suggests, integrating people's knowledge with scientific expertise can result in climate-resilient solutions that serve both people and nature (Intergovernmental Panel on Climate Change, 2023). In much of the world, women do more than fetch water, they also assist in deciding its use. Women are engaged far beyond the daily chores, taking on planning water allocation and ensuring water quality. Projects empowering women, such as water quality testing and home treatment skills, tend to improve public health as well as foster gender equality. These initiatives also highlight, in general, the need for incorporating the people who work with water on a daily basis, supporting evidence of the disastrous impact water-related issues can have on communities (Christopher et al., 2022). At other times, successful water management owes more to its strong social bonds than to any secret. Neighbors informally exchange resources, ideas, and best practices in local networks, resulting in more resilient systems, even when faced with unforeseen water shortages. It is when local governments, NGOs, and residents blend their efforts that the outcome is not always by the book but is effective enough to cope with capricious climate changes. By promoting a nonchalant, collaborative attitude to managing water, communities not just enhance water availability and quality but also establish an atmosphere of responsibility shared among themselves. This carefree attitude genuinely emphasizes how localized cooperation can confront intricate water matters while ensuring the participation of everybody involved (Intergovernmental Panel on Climate Change, 2023).

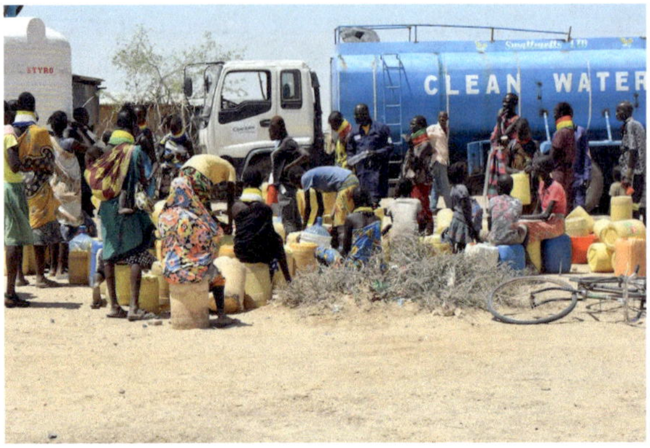

Source: Concern Worldwide. (n.d.). *Water Truck Delivering Clean Water in Kenya.*https://concernusa.org/uploads/concern-rs75206-kenya-water-truck.webp.

10.5.1. Grassroots Initiatives Led by Women

Thousands of communities experience firsthand change when women, who typically make the daily water rounds, take leadership roles and drive local initiatives that address day-to-day water challenges. These women, faced with everything from water scarcity to its contamination, often end up naturally taking responsibility. Their day-to-day work makes them visible at home and even enables them to contribute to bigger water decisions. At times, people's own initiatives on the ground to utilize water more sustainably add technical training and useful inputs that strengthen their capacities. When communities embrace the expertise and tenacity of women, they all end up distributing the burden and collaborating on water management. This not only conserves water but also enhances women's autonomy to take on health risks and inequalities associated with access. Meanwhile, most of these women endure difficult challenges during their water trips, leading initiatives that target precisely constructing the required infrastructure. In much of the world today, unsafe water subjects women and children to danger, frequently triggering disease emergencies. So, women-oriented projects often bring water points to the doorstep and renovate sanitation facilities, shortening those exhausting, long water treks. By placing these needs foremost, women can reclaim the time they'd otherwise lose, the time they now spend in school, working, or just engaging in their communities. This type of ripple effect demonstrates that by increasing women's participation in water issues, we're not only energizing individual change—but we're also weaving stronger, more resilient communities. Essentially, these initiatives demonstrate that combining gender lenses into water policies is essential if we're to tackle the numerous challenges that emanate from water inequality. Other than that, the empowerment of women in water management resonates with deeper social and economic issues. Grassroots leaders such as these tend to advocate for equitable access and are not afraid to speak out against entrenched disparities. In all but a few instances, experiential projects addressing water-related issues demonstrate a close connection between defending nature and advocating for gender equity. Take, for instance, the case of women's role in controlling Peste des petits ruminants (PPR); there, they become involved in animal health and, as a result, ensure food availability—allegedly demonstrating how disassembling barriers at the community level is vital (Hungerb et al., 2025). And let's be honest, climate change, with its attendant droughts or floods, makes life even more challenging, particularly for women who are already disadvantaged (Gao, 2025). Addressing these challenges through local initiatives not only supports women's leadership but also initiates community responses toward long-term, sustainable solutions.

10.5.2. Role of Education in Promoting Equitable Water Access

Education is among those fundamental resources that not only assist individuals with water issues but also renders the access to water more equitable. When people understand more, they're usually in a better place to advocate for water policies that endure, particularly in areas where gender disparities remain an issue. Many times, women bear the burden of managing household water, and if they are educated, they can challenge existing systems and take a more active role in making water resource decisions. Incorporating gender discussions into school curricula can organically increase women's participation in designing projects that impact water supply and quality. In most instances, these measures not only address current water challenges; but they establish a sort of foundation for future social equity and more secure water management habits (OECD, 2021). It's also apparent that when water is not properly managed, the issues bleed into health. Bad water habits bring the whole mess of complications, such as waterborne diseases that strike women and children particularly severely. That's why it is important to educate individuals on hygiene, sanitation and water-saving tips—having that extra bit of know-how regarding the safety of the water can significantly reduce disease and enhance overall community health. It is particularly critical in areas where natural resources have been eroded over time, something that history teaches us has the potential to jeopardize public health (Sandra Díaz et al., 2019). Overall, placing some emphasis on health-related water problems with education is the idea that people not only learn to know about their rights and responsibilities but also acquire hands-on skills to build healthier environments. Another approach is that education can instigate a transformation in the way communities deal with water problems. As individuals become better aware of the ways water, gender, and sustainability blend together, they will begin to demand approaches that respect everyone's needs. This mental shift is central to repairing the water deficits that most frequently omit women and other marginalized individuals. By integrating gender-sensitive concepts into the education curriculum, a more organic comprehension of the intricate social and economic relationships informing water allocation arises. These types of learning initiatives can mobilize individuals to collaborate, creating the type of partnerships that advocate for equitable access to water and more resilient local systems (OECD, 2021). Overall, education not only addresses everyday water issues but also shifts the narrative on who has a voice in water management, setting the stage for a more equitable future (Figure 10.8).

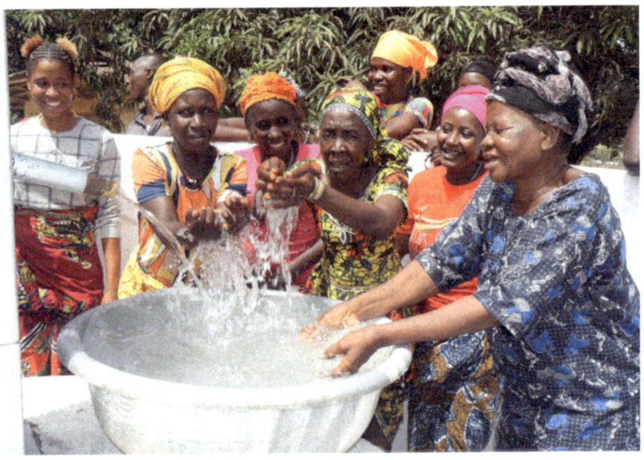

Figure 10.8. Community members happily splashing clean and safe drinking.

Source: The Water Project. (2023). *Community Members Happily Splashing Clean and Safe Drinking Water in Sangoya Community, Sierra Leone.*

10.5.3. Collaboration Between Genders in Water Management Strategies

Water management is not a tidy affair, it's an involved one that tends to reveal stark gender differences. Women in most areas end up doing the bulk of water fetching, a task that not only puts their health at risk but also generates daily obstacles, especially when climate fluctuations render water supplies changing. This onerous task, most would attest, can easily prove too much for them, especially in our warming climate. When everyone across both genders contributes, the scene is altered: choices become less about checking boxes and more about genuine needs, and plans begin to respond to the specific issues confronted by women and other marginalized groups (Wilbur et al., 2024). Let's point out that working together isn't merely about dividing work in half. In most communities, men will tend to make the decisions and control resources and women's ideas tend to lead the efforts toward improving water and sanitation. Usually, however, these are not fixed roles; genuine dialogue—sometimes even in informal, spontaneous meetings—enables each group to infuse its own brand of wisdom. In general, when both parties are contributing, a more integrated strategy comes into place, one that's better equipped to handle water emergencies fueled by climate changes, stimulating local innovative thinking in solving problems that have existed for centuries (Cenedesi et al., 2024). Even more so, emphasizing gender cooperation in managing water can ignite real change in public health and overall development. Clean water access impacts all: the health of individuals, education, and even employment opportunities, especially among women and girls. When everyone is included in strategies, surprising solutions tend to emerge, such as technologies that increase water use efficiency and reduce health hazards associated with inadequate sanitation. For example, allowing women to be in the lead when designing rainwater systems at times leads to solutions that are both functional and resonant with local culture. In the long term, these role and voice realignments can push apart long-standing power balances, creating the space for a more equitable and healthier overall climate (Wilbur et al., 2024).

SUMMARY

Water management and gender concerns merge together in a manner that demonstrates why we need to address these issues head-on. Women throughout much of the world – particularly in low- and middle-income regions – endure dramatic risks when water is limited or not safe. Much of the time, they must spend extensive amounts of time carrying water, which can result in physical injury as well as profound emotional exhaustion. It's not merely an urgent health risk either; these issues reverberate out, exacerbating social and economic inequalities. Attending to these daily burdens enables local groups and policymakers to begin crafting wiser, more inclusive water policies that respect the important role women play. Numerous communities also grapple with entrenched disparities that complicate women's adaptation when climate change and resource shortages strike. Climate change typically makes water problems worse – quality and availability decrease, and consequently, people face heightened health concerns such as reproductive problems and mental strain. Women naturally end up in caregiving positions in most places, bearing additional burdens when resources become scarce. That combination of factors necessitates the layered response; programs should integrate gender issues into water management programs. On most occasions, when women have improved access to resources, education, and decision-making forums, communities are more able to manage water issues while advocating for equity. Taking the bigger picture into consideration, equitable water management involves a strong grasp of gender's role in water issues. In general terms, the effects of climate change on water security highlight the necessity for holistic policies with specific vulnerabilities in mind. Enhancing women's participation in these initiatives not only mitigates short-term health consequences but also sets the stage for long-term community resilience. It requires all the collaborative efforts of the local voices, policymakers, and all other stakeholders joining hands – even if at times the nitty-gritty may get a little complicated – in coming up with adaptive strategies that are inclusive. Ultimately, making the link between water, health, and gender sets the stage for the way toward a sustainable and equitable future for all (Anjum et al., 2025; Gao, 2025).

Women in most societies are left with most of the complex wreckage when water management is substandard, and that's not necessarily about having no clean water, it's about risking health and splitting deep social divisions that just continue on. Studies indicate that when water supply and sanitation deteriorate, it's usually the women who end up bearing the brunt, affecting both their physical condition as well as what society perceives about them. They should typically be the ones tasked with fetching water, and in times of low access, they have longer walks and lesser-quality water—making their workloads heavier and health risks more common. This imbalance over time carries over into education and opportunities for jobs as well, and should typically make these imbalances worse. In most instances, considering water and gender side by side explains why intervention must be constructed around women's everyday lives, paving the way for policies to support more equitable resource governance (Fisher & Mohun, 2015). Considering farming practices and local solutions enters another layer into the mix, as mixing down-to-earth community experience with scientific concepts can sort out water-related issues. Small-scale farmers, particularly in sub-Saharan West Africa, rely heavily on what is available in the local environment, but they're being pinched by increasing pressures from climate change and unsustainable agriculture. Studies comparing farm approaches—traditional, GMO or purely organic farming—indicate that cooperative, cross-disciplinary approaches appear to be the key to managing both environmental and social equity. Technically, when societies wed new methods with the lessons they've accumulated over the years, they can weather climate fluctuations more effectively as well as safeguard their food store. It's a complex, but necessary crossroads at which water management intersects with agriculture, one that truly demands increased resilience while pushing forward with gender equity (Nicolay & Fliessbach, 2012). Understanding how water management influences gender roles can broaden our perspective on how to frame policies. In general, since climate change is likely to affect women more than most, it's become pretty much necessary that water and climate policy require an added sprinkle of gender sensitivity. When such gender-sensitive strategies are integrated into policy, they manage to cushion the impact of unpredictable climate events and invite greater participation and empowerment among women. Of course, if these values are not respected, the vulnerabilities become only deeper—prolonging poverty and inequality cycles that are difficult to escape. Therefore, working toward increasing water access and sanitation means placing gender equity at the very center of things, not merely because it's the right thing to do, but also because it's essential for good resource management and community building (Fisher & Mohun, 2015).

KEY TERMS FROM THIS CHAPTER

- Water collection
- Water management habits
- Water-related issues
- Capacity-building activities
- Colonial power
- Community groups
- Community-based initiatives
- Conservation programs
- Diarrhea
- Gender equity
- Health-related water problems
- Resilient local systems
- Social equity
- Water access
- Water management
- Water-fetching burden
- Antibiotic resistance
- Cholera
- Community existence
- Community solutions
- Community-centric strategies
- Decision-making process
- Environmental conservation
- Gender-sensitive policies
- Inclusive strategies
- Short-term health consequences
- Social justice

CLOSER LOOK

WATER AND GENDER

Without safe water, sanitation and hygiene (WASH) services, women and girls face higher risks of abuse, attack and disease, impairing their capacity to learn, work and live with dignity. WASH improvements in the home, school, workplace and public areas promote gender equality. Women and girls should be at the center of designing and delivering solutions to ensure that services meet their particular needs.

The Issue Explained:

- Women and girls usually have the responsibility of fetching water. This can be a dangerous, time-consuming and physically demanding task. Long journeys by foot, often more than once a day, can leave women and girls vulnerable to attack and often preclude them from school or earning an income.
- For women and girls, sanitation is about personal safety. Having to go to the toilet outside or sharing facilities with men and boys puts women and girls at increased risk of abuse and assault.
- Women and girls have specific hygiene needs. A clean, functional, lockable, gender-segregated space is needed, with access to sanitary products and disposal systems, for women and girls to manage menstrual hygiene and pregnancy.
- Lack of safely managed water and sanitation is an equality issue. Women and girls are disproportionately affected by poor water, sanitation and hygiene services and facilities. However, their voices and needs are often absent in the design and implementation of improvements, thereby ensuring their continued marginalization.
- By failing women and girls, we risk the 2030 Agenda. Access to water and sanitation are human rights. Where females are unable to enjoy those rights, their health is profoundly affected, curtailing their educational and economic opportunities, and denying them their full role in society.

The Way Forward:

- WASH needs to be addressed from a gender perspective. Policies and action plans need to address the needs of women and girls by engaging them in planning, decision-making and governance of services.
- Gender-responsive WASH is essential to the 2030 Agenda. Integrating gender equity into policy at every level will be important to ensuring water and sanitation for all, which will, in turn, contribute to developing many other aspects of the SDG agenda, especially poverty reduction, health, education, and work.

References

1. Amorim-Maia, A. T., Anguelovski, I., Chu, E., & Connolly, J. J. (2021). Intersectional climate justice: A conceptual pathway for bridging adaptation planning, transformative action, and social equity. *Urban Climate, 41*, 101053. https://doi.org/10.1016/j.uclim.2021.101053.
2. Anjum, G., & Aziz, M. (2025). Climate change and gendered vulnerability: A systematic review of women's health. *Women's Health, 21*. https://www.semanticscholar.org/paper/2a6d52d50856459296e1c91b78e6e0a7c9591db2 (accessed on 14 May 2025).
3. Calvin, K., Dasgupta, D., Krinner, G., Mukherji, A., Thorne, P., Trisos, C. H., Romero, J., et al. (2023). *Climate Change 2023: Synthesis Report. Contribution of Working Groups I, II and III to the Sixth Assessment Report of the Intergovernmental Panel on Climate Change* (Core Writing Team, H. Lee & J. Romero, Eds.). IPCC. https://doi.org/10.59327/ipcc/ar6-9789291691647.
4. Cenedesi Júnior, M. A., Rodrigues, D. P. V., Merege, M. C., Schwarz, F. S., Gomes, G. S. B. F., Vasconcelos, J. L. de A., Melo, J. L. do N., de Amorim, K. T., da Silva, K. C. R., Araújo, M. A. de A., Platon, N. de S., de Moraes, R. G. C., Pinto, P. R. F., Martins, S. R., & Malta, A. do M. M. (2024). The challenges in rebuilding a quality public health in Brazil. *OBSERVATÓRIO DE LA ECONOMÍA LATINOAMERICANA, 22*(2), e3219. https://doi.org/10.55905/oelv22n2-088 (accessed on 14 May 2025).
5. Díaz, S., Settele, J., Brondízio, E. S., Ngo, H. T., Agard, J., Arneth, A., Balvanera, P., et al. (2019). Pervasive human-driven decline of life on Earth points to the need for transformative change. *Science, 366*. https://doi.org/10.1126/science.aax3100.
6. Dwivedi, Y. K., Hughes, L., Baabdullah, A. M., Ribeiro-Navarrete, S., Giannakis, M., Al-Debei, M. M., Dennehy, D., et al. (2022). Metaverse beyond the hype: Multidisciplinary perspectives on emerging challenges, opportunities, and agenda for research, practice and policy. *International Journal of Information Management, 66*, 102542. https://doi.org/10.1016/j.ijinfomgt.2022.102542.
7. Eriksen, S., Schipper, E. L. F., Scoville-Simonds, M., Vincent, K., Adam, H. N., Brooks, N., Harding, B., et al. (2021). Adaptation interventions and their effect on vulnerability in developing countries: Help, hindrance or irrelevance? *World Development, 141*, 105383. https://doi.org/10.1016/j.worlddev.2020.105383.
8. Nicolay, Gian L. and Fliessbach, Andreas (2012) Production of Innovations within Farmer–Researcher Associations Applying Transdisciplinary Research Principles. In: *International Conference on Research for Development (ICRD 2012). Research for Global Transformation, Theme 4: Enabling Research in Global Transformation Session 26: Integrated Development Research Approach*, NCCR North-South Dialogue, no. 44, p. 164. (accessed on 14 May 2025).
9. Folke, C., Polasky, S., Rockström, J., Galaz, V., Westley, F., Lamont, M., Scheffer, M., et al. (2021). Our future in the Anthropocene biosphere. *AMBIO, 50*, 834–869. https://doi.org/10.1007/s13280-021-01544-8.
10. Gamage, A., Gangahagedara, R., Gamage, J., Jayasinghe, N., Kodikara, N., Suraweera, P., & Merah, O. (2023). Role of organic farming for achieving sustainability in agriculture. *Farming System, 1*, 100005. https://doi.org/10.1016/j.farsys.2023.100005.
11. Gao, X. (2025). Climate change and the poor: Reasons, impacts, inequities, and sustainable

solutions. *Applied and Computational Engineering*. https://www.semanticscholar.org/paper/5b604b334d29732b0a6a5e4ab0206706b26ca226 (accessed on 14 May 2025).

12. Paolo Galizzi & Alena Herklotz, Missing in Action: Gender in International Environmental Law, in Powerful Synergies: Gender Equality, Economic Development and Environmental Sustainability (UNDP: 2012).. (accessed on 14 May 2025).
13. Hungerbühler,Valerie and Barkadle,Buckary and Hussein,Amina Mohamed and Zambrano,Sofia C. and Digale,Mohammed and Belay,Kebadu Simachew and Derungs,Flurina and Dürr,Salome, cabionehealth.2025.0010, CABI One Health, doi:10.1079/cabionehealth.2025.0010, CABI, Women's experiences and perspectives on livestock management and empowerment in PPR vaccination in the Somali region, Ethiopia, (2025) (accessed on 14 May 2025).
14. Intergovernmental Panel on Climate Change. (2023). *Climate Change 2022–Impacts, Adaptation and Vulnerability*. https://doi.org/10.1017/9781009325844.
15. Macura, B., Del Duca, L., Espinoza Soto, A. E., Carrard, N., Gosling, L., Hannes, K., Thomas, J., et al. (2021). PROTOCOL: What is the impact of complex WASH interventions on gender and social equality outcomes in low- and middle-income countries? A mixed-method systematic review protocol. *Campbell Systematic Reviews, 17*, e1164. https://doi.org/10.1002/cl2.1164.
16. Marselle, M., Hartig, T., Cox, D. T. C., de Bell, S., Knapp, S., Lindley, S., Triguero-Mas, M., et al. (2021). Pathways linking biodiversity to human health: A conceptual framework. *Environment International, 150*, 106420. https://doi.org/10.1016/j.envint.2021.106420.
17. Menton, M., Larrea, C., Latorre, S., Martínez Alier, J., Peck, M., Temper, L., & Walter, M. (2020). Environmental justice and the SDGs: From synergies to gaps and contradictions. *Sustainability Science, 15*, 1621–1636. https://doi.org/10.1007/s11625-020-00789-8.
18. Fisher, S. and Mohun, R. 2015. Low carbon resilient development and gender equality in the least developed countries. IIED Issue Paper. IIED, London.(accessed on 14 May 2025).
19. Murray, C. J. L., Ikuta, K. S., Sharara, F., Swetschinski, L. R., Robles Aguilar, G., Gray, A. P., Han, C., et al. (2022). Global burden of bacterial antimicrobial resistance in 2019: A systematic analysis. *The Lancet, 399*, 629–655. https://doi.org/10.1016/S0140-6736(21)02724-0.
20. Tripathi, Ruchi, Chung, Youkin B Deering, Karl. Marina Publisher(s). (2012). *What Works for Women: Proven Approaches for Empowering Women Smallholders and Achieving Food Security*. OXFAM. https://core.ac.uk/download/75780841.pdf (accessed on 14 May 2025).
21. UNDP. (2016). *Scaling Up Climate Action to Achieve the Sustainable Development Goals*. https://core.ac.uk/download/75760930.pdf (accessed on 14 May 2025).
22. Newell, P., Srivastava, S., Næss, L. O., Torres Contreras, G. A., & Price, R. (2021). Toward transformative climate justice: An emerging research agenda. *Wiley Interdisciplinary Reviews: Climate Change, 12*, e733. https://doi.org/10.1002/wcc.733.
23. OECD. (2021). *Women in Infrastructure*. Public Governance Policy Papers. https://doi.org/10.1787/9eab66a8-en.
24. Pörtner, H. O., Roberts, D., Parmesan, C., Adams, H., Adelekan, I., Adler, C., Adrian, R., et al. (2023). *Technical Summary*. Cambridge University Press eBooks. https://doi.org/10.1017/9781009325844.002.
25. Radics, A., Vásquez, F., Pérez Benítez, N., & Ruelas, I. (2023). *Outlook of Fiscal Relations Among Government Levels in Latin America and the Caribbean*. https://doi.org/10.18235/0004708.

26. Shulla, K., Voigt, B. F., Cibian, S., Scandone, G., Martinez, E., Nelkovski, F., & Salehi, P. (2021). Effects of COVID-19 on the Sustainable Development Goals (SDGs). *Discover Sustainability, 2*. https://doi.org/10.1007/s43621-021-00026-x.

27. Thomas, K. A., Hardy, D., Lazrus, H., Méndez, M., Orlove, B., Rivera-Collazo, I., Roberts, J. T., et al. (2018). Explaining differential vulnerability to climate change: A social science review. *Wiley Interdisciplinary Reviews: Climate Change, 10*, e565. https://doi.org/10.1002/wcc.565.

28. Wilbur, J., Ruuska, D., Nawaz, S., & Natukunda, J. (2024). *Climate Risks to Water, Sanitation and Hygiene Services and Evidence of Inclusive and Effective Interventions in Low and Middle-Income Countries: A Scoping Review*. https://www.semanticscholar.org/paper/55868cc99b6d1ccf5fb604333261e04880f982cc (accessed on 14 May 2025).

29. Yoshikawa, H., Wuermli, A. J., Britto, P. R., Dreyer, B. P., Leckman, J. F., Lye, S. J., Ponguta, L. A., et al. (2020). Effects of the global Coronavirus disease-2019 pandemic on early childhood development: Short- and long-term risks and mitigating program and policy actions. *The Journal of Pediatrics, 223*, 188–193. https://doi.org/10.1016/j.jpeds.2020.05.020.

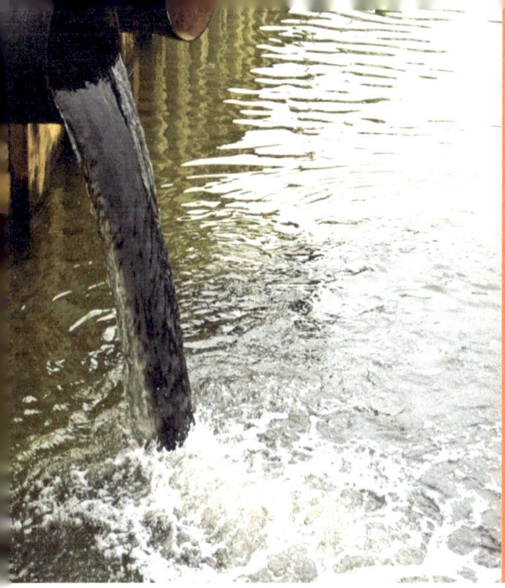

Chapter 11

WATER QUALITY AND ENVIRONMENTAL POLLUTANTS

Contents

Introduction

The intricate relationship between water quality and environmental pollutants is a matter of increasing concern globally, with consequences for both ecosystem integrity and human health. Agriculture, industry, and urbanization have introduced a variety of pollutants into water systems, leading to reduced water quality. Pollutants can be from a variety of sources, including effluent, agricultural runoff, and atmospheric deposition, all exacerbated by poor regulatory frameworks. As these pollutants accumulate, they have extremely detrimental effects on aquatic life, causing biodiversity loss and disruption to natural processes. Further, water-quality degradation impacts human communities that depend on these sources for drinking water and crop production, reinforcing the essential link between public welfare and environmental health. Much attention has been given to farm practices, specifically the application of pesticides and fertilizers, which have been termed as the main sources of water pollution. Chemical runoff is prevalent and contributes to water body overloads of nutrients, bringing about hypoxic conditions that are harmful to aquatic plants and animals. Contemporary farming methods, though important for production, have tended to sacrifice high-volume yields in the short term at the expense of long-term ecosystem sustainability.

A paradigm shift toward organic agriculture, as proposed by recent studies, would help lessen some of these negative impacts through decreased use of synthetic chemicals. As (Gamage et al., 2023) points out, the incorporation of organic practices into agriculture not only ensures environmental well-being but can also increase the overall quality of agricultural crops, creating a healthier agricultural environment. The toxicological effects of heavy metals, a ubiquitous yet underappreciated contaminant in water systems, further complicate the challenge of having clean water. Heavy metal pollution is caused by industrial effluent, urban runoff, and even geological occurrences in nature, posing enormous consequences to ecosystems as well as public health. Heavy metals are capable of bioaccumulation, giving rise to long-term environmental effects as well as grave health consequences for people who depend on contaminated water sources. As highlighted in (Aziz et al., 2023), understanding the sources and mechanisms of heavy metal contamination is key to guiding proper remediation interventions. Implementation of cost-effective technologies for removing such pollutants from water can prove to be a key driver in ensuring water quality and obtaining the security of water resources for generations to come. Through an integrated approach with technology, policy reform, and sustainable strategies, it is highly possible to address these pressing water quality issues.

Importance of Clean Water for Ecosystems and Human Health

The interplay between clean water and ecosystem health cannot be overemphasized because aquatic environments represent vital habitats for thousands of species. With degrading water quality due to the presence of pollutants such as heavy metals and agricultural runoff, ecosystems inevitably face critical disruptions. These contaminants cause bioaccumulation in water organisms, thus injuring flora and fauna and, ultimately, destabilizing food chains. For example, heavy metal-exposed fish can suffer from compromised reproductive functions and higher mortality rates, causing fish populations to reduce that many species, including human beings, depend on for food. Furthermore, water quality degradation has a direct impact on ecosystem services such as natural purification processes and the maintenance of habitats, citing the necessity for strict measures of pollution control to guarantee the protection of these valuable water resources and the biodiversity they rely upon. Equally so, apart from its ecological significance, pure water is totally critical to human health and well-being. Contaminated water sources expose residents to different types of health risks, ranging from gastrointestinal disease to chronic diseases like cancer. Research indicates that chemicals in contaminated water such as industrial contaminants and pesticides bioaccumulate in the food chain, thus exposing man to toxic carcinogens (Smith et al., 2023). The effects of chronic exposure to such substances not only carry health risks to an individual but can also trigger widespread public health issues, especially for underprivileged communities with reduced access to clean sources of water. This supports the importance of universal public health policy with a focus on access to clean water first, again linking health in the environment and health outcomes in human beings. Initiatives to improve the quality of water have launched, spurred on by government backing and grassroots movements. For example, the United Nations Environment Programme (UNEP) considers the link between water quantity and quality a cause for increased investment and public consciousness toward the issues of water (Palaniappan et al., 2010). High-technological purification methods are only one extreme; more rigid regulations for industrial waste treatment and agricultural activities can also contribute. Conservation of water sources by using effective methods to respond to pollution can thus support ecological integrity and enhanced public well-being. Through concerted action at the local, national, and global levels, sustainable water management can be achieved, demonstrating that clean water is not only a resource but a critical foundation for healthy ecosystems and thriving communities.

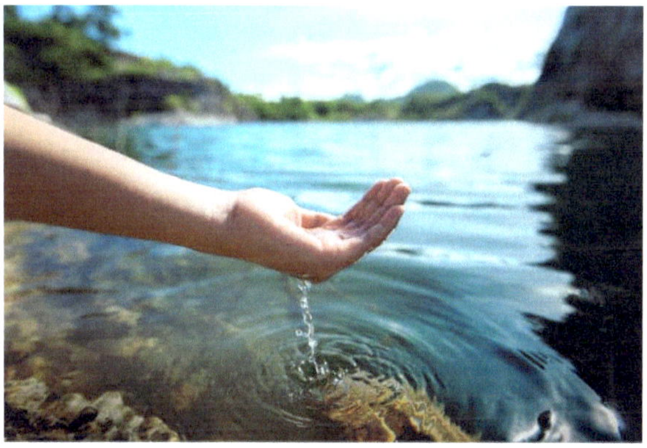

Overview of Major Pollutants Affecting Water Quality

The understanding of water quality impairment requires acknowledging the vast array of pollutants that impair aquatic ecosystems. Industrial pollution ranks as one of the most alarming types, typically in the form of discharging harmful chemicals and heavy metals into water sources (Figure 11.1). Industrial plants tend to release partially or untreated wastes, resulting in high levels of substances harmful to human health as well as ecological integrity. Heavy metals such as lead, mercury, and cadmium can bioaccumulate and bio-magnify marine life, leading to severe consequences for the environment and human health. The consequences are severe, with widespread effects on biodiversity and causing significant health risks to people who use contaminated water sources for drinking and irrigation. The need for regulation and better treatment processes is highlighted by research indicating high levels of contamination linked to industrial discharges requiring comprehensive approaches to protect water quality in the affected areas. Runoff from agriculture is another major pollutant to water quality, frequently heightened by widespread farming practices. Overapplication of fertilizers results in nutrient runoff, mainly nitrogen and phosphorus, which may trigger harmful algal blooms in aquatic systems. These blooms not only deplete oxygen levels in the water but also produce toxins that threaten aquatic life and human health. The runoff can transport pesticides, which, while intended to manage agricultural pests, have unforeseen effects on non-target organisms and general ecosystem balance. Testimony from several studies shows that those jurisdictions with high-intensity agricultural production commonly observe drastically lowered water quality, resulting in heightened monitoring and the adoption of best management practices (BMPs) to reduce the effects of agricultural runoff. These preventive measures are necessary to maintain both water quality as well as agricultural productivity in the future. Moreover, the role of urbanization and wastewater cannot be overlooked while evaluating water quality pollutants. Urban areas tend to impact water quality issues with stormwater runoff as well as inadequate wastewater infrastructure. Urban runoff carries various contaminants, including oils, heavy metals, and pathogens, into neighboring water bodies, contributing to further water quality issues. Contamination can affect both surface and groundwater, not just the aquatic environment but also water sources that humans drink from. Seasonal changes, as found in research that examined the Tamiš River, show that urban runoff increases during rainfall events, leading to heightened contamination levels. Successful measures, including better stormwater control, upgraded wastewater facilities, and citizens' participation in pollution mitigation, are essential in safeguarding water resources. The resolution of these multi-causal causes of pollution is imperative to the sustenance of vital water infrastructure.

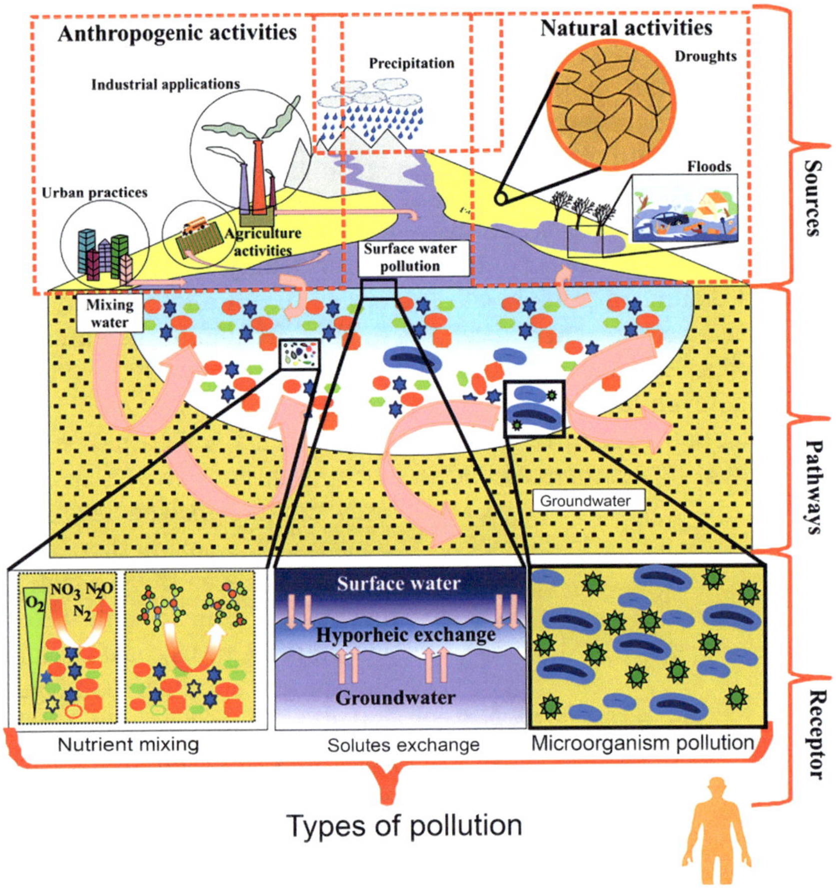

Figure 11.1. Causative agents for water pollution.

Source: Akhtar N, Syakir Ishak MI, Bhawani SA, Umar K. Various Natural and Anthropogenic Factors Responsible for Water Quality Degradation: A Review. *Water*. 2021; 13(19):2660. https://doi.org/10.3390/w13192660

11.1. Industrial Pollution

Water quality degradation, which is a critical problem of global concern, is mainly fueled by industrial pollution. Industrial effluents tend to discharge a mixture of toxic waste into aquatic ecosystems, leading to ecosystem degradation. The effluent might contain an assortment of toxic waste ranging from heavy metals, solvents, to other industrial chemicals that have devastating effects on both aquatic and human life (Figure 11.2). Specifically, mercury and lead have been identified as key pollutants linked with industrial processes, resulting in bioaccumulation within aquatic life. The consequences are far-reaching, impacting not only direct water sources but also ecosystems and food webs. Furthermore, industrial pollution has a way of exacerbating current environmental issues, and therefore proper regulation and monitoring to control sources and discharge quality into water bodies (Syafrudin et al., 2021). Industrial pollution has an impact on much more than the surrounding area of the point of discharge. Pollutants are carried along rivers and waterways, eventually impacting far-off ecosystems and communities that use such water sources for drinking, recreation, and sustenance. The combined impacts of pollutants contribute to serious public health problems, as seen in the increased rates of waterborne diseases and other health afflictions in communities that have been subjected to contaminated water. Long-term exposure to these industrial contaminants has been associated with numerous health problems, such as neurological impairment and reproductive disorders. Mitigation of this dire dimension of industrial pollution is significant in guarding the well-being of humans and in securing the sustainability of water resources. Successful interventions need to include industrial regulation, frequent monitoring of water quality, and the adoption of cleaner technologies to reduce effluent discharge (Syafrudin et al., 2021). Reduction of industrial pollution impacts requires a multi-level approach that involves legislation, public participation, and technology. Regimes must have strict legislation against wastage releases, coupled with promoting best management practices in waste management among industries. Investment in advanced water treatment technologies can also play a significant role in reducing the entry of poisonous pollutants into water bodies. Community action is also essential; mass campaigns for awareness can lead individuals to pressurize governments to provide cleaner water and pressure the industry to conserve the environment. Government-industry-civil society tripartite collaboration can enhance the creation of more environmentally friendly approaches that conserve water quality. All these attempts not only ensure the health of water ecosystems but also the people dependent upon them, rendering it a vital approach toward the conservation of our valuable water resources (Philip et al., 2020).

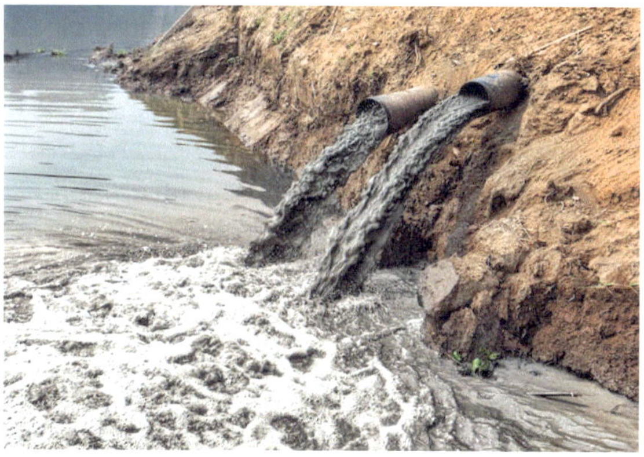

Figure 11.2. Industrial liquid waste.

Source: Aquaread (2022). *Water Pollution Runoff in a River*.

https://www.aquaread.com/blog/wp-content/uploads/2022/07/water-pollution-runoff-river.jpeg.

11.1.1. Sources of Industrial Pollutants

Industrial activity intersection with water quality is a typical example of an intricate network of environmental issues. As industries grow and mature, they tend to release all kinds of pollutants directly into water bodies, heavily reducing the integrity of the ecosystems. Chemical processing, metal processing, and plastic manufacturing factories help fill the flow of toxic waste, which may leach toxic substances into adjacent rivers and lakes. This unregulated emission of contaminants not only has serious effects on aquatic life but also poses serious health concerns to the communities that depend on these bodies for drinking and recreational purposes. Many industries, thus, avoid compliance with regulations even after their implementation. This attains a level of importance demanding strict oversight and innovative solutions in managing industrial waste effectively. Agricultural practices, thus, play a critical role in food production, which cannot be kept outside the consequences of industrial pollutants. The application of fertilizers, pesticides, and herbicides has promoted runoff of poisonous chemicals that flow into water bodies, promoting a rise in the level of pollution. Present agricultural practices, including conventional farming, focus more on production rather than environmental sustainability, creating too much nutrient loading in water systems. The induced eutrophication produces algal blooms that lower oxygen levels, resulting in dead zones detrimental to aquatic life. However, the integration of practices of organic farming has proved itself to be a viable counter-strategy, promoting biodiversity and reducing reliance on chemical inputs. By embracing these sustainable agronomic practices, the agricultural sector can reduce its role in water pollution, exhibiting the potential for systemic change. Heavy metals resulting from industrial activity constitute another critical water pollution element. Industrial processes, ranging from mining to manufacturing, tend to bring in such toxic elements into the environment. Heavy metal contamination is subtle, as the metals do not easily degrade and bioaccumulate in aquatic life, posing long-term health consequences for wildlife as well as humans. The consequences are far-reaching, affecting neurological, hepatic, and reproductive systems, among others. Mitigating heavy metal contamination not only calls for groundbreaking remediation techniques, including the application of advanced oxidation processes (AOP) and biochar adsorption but also stringent policies governing industrial operations. With growing awareness of the toxicity of heavy metals, even more imperative is the need for effective remediation techniques, as this underscores the importance of achieving equilibrium between the progress of industries and environmental stewardship.

11.1.2. Impact of Industrial Waste on Water Bodies

The impact of industrial wastes on water ecosystems is enormous since the release of toxic substances often pollutes water bodies and destabilizes the balance of nature. Such pollution not only undermines the recreational and aesthetic value of water resources but also presents substantial risks to the health of people. Heavy metals, solvents, and petrochemicals are among the toxins that have been found to bioaccumulate and bio magnify in aquatic animals' tissues, leading to their accumulation in the food chain. Through their slow penetration into the environment, they can damage aquatic and terrestrial life, later extending to human health by being ingested through fish and shellfish. In response to these damaging effects, there is a need to address the complex interactions between industrial waste and water systems in an effort to create proper remediation methods. Among the most pressing issues involving industrial pollution is the function of runoffs containing pesticides and heavy metals, which overwhelm localized water bodies. Their introduction into water bodies could be the outcome of both farm operations and urban industrial activities, thus entangling a web of causality making it challenging for water quality management. Pesticides, commonly applied in agricultural settings, flow into adjacent streams and rivers during rainfalls, with industrial effluent providing an additional source of pollution by toxic chemicals. Research has established how these contaminants impair water quality, leading to unwanted shifts in aquatic environments, including algal blooms and hypoxia. Investigations have established that more than 80% of ocean pollution originates from terrestrial sources, which highlights the importance of widespread surveillance and control strategies to keep these effects under check (Philip et al., 2020). To successfully address the ill effects of industrial waste on water bodies, integrated approaches need to be adopted. Methods like tight controls on industrial effluents, improved planning of urban areas, and enhanced waste treatment technologies are needed to reduce the hazards associated with contaminants. On the other hand, the implementation of AOPs is a potential solution to controlling pesticide contamination since it provides a more environmentally friendly method for treating recalcitrant contaminants (Syafrudin et al., 2021). By placing emphasis on sustainable practices and robust regulation mechanisms, communities can strive toward the restoration of water quality and building the resilience of ecosystems. Finally, coordinated efforts from policymakers, industry players, and the general public are crucial for safeguarding critical water resources from the harmful impacts of industrial pollution.

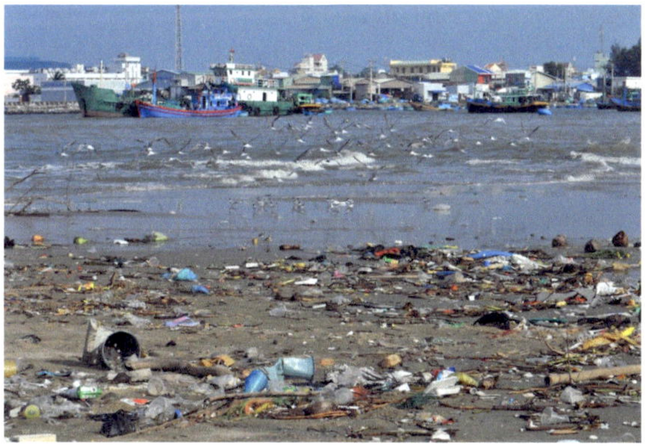

Source: Nguyen, Q. H (2021). *Photograph of Environmental Impact in Vietnam*. Earth.org. https://earth.org/wp-content/uploads/2021/08/rsz__nguyen_quoc_huy_2-1200x800.jpg.

11.1.3. Regulatory Measures to Control Industrial Pollution

The increasing trend in industrial pollution renders it crucial to have an effective system of control regulations for guaranteeing water quality. One of the main pillars of the regulations is the implementation of discharge permits that stipulate the limits of the allowable levels of introduced pollutants that enter the water bodies (Figure 11.3). Through setting up monitoring and reporting of emissions by industries, stakeholders are better able to see the impacts of industrial processes on aquatic systems. This system not only requires compliance but also causes firms to adopt cleaner practices and technologies. Further, it is policies driven by transparency in reporting that help to establish public trust, leading to public involvement in environmental responsibility. But without the enforcement clauses, the same could fail to be effective, which underscores the significance of perpetual monitoring and revision of standards following technological developments and environmental knowledge (Smith et al., 2023). Besides permits, regulatory frameworks in many cases include pollution prevention methods that are being encompassed around source reduction of contaminants. By promoting BMPs and encouraging the use of environmentally friendly alternatives, these measures promote sustainable industrial operation. Joint initiatives between governments, industries, and environmental groups can further enhance the efficacy of these strategies. For example, programs that provide fiscal rewards for businesses to invest in cleaner technologies not only encourage regulatory compliance but also strengthen corporate responsibility. This combined approach ensures that industries not only get punished for pollution but are also inspired to innovate toward a minimal environmental footprint, ultimately ending up with cleaner water resources (Smith et al., 2023). The dynamic processes of industry necessitate an ongoing evaluation of current regulatory frameworks to ensure that they become relevant and effective. Integration of science into policy-making enables regulators to respond to new threats from emerging pollutants, such as microplastics and pharmaceuticals, that were perhaps not envisioned in prior regulations. In addition, pursuing international cooperation can enable nations to combat transboundary pollution challenges since water bodies often cut across state boundaries. Through approaches like the Water Framework Directive from the European Union, countries can exchange best practices and technologies to increase regulatory cohesion and effectiveness. With changing industrial activity, so do the strategies formulated to contain their environmental impact, guaranteeing continued protection of critical water resources (Yadav, 2024).

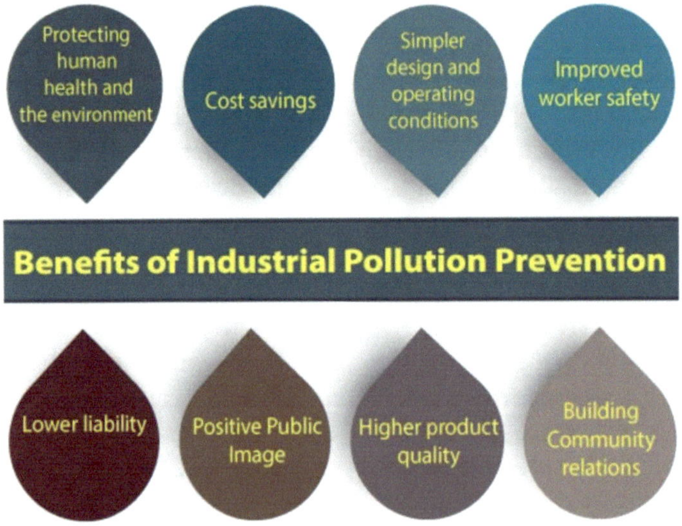

Figure 11.3. Benefits of industrial pollution prevention.

Source: ERA Environmental (2022). *Benefits of Industrial Pollution Prevention*.

11.2. Agricultural Runoff

The complex interaction between water quality and farm practices is illustrated in the case of agricultural runoff, which is becoming widely acknowledged as a major factor in water pollution (Figure 11.4). Nutrients like nitrogen and phosphorus, which are usually contained within fertilizers, are carried from fields to adjacent water bodies during rainfall or irrigation runs. This movement not only has an impact on the surrounding ecosystem but also translates into wider environmental issues, such as eutrophication, with its defining feature being the excessive growth of toxic algal blooms. These blooms use up oxygen and release toxins that are harmful to aquatic organisms, eventually affecting the quality of drinking and recreational water resources. To solve this problem, there has to be understanding and solutions that combine agricultural operations with environmental conservation to reduce the adverse effects of runoff on water bodies. Strategies to fight agricultural runoff focus on using new management strategies that seek to minimize nutrient loss. The application of practices such as the "4R" strategy—right rate, right time, right source, and right placement of nutrients, is equally efficient in minimizing runoff without compromising crop yield. Research has shown that surface runoff is minimized by source reduction measures, along with enhancing the overall environmental well-being of agricultural watersheds (Kumwimba et al., 2023). Bringing these practices together with cutting-edge technologies, such as stabilized fertilizers that slowly release nutrients, further maximizes the management of nutrients and reduces environmental pollution. This holistic strategy illustrates the potential for agricultural systems to become more sustainable while at the same time protecting freshwater ecosystems, highlighting the necessity for continuous research and study into these methods.

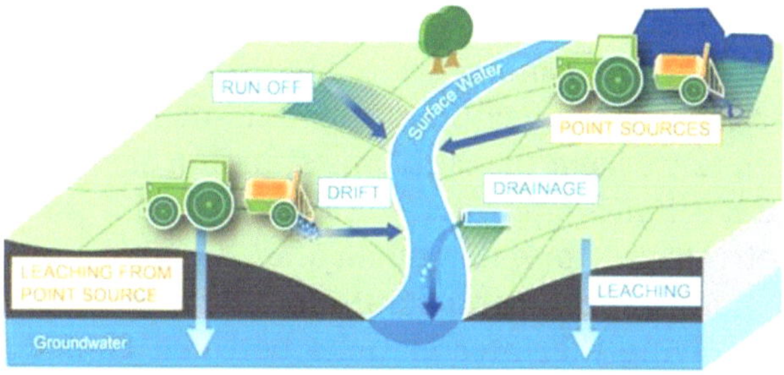

Figure 11.4. The schematic map of agricultural pollution for water sources.

Source: Ebadi, A., et al (2020). *The Schematic Map of Agricultural Pollution for Water Sources of Iran* [Map]. In *A Brief Overview on Current Environmental Issues in Iran*. Cajesti – Cas Press.

The search for solutions to farm runoff requires a thorough analysis of the processes involved in diffuse pollution since the effects of agricultural activity go beyond nutrient runoff alone. Both historical and current analysis shows that excess nutrient loads can greatly hamper attempts to attain desirable environmental conditions in aquatic ecosystems (Kumwimba et al., 2023). The complementarity between efficient nutrient recycling and the rehabilitation of eutrophic water bodies is at the core of improving water quality. In addition, combining constructed wetlands with traditional pollution control technologies is a promising route to improve pollutant retention and purification processes. By optimizing agroecosystem regulating services, we are able to best counter the disservices presented by agricultural runoff, opening the door to ecological balance and sustainable methods that help safeguard critical water resources (Figure 11.5).

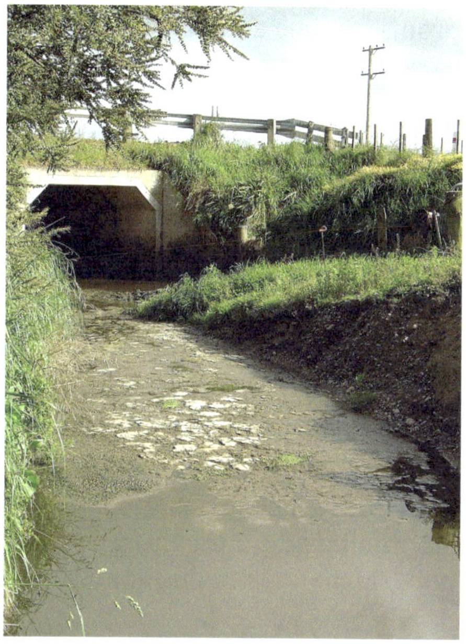

Figure 11.5. Water pollution due to dairy farming.

Source: Wikipedia contributors. (n.d.). *Water Pollution in the Wairarapa*. Wikipedia. https://upload.wikimedia.org/wikipedia/commons/thumb/d/da/Water_pollution_in_the_Wairarapa.JPG/800px-Water_pollution_in_the_Wairarapa.JPG.

11.2.1. Causes of Agricultural Runoff

The relationship between farming activities and water quality is intricate and substantial, giving rise to a host of environmental issues. The intensive farming practices widely depend on artificial fertilizers and pesticides to gain more yield from crops. During rains, these chemicals will run off easily into adjacent water bodies, leading to nutrient pollution and toxic algal blooms. Excess nitrogen and phosphorus not only reduce oxygen levels in water bodies but also lead to severe threats against aquatic ecosystems and public health. This runoff, along with sediment erosion from plowed land, can further contaminate the water quality, and so it is important to know the sources and effects of agricultural pollutants on our water infrastructure, as emphasized in studies on water pollution in contexts such as Nigeria, which reports that agricultural chemicals are main sources of this issue (Vosa et al., 2025). Another critical aspect is the misuse or overuse of agrochemicals, leading to higher runoff rates. The farmers themselves could use the chemicals without necessarily understanding the appropriate time and amounts to use for effective utilization. Poor management practices, such as the lack of buffer strips around farms and water bodies, fuel this issue. Water not only carries these pollutants into aquatic ecosystems but also transforms them into poisonous byproducts that will last and build up in ecosystems. All of these are indications toward the need for improved agricultural practices based on preventing water pollution. For instance, benefits from implementing integrated pest management (IPM) and crop rotation can profoundly limit chemical reliance and thus decrease levels of pollution (Baba, 2024). Lastly, climate change is increasingly affecting the nature and extent of agricultural runoff. Precipitation and temperature changes can drive more intense and frequent rain events, which in turn raise the risk of runoff polluted with contaminants moving into water bodies. Drought, too, could force farmers to use more amounts of irrigation water, which has the potential to release resident pollutants from the soil. This situation serves to show the way climate variability introduces a second level of complication into the situation since agricultural runoff becomes less predictable and detrimental to water quality. As the ecological and health consequences escalate, it becomes ever more important to create measures not only aimed at minimizing agricultural runoff but also at solving the interrelations between climate, agriculture, and water management regimes (Vosa et al., 2025).

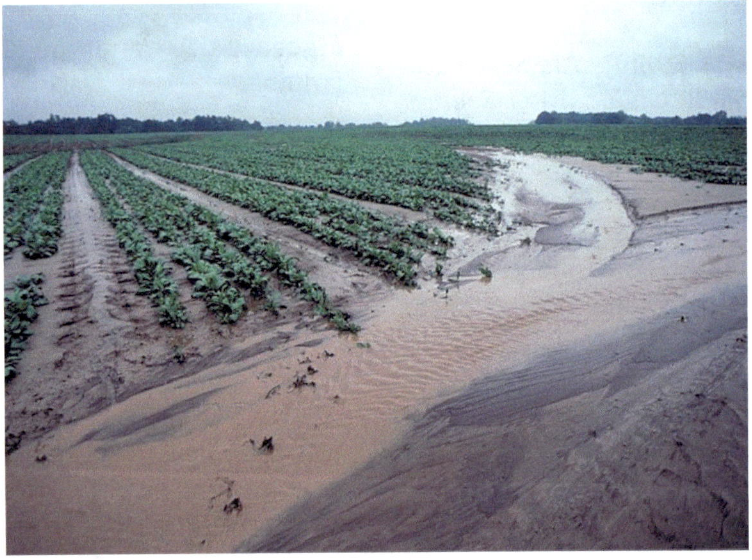

Source: Natural Resources Conservation Service. (2016). *Sediment Runoff from an Agricultural Field.* U.S. Department of Agriculture.

11.2.2. Effects of Runoff on Local Water Systems

Runoff is also an important aspect affecting the quality of local water systems since it can carry a range of pollutants from agricultural and urban areas into surrounding water bodies. Runoff from cities tends to consist of chemicals found in fertilizers, heavy metals, and oil, which pollute water bodies and damage aquatic environments. For instance, rainfall can wash them into storm drains, which will eventually release them into rivers and lakes without being filtered. As a result, such a transfer of contaminants disturbs the natural chemical equilibrium, resulting in problems like eutrophication, where levels of nutrients skyrocket, causing high growth of algae. The effects go beyond water quality, as such alterations can pose a threat to aquatic biodiversity, severely hindering local fisheries and leisure zones, and degrading the usability of waters for agricultural and domestic purposes (Hou, 2023). Runoff from agriculture, on the other hand, is another type of problem, one caused mainly by the widespread use of pesticides and fertilizers in farming. When rain occurs, the surplus nutrients and agrochemicals are being leached from farms and into nearby water bodies, harming the aquatic ecosystem. For instance, it has been established in research that very limited amounts of fertilizers are absorbed by crops, while the rest is transported into surface water, thus elevating nutrient loading that promotes algal blooms (Gamage et al., 2023). This effect not only contaminates water quality but also presents health hazards to communities that source water from these water bodies for domestic consumption. Furthermore, the integration of these farming activities with land erosion maximizes the runoff situation, creating sedimentation that further degrades water quality and aquatic ecosystems. Runoff's ecological as well as health consequences, spurred by industrial as well as agricultural activities, establish the urgency for sustainable water management strategies. One of the best ways is to establish buffer belts of vegetation alongside streams and rivers to absorb excess nutrients and pollutants prior to entering the water bodies. Organic farming is also a farming practice that can be utilized to mitigate runoff effects. Through minimizing the use of synthetic fertilizers and pesticides, organic farming can maintain soil health and reduce pollution inputs (Gamage et al., 2023). Tightening regulatory policies, in conjunction with society's awareness of the need for water conservation as well as sustainable farming practices, can further abate the adverse effects of runoff as well as promote improved local water systems for future generations (Hou, 2023).

11.2.3. Best Management Practices to Mitigate Runoff

Sensible use of farming practices is crucial in mitigating runoff and ensuring water quality. Implementation of practices such as no-till farming, cover crops, and precision application of fertilizer can significantly mitigate the negative effects of nutrients and sediments in water bodies. No-till agriculture mitigates soil disturbance, hence preventing the loss of soil structure and enhancing water infiltration, minimizing surface runoff. Cover crops have two functions, nevertheless: they improve the quality of the soil in addition to acting as sedimentation and nutrient barriers that won't be washed away by rain. Precision fertilizer application enables farmers to apply fertilizers with greater precision, minimizing excessive application that would lead to nutrient runoff. As indicated in (Marshall et al., 2008), compliance with these BMPs is key to the development of sustainable agricultural systems that focus on ecological balance and protection of water. Urban areas also need specific BMPs to effectively deal with runoff, especially by utilizing Sustainable Drainage Systems (SUDS). The SUDS method promotes a paradigm shift from conventional drainage practices, which tend to be ineffective in handling water quality issues. Through the establishment of drainage systems that mimic the natural process of drainage, SUDS attempts to treat and handle polluted runoff where it occurs. Techniques included in this approach, like rain gardens and permeable pavements, encourage stormwater filtration, storage, and infiltration. The emphasis on source control is increasingly embraced in policy regulations, as seen in (Duffy et al., 2013), where it is reported how some guidelines have facilitated the adoption of SUDS in urban planning. With increased urbanization, and urban growth, adopting these innovative drainage solutions becomes essential in enhancing city resilience to flooding and water quality maintenance. In addition to agricultural and urban practices, community education and participation are essential components of effective runoff management initiatives. By educating people on the effects of runoff on nearby water bodies, communities can create a culture of stewardship that promotes prudent land use practices. Training residents to maintain natural vegetative buffers on rivers and streams can lead to enhanced protection from potential pollutants. Workshops, clean-ups, and partnerships with local governments can be employed to introduce the required behavioral change that translates into water quality improvement. As a unit, communities will be better placed to implement BMPs that guarantee runoff reduction. The promotion of local initiatives is thus in harmony with the common desire to reduce environmental pollutants and make water resources more sustainable, hence highlighting the role of grassroots in this significant undertaking.

11.3. Pesticides

The negative effects of farming systems based largely on pesticides cannot be overemphasized, particularly in terms of water quality and ecosystem health. Since the chemicals leach into adjacent environments through runoff, they pollute adjacent water bodies, resulting in harmful effects on aquatic communities. The introduction of such chemical compounds changes the biodiversity in these systems, degrading trophic relationships and causing population decreases in sensitive organisms. In addition, the buildup of these pesticides will cause bioaccumulation and biomagnification in food webs, further elevating the toxicity risk for higher trophic levels, including humans. Through research, it is established that not only do pesticides attack organisms but also non-target organisms, thereby escalating ecological imbalances and causing challenges in sustainable agricultural practices (Alengebawy et al., 2021). In addition to water pollution, soil contamination by pesticides affects crop yields as well as microbial diversity, which is responsible for maintaining a healthy ecosystem. The ongoing application of the chemicals may alter soil chemistry, which affects soil structure, nutrient level, and overall quality of the soil, leading to decreased soil quality. Pesticides may directly destroy soil microorganisms, which play important roles in the decomposition activities of organic matter and nutrient cycling. The resultant long-term effects of the impacts are diminished agricultural productivity and increased dependence on chemicals, creating a cycle of economic instability and environmental degradation. Such problems reinforce calls for more efficient farming practices that reduce the application of pesticides while encouraging IPM strategies that utilize biological control and habitat manipulation (Sara et al., 2021). As much as the immediate benefits in crops following the use of pesticides in farming are apparent, their long-term consequences raise serious questions regarding environmental sustainability. The interactive toxicological effects of the synergism among pesticides and other contaminants, like heavy metals, add to the problem, causing intricate combinations that reinforce their toxicological effects on plants and soils (Alengebawy et al., 2021). Minimization of these factors requires a multidirectional approach that involves policy reform, increased public visibility, and advances in technology to reduce dependency on poisonous chemicals. Encouragement of practices such as organic farming, precision agriculture, and the use of less toxic substitutes can offset the adverse effects of pesticides on water quality and overall environmental health. Together, these steps can help to build stronger ecosystems and preserve our valuable water resources for the future (Sara et al., 2021).

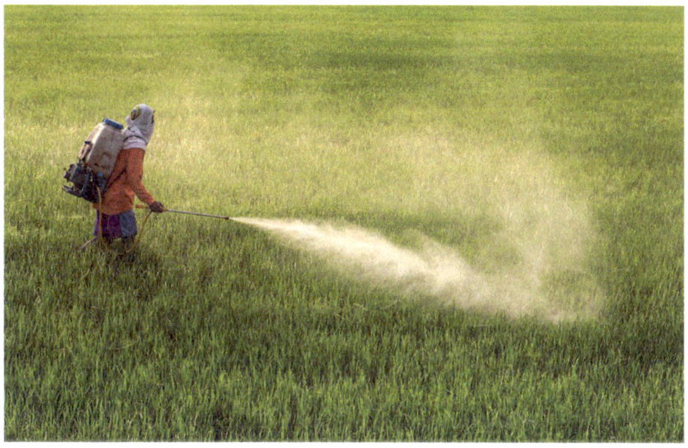

11.3.1. Types of Pesticides Commonly Used in Agriculture

Within the intricate mechanisms of modern agriculture, the extensive usage of pesticides is key to improving crop yield and pest control (Figure 11.6). Amongst the most significant categories are insecticides, herbicides, and fungicides, each with a targeted crop issue in mind. Insecticides are applied to deal with pest infestations that would otherwise destroy crop integrity, having a huge impact on the yield. Herbicides, nonetheless, seek to eliminate invasive weeds, which might hamper crops' access to essential resources like water and nutrients.

Fungicides, in contrast, combat fungal infectious diseases that have the potential to devastate plant health and production. A thorough understanding of such pesticides is required, not only to maximize agricultural production but also to minimize their broader environmental effects, as reflected in the emerging problems of water quality and pollution levels. Greater dependence on these chemical fix-it's has fueled great controversy over their effects on both human health and environmental ecosystems. Research has shown that the residues from the chemicals can last in agricultural runoff and end up contaminating surrounding water sources and harming aquatic organisms and human health. As crop varieties like glyphosate and neonicotinoids become more infamous for their harmful impacts, the agricultural industry is brought to a boil over its sustainability standards. In addition, the process of bioaccumulation is alarmingly toxic because the concentration of harmful substances in living things accumulates over time. Not only is biodiversity jeopardized but also food safety is at stake, prompting a critical consideration and regulation of the use of pesticides. The subtleties involved in these toxicants call for a more rigorous inspection of their implications on agriculture as well as the environment at large. In addition, the social effects of pesticide application go beyond environmental issues, entangling with agricultural policy and regional economies. Agriculturalists tend to be trapped in a cycle of reliance on chemical measures for increasing output while the long-term effects are under-explored. As industrial pollution and climate change magnify stress on agricultural systems, the dependence upon pesticides as a band aide solution to problems worsens issues, especially in areas already contending with degraded water quality. To manage these multifactorial stress combinations, strong agricultural strategies that position environmental health as equally important with productivity are needed. Increased education and promotion of organic methods of farming, decreased chemical reliance, and IPM represent possible avenues of enhancing agricultural resilience and the increasing awareness of the interdependence between human and environmental health in sustainable agriculture, as seen in numerous studies investigating the toxic impact of agricultural pollutants (Alengebawy et al., 2021; Sara et al., 2021).

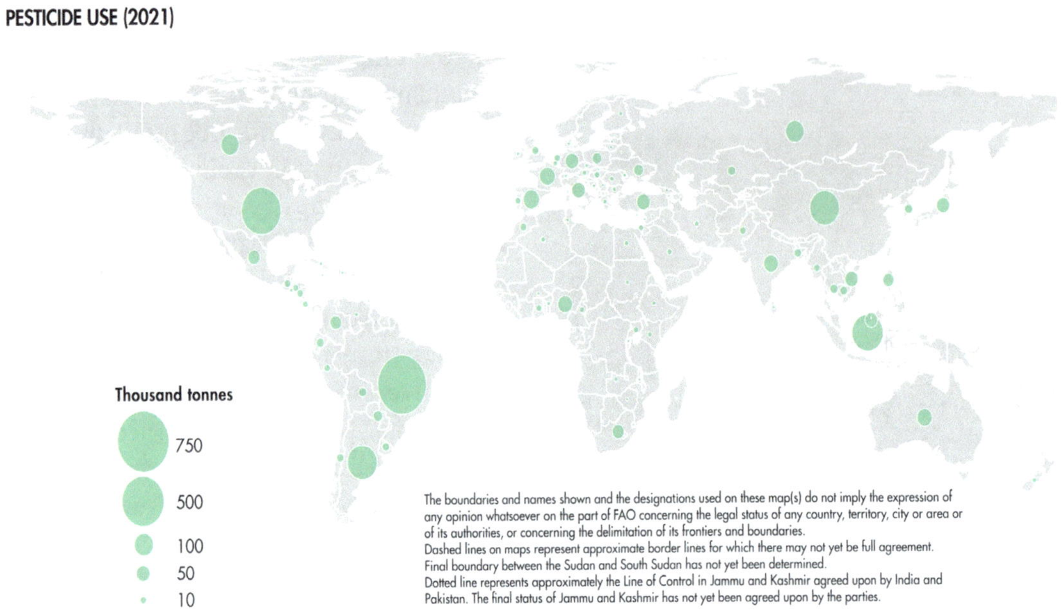

Figure 11.6. 8 Different types of pesticides used in agriculture.

Source: By FAO - https://www.fao.org/documents/card/en/c/cc8166en , File:World Food and Agriculture - Statistical Yearbook 2023.pdf, CC BY-SA 3.0 igo, https://commons.wikimedia.org/w/index.php?curid=142156127

11.3.2. Pathways of Pesticide Contamination in Water Sources

The complex relationships that control pesticide pollution underscore the various facets of agricultural operations and their influence on water quality. With the growing use of chemical inputs in contemporary agriculture, precipitation runoff can carry pesticides directly from fields to surrounding water bodies. This is a high-risk pathway because pesticides become persistent in water bodies, settling in sediments and impacting biodiversity. Research has shown that not only is pesticide runoff responsible for acute toxicity in aquatic life, but long-term ecological disruptions are also possible. Here, knowing the routes of pesticide transfer to water bodies is important to formulate effective mitigation measures that take into account agricultural productivity and environmental protection, ensuring thereby a sustainable equilibrium between human requirements and ecological well-being (El-Sharkawy et al., 2025). Additionally, the contribution of urbanization and poor wastewater management cannot be underestimated in the pesticide contamination pathways discussion. Urban runoff has the potential to add to the pesticide burden in water systems, especially in peri-urban areas where agricultural and urban development's intermingle. The mixture of stormwater runoff, typically laden with many types of pollutants, and mixed landscape characteristics makes water quality management more difficult. An example is research on urban streams that has found high levels of pesticides in rivers along agricultural fields, which is attributed to agricultural practice runoff and household product leachate with the same chemicals. The intricacies brought by urbanization call for holistic measures that involve both agricultural and urban planning to effectively curtail pesticide contamination (Milija et al., 2025). Lastly, pesticide transport via soil and groundwater interactions presents another level of intricacy in understanding contamination routes. Subsurface leaching can ease the transport of pesticides into aquifers, which represents a critical threat to drinking water sources and aquatic environments. According to research, it has been found that some types of soils, especially the highly permeable ones, are prone to leaching of pesticides, which results in spatial variability in contamination. As a result, targeted management practices like buffer zones and cover crops can be put in place to reduce pesticide runoff and increase the capability of the soil to retain. By taking an integrated and holistic approach to water and land management, it is possible for stakeholders to respond more effectively to pesticide contamination and protect critical water resources for both ecosystem and human health (El-Sharkawy et al., 2025) (Figure 11.7).

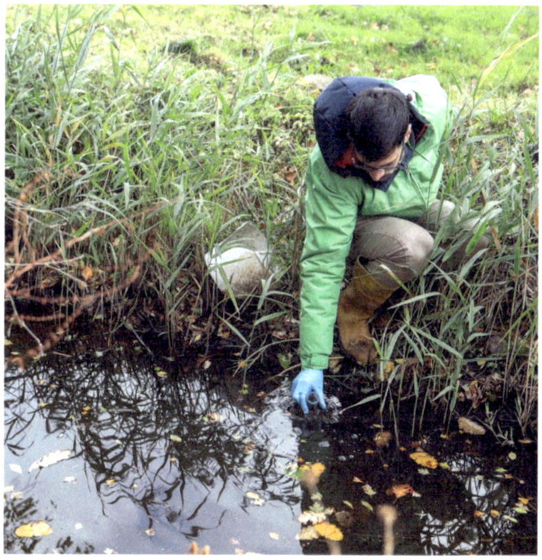

Figure 11.7. Collecting water sample from a stream.

Source: Liefting, A. (2003). *Water Pollution in the Wairarapa*. Wikimedia Commons.

11.3.3. Long-Term Effects of Pesticide Exposure on Aquatic Life

The subtle interaction of aquatic and agricultural ecosystems is significantly affected by pesticide use. When pesticides are sprayed or sprinkled over crops, rainwater can lead to runoff, ultimately polluting adjacent water bodies on a large scale. Pesticides can emit poisonous substances in aquatic ecosystems, disturbing local ecosystem equilibrium. Aquatic organisms like fish and invertebrates can face acute and chronic toxicity due to continuous exposure to the chemicals. The toxic impacts are not only reflected in death rates but also in reproduction success and growth rates among such organisms, which can lead to loss of biodiversity. Therefore, the effects of pesticide exposure are not limited to one species but extend to entire food webs and ecosystem functioning, thereby posing a threat to freshwater systems' ecological integrity. Apart from direct toxicity, exposure to pesticides over the long term may lead to bioaccumulation in water organisms (Figure 11.8). Bioaccumulation is the process through which organisms take up toxic substances at a rate higher than they are removed, causing their concentration to increase in their bodies over time. This process directly threatens species across multiple trophic levels, from producers to top predators, by interfering with higher concentrations necessary for biological processes that are critical for growth and reproduction. Additionally, humans indirectly come into contact with them by eating contaminated aquatic organisms, which can cause health complications such as cancer and compromise of the immune system. Hence, agricultural runoff that inputs pesticides into aquatic ecosystems contributes to a cycle of poisoning that radiates horizontally across ecosystems and upwards into the human food chain. Mitigating the long-term consequences of pesticide exposure on aquatic organisms requires all-encompassing regulatory policies and campaigns aimed at agricultural activities. Enhanced knowledge of the mechanisms of action through which pesticides affect aquatic ecosystems is crucial for the establishment of effective measures to abate these threats. The solutions would lie in the promotion of IPM practices that ensure the reduction of chemical pesticide use, as well as the creation of buffer zones to trap runoff into water bodies. As emphasized by latest studies, farmers, policymakers, and scientists should join forces in advocating for sustainable agricultural methods that protect aquatic life and water quality. Through such practices, the likelihood of contaminants to harm freshwater ecosystems can be reduced, creating cleaner habitats for today and tomorrow's generations.

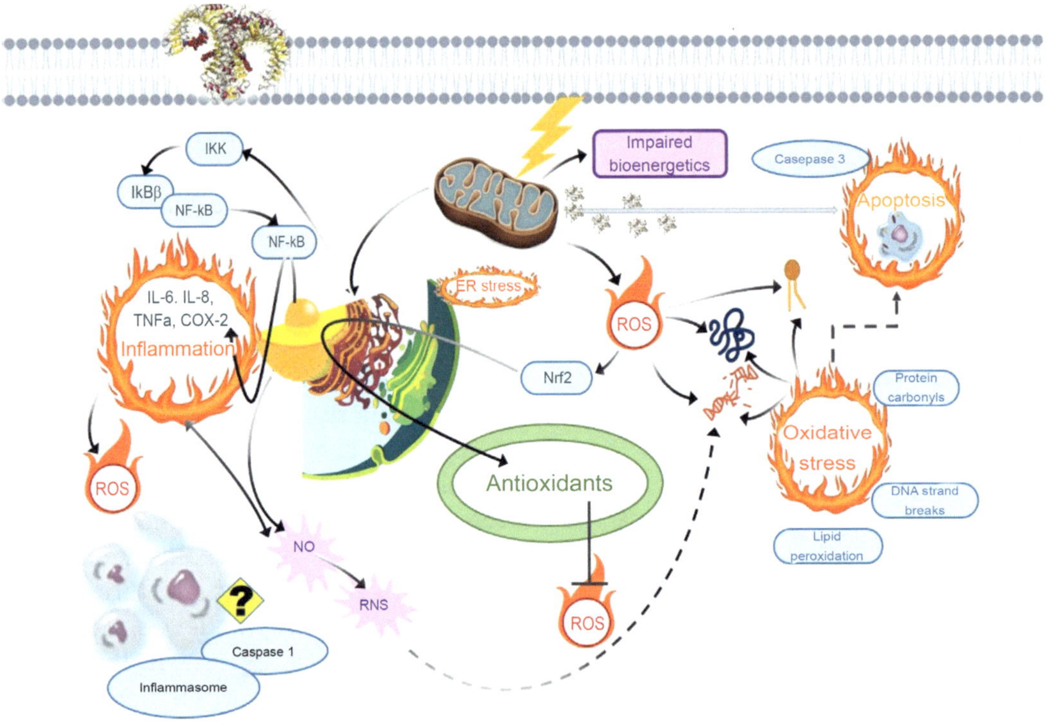

Figure 11.8. Impact of herbicide/insecticides in aquatic ecosystem.

Source: Khatib I, Rychter P, Falfushynska H. Pesticide Pollution: Detrimental Outcomes and Possible Mechanisms of Fish Exposure to Common Organophosphates and Triazines. *Journal of Xenobiotics*. 2022; 12(3):236-265. https://doi.org/10.3390/jox12030018

11.4. Heavy Metals

The occurrence of heavy metals in water sources presents a major threat to both environmental systems and human life. The poisonous elements such as lead, mercury, cadmium, and arsenic commonly originate from industrial effluents, mines, and agricultural activities. Upon release into the environment, heavy metals have the potential to be accumulated by aquatic animals, resulting in bioaccumulation and biomagnification in the food web. Research shows that even at low levels, these metals can cause adverse physiological effects such as neurotoxicity and developmental diseases in humans as well as wildlife. Additionally, long-term exposure to heavy metals has been associated with different health conditions such as cancer, cardiovascular diseases, and weakening of the immune system. Combating these threats requires effective systems of monitoring and management that bridge the link between environmental science and public health policy, enhancing the vital connection between water quality and society's health and well-being. Countermeasures against heavy metal water pollution should aim at industrial and agricultural change. Industry must adopt cleaner production techniques, such as the application of closed-loop systems to minimize discharges of waste. By using advanced filtration technologies and proper waste management practices, heavy metal discharge can largely be avoided. Furthermore, agriculture must rethink its utilization of particular fertilizers and pesticides leading to heavy metal runoff into local water bodies. Organic farming technologies and the use of bioremediation technologies are crucial in minimizing the heavy metal burden of soils, thus restricting their leaching into aqueous systems. Strategies deliberated at global forums, like the United Nations Climate Change Conference, emphasize cooperation among countries to enact tight controls and promote green practices in industry and agriculture to effectively conserve water resources and lower levels of pollution (Calvin et al., 2023).

Education and community engagement are important in mitigating the prevailing issue of heavy metals in water. Educational programs enlightening individuals on sources of heavy metal contamination and their health impacts can empower communities to take action. Local campaigns emphasizing regular water testing and reporting systems against pollution incidents can promote action-driven means in safeguarding public health. Also, public engagement via environmental activism can lead to effective policy frameworks upholding clean water interventions. The integration of the community's voice into the policy-making process enhances the efficiency of actions against pollution. By instilling a sense of collective responsibility for the purity of the water, communities can drive meaningful change, bridging local action with more general environmental goals, leading ultimately toward more sustainable systems and healthier communities (Chen et al., 2022).

11.4.1. Common Heavy Metals Found in Water Sources

Heavy metal presence in aquatic organisms has emerged as a pressing problem, largely because of human activities. Lead, mercury, cadmium, and arsenic are commonly present in contaminated water sources, which originate from industrial effluent, mining operation, and agricultural drain. Each metal is related to certain health risks, influencing both humans and aquatic organisms. For instance, lead has been linked to neurological deficiencies and developmental issues in children, while mercury is notorious for its insidious effects on the nervous system. Both metals inevitably find their way into drinking water supplies, laying the groundwork for the acute necessity of stringent monitoring and control systems. Tackling these pollutants calls for comprehending their entry routes to water bodies and the impact they have on water quality and human health, calling for strategized intervention and remediation in affected territories (Khan et al., 2025). The literature shows that heavy metal pollution severely degrades water quality and ecosystem condition. An example of this phenomenon is given through a study carried out on the Ichu River that showed alarming levels of heavy metals like arsenic, lead, cadmium, and chromium that surpassed World Health Organization (WHO) limits. Heavy metal contamination can be traced to industrial wastewater effluent discharge and agriculture, which aggravate the situation through runoff. The synergistic effect of heavy metals in combination with microbial contamination emphasizes a pressing danger to both environmental integrity and human health. Monitoring parameters like turbidity and dissolved oxygen have been found to have a correlation with higher levels of heavy metals, indicating a complicated interaction that enriches total water pollution. These findings indicate the necessity of immediate intervention and strengthened management procedures in order to arrest the ongoing loss of vital water resources (Zarate-Cáceres et al., 2025). Long-term exposure to heavy metals in water sources necessitates integrated remediation measures to minimize their impact on ecosystems and human health (Figure 11.9). Traditional methods are often ineffective and can create secondary pollutants. Emerging technologies such as bioremediation, in which microorganisms are employed to remove pollutants, and nanotechnology for enhanced adsorption of heavy metals are gaining traction. Secondly, the integration of green policies and policy-based approaches, including community-level awareness programs and robust regulatory systems, will also prove useful in enhancing water quality governance. Scientists, regulatory bodies, and local communities must work together to evolve and implement sustainable solutions. Through enhanced innovation and adherence to green legislation, societies can open the doors to cleaner water sources and safeguard vulnerable ecosystems from the widespread menace of heavy metal pollution (Khan et al., 2025).

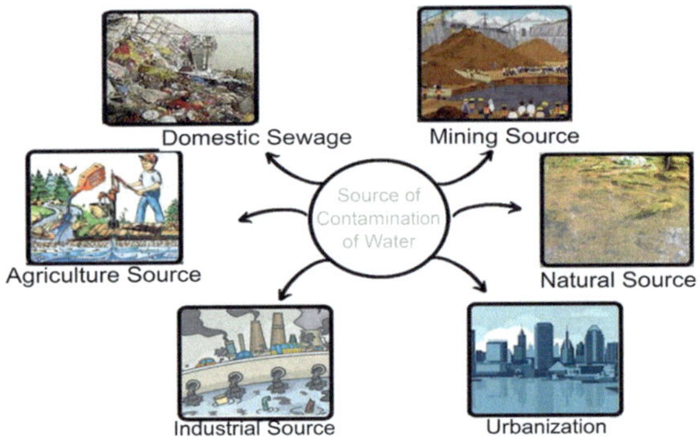

Figure 11.9. Different sources of heavy metal contamination in water and aquaculture.

Source: Singh A, Sharma A, K. Verma R, et al. (2022) Heavy Metal Contamination of Water and Their Toxic Effect on Living Organisms. The Toxicity of Environmental Pollutants. IntechOpen. Available at: http://dx.doi.org/10.5772/intechopen.105075.

11.4.2. Sources of Heavy Metal Contamination

The complex relationships between different human activities and heavy metal pollution have posed serious environmental issues. Mining, manufacturing, and chemical processing industries are among the major offenders in terms of releasing toxic metals like lead, cadmium, and mercury into aquatic systems. These metals typically find their way into water bodies in the form of wastewater discharges, where they remain for long periods of time because of their degradability. Urbanization also amplifies the issue; more construction and infrastructure development create greater runoff rates, transporting contaminants to nearby streams and rivers. The prospects for damage to aquatic environments and human health are catastrophic, making long-term approaches necessary to address this widespread problem (Gamage et al., 2023). Farming practices are another primary contributor to heavy metal contamination, fueled chiefly by the application of synthetic fertilizers and pesticides. Although such chemicals are designed to increase crop yield, their ingredients contain trace amounts of heavy metals that seep into the soil and water bodies. With time, runoff on agricultural fields carries such pollutants into surrounding water bodies and threatens aquatic life and also threaten the safety of drinking water. In addition, the long history of application of lead-based pesticides as well as other conventional farming practices has resulted in cumulative contamination, making it difficult to restore the environment. Other methods, like organic agriculture that reduces dependence on chemical inputs, can provide a potential remedy to decrease the exposure of heavy metals in water (Gamage et al., 2023). Natural sources like geological structures and weathering also find their way into the heavy metal pollution. Substances like arsenic and mercury can leach into groundwater due to the natural erosion of mineral deposits. Human activities such as mining and drilling can also mobilize naturally occurring metals, further increasing their occurrence in both surface and groundwater sources. The interaction between human impacts and natural factors makes the evaluation and management of water quality challenging. Since heavy metals tend to bioaccumulate along the food chain, the ecological and health effects of this pollution can be widespread (Figure 11.10). Interventions to counter these sources of pollution are important for both environmental sustainability and human health (Aziz et al., 2023).

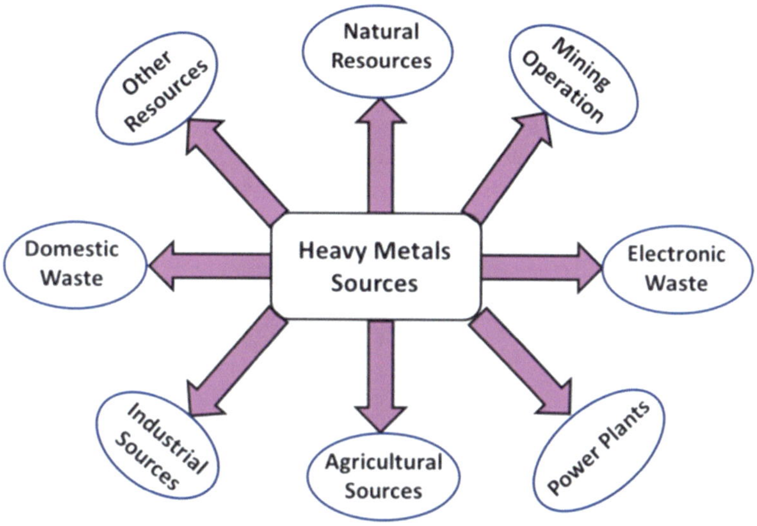

Figure 11.10. Heavy metal pollution source.

Source: Das TK, Poater A. Review on the Use of Heavy Metal Deposits from Water Treatment Waste towards Catalytic Chemical Syntheses. *International Journal of Molecular Sciences*. 2021; 22(24):13383. https://doi.org/10.3390/ijms222413383

11.4.3. Health Risks Associated with Heavy Metal Exposure

The recurring occurrence of heavy metals in water bodies has become a serious public health issue, with the major factors being industrial contamination and urban runoff. Such poisonous materials like lead, mercury, and cadmium have the ability to be stored in the food web, finally causing severe health effects in both wildlife and humans. These metals are not readily degradable and can persist in ecosystems for long durations, causing bioaccumulation and biomagnification. Consequently, populations using polluted water sources can experience elevated cases of neurological diseases, childhood development problems, and a host of chronic ailments. Realization of these threats emphasizes the imperative for all-inclusive methods to curtail industrial emissions and improve water quality, an effort backed by global environmental policies aimed at safeguarding public health (Calvin et al., 2023). The association between heavy metal exposure and health effects goes beyond acute toxicity; it also considers long-term chronic disorders. It is assumed that trace concentrations of metals can cause some complications like cardiovascular disease, kidney impairment, and cancers. High-risk groups, that is, children and expectant mothers, are especially sensitive, as their evolving systems are more vulnerable to adverse constituents (Figure 11.11). Community-based educational programs can help raise awareness of such risks and the necessity for pure water resources. These programs can educate local communities to become conscious and capable of influencing governments to have stricter regulations on industrial contaminants, making the environment cleaner. Installation of systems to regulate heavy metals in drinking water is also necessary for identifying and solving health threats posed by exposure (Syafrudin et al., 2021). In order to control the risk caused by heavy metal contamination, master plans should be enforced with a focus on prevention and decontamination. Effective methods for controlling pollution must be directed at reducing industrial emissions and implementing strict waste management strategies. Moreover, newer technologies such as bioremediation can prove beneficial in cleaning up polluted areas without introducing additional contaminants. Public policy also has its part to play; legislation that supports sustainable agriculture and regulates industrial waste will do much to reduce the heavy metal runoff into the water systems. Investment in education and community participation not only helps generate awareness but also builds a sense of community responsibility toward water quality. The joint efforts of government and non-governmental organizations (NGOs) are crucial in protecting health and providing access to safe drinking water (Calvin et al., 2023).

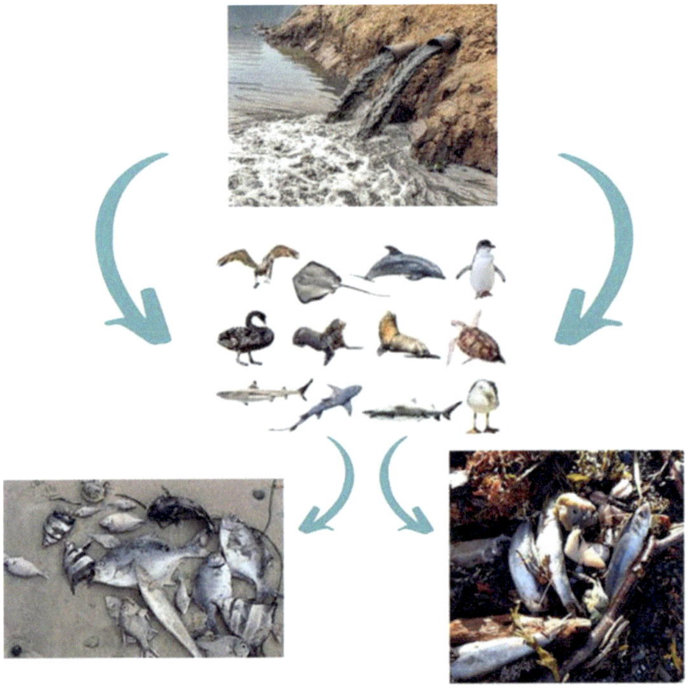

Figure 11.11. Impacts of heavy metals toxicity on human health.

Source: Singh A, Sharma A, K. Verma R, et al. (2022) Heavy Metal Contamination of Water and Their Toxic Effect on Living Organisms. The Toxicity of Environmental Pollutants. IntechOpen. Available at: http://dx.doi.org/10.5772/intechopen.105075.

11.5. Strategies for Reducing Pollution

The pressing need to counter increasing levels of pollution requires a polyphony of measures, specifically in the area of water quality conservation. New-fangled practice like AOPs are becoming increasingly popular as efficient modes for the treatment of pesticide-polluted water. Traditional methods of treatment carry a high cost of operation and risk of secondary pollution, pointing toward an imperative to use a newer technology with fewer drawbacks. AOPs with their ability to degrade recalcitrant substances provide a good option not only for remediating pesticides but also for decontaminating a variety of residues resulting from industrial effluents. As an adjunct to this, intensive monitoring systems must be implemented to assess the effectiveness of these methods in real-time so that water quality improvements are both sustainable and effective in preventing health hazards from polluted sources (Syafrudin et al., 2021). In addressing the impacts of agricultural runoff, the application of BMPs has emerged as a primary strategy for pollution prevention. These practices range from promoting organic farming practices to promoting controlled use of fertilizers. By adopting BMPs, farmers can reduce the fertilizers and pesticide runoff into adjacent water bodies, thus safeguarding aquatic environments and safeguarding sources of drinking water. Moreover, building buffer zones—vegetation-lined strips along water bodies, can serve as a good bulwark against rain-swept pollutants. Not only does it enhance biodiversity along the riparian zones, but it also plays a key role in sedimentation retention, illustrating how agricultural reforms can lead to broader environmental advantages (Philip et al., 2020). Public policy is also used to enable programs to restrict water pollution. Regulatory laws reducing industrial discharge, combined with incentives to upgrade treatment plants, can go far to improve the quality of the water. Policies to remove hazardous substances, such as persistent organic pollutants, demonstrate a proactive commitment to environmental and public health protection. Furthermore, raising awareness among community stakeholders of the effects of pollution on water quality has the potential to stimulate communal activism calling for policy reform. Joint implementation among government agencies, non-governmental organizations, and the private sector has the potential to strengthen sound pollution prevention strategies. Keeping these different approaches from one another not only enhances the quality of water but also underscores the significance of collaboration in the alleviation of the intricate implications of water pollution (Syafrudin et al., 2021).

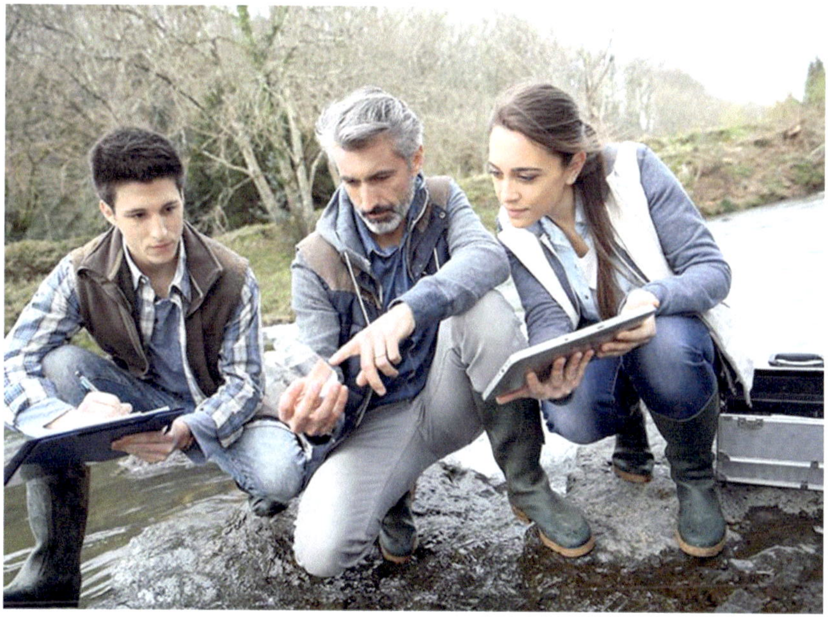

Source: IndiaCelebrating.com. (n.d.). *How to Control Water Pollution.* https://www.indiacelebrating.com/wp-content/uploads/How-to-Control-Water-Pollution.jpg.

11.5.1. Technological Innovations for Water Treatment

Recent developments in water treatment technologies play a central role in responding to the increasing pressures on freshwater supplies driven by industrial and agricultural contamination. The methods of purifying water are evolving at a rapid pace with an emphasis on optimum efficiency and minimum environmental impact. For instance, reverse osmosis desalination has emerged as a preponderant technique, effectively transforming seawater and brackish water into potable water. The process, apart from accommodating the growing demand for purified water, also integrates harmoniously into comprehensive strategies of sustainable water management. Other approaches such as governance centrally and improved infrastructure are important in the successful implementation of these technologies to ensure the benefits of new treatments are delivered to vulnerable populations (Shemer et al., 2023).

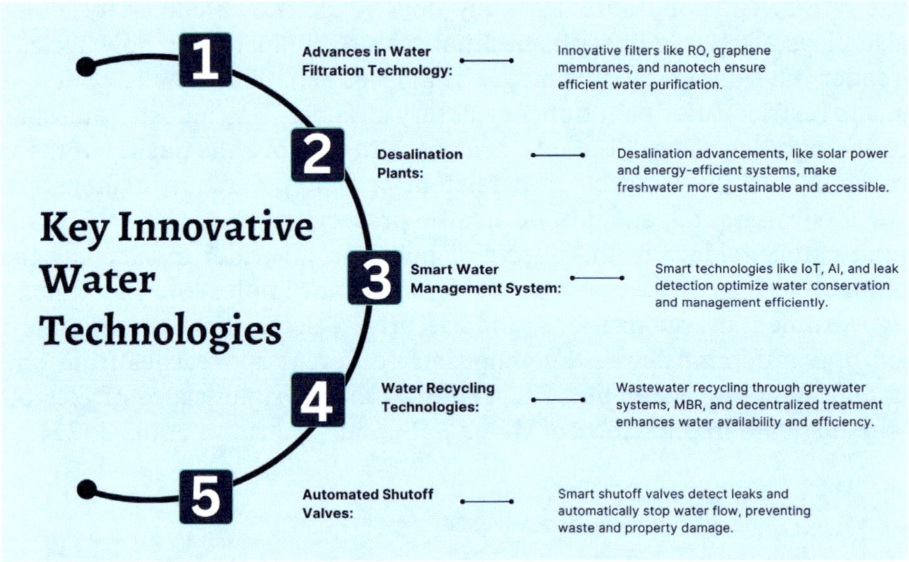

Figure 11.12. Key innovative water technologies.

Source: H2O Global News. (2023). *Key Innovative Water Technologies.* https://h2oglobalnews.com/wp-content/uploads/2023/09/Key-Innovative-Water-Technologies-1536x864.webp.

At the same time, utilizing farm waste as a resource to treat water is being increasingly accepted as a novel method of averting pollution. Traditional practices of waste management tend to be responsible for environmental degradation by overlooking the potential of biomass produced in crop production. Through the utilization of agricultural residues as adsorbents, scientists are seeking the potential for efficient removal of contaminants, such as heavy metals and pesticides, from wastewater. Biomass-derived materials can be converted into engineered bio-sorbents by certain processes such as carbonization, highlighting the double benefit of waste minimization and water purification. This holistic-engineering strategy provides a sustainable approach to prevent environmental pollution, which not only emphasizes the beneficial role of *in-situ* resources in combating water contaminant concerns (Nataša Karić et al., 2021), but also ensures proper investment in innovative treatment technologies for the adjustment to the nuances of new contaminants that continue to pose challenging concerns in established water quality standards. Technologies such as AOPs and biofiltration systems are applied to treat pollutants that traditional treatments often overlook (Figure 11.12). These technologies tap multiple chemical and biological processes for delivering advanced purification needs, ensuring that the treated water is safe to be used in industry and agriculture. Integrating these advanced techniques with traditional techniques offers increased resistance to the complexity of pollution sources, from agricultural runoff to industrial effluents. Therefore, the ongoing advancements in water treatment technologies place them at center stage in the overall strategies toward protecting water resources and enhancing the overall water quality (Shemer et al., 2023).

11.5.2. Policy Initiatives Aimed at Reducing Water Pollution

The control of water pollution through sound policy interventions has been attracting increasing interest worldwide, especially in the face of mounting environmental pressure. Governments and institutions have developed sophisticated systems for regulating industrial effluents, promoting environmentally friendly farming, and enhancing overall water quality. These interventions generally include imposing rigorous standards for contaminants such as heavy metals, nitrates, and pesticides, which have long-term implications on human health as well as aquatic ecosystems. Initiatives geared toward encouraging compliance by industries, and educational campaigns for farmers on sustainable practices, have been helpful. Further, putting in place regulations for detecting and monitoring water quality can act as early warning systems to detect problems ahead of time. Policies can hence revolutionize the face of water resource management to make preventive measures possible instead of reactive ones, leading to healthier ecosystems and communities. In farm environments, the major contribution toward groundwater contamination comes from runoff rich with fertilizers and pesticides. Efficient policy measures are currently being formulated to regulate such runoff by using BMPs and IPM measures that ensure minimal chemical use. Evidence shows that training regarding sustainable soil management is instrumental in helping decrease the use of synthetic fertilizers, which subsequently reduces nutrient runoff into water bodies. Policymakers are considering subsidies and grants to farmers who use eco-friendly practices that enhance soil health while saving water resources.

It is critical for the government agencies, agricultural scientists, and farmers to join hands in formulating and applying these measures in a beneficial way. Ultimately, strong policies promoting sustainable agriculture can reduce the negative impacts of agricultural runoff on water quality and lead to a more resilient ecosystem. Marine ecosystems are also severely threatened by water pollution, which has led to global debate over efficient policy intervention. Pollution reduction measures aimed at land are critical, countering the upstream causes of ocean pollution. The integration of laws outlawing the dumping of harmful wastes and promoting cleaner methods of production is essential to improving coastal water quality. Monitoring and evaluation programs for marine pollution are also increasingly important, providing necessary information back into policy changes for the future. Initiatives that raise the awareness of the public and community involvement in the fight against marine pollution have shown promise toward the establishment of a culture of water resource stewardship. Focused interventions, like the proclamation of Marine Protected Areas (MPAs), can help nations safeguard key aquatic habitats without losing out on the long-term benefit of improved water quality and public health. The multi-threat approach embraced in the policy measures reflects a growing recognition of the interdependence between human health and environmental integrity, with a stress on the necessity of holistic measures addressing water pollution (de Lima et al., 2008; Landrigan et al., 2020).

11.5.3. Community Engagement and Education on Water Conservation

Engaging communities in water conservation is crucial in the development of environmentally sustainable bad habits. Effective initiatives typically lie on the shoulders of community participation and awareness-raising, which may significantly enhance public knowledge about water issues and their consequences. Education programs and workshops enable communities to discover the complex relationships between sources of water pollution, like industrial effluent and agricultural runoff, and how they directly affect local environments. Once people are informed about their responsibility for water conservation and the impact of doing nothing, they will be more likely to embrace positive behavior change. Further, hands-on experience programs, such as community clean-up drives and tree planting, can instill a feeling of ownership and responsibility toward local water resources. According to available literature, enhanced community participation is also important in strengthening the effectiveness of water conservation programs (Ewim et al., 2023a).

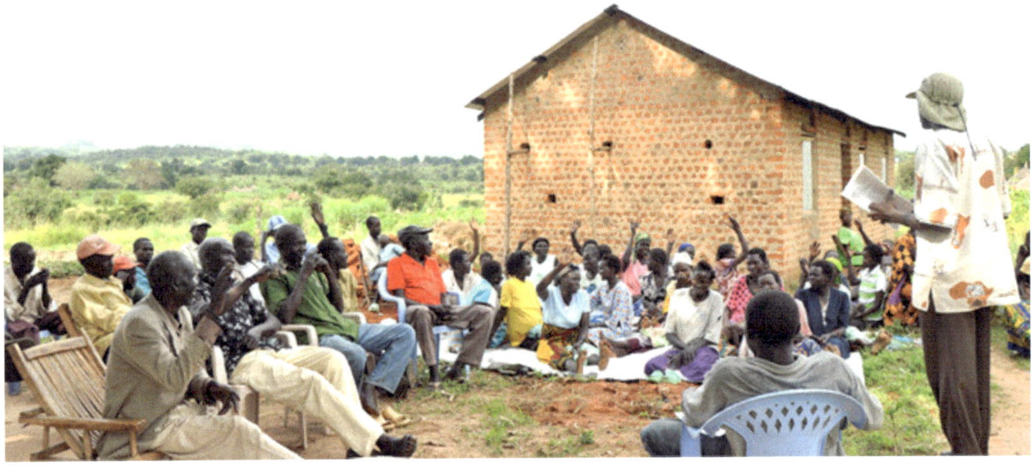

Source: The Water Project. (n.d.). *Community Members Receiving Clean Water.* https://thewaterproject.org/images/community_help.jpg.

In effective implementation of education programs, one must customize programs based on the unique demands and challenges of a specific community. Heterogeneous communities are likely to have differing levels of access to information and varying cultural beliefs on water use. Therefore, the utilization of culturally relevant material and presentation modes of information can encourage more understanding and involvement. Alliance with leaders and organizations from within the community can also facilitate louder voices, ensuring that education work resonates deeper. This local method can correct water conservation misconceptions so that communities can address their local environmental challenges while focusing on mutual effort. This approach is compatible with suggestions from environmental science, where stakeholder involvement ensures stronger feedback loops and sustainable processes (Ewim et al., 2023b). In addition, sustainable water management requires continued community engagement beyond the initial level of education. Long-term partnerships between schools, municipalities, and community organizations can foster continued exchange and adaptive learning. Through such partnerships, there are opportunities for the exchange of resources and information, and more integrated water management plans can be devised that are optimally adapted to specific geographic contexts and socio-economic settings. Continuous evaluation and public participation can allow educational programs to be enhanced and issues in the making identified, which is critical in providing long-term sustainability. Significantly, fostering a culture of conservation can allow communities to advocate for policy reforms that protect their water supplies, thus becoming resistant to many contaminants and environmental risks. Therefore, constant education and outreach activities are crucial in cementing community dedication to water conservation (Ewim et al., 2023a).

11.6. Protecting Water Sources

The pressing necessity of efficient measures to safeguard water resources has become increasingly pressing owing to the complex challenges presented by pollution (Figure 11.13). Several pollutants, such as heavy metals and agricultural runoff, have emerged as major sources of threats to water quality, with negative effects on ecosystems and human health. The Saraswati River case is a prime example of the ramifications of unbridled pollution—where industrial waste and urban runoffs resulted in extreme contamination as indicated by the presence of an extensive array of pathogenic microbial species and increased concentrations of harmful substances such as heavy metals and pesticides (Dutta et al., 2025). Utilizing sustainable recovery measures is needed. These involve updating waste management infrastructure and using newer geospatial technology to monitor water quality so that interventions can be implemented on time to handle pollution sources before they worsen. Good governance is the key to the struggle to prevent water resources from being contaminated. Policy frameworks for stakeholder engagement, regulatory requirements, and international cooperation are critical aspects of preventing water pollution (Baba, 2024). Laws must not only increase regulations but also promote societal awareness of the health and environmental consequences of pollution. For instance, official environmental impact assessments (EIAs) with water pollution considerations in mind can provide a comprehensive appreciation of potential ecological consequences and enhance better decision-making. Strengthening these governing frameworks can allow a more collaborative method to water quality assurance, reconciling economic growth with the protection of the environment, thus guaranteeing the sustainability of water supplies for future generations. Furthermore, applying new farming methods can significantly reduce the impact of agricultural runoff on water quality. Precision farming and IPM are methods that reduce the chemical application of fertilizers and pesticides, thus limiting their leaching into water bodies. Wetland restoration and conservation of natural buffers along water courses are essential in filtering out contaminants before their entry into aquatic ecosystems. It is important that policymakers sanction these practices with economic incentives and education programs for sustainable land use (Baba, 2024). Together, all these efforts will not only help in curbing pollution but also develop the resilience of water sources so that a safe and reliable supply can be ensured for communities and ecosystems.

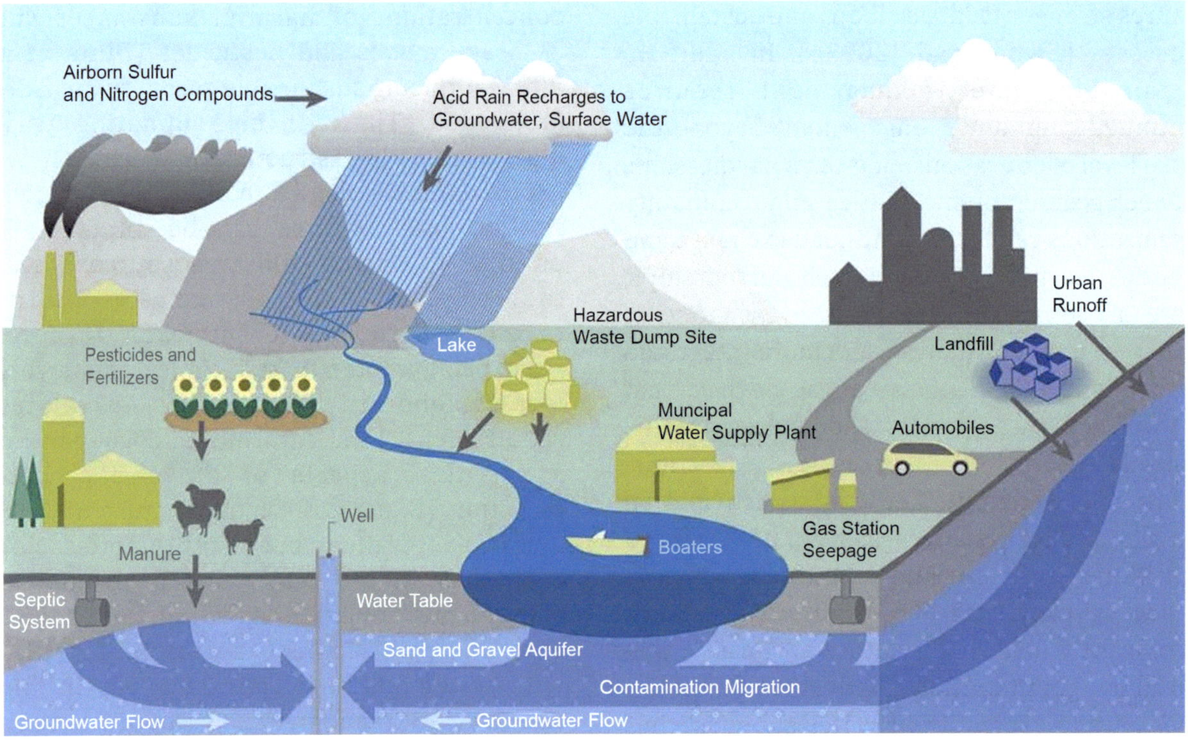

Figure 11.13. Source water protection.

Source: IntechOpen. (n.d.). *Human activities affecting source water.*

https://images.squarespace-cdn.com/content/v1/583ca2f2d482e9bbbef7dad9/1485468971436-NTZNNFI2B6K1LGZ7QJLU/Human+Activities+Affecting+Source+Water.

11.6.1. Importance of Watershed Management

Good management of watersheds is very important in dealing with a myriad of water quality problems originating from environmental contaminants. The interaction between land use management and water bodies plays a vital role in determining the quality of water resources. For example, agricultural runoff is one of the main causes of water pollution, depositing toxic pesticides and fertilizers into water bodies. These compounds not only pollute water quality but also represent serious human health hazards through bioaccumulation in aquatic life and ultimately, humans. Research indicates that pesticides can be accumulated in sediments and organisms, indicating the need for urgent watershed management practices that reduce these effects on water quality (Syafrudin et al., 2021). Through the use of improved land management practices, such as sustainable agriculture, runoff is minimized and water sources cleaned up, leading to better public health and ecosystem resilience. In addition, watershed management plays an essential role in sustaining soil erosion controls, which affect water quality directly (Figure 11.14). Human activities such as deforestation, urbanization, and industrialization may lead to tremendous sedimentation in proximal water bodies. This sediment holds various visible and chemical pollutants that contribute to surface water degradation (Issaka et al., 2017). Effective watershed management includes erosion control measures, which not only preserve soil but also maintain water quality through the regulation of sediment transport into rivers and lakes. Taking practices like reforestation, buffer strips, and contour farming not only saves soil but also enables the natural filtering of pollutants before they enter water bodies. Integrated watershed management thus proves useful to save both terrestrial and aquatic environments. Besides, watershed ecosystems require a multidisciplinary approach in their management. Practical plans must balance the environmental, social, and economic factors in consideration of the tendency for human activities to be the core of the degradation of watersheds. Coordinated efforts between government, local communities, and industries can offer comprehensive frameworks for pollution control and conservation. By giving paramount importance to education and sensitization, stakeholders can forge a culture of custodianship of water resources. Furthermore, contemporary technologies for pollutant detection and remediation, such as new filter systems or constructed wetlands, can be added to these systems to enhance water quality (Issaka et al., 2017; Syafrudin et al., 2021). Finally, integrative watershed management not only solves the immediate problems of industrial contamination and agricultural runoff but also facilitates sustainable measures that preserve valuable water sources for generations to come.

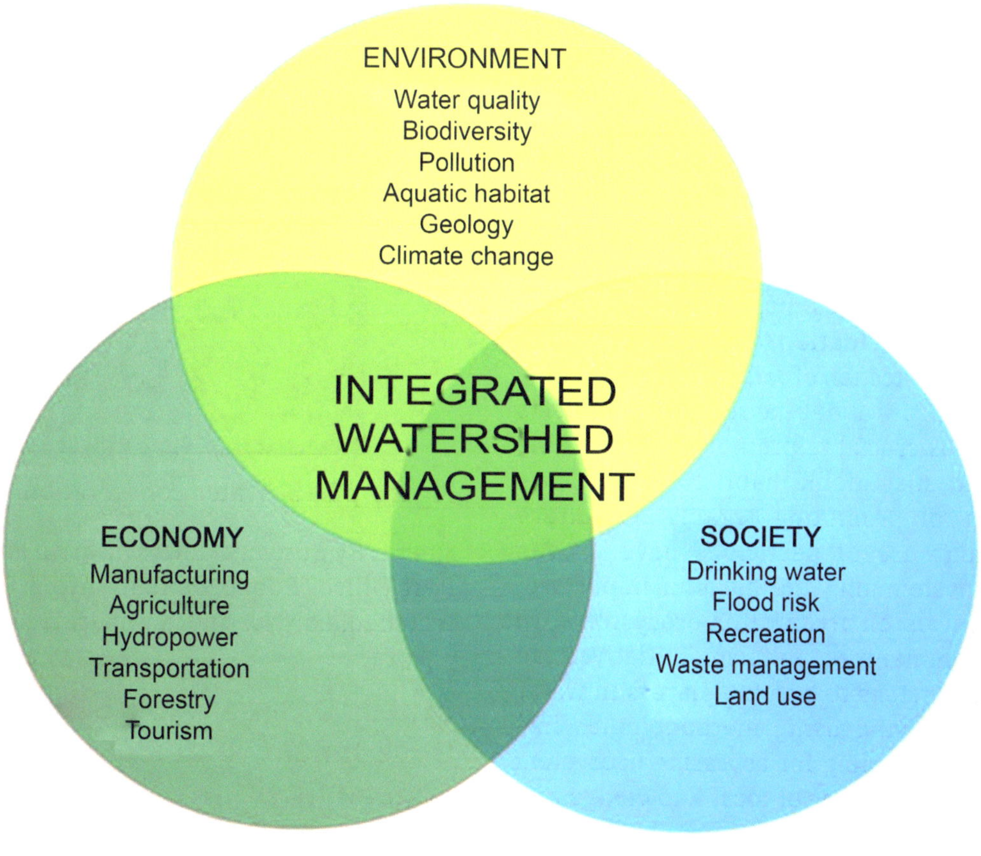

Figure 11.14. Processes influencing the process of watershed management.

Source: Tang X, Adesina JA. Integrated Watershed Management Framework and Groundwater Resources in Africa—A Review of West Africa Sub-Region. *Water*. 2022; 14(3):288. https://doi.org/10.3390/w14030288

11.6.2. Role of Conservation Practices in Protecting Water Quality

The complex interrelationship between water quality and conservation methods indicates a deeper commitment to environmental sustainability and well-being. Tackling the threat of industrial effluent and farm run-off, for example, are several measures, including riparian buffer strips, wetland reclamation, and no-till agriculture. Riparian buffers, for example, are natural buffers that capture sediment and nutrients before reaching water bodies, thus absorbing the negative impacts of agricultural operations. Additionally, incorporating better wastewater treatment systems is essential in minimizing the pollutants that find their way into waterways. Prioritizing these conservation efforts will help communities increase ecosystem resilience and water quality, essentially mitigating the effects of pollution while protecting precious water resources for future use (Figure 11.15). Apart from physical conservation measures, public awareness and community participation are also crucial in ensuring the protection of water quality. Teaching local communities about the sources and effects of pollution is crucial to promoting responsible actions and sustainable habits. For instance, campaigns for promoting organic agriculture and prudent use of pesticides have proven effective in stemming the harmful impacts of farm chemicals on freshwater ecosystems. In addition, community monitoring initiatives can also enable citizens to become players in water quality monitoring using methodologies like zooplankton sampling for assessing ecosystem health. With the power of local knowledge and expertise, such programs can instill a sense of ownership that encourages people to participate in conserving, thereby realizing better water quality results in their area. The imperative for holistic water management strategies cannot be overemphasized, particularly in environments dominated by climate change as well as rising pollution levels. Multi-pronged strategies marrying conservation practices with regulatory policies are vital for tackling the complex challenges to water quality. The results from investigations such as for the Tamiš River illuminate the value of seasonal surveys and ongoing surveillance in mirroring the need for shifting conservation regimes responding to dynamic changes in environment conditions. Sensitization about water quality-habitable links of urban design, agricultural catchment areas, and industrial activities will promote enhanced enforcement of policy responses. When pollutants from multiple sources tend to aggregate in freshwater ecosystems, it becomes essential to have a comprehensive understanding of the conservation practices in order to sustain water quality and ensure the sustainability of vital water resources in a rapidly evolving world.

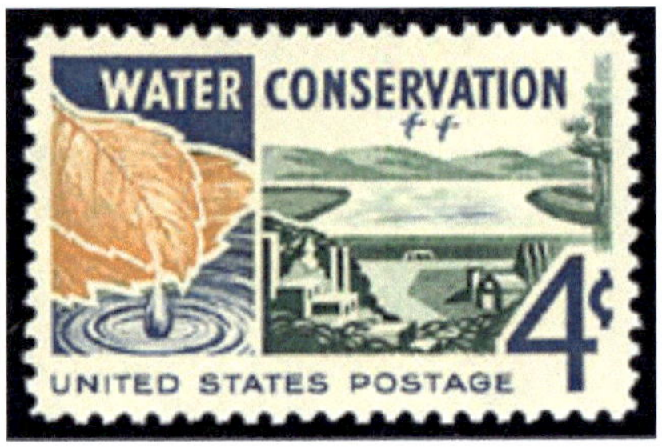

Figure 11.15. Water conservation.

Source: By Bureau of Engraving and Printing - U.S. Post Office, Public Domain, https://commons.wikimedia.org/w/index.php?curid=2929522

11.6.3. Collaboration Between Government, Industry, and Communities

It depends largely on the successful partnership between industries, local communities, and government agencies to respond to environmental pollutants. Such partnership promotes resource and knowledge sharing that is crucial in building overall strategies for combating water quality deterioration. For example, local governments can offer regulatory standards that promote industries to use environmentally friendly technologies while building community responsiveness through educational initiatives. This collaboration is crucial while dealing with the complex problem of water pollution, as it involves contributions from various stakeholders who have exclusive ideas about regional environmental situations. Studies emphasize the importance of incorporating public consciousness into these activities, which can help communities play an active part in safeguarding water supplies and promoting sustainable practices (Sahoo et al., 2023). The contribution of industry toward collaboration cannot be downplayed since private firms usually have advanced technologies that can make a substantive contribution to minimizing water pollution. Through collaboration with governmental agencies, industries can adopt environmentally friendly technologies geared toward reducing their environmental impact while remaining economically viable. For instance, sectors can create and utilize innovative filtration techniques to deal with pollutants like heavy metals and pesticides, thereby enhancing water quality. Joint initiatives also open up avenues for common research and development programs that aim to find new solutions to long-standing issues like farm runoff. This collective strategy promotes a culture of accountability and responsibility among all stakeholders so that the overall objective of clean water for the generations to come remains within reach (Rolnick et al., 2022). Community participation is important in promoting accountability and instilling sustainable behaviors at the grassroots level. Public behavior toward water conservation and avoidance of water pollution can be positively affected by local awareness campaigns organized by the community organizations. These campaigns tend to bridge the gap between scientific information and common practices, empowering citizens with the weapons required to fight for their environmental rights. Moreover, local communities can be instrumental in water-quality monitoring and reporting, further strengthening cooperative frameworks. Where communities are empowered and educated, they are essential stakeholders in efforts to conserve water sources, hence developing a comprehensive strategy for water quality management that suits all concerned parties (Sahoo et al., 2023).

11.7. Public Health Implications

Water quality is closely related to public health because the contaminants pose a significant risk to human populations. The occurrence of industrial pollutants in water bodies can result in a range of health consequences, from respiratory diseases and neurological disorders. Vulnerable populations and children are especially susceptible, making it crucial to have interventions designed to avert these risks. In addition, long-term exposure to heavy metals contained within contaminated waterways has been linked with chronic disease, hence emphasizing the need for strict regulatory policies to control water quality. Public health interventions must not only focus on diminishing contaminants but also on educating populations on the associated health hazards with contaminated water supplies.

Additionally, agricultural runoff only worsens the issues surrounding water quality and public health. Runoff with pesticides and fertilizers flows into water bodies around them, promoting the development of harmful algal blooms that produce toxins harmful to human health. These toxins result in gastrointestinal diseases, liver injury, and even neurological impacts in people. Public health measures should therefore emphasize tracking farming activities and encouraging sustainable practices that minimize runoff. Including these practices within policy structures may not only protect water quality but also improve health in the community. Since waterborne diseases still linger as threats, tackling agricultural runoff is important within the larger context of public health and environmental stewardship.

To the extent that the interaction between water quality and public health is complicated, new approaches are gaining attention. Nature-based approaches are an exciting opportunity to enhance water quality while also solving health-related issues. Through the restoration of ecosystems, like wetlands and riparian corridors, communities are able to improve their water filtration capabilities as well as lower pollutant loads. This strategy not only addresses the risks of contaminated water but also promotes healthier contexts for local communities. Additionally, the variety of benefits of these solutions, such as increased community resilience and better mental health, highlight their potential as successful public health interventions. As solutions continue to develop, stakeholder collaboration will be important in adjusting solutions to suit local contexts and achieving long-term public health outcomes.

11.7.1. Health Risks Associated with Contaminated Water

The complex association between contaminated water and public health gives strength to the enormous issues in communities globally. Significantly, poor sanitation, industrial effluent, and agricultural runoff cause a range of waterborne diseases that can have a drastic impact on populations. Pathogens and heavy metals contaminate water bodies, presenting serious health consequences, especially in vulnerable areas. The consequent rise in diseases such as cholera, typhoid, and dysentery underscores the need to address issues concerning water quality (Figure 11.16). In addition, the long-term implications of these pollutants pass beyond the realm of acute health issues, with possibilities for long-term conditions like cancer and neurodegenerative diseases. An awareness of these hazards is important in developing suitable public health interventions to protect populations from the widespread menace of contaminated water.

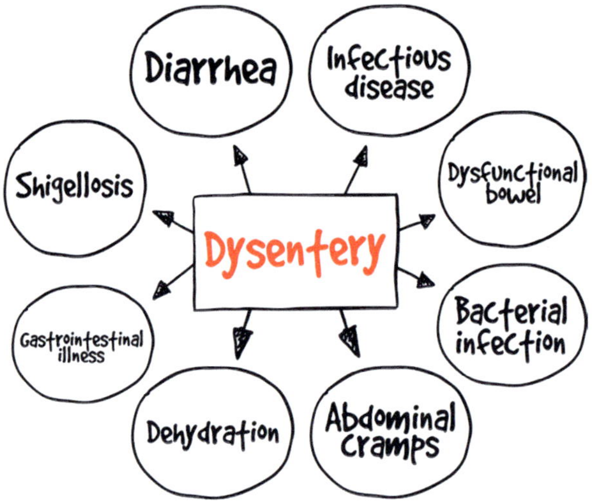

Figure 11.16. Dysentery.

Source: https://t3.ftcdn.net/jpg/07/36/66/80/360_F_736668002_FFI5RJT21ropPKEepjfBmIpUOquJ6CBH.jpg.

Industrial waste management approaches in most areas have not done enough to mitigate the hazards caused by pollutants entering water bodies. Heavy metals and organic pollutants, commonly present in factory process effluents, can bio-accumulate in aquatic environments and later migrate into the food chain for humans. The health effects are immense, as humans using contaminated food and water are likely to be affected by numerous diseases, ranging from neurological impairment and reproductive problems. In addition, agricultural runoff tends to compound the issue by depositing pesticides and fertilizers into water supplies, further deteriorating water quality. This intricate interaction between industrial contamination and farming practices calls for enacting full-scale regulatory initiatives that can guarantee the safety of water sources both for human use and for agriculture. Effective measures should not only emphasize swift remediation efforts but also long-term prevention in the context of stricter industry regulation and more sustainable farming practices.

A concerted effort between governments, communities, and health organizations is needed to address the cross-cutting health threats of dirty water. Public awareness campaigns are key in educating people on the risks of consuming dirty water and calling for sustainable use of water in industries and agriculture. Highlighting the need for clean sources of water can galvanize community action to push for clean water and sanitation. Moreover, improving monitoring mechanisms for water quality can detect sources of contamination so interventions can be made on time. Improving water treatment technologies should also be given priority to guarantee access to clean drinking water, especially where there is high pollution potential. In the end, an integrated approach that harmonizes policy, education, and community involvement is crucial to addressing the health consequences of polluted water and promoting the overall health of impacted communities.

11.7.2. Vulnerable Populations Affected by Water Pollution

The disproportionate burden of water pollution borne by marginalized communities demonstrates the stealthy character of environmental injustice. Low-income and marginalized communities in many areas are frequently subjected to industrial pollution and agricultural runoff, which result in major public health problems. For example, these groups often reside close to polluted water sources that subject them to various toxic metals, pesticides, and pathogens that weaken their health and wellbeing. It is especially worrying for children and pregnant females, who stand a greater chance of suffering from developmental impairments and other serious health complications. This pattern not only emphasizes the inequality inherent in environmental policy but also the imperative to introduce specific public health interventions to mitigate these inequalities, as the findings of water quality evaluations from across the world elaborate.

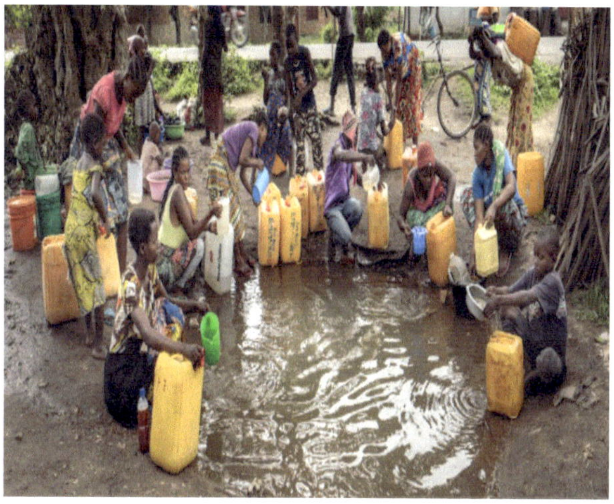

Source: https://acnudh.org/wp-content/uploads/2021/03/image1170x530cropped.jpg.

The socioeconomic effects of contaminated water surpass direct impacts on the health of individuals, echoing throughout communities. Degraded water quality typically thwarts economic prospects by degrading local fisheries and agriculture, upon which many vulnerable groups are dependent for their survival. These industries' collapse devastates food security and raises dependency on costly imported commodities further, further compounding poverty levels. In addition, people who are impacted by water pollution often bear heavy healthcare expenses as they struggle with long-term diseases related to prolonged exposure to pollutants. This environmental degradation and economic suffering are not solitary incidents but rather representative of deeper systemic injustices that aggravate health disparities and undermine community resilience. Multifaceted public health interventions that address these interrelated issues effectively are crucial in building sustainable development among vulnerable communities.

Involvement of impacted communities in developing and applying public health interventions may result in more appropriate and effective measures for preventing the effects of water pollution. Involving local perspectives allows policymakers to get a better understanding of the specific issues these people encounter and develop interventions that can be applicable to their individual needs. Such a community-focused strategy has the potential to empower residents to make claims for their right to clean water and healthy surroundings, resulting in a sense of agency that such groups tend to lack. In addition, national and global organizations need to invest money primarily in programs related to monitoring the quality of water and eradicating sources of pollution. Encouraging education and awareness of the dangers of water pollution can not only improve community resilience but also stimulate community action against industrial and agricultural processes that threaten public health.

11.7.3. Economic Costs of Waterborne Diseases

The complex relationship between economic stability and water quality is highlighted starkly by the incidence of waterborne diseases. These diseases, which are brought on by polluted water sources, place a major financial burden on healthcare systems, households, and national economies. The economic cost of waterborne diseases to the global economy has been estimated to be more than hundreds of billions of dollars every year. This estimate includes direct medical costs, lost labor productivity, and wider social consequences, such as poorer educational achievement in infected children. The economic burden is especially severe in low- and middle-income countries (LMIC), where the absence of clean water and sanitation heightens susceptibility to these diseases, perpetuating poverty cycles and restricting economic development. The economic effects of waterborne disease therefore highlight the need for contaminant control reform and public health infrastructure investment.

The interdependence between industrial pollution and waterborne disease further complicates economic difficulties. Industries frequently release untreated wastewater into bodies of water, drastically elevating the potential for contamination. This run-off from industry, charged with toxic chemicals and pathogens, not only compromises public health, but it also disproportionately affects economically disadvantaged groups. These groups have fewer resources available for proper healthcare and are more apt to endure drastic economic losses from disease. A research established a connection between water quality problems and increased healthcare expenses and reduced workforce productivity, exemplifying the cascading effect industrial pollution has on local economies. Further, the long-term consequences involve the curtailment of local economic activities that depend on clean water, driving communities further into economic hardship. Counteracting this problem requires stronger regulatory environments and preventative measures for reducing industrial pollutants.

Public health interventions are a key counteraction to the economic burden of waterborne diseases. The interventions are varied, involving sanitation facility upgrades, hygiene practice education, and ready access to healthcare for treatment of those infected. Investing in these interventions allows countries to dramatically lower the occurrence of waterborne diseases, the resulting reduced healthcare costs, and enhanced labor productivity. For example, good sanitation and hygiene interventions can reduce morbidity rates, leading to healthier populations and improved economic performance. In addition, investment in clean water programs not only solves short-term public health issues but also builds long-term economic resilience. Studies have indicated that communities with strong public health systems have better educational outcomes and higher workforce participation, highlighting the interdependence of water quality, health, and economic well-being. These results demonstrate that focusing on the economic costs of waterborne diseases is essential for the attainment of sustainable development goals and promoting proactive policy measures.

SUMMARY

The complex interface between water quality and environmental contaminants highlights the need to combat the complex problems posed by industrial pollution, farm runoff, and the widespread use of toxic chemicals like pesticides and heavy metals. Knowing the causes and effects of these contaminants is essential to designing sustainable solutions. A comprehensive strategy entails not only the adoption of new technologies but also a dramatic change in farming practices toward greener approaches. The application of green technologies, particularly in the production and application of fertilizers and pesticides, is the cornerstone of minimizing environmental degradation while keeping agriculture productive. Therefore, advancing expertise in environmental sciences must be balanced by practicality with a focus on the health of the ecosystem and public safety. Efforts to reduce pollution and retain water supplies grow more urgent. The discovery of the detrimental effects of pesticides on aquatic organisms as well as human health further necessitates the importance of proper measures of management. For instance, the widespread use of pesticides has led to their accumulation in water bodies, disrupting aquatic life as well as polluting sources of drinking water. Conventional treatment methods are normally deficient, with limitations such as high costs and secondary pollution risks. Hence, probing more sophisticated water purification technology, such as AOPs, deserves keen attention. The technologies not only enhance the elimination of recalcitrant contaminants but also address a general trend toward cleaner, more efficient water treatments in line with global sustainability aims. In essence, an integrated approach to facing the crisis driven by environmental contaminants is required for safeguarding water quality. Interdisciplinary collaboration among stakeholders such as policymakers, farmers, and environmental experts must go into the development and application of creative solutions in varied contexts. The use of green technologies and nanomaterials is a chance to transform conventional farming technologies while solving long-standing water quality problems. In addition, ongoing research on how pollutants move into aquatic environments will guide more efficient management and inform public health measures. Ensuring a cleaner, healthier environment, our commitment to protecting water sources will continue to be a foundation for sustainable development and environmental responsibility.

Industrial contamination and water quality converse in a shocking manner where industries frequently release poisonous products into bodies of water that affect ecosystems and human health. Industrial waste chemicals, heavy metals, and other toxic chemicals are some of the primary factors contributing to water contamination. Industrial contaminants tend to disrupt aquatic life and worsen biodiversity. Moreover, the health effects on water-depending populations of polluted water sources are gigantic in nature, manifesting themselves in the form of endemic and chronic diseases. The problems necessitate not only stringent regulation but also the adoption of state-of-the-art technologies designed to avoid water pollution. It is thus important to understand the cause and type of industrial waste to develop effective strategies that guarantee water resources are saved for the future. Run-off from farms also aggravates the water quality issues, where pesticides and fertilizers leach into water bodies. Run-off from farms is at times high in nitrogen and phosphorus, both of which cause eutrophication—a process that absorbs oxygen from water and causes death among aquatic life. And indiscriminate use of chemical pesticides is a threat to aquatic and terrestrial ecosystems by releasing toxic chemicals that affect non-target organisms. As mentioned, incorporating organic farming practices will drastically minimize the environmental impact linked with conventional agriculture. Organic farming can help to restore natural nutrient cycles, improve soil health, and ultimately encourage better water quality by minimizing the use of chemical fertilizers and pesticides. This transition is critical in sustaining agricultural landscapes as well as protecting water resources from ongoing pollution (Gamage et al., 2023). In addition to industrial pollution and farm runoff, the role of heavy metals in water quality is an important area of concern. Toxic heavy metals such as lead, mercury, and cadmium have cumulative effects on the environment and exert severe ecological and health impacts. Contamination is often the outcome of industrial processes, improper disposal of wastes, and mining activity. The synergistic effect of these metals is of serious concern not only to aquatic organisms but also to human health, particularly to vulnerable populations. To combat these challenges, it is necessary to develop extensive pollution control measures using innovative technologies and environmentally friendly practices. For example, using machine learning methods can enhance the optimization of resource utilization and help with monitoring and controlling pollution rates, which in turn will lead to an improved environment and better water quality (Rolnick et al., 2022).

KEY TERMS FROM THIS CHAPTER

- Advanced oxidation processes (AOP)
- Agricultural runoff
- Aquatic organisms
- Bioaccumulation
- Chemical processing industries
- Ecological integrity
- Environmental situations
- Geological occurrences
- Heavy metals
- Industrial pollution
- International cooperation
- Neonicotinoids
- Polluted water sources
- Sustainable drainage systems (SUDS)
- Water framework directive
- Agricultural ecosystems
- Aquatic ecosystems
- Best management practices (BMPs)
- Biomagnification
- Critical water resources
- Environmental pollutants
- Environmental stewardship
- Government agencies
- Industrial effluents
- Integrated pest management (IPM)
- Natural purification processes
- Pesticide
- Recalcitrant contaminants
- Wastewater infrastructure,
- Water organisms

CLOSER LOOK

INDUSTRIAL EFFLUENTS AND URBAN WATER SAFETY

Factory effluents or industrial wastewater not only threaten urban water safety by injecting pollutants such as heavy metals, toxic chemicals, and organic waste into water bodies but also lead to disruptions of aquatic ecosystems, harm to human health, and contamination of drinking water supplies. It is therefore imperative that proper treatment of industrial effluents reduces these effects to ensure urban water resource safety.

Impacts of Industrial Effluents:

- **Water Pollution:** Untreated or partially treated industrial effluents can contaminate Rivers, Streams, And Groundwater, Rendering Them Unsafe For Drinking, Irrigation, And Aquatic Life.
- **Ecosystem Disruption:** Toxic Chemicals In Industrial Runoff Can Accumulate In Aquatic Organisms, Disrupting Their Natural Balance And Affecting Their Growth, Reproduction, And Even Causing Death.
- **Human Health Risks:** Contaminated Water Sources Can Lead To Various Health Issues, Including Organ Damage, Developmental Disorders, And Cancer, Especially For Communities Reliant On Those Water Bodies For Their Daily Needs.
- **Eutrophication And Algal Blooms:** Industrial Wastewater Can Contain High Levels Of Nutrients, Like Nitrogen And Phosphorus, Which Can Cause Excessive Plant Growth, Leading To Algal Blooms And Oxygen depletion in aquatic ecosystems, further impacting water quality.

Challenges and Solutions:

- **Insufficient Treatment:** Many industries discharge untreated or partially treated effluents due to factors like cost, lack of infrastructure, and insufficient regulations.
- **Lack of Awareness:** There may be a lack of awareness among communities about the potential health and environmental risks of industrial effluents, hindering their engagement in advocating for better waste management.
- **Effective Treatment:** Implementing robust industrial wastewater treatment technologies, including physical, chemical, and biological methods, is crucial to remove harmful pollutants before they are released into water bodies.
- **Regulation and Enforcement:** Strengthening environmental regulations, enforcing compliance, and implementing social awareness programs can help ensure that industries adhere to responsible waste management practices.
- **Technological Advancements:** Exploring innovative treatment technologies, like membrane filtration using metal-organic frameworks (MOFs), can provide more efficient and sustainable solutions for removing pollutants from industrial effluents.

References

1. Alengebawy, A., Abdelkhalek, S. T., Qureshi, S. R., & Wang, M. Q. (2021). Heavy metals and pesticides toxicity in agricultural soil and plants: Ecological risks and human health implications. *Toxics, 9*(3), 42. https://doi.org/10.3390/toxics9030042.
2. Meena Palaniappan, Peter Gleick, Lucy Allen, Michael Cohen, Juliet Christian-Smith and Courtney Smith (2010). *Clearing the Waters: A Focus on Water Quality Solutions*. https://pacinst.org/publication/clearing-the-waters-focus-on-water-quality-solutions/ (accessed on 14 May 2025).
3. Arsanov, M., Tokaeva, M. A., & Bamatov, D. (2024). Mitigating climate impact through stabilized fertilizers: Enhancing agricultural sustainability. *E3S Web of Conferences*. https://www.semanticscholar.org/paper/4c348af6de03d9b430a0c8702c5c842d13b843ed (accessed on 14 May 2025).
4. Aziz, K. H. H., Mustafa, F. S., Omer, K. M., Hama, S., Hamarawf, R. F., & Rahman, K. O. (2023). Heavy metal pollution in the aquatic environment: Efficient and low-cost removal approaches to eliminate their toxicity: A review. *RSC Advances, 13*(30), 17595–17610. https://doi.org/10.1039/d3ra00723e.
5. Baba, F. A. M. (2024). Water pollution: Causes, impacts, and solutions: A critical review. *Journal of Sciences and Humanities – College of Arts and Sciences – Marj* DOI:10.37376/jsh.vi76.5785 (accessed on 14 May 2025).
6. Bahrulolum, H., Nooraei, S., Javanshir, N., Tarrahimofrad, H., Mirbagheri, V. S., Easton, A. J., & Ahmadian, G. (2021). Green synthesis of metal nanoparticles using microorganisms and their application in the agrifood sector. *Journal of Nanobiotechnology, 19*, Article 159. https://doi.org/10.1186/s12951-021-00834-3.
7. Duffy. A., Berwick, N., D'Arcy, B., Wade, R., Jose, R., (2013), A rapid review of the background to source control, CRWRR006 (CD 2012 27 R1). Available online at: crew.ac.uk/publications (accessed on 14 May 2025).
8. Calvin, K., Dasgupta, D., Krinner, G., Mukherji, A., Thorne, P., Trisos, C. H., Romero, J., et al. (2023). *Climate Change 2023: Synthesis Report. Contribution of Working Groups I, II and III to the Sixth Assessment Report of the Intergovernmental Panel on Climate Change* [Core Writing Team, H. Lee & J. Romero (Eds.)]. IPCC. https://doi.org/10.59327/ipcc/ar6-9789291691647.
9. Chen, L., Msigwa, G., Yang, M., Osman, A. I., Fawzy, S., Rooney, D. W., & Yap, P. S. (2022). Strategies to achieve a carbon neutral society: A review. *Environmental Chemistry Letters, 20*, 2277–2310. https://doi.org/10.1007/s10311-022-01435-8.
10. Dutta A, Karmakar S, Das S, Banerjee M, Ray R, Hasher FFB, Mishra VN, Zhran M. Modeling the River Health and Environmental Scenario of the Decaying Saraswati River, West Bengal, India, Using Advanced Remote Sensing and GIS. *Water*. 2025; 17(7):965. https://doi.org/10.3390/w17070965 (accessed on 14 May 2025).
11. El-Sharkawy M, Alotaibi MO, Li J, Du D, Mahmoud E. Heavy Metal Pollution in Coastal Environments: Ecological Implications and Management Strategies: A Review. *Sustainability*. 2025; 17(2):701. https://doi.org/10.3390/su17020701(accessed on 14 May 2025).
12. Ewim, D. R. E., Orikpete, O. F., Scott, T. O., Onyebuchi, C. N., Onukogu, A. O., Uzougbo, C. G., & Onunka, C. (2023a). Survey of wastewater issues due to oil spills and pollution in the Niger

Delta area of Nigeria: A secondary data analysis. *Bulletin of the National Research Centre, 47*, Article 90. https://doi.org/10.1186/s42269-023-01090-1.

13. Ewim, D. R. E., Orikpete, O. F., Scott, T. O., Onyebuchi, C. N., Onukogu, A. O., & Onunka, C. (2023b). Survey of wastewater issues due to oil spills and pollution in the Niger Delta area of Nigeria: A secondary data analysis. *Research Square*. https://doi.org/10.21203/rs.3.rs-2895102/v1.
14. Gamage, A., Gangahagedara, R., Gamage, J., Jayasinghe, N., Kodikara, N., Suraweera, P., & Merah, O. (2023). Role of organic farming for achieving sustainability in agriculture. *Farming System, 1*, 100005. https://doi.org/10.1016/j.farsys.2023.100005.
15. Hou, D. (2023). Soil health and ecosystem services. *Soil Use and Management, 39*(4), 1259–1266. https://doi.org/10.1111/sum.12945.
16. Issaka, S., & Ashraf, M. A. (2017). Impact of soil erosion and degradation on water quality: A review. *Geology, Ecology, and Landscapes, 1*(1), 1–11. https://doi.org/10.1080/24749508.2017.1301053.
17. Karić, N., Maia, A. S., Teodorović, A., Atanasova, N., Langergraber, G., Crini, G., Ribeiro, A. R., et al. (2021). Bio-waste valorisation: Agricultural wastes as biosorbents for removal of (in)organic pollutants in wastewater treatment. *Chemical Engineering Journal Advances, 9*, 100239. https://doi.org/10.1016/j.ceja.2021.100239.
18. Khan, F., Tehseen, M., Ali, S., Ali, B., Fatima, K., Khaliq, H., Chohan, A. A., et al. (2025). Environmental toxicology of heavy metals: Chemical strategies for mitigation. *Kashf Journal of Multidisciplinary Research, 2*(02), 1-17. https://doi.org/10.71146/kjmr253 (accessed on 14 May 2025).
19. Sanjay Koushal, Devesh Arya, S. Anbarasan, Dipankar Haloi, Rashmi M, et al.. Soil Pollution: Sources, Effects, and Mitigation Strategies. Asian Journal of Soil Science and Plant Nutrition, 2025, 11 (1), pp.280-290. ⟨10.9734/ajsspn/2025/v11i1480⟩. ⟨hal-05050968⟩(accessed on 14 May 2025).
20. Nsenga Kumwimba M, Zhu B, Stefanakis AI, Ajibade FO, Dzakpasu M, Soana E, Wang T, Arif M, Kavidia Muyembe D and Agboola TD (2023) Advances in ecotechnological methods for diffuse nutrient pollution control: wicked issues in agricultural and urban watersheds. Front. Environ. Sci. 11:1199923. doi: 10.3389/fenvs.2023.1199923 (accessed on 14 May 2025).
21. Landrigan, P. J., Stegeman, J. J., Fleming, L. E., Allemand, D., Anderson, D. M., Backer, L. C., Brücker-Davis, F., et al. (2020). Human health and ocean pollution. *Annals of Global Health, 86*(1), 151. https://www.semanticscholar.org/paper/80d17026d31d2c4ba0e126620605ae631704aa98(accessed on 14 May 2025).
22. Javier Mateo-Sagasta (IWMI), Sara Marjani Zadeh (FAO) and Hugh Turral More people, more food, worse water? A global review of water pollution from agriculture. Published by the Food and Agriculture Organization of the United Nations Rome, 2018 and the International Water Management Institute on behalf of the Water Land and Ecosystems research program of the CGIAR Colombo, 2018. https://core.ac.uk/download/159238492.pdf (accessed on 14 May 2025).
23. Marshall, L., & Sugg, Z. (2008). Finding balance: Agricultural residues, ethanol, and the environment. https://core.ac.uk/download/71351310.pdf (accessed on 14 May 2025).

24. Milijašević Joksimović, D., Jakovljević, D., & Jojić Glavonjić, T. (2025). Evaluation of water quality in the Tamiš River in Serbia using the Water Pollution Index: Key pollutants and their sources. *Water.* https://www.semanticscholar.org/paper/99e31e363e9a9eecf15931e4e98f29f49919aed0 (accessed on 14 May 2025).

25. de Lima, A.C.R., Hoogmoed, W. and Brussaard, L. (2008), Soil Quality Assessment in Rice Production Systems: Establishing a Minimum Data Set. J. Environ. Qual., 37: 623-630. https://doi.org/10.2134/jeq2006.0280 (accessed on 14 May 2025).

26. Rolnick, D., Donti, P. L., Kaack, L. H., Kochanski, K., Lacoste, A., Sankaran, K., Ross, A. S., et al. (2022). Tackling climate change with machine learning. *ACM Computing Surveys, 55*(1), 1–96. https://doi.org/10.1145/3485128.

27. Sahoo, S. K., & Goswami, S. S. (2023). Theoretical framework for assessing the economic and environmental impact of water pollution: A detailed study on sustainable development of India. *Journal of Future Sustainability, 4*, 23–34. https://doi.org/10.5267/j.jfs.2024.1.003.

28. Sharma, R., Singh, S., & Reddy, P. B. (2025). Effects of water quality and seasonality on zooplankton responses. *World Journal of Biology Pharmacy and Health Sciences.* https://www.semanticscholar.org/paper/23f94f71e759a66349d6050e8a39cf72ecb95886 (accessed on 14 May 2025).

29. Shemer, H., Wald, S., & Semiat, R. (2023). Challenges and solutions for global water scarcity. *Membranes, 13*(6), 612. https://doi.org/10.3390/membranes13060612.

30. Smith, I. (2023). Water pollution and cancer: An updated review. https://core.ac.uk/download/591386665.pdf (accessed on 14 May 2025).

31. Syafrudin, M., Kristanti, R. A., Yuniarto, A., Hadibarata, T., Rhee, J., Al-onazi, W. A., AlGarni, T. S., et al. (2021). Pesticides in drinking water—A review. *International Journal of Environmental Research and Public Health, 18*(2), 468. https://doi.org/10.3390/ijerph18020468.

32. Vosa , O., Salibi, G., & Tzenios, N. (2025). Water pollution and its impact on human health in Nigeria. *Special Journal of the Medical Academy and Other Life Sciences., 3*(2). https://doi.org/10.58676/sjmas.v3i2.110 (accessed on 14 May 2025).

33. Yadav, S. C. (2024). Water Pollution: The Problems and Solutions. Science Insights, 44(2), 1245–1251. https://doi.org/10.15354/si.24.re905 (accessed on 14 May 2025).

34. Zandalinas, S. I., Fritschi, F., & Mittler, R. (2021). Global warming, climate change, and environmental pollution: Recipe for a multifactorial stress combination disaster. *Trends in Plant Science, 26*(6), 588–599. https://doi.org/10.1016/j.tplants.2021.02.011.

35. Zarate-Cáceres, C.R.; Iparraguirre-Meza, M.; Pérez-Venegas, C.J.; Picoy-Gonzales, J.A.; Ordoñez-Ccora, G.; Lacho-Gutiérrez, P.; Riveros-Laurente, K.Y.; Diaz-Aranda, D.L.; Gutiérrez-Iparraguirre, G.G.; Huarcaya-Taype, R.; et al. Integrated water quality assessment and health risk analysis of heavy metal and microbial contamination in the Ichu River, Peru. *F1000Research* **2025**, *14*, 384, https://doi.org/10.12688/f1000research.162022.1. (accessed on 14 May 2025).

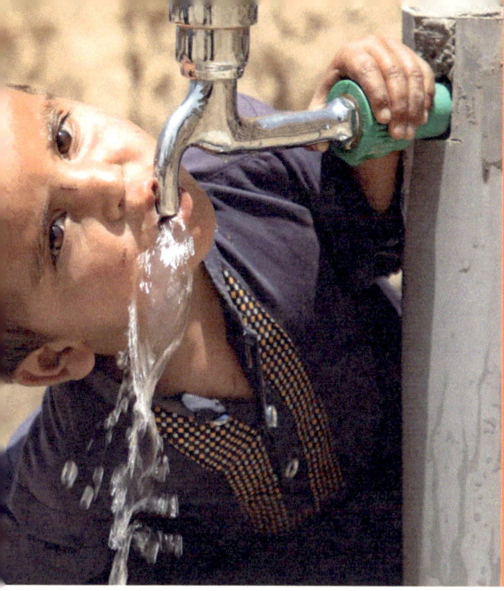

Chapter 12

GLOBAL WATER AND SANITATION POLICIES

Contents

Introduction

International water and sanitation problems are over-layered in complexities that impact health and development in unforeseeable ways. Water is an essential need—something most of us take for granted—yet its governance leaks over into an extended social and economic cocktail that's not always tidy. Clean water and correct sanitation reduce waterborne disease, and while it sounds easy, getting everyone access isn't a stroll in the park. Organizations such as USAID, for instance, have thrown together strategic frameworks (their 2013–2018) Water and Development Strategy is one good example (WSP, 2011; WHO, 2015) that attempt to align different projects with overarching water objectives. Essentially, these guidelines suggest that maintaining an open, if somewhat chaotic, conversation among all the various actors is the key to addressing the challenges head on. In most of the world, however, gaps in research obstinately stand in the way of good policy. A consultancy investigating Malawi revealed gaps in environmental health research on a serious scale—a indicator that a certain, action-oriented strategy is required. For the most part, when data and knowledge lack, thorough water and sanitation policy falters. Research focus can ensure an intelligent way to make decisions and nudge organizations toward a feeling of responsibility (Morse et al., 2010).

A measured, occasionally uneven examination of existing frameworks can uncover underlying problems, bringing possibly necessary reforms. And when policymakers go out of their way to listen to local communities and specialists, even if the process becomes a little complex, they are more likely to develop solutions that fit the actual-world, diverse needs of various areas. No water and sanitation progress is achieved without a healthy measure of collaboration. Government agencies, NGOs, and even the academic community can, most times, spur innovation and exchange ideas when they work together in a less formal, sometimes dialogue-and-counter-dialogue fashion. Such collaborative efforts tend to impact measurably in places burdened with both water shortage and inadequate sanitation facilities. Including strategies for climate resilience can further increase the impact, working to protect vulnerable individuals from the harsh blows of climate change. Because a lot of communities continue to wrestle with reliable water supplies, maintaining water resources in good order is nothing less than critical. In the end, when citizens' voices make it into the policy mix, the mess of social, environmental, and economic considerations gets a more well-rounded view—a complex but real assessment of what it takes to get things rolling internationally.

Definition of Water and Sanitation Policies

In the world today, when everything is uncertain, water and sanitation issues keep changing, and we literally need policies that get right to the point—guaranteeing everyone access to safe drinking water and good sanitation. You may discover that these agendas are not merely a neat list of guidelines and protocols; rather, they blend into each other diverse strategies that deliver more than just access. Sometimes they attempt to integrate health themes as well, because the connection between polluted water and mass disease is difficult to deny, and, more often than not, inadequate sanitation can hinder economic development. Local insights matter a great deal—policymakers, through involving communities and tailoring concepts to suit particular cultural and socio-economic contexts, can address the underlying causes of water insecurity while keeping equity and the environment in mind, although the strategy at times seems a little all over the place. Water and sanitation planning also relies on international standards and familiar best practices, aligning with large goals such as those defined by the Sustainable Development Goals (SDGs), particularly Goal 6, which mandates managing water and sanitation sustainably for all by 2030. If you read through several reports, you will see that gaps in access tend to coincide with economic issues and deteriorated infrastructure. Recent surveys from low- and middle-income countries, for example, show that even the most simple water facilities are not accessible to many locations, with some 38% of healthcare centers having improper sanitation facilities. These figures, if you consider them, cry out for an immediate, concerted effort by international agencies, governments, and many other players, all unveiling evidence-based policies to tackle these causes (Lief et al., 2009; WSP, 2011; WHO, 2015). It's easy to lose sight of the fact that water and sanitation policy isn't just administrative mumbo-jumbo, it sounds out what society cares about regarding health and rights. A good policy is not only about pledging access; it must also ensure quality, safety, and long-term viability in terms of water management. The price of neglect can be dire, with poor access upsetting public health, particularly as urbanization and climate change create additional stress. That's why these policies must have a little bit of a flexible, adaptable edge, prepared to act whether in crowded city centers or outlying areas. Frequently, a little additional local coordination creates creative solutions and makes everything more manageable. Eventually, water and sanitation done correctly is the key to increasing public health, encouraging social equity, and preserving the environment, a true cornerstone of wider global development initiatives.

Importance of Water and Sanitation for Public Health

Clean water and sanitation are at the very center of public health—in a great number of ways, they keep people and populations alive. When these essential services fail, all manner of issues arise: waterborne diseases such as cholera and dysentery tend to affect the most vulnerable most severely. In some cases, poor sanitation even stops the body's ability to take in the nutrients it needs, which can worsen malnutrition and other health issues. You'll notice that in several countries, mixing water and sanitation projects with healthcare and nutrition support has shown some real promise; case studies from around the world generally back up this less systematic, more integrated approach. Not only do they address short-term health issues, but they drive forward wider development goals, illustrating that when world water and sanitation policies align strongly, communities win big time (WSP, 2011; WHO, 2015). And that's not all—water and sanitation have a significant part to play in gender equality too, something often forgotten. Women and girls traditionally carry the added burden when these services are not available; for instance, they may spend so much time collecting water that it takes away from school or job time, which in turn perpetuates cycles of poverty and injustices. It appears that empowering women through involvement in water decision-making brings new insights and more sustainable approaches. With rare exceptions, providing women an opportunity to contribute an opinion helps to achieve healthier outcomes while contributing to a more just society as a whole (WSP, 2011; WHO, 2015). Apart from the direct health issues, the ripple effects of poor water and sanitation can strike a community's economy severely. Poor sanitation typically translates to increased healthcare costs and lost productivity as individuals are absent from work due to disease. Conversely, investing in good water and sanitation infrastructure normally pays off; healthier citizens can work longer and harder to contribute to economic growth, and obscuring disease prevention saves costs and even enhances quality of life. This sort of virtuous cycle, even if it sounds a tad circuitous—makes communities more resilient against threats such as climate change and natural disasters. All these factors combined illustrate how important it is to integrate water and sanitation into wider public health policies so that international policies take these interrelated issues into account as a whole (WSP, 2011; WHO, 2015).

Overview of Global Challenges in Water and Sanitation

Water and sanitation problems aren't so straightforward as they may appear. There's a crazy combination of problems—climate change, exploding populations, growing cities—all fighting around and straining the old infrastructure. The more people move into the cities, the more demand there is for clean water and good sanitation, and sometimes, the infrastructure just can't keep up. Where water is already in short supply, external pressures just worsen. Generally speaking, it's important to look at all these factors together if we're going to shape policies that work in the long run. Some recent studies even suggest that solutions really need to be tailored region by region, because what works in one spot might not do the trick somewhere else (WWAP Report, 2012). Overall, new, innovative thinking is required to deal with today's challenges and prepare for impending threats to access to and the quality of water. While seeking improved sanitation, discussions across the globe have suggested speed bumps that impede progress. The first Unclogging the Blockages conference, for example, generated robust demands for collaboration to overcome these obstacles. Some of the learnings from that conference highlighted that relying on market-based solutions is, for the most part, central to overcoming the major barriers in scaling up sustainable sanitation. Sometimes there were discussions about combining sanitation with wider sectors such as housing or health in order to develop solutions that really suit urban contexts. One creative proposal was to initiate a Global Sanitation Financing Alliance, designed to mobilize resources and trigger innovations to make sanitation infrastructure more resilient. These strategies highlight the connection of sanitation to economic development and push policymakers to reconsider finance policies that support sustainable practices (Narracott et al., 2014). Providing water and sanitation to all is more than just repairing pipes, it's also about equity. Women and the poor often find themselves shouldering the effects of lack of sanitation, which can damage their well-being, security, and even school opportunities. Filling these gaps is typically viewed as an absolute requirement if we are to achieve the global sustainability goals outlined by the United Nations SDGs. Even some regional research indicates that when water and sanitation policy addresses gender, services improve and people get more engaged. Suggestions are circulating to increase women's participation in making water and sanitation choices, which has the potential to enhance family life and create more resilient, better communities. As policies continue to change, maintaining inclusivity as the central focus could be just what gets us through these hurdles and ensures that everyone can count on vital services (WWAP Report, 2012).

12.1. Historical Context

International water and sanitation networks have developed in ways that aren't necessarily clear at first view. In the 19th century, sanitation suddenly came into the foreground—cholera epidemics brought a new consciousness regarding disease transmission. Cities began to assemble sewer systems and providing clean water supplies, which merged public health interests with daily life. Urban expansion at high speed meant waste management and offering potable water weren't optional any longer; governments noticed and intervened, sometimes in unexpected ways, to bridge the gap. Global health and human rights debates eventually started treating water and sanitation as fundamental rights, initiating the policies we rely on today. As we continue to update sanitation methods, the tale remains complex with socio-political strings. In most developing nations, legacies of colonization and economic inequalities have left strong imprints on water distribution and infrastructure. Studies such as the Global Economic and Sector Work (ESW) Political Economy of Sanitation study in Brazil, India, Indonesia, and Senegal by the Water and Sanitation Program (WSP) and World Bank (WSP, 2011; WHO, 2015) typically indicates how local interests and self-interests tend to influence sanitation investment decisions—assuming the costs by marginalized groups. From a certain point of view, comprehending these cyclical patterns is quite central to designing policies that fill in systemic water and sanitation gaps. And then there's the bonus complication of climate change, which throws the entire narrative into even darker waters. In sub-Saharan Africa, for instance, smallholder farmers continue to use local know-how and resources, so the integration of this knowledge with scientific disciplines nearly becomes imperative (Nicolay & Fliessbach, 2012). This combination not only increases agricultural yields but also serves to streamline water management and sanitation habits, although the answers aren't always tidy. As countries struggle with unpredictable weather conditions and changing climates, historical lessons on community cooperation remain relevant. In the majority of situations, possessing a wide perspective that includes history, politics, and environmental shifts is crucial for the development of resilient water and sanitation policies that are equitable as well (Figure 12.1).

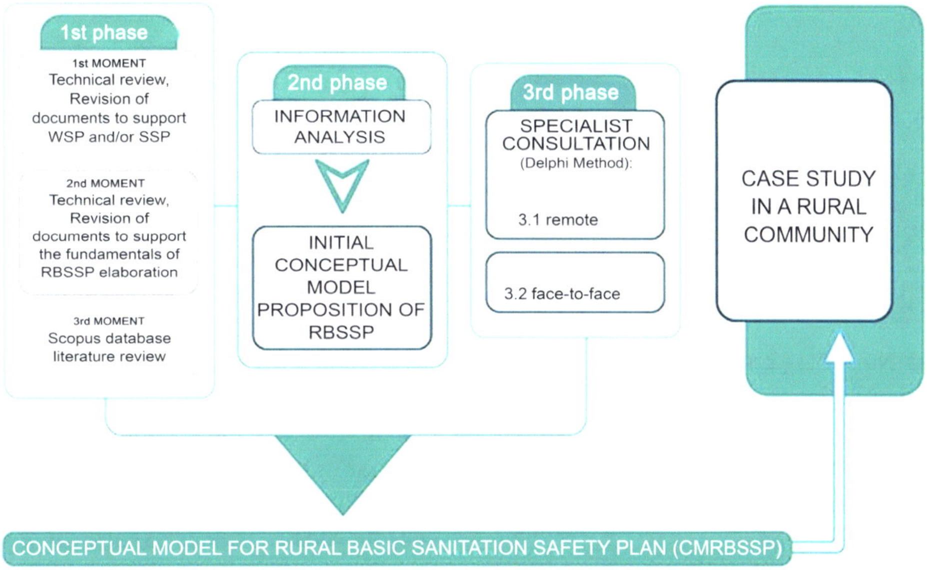

Figure 12.1. Conceptual framework of the national rural water supply and sanitation program.

Source: Baracho RO, Bezerra NR, Scalize PS. Proposition and Application of a Conceptual Model for Risk Management in Rural Areas: Rural Basic Sanitation Safety Plan (RBSSP). *Resources*. 2024; 13(7):90. https://doi.org/10.3390/resources13070090

12.1.1. Evolution of Water and Sanitation Policies Over the Decades

Water and sanitation policies have evolved significantly over the decades under the influence of a combination of social and economic pressures. In the mid-1900s, the government would typically intervene with large public works to enhance water infrastructure. However, with cities expanding and populations swelling, the initial plans began to fail, particularly in regions with limited development. Individuals started realizing that merely increasing pipes was not sufficient; solutions increasingly involved everybody having a stake in them. In most instances, diverse local water problems compelled various groups to collaborate in manners that ultimately paved the way for more holistic management strategies. As the latter half of the 20th century arrived, environmental concerns suddenly began to have a greater influence on water policies. In general, the emergence of sustainable development caused governments and organizations to take a step back and reconsider their previous strategies, attempting to incorporate ecological issues into current plans. International treaties, for example, the Dublin Principles in 1992—were intended to remind us that water is not merely about supply, but about equitable distribution and long-term stewardship. Some accounts even point out how external factors can interfere with water supplies, emphasizing the need to manage water with uncertainty and risk in mind (WWAP Report, 2012).

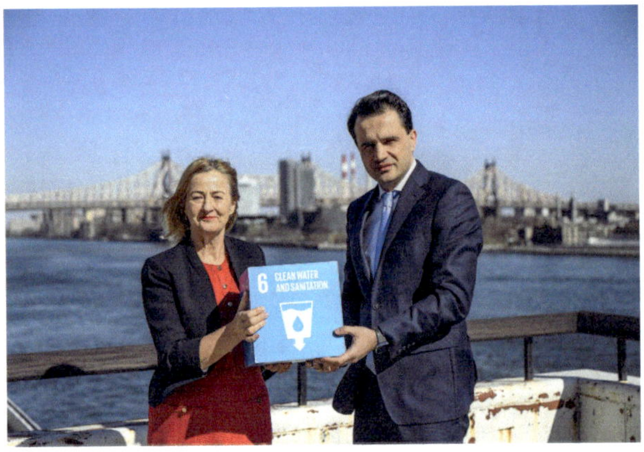

Source: United Nations. (2023). *Co-hosts*. United Nations Sustainable Development. https://www.un.org/sustainabledevelopment/wp-content/uploads/2023/02/co-hosts-scaled.jpg.

It was apparent that successful policies must not only address how water is distributed but also its overall environmental impact and fairness to the community. With the transition to the 21st century, all these developing concepts have been tried to bring together into more harmonized paradigms, particularly with worldwide programs such as the SDGs (SDGs) on the agenda. New policies today set out to rectify the frailties of older systems, such as relying on archaic public standpipes or on-site providers who simply weren't able to supply enough (Dagdeviren et al., 2009). This newer philosophy views water supply, health, and hygiene as facets of a complex problem, requiring solutions that bring in specialists from all types of disciplines. Also, the recent explosion in water management technology has produced data-driven decision-making, which assists in developing strategies that function today and can adapt to tomorrow's changes in climate and population. In the majority of instances, these developments enable policymakers to introduce policies that right human needs even if the process becomes somewhat complex occasionally.

12.1.2. Key International Agreements and Their Impact

International water and sanitation policy has evolved across history through international agreements that, candidly, continuously change. In 1992 – when a large United Nations Conference on Environment and Development was held – nations began coordinating in a manner that subsequently flourished into the Millennium Development Goals, establishing a loose framework for a common objective of clean water and good sanitation. These pacts, which emphasize that countries are held together by transnational water concerns, continue to remind us that justice for marginalized communities counts a great deal. With climate change, you see, increasing the pressure on water supplies, these pledges have come to the fore, catalyzing collaborative initiatives that create resilience against water scarcity and pollution. More often than not, the humble beginnings of simple guidelines now serve as essential triggers for the emergence of new policies. The SDGs sort of top them all in this area, particularly Goal 6, which is largely all about having water accessible and sustainably maintained for all. By integrating water and sanitation requirements into overall development schemes, it's obvious that clean water access has a direct impact on health, education, and economic progress. This concept pushes governments to spend resources prudently and implement far-reaching reforms, thus making them, in essence, more accountable to the people they govern. And, with systems designed to monitor progress, the SDGs automatically promote the exchange of best practices and creative ideas as well as international partnerships that enlarge their global impact. And then there are slums, which have their own range of challenges in water and sanitation—challenges exacerbated by disjointed infrastructure and often fragile legal support. About a billion people, largely residents of low- and middle-income zones, live without basics such as piped water or decent sanitation facilities. In recent times, global pacts, even those specifically targeting climate resilience—have begun giving greater emphasis to these at-risk populations. Some policy guidelines, for example, now combine short-term water solutions with longer-term climate adaptation measures with the ongoing effect of climate change on these populations in mind. Local governments and institutions are increasingly being pressured, sometimes in surprising ways, to collaborate on the upgrading of basic services, thus setting the stage for a more integrated strategy to enhance the living conditions of the urban poor (Satterthwaite et al., 2020Intergovernmental Panel on Climate Change, 2023).

12.1.3. Case Studies of Successful Historical Policies

International water and sanitation initiatives sometimes appear in subtle forms. In the Netherlands, for instance, when serious flooding threatened everyday life, authorities drew upon concepts from everywhere. They didn't merely tackle the immediate water problems, they also initiated a system that promoted improved long-term water behavior. Various communities found themselves conversing and collaborating shoulder to shoulder, which not only addressed the flood threats but also increased local resilience and concern for nature.

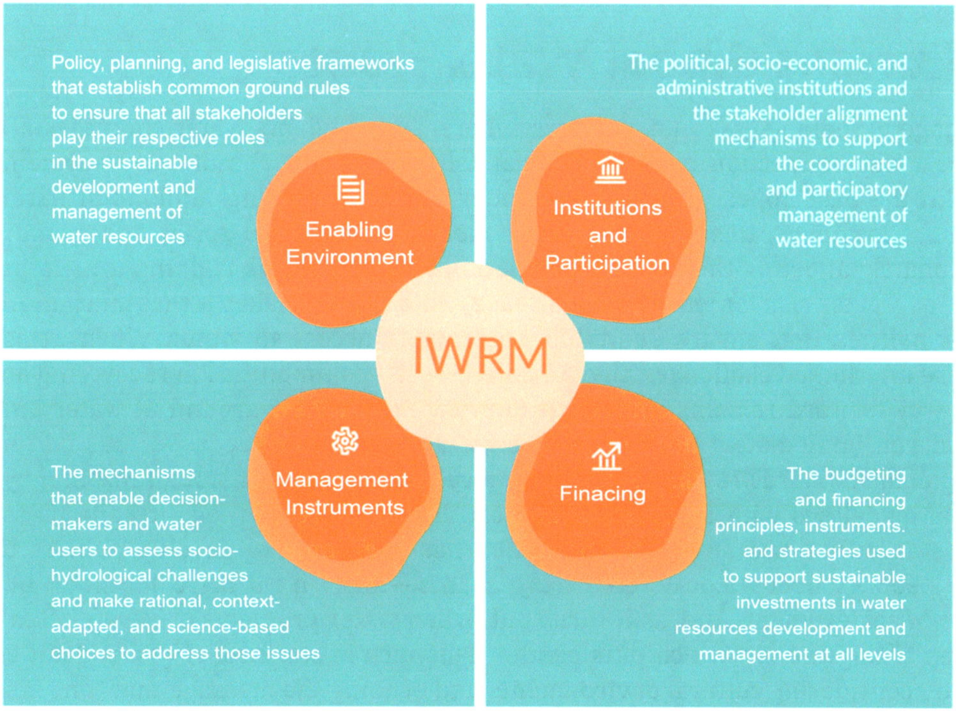

Figure 12.2. IWRM action framework.

Source: IWRM Action Hub. (2022). *GWO Toolbox.*

https://iwrmactionhub.org/system/files/2022-08/GWO%20toolbox%20figure2.png.

The Dutch strategy, referred to more generally as Integrated Water Resources Management, is a reminder that when policies integrate nature, people, and the economy, they are more likely to function coherently instead of colliding (Figure 12.2). Consider Singapore, where sparse natural resources required some creative innovation. The city-state did not fall back on a single strategy; rather, it diversified with strategies such as purifying saltwater into fresh water, harvesting rain, and reusing water. This sort-of high-technology, grassroots movement alleviated water shortages without undermining urban life sustainability. They generated buzz through public campaigns and even spent money on research and development. Overall, their experience teaches us that the combination of smart technology and collective effort can work to address water issues in the world today. Moving into sanitation, Brazil's Bolsa Família program offers us a glimpse of closing the rural-urban gap for health access. Here, distributing cash was linked to fulfilling minimum hygiene standards, a smart incentive for poor households to improve their everyday living. This arrangement enhanced household cleanliness and, by extension, overall public health, proving the coherence between money and healthier habits. How Bolsa Família was designed and implemented illustrates that locally driven, targeted policies can effect meaningful gains in access to water and sanitation. If we step back and look at these examples, they encourage us that innovative solutions can create systems that are both equitable and resilient, especially given the imperative for this in our fast-changing climate environment (Calvin et al., 2023; Intergovernmental Panel on Climate Change, 2023).

12.2. Current Global Water Issues

Climate change is shaking governments everywhere, and suddenly water shortages are a crisis to fear. It's not a tidy connection between eco-vandalism and taps running dry—systems that have functioned in the past appear to fall apart under duress, depriving millions of barely sufficient water. In most instances, this water shortage merely exacerbates social and economic divides, disproportionately affecting the poorest populations. Freshwater is running low, so people at the margins are at greater risk for waterborne disease, which really makes it that much more important to establish policies that ensure equitable, sustainable access to water. When decision-makers address these interlinked challenges, they're able to assist communities in recovering and adapting, even if the way forward remains somewhat uneven. Take a view around at water and sanitation policies, and you immediately notice one-size-fits-all just won't cut it. Various cultural contexts mean that global standards regularly require a local adaptation. Consider Tanzania: by combining international guidelines with measures that work in the context of local traditions (some would even say it's a decolonized strategy), the nation has been able to develop policies that directly address its people's needs. Local voice truly counts—this isn't a mere footnote, but an actual cornerstone of achievement. And, as it turns out, when water problems arise, it's often the women who wind up taking the hit, which puts gender dynamics in stark relief (Thibodeau et al., 2023). Ultimately, by considering cultural environments and echoing the message that "one size doesn't fit all," development agencies can construct targeted, effective solutions. Life during a period of mass industrialization and urban spread gives a whole other dimension to the management of water resources. Higher demand and additional pollution have made countries such as Brazil and Portugal balancing growth aspirations with ensuring water use remains sustainable (Figure 12.3). The entire picture changes radically based on each nation's economic landscape, with the legal regulations influencing how farms, cities, and businesses draw on water sources. A brief SWOT-kind of view at these examples reveals a combination of strengths, weaknesses, opportunities, and threats that is far from straightforward. Digital tools are beginning to assist in streamlining things—but there is no silver bullet. Whenever different case studies and studies are combined, a better picture is formed that can guide the development of sustainable practices balancing ecological health along with societal requirements (Carvalho et al., 2023).

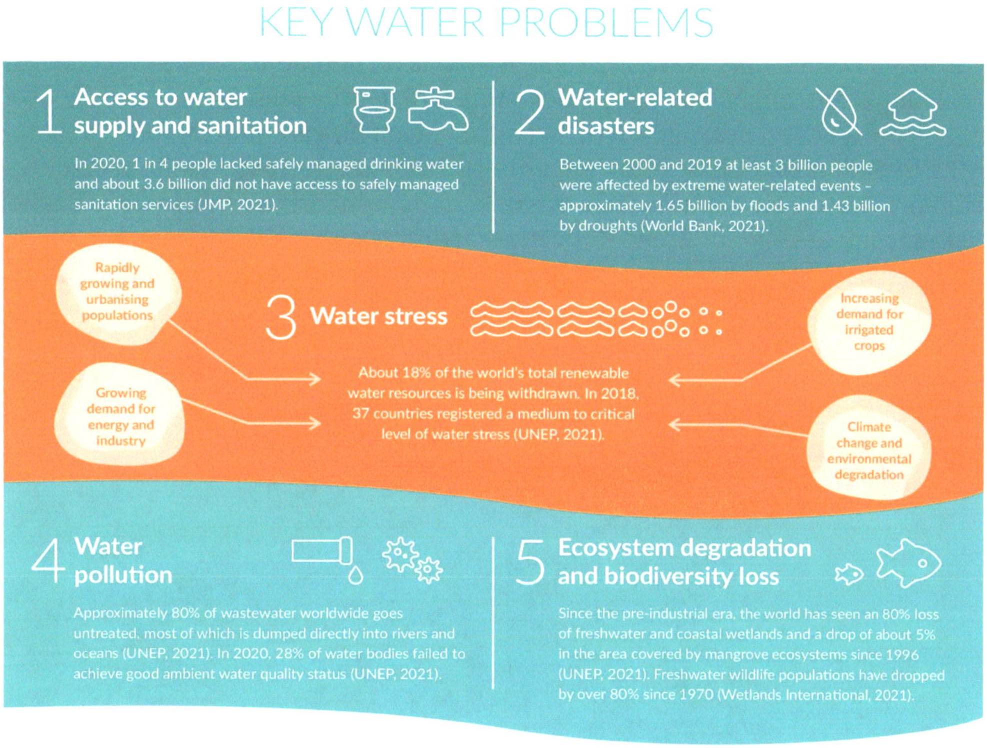

Figure 12.3. Key water challenges.

Source: IWRM Action Hub. (n.d.). *IWRM Explained.*

https://iwrmactionhub.org/about/iwrm-explained.

12.2.1. Water Scarcity and Its Implications

Water scarcity truly hits home in so many unexpected places. In areas where agriculture is more than a means to a meal on the plate, it's the foundation of the regional economy—such scarcity has its impact (Figure 12.4). Consider India, for instance; poor water management in rural communities makes food security a constant concern, particularly when monsoon trends control it all. Tensions usually boil over when various groups and areas fight for the same scarce resource. Some think a new examination of policies, perhaps even the introduction of some contemporary technology like artificial intelligence, could make the water flow more smoothly and preserve what little we have (Singh et al., 2025). Pollution heaping on top of diminishing supplies of water makes an already sticky predicament even more complicated. Clean water grows scarcer by the day, primarily in the developing world where approximately 80% of wastewater is dumped untreated into rivers and lakes—not exactly the best recipe for a drink or a clean swim. In most African countries, for example, nearly 319 million people continue to have difficulty finding water that won't poison them. This is not solely an issue of health; it interferes with ecosystems and agriculture as well, initiating a vicious cycle of deficit and deterioration. In most cases, addressing such issues requires a pragmatic policy that reduces pollution while involving local populations in participation, which would consequently enhance overall well-being and bring us nearer to the UN's SDGs (Ariho et al., 2024). In addressing water scarcity, it is not sufficient to repair only a segment of the problem. The problems of water waste and contamination, as it happens, are inextricably linked, requiring a blended strategy. Rather than adhering to strict plans, subtle adjustments such as conservation tillage or rotating crops might manage water more efficiently, allowing nature to do its work a little better. Local expertise, seasoned with scientific acumen, can inform policies suitable for the spaces they're intended to assist—most situations, they require that human element. Partnering with government, NGOs, and community organizations appears nearly indispensable to create a genuine all-encompassing solution. Collective action and on-the-ground awareness-building campaigns, in a sense, may just lead us toward a more stable, equitable water future (Ariho et al., 2024; Singh & Goyal, 2025).

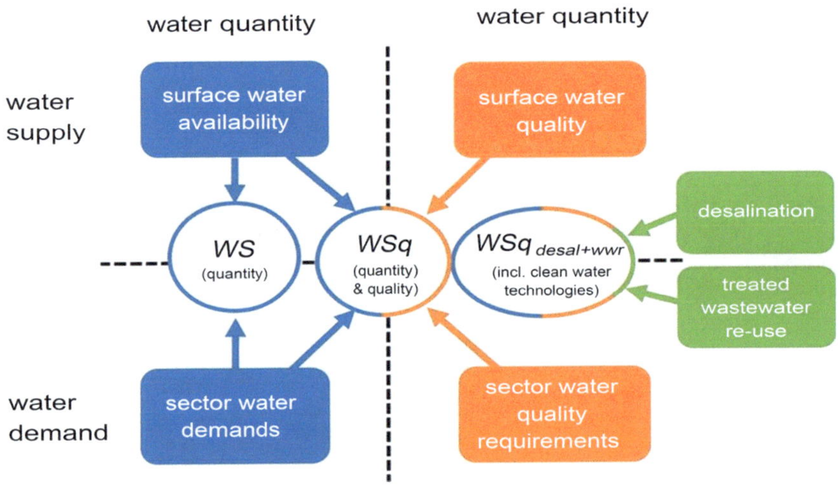

Figure 12.4. Water scarcity framework and three water scarcity indicators: 1. Water scarcity based on only quantity (WS), 2. Water scarcity including both water quantity and water quality (WSq); and 3. Water scarcity based on both water quantity and quality, and including desalination and treated wastewater reuse.

Source: Michelle T H van Vliet et al 2021 Environ. Res. Lett. 16 024020 DOI 10.1088/1748-9326/abbfc3

12.2.2. Pollution and Its Effects on Water Quality

Water quality is suffering due to pollution, and this clean-up is interconnected with worldwide sanitation problems in ways that are not immediately apparent. Factories that emit waste, farm runoff, and city garbage all leach into rivers and lakes, disrupting both sensitive ecosystems and human health (Figure 12.5). Several studies emphasize that the pollutants not only render drinking water unsafe but also pose threats to aquatic life by disturbing food webs and eroding biodiversity.

It's a true balancing act for communities, particularly in developing areas where poor infrastructure complicates matters even further. All these problems compel policymakers to seek more holistic solutions addressing pollution control and enhancing water quality, especially where the most vulnerable citizens reside. In most instances, if left untreated with timely and effective intervention, our capacity to protect both citizens and nature will be gravely threatened (Intergovernmental Panel on Climate Change, 2023). Informal settlements everywhere indicate the severity of the impacts of water pollution. Placed here and there in unsafe locations, these settlements lack proper sanitation facilities, further increasing their vulnerability to water-borne diseases. An estimated 1 billion individuals residing in informal settlements use tainted water for basic needs, exponentially increasing their health risks. Recent research informs us that insufficient piped water and adequate waste management make these individuals particularly vulnerable to climate-induced emergencies, entrapping them in poverty and constant ailments. International water and sanitation policies need to catch up with reality, demanding infrastructure investments that reduce pollution and improve water safety. Through community-driven action and more robust local control, there is a chance to mitigate these severe effects and enhance resilience within vulnerable groups (Satterthwaite et al., 2020). Unraveling the intricate connection between pollution and water quality requires a multi-layered strategy that artfully combines existing scientific understanding and visionary policy. The IPCC emphasized that comprehensive, integrated solutions whereby water management becomes married to strategies for adapting to climate change are necessary. Controlling entire watersheds or targeting contamination at its origins may alleviate harm to aquatic organisms while also fortifying community strength. Green infrastructure and sustainable practice investments can do more than replenish water quality; they can also unlock cleaner water sources for those who most need them. In the majority of instances, worldwide policies must tilt toward strategies that combine economic growth with care for the environment, even when the implementation at times becomes somewhat patchy. Collating these concepts can take countries to a more equitable future where clean water is the norm for all (Intergovernmental Panel on Climate Change, 2023).

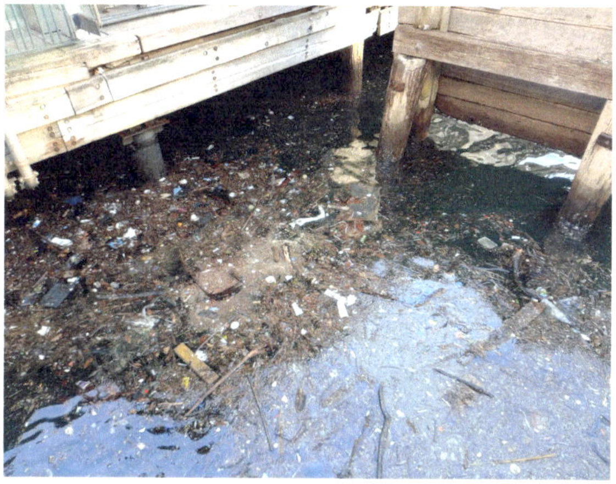

Figure 12.5. Pollution sources that affect water quality.

Source: By MrActiniuM - Own work, CC BY-SA 4.0, https://commons.wikimedia.org/w/index.php?curid=167108453

12.2.3. Climate Change and Its Impact on Water Resources

Climate change is interfering with our water sources in ways that are not so easy to overlook. Increasing temperatures are disrupting rain patterns and accelerating evaporation so that areas formerly graced with seasonal rains now sometimes experience a severe drought, while other parts of the world receive pounded-by-the-storm flooding. This kind of volatile change disrupts agriculture and has communities scrambling to find clean drinking water, further exacerbating the disparity in access to water. Too often, it's the most vulnerable populations, usually women in low- and middle-income areas—who bear most of the cost, resulting in a chain of health consequences and increasing water insecurity (Anjum et al., 2025). Water isn't all about how much there is; its quality is suffering as well. Floodwaters have the potential to blend in unwanted contaminants with local water sources, which creates public health concerns, and in addition to that, warmer temperatures can contribute to problematic algae blooms and disease-causing microbes spreading. All things considered, these water quality issues, in combination with the climate debacle, are real barriers to achieving global water and sanitation goals, such as those in the SDGs (Obringer et al., 2024). What happens is that addressing these problems means policymakers must look beyond, integrating measures that respond to the unpredictable impacts of climate on available water and its safety. Meeting these threats head-on requires us to implement wiser adaptation and mitigation strategies. Much of that is improved, more localized climate impact assessments so local communities can truly grasp the specific ways their water systems are threatened. Leaning on sophisticated tools, such as AI-based models—we can get a clearer picture of just how climate change may be disrupting supply and quality (Obringer et al., 2024). Also, putting an extra layer of gender-sensitive policies into water management (keep in mind, women tend to bear the biggest burden) can ensure that the actual needs of all are heard. For the most part, when communities embrace a holistic strategy that integrates both climatic concerns and social disparities, they are more likely to keep their water secure and sustainable over the long term.

12.3. Global Sanitation Challenges

Water, sanitation, and social issues all blend together in ways we sometimes forget. Poor sanitation merely adds to issues such as poverty, inequality, and environmental disrepair, where finances are limited. Consider eThekwini, for instance – by the year 2020 almost 27% of households lacked even the most fundamental facilities, indicating just how resilient these issues are when attempting to meet targets such as SDG6. It's not just about health, you see; a failure of sanitation eats away at people's dignity and can even disunite communities. Addressing such ingrained problems requires local policies that understand what every community needs and is inclined to push for solutions that increase gains in many areas (Carbonell et al., 2022). Sanitation's relationship to nutrition isn't a minor issue either – studies continue to indicate that it's something that really warrants some serious consideration in international policy. Looking over the research easily reveals that improving water and sanitary habits really can assist in reducing undernutrition, especially among vulnerable populations. You find that trend all over the globe, in countries like Bangladesh, where extensive reviews have been conducted (Mahmud & Mbuya, 2016). It seems too frequently that if policymakers, nutritionists, and health advocates all get in on the conversation, they could create schemes that address both the so-called obvious and not-so-obvious effects of poor sanitation , such as staggered effects on the development of children and even long-term community productivity. Policymakers are attempting to close the gap between sustainable development and sanitation concerns by seeking benefits that intersect in various sectors. In eThekwini, for example, individuals are examining how sanitation activities can be connected to a number of sustainable objectives, creating opportunities to exchange resources more intelligently. One fascinating concept is the reuse of untreated wastewater as energy or even fertilizer; it's a new spin on repairing infrastructure issues while bringing in the involvement of resource circularity. Even so, reaching these lofty targets involves engaging the community in decision-making so that they really do feel invested , and ensuring that groups on the periphery are not forgotten, lest new inequalities be unintentionally reinforced (Carbonell et al., 2022). Balancing the public's input with concern for the environment may well be the path to destroying barriers to access for all in most instances.

12.3.1. Access to Sanitation Facilities Worldwide

Clean and accessible sanitation pervades every aspect of our lives. Its lack does not only impair physical health, it also reduces the opportunities for learning and making a good living, particularly for vulnerable individuals. Numerous communities struggle with poor sanitation daily, and this often translates into more responsibility for women and girls, who get sicker and have less opportunity to go to school. Occasionally, a combined effort from local authorities, community organizations and even private enterprise is quite simply what's required to turn things around; a shared, hands-on approach can change the status quo for those without access to basic facilities (WSP, 2011; WHO, 2015).

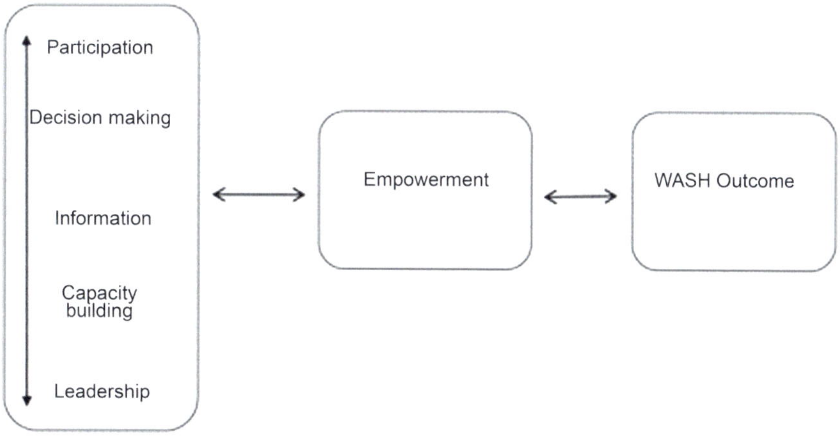

Figure 12.6. The combination of factors or parameters that need to synchronize for improving WASH facilities across all communities.

Source: By Florence Dery; Elijah Bisung; Sarah Dickin; Michelle Dyer - Understanding empowerment in water, sanitation, and hygiene (WASH): a scoping reviewhttps://doi.org/10.2166/washdev.2019.077, CC BY 4.0, https://commons.wikimedia.org/w/index.php?curid=144495294

Without proper sanitation, it tends to ripple out well beyond individual homes, impacting whole communities in unexpected ways. A number of studies indicate that breaking with open defecation toward better sanitation reduces diseases that strike young children hardest. Spending on solid sanitation infrastructure makes a significant impact as a public health measure, especially in rural areas where access is usually limited. When policymakers adopt a community-focused strategy, they manage to curb health threats and systematically elevate the overall standard of living for all parties involved (Andres et al., 2014). It's difficult to discuss social and economic advancement without bringing up sanitation. Nations that place significant value on fundamental sanitation appear to reap rewards that spill over into their economies and social lives—rewards that accumulate slowly into stronger communities. Typically, good leadership and consistent momentum in policy-making are essential to implementing sanitation interventions that suit local contexts (Figure 12.6). By providing equitable access to quality sanitation, the poor and vulnerable populations have an opportunity to escape the poverty trap and construct stronger, more resilient lives. In a sense, improved sanitation isn't merely about avoiding disease; it's an investment that supports wider advancement and equality (WSP, 2011; WHO, 2015).

12.3.2. Health Risks Associated with Inadequate Sanitation

Expanding city populations make maintaining things sanitary a headache. Inadequate sanitation creates a chain of public health issues that, quite frankly, take the hardest hit on the most vulnerable, often children (Figure 12.7).

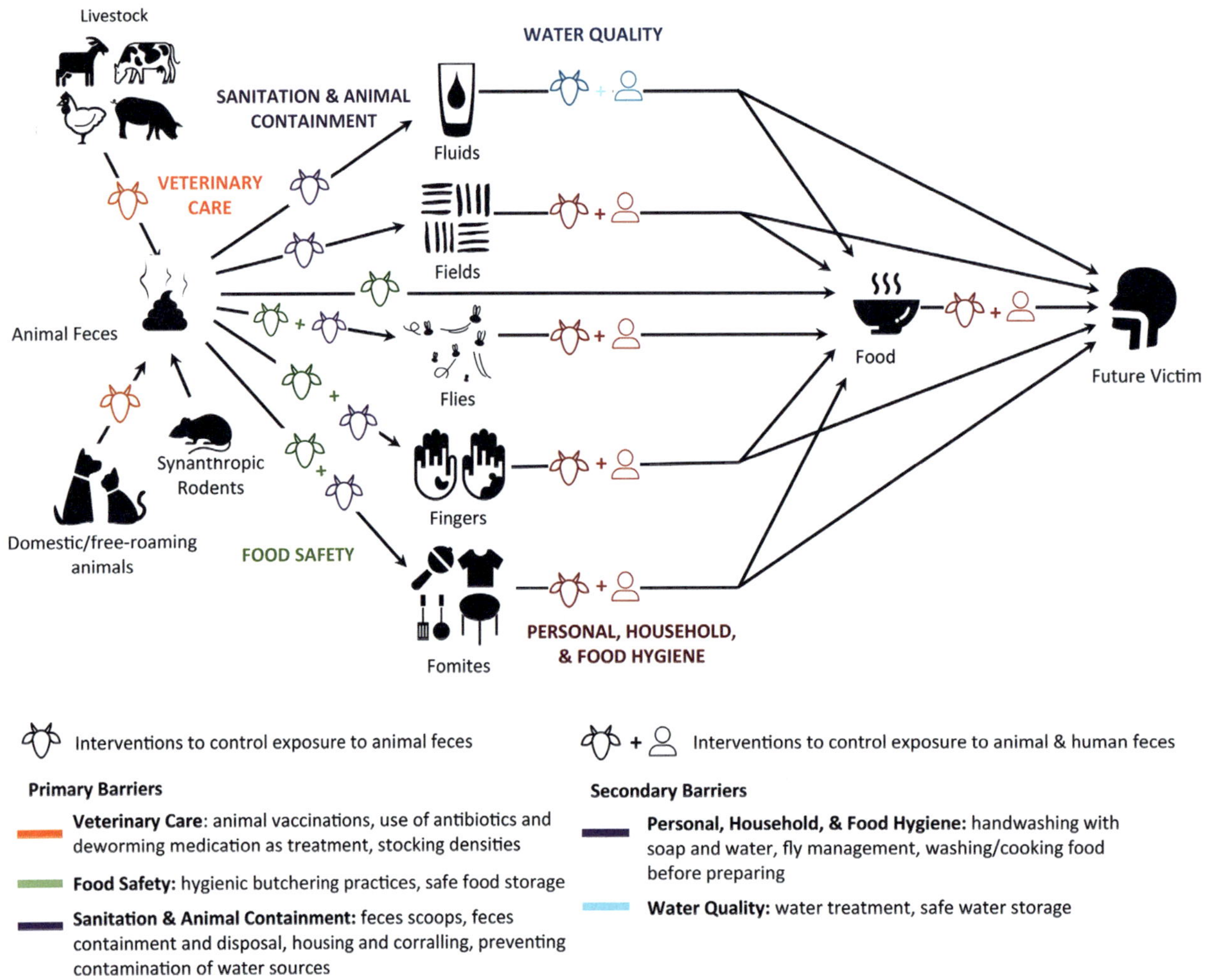

Figure 12.7. The health impacts from unsafe sanitation through various transmission pathways.

Source: By Gauthami Penakalapati , Jenna Swarthout, Miranda J. Delahoy, Lydia McAliley, Breanna Wodnik, Karen Levy, and Matthew C. Freeman* - http://pubs.acs.org/doi/10.1021/acs.est.7b02811, CC BY-SA 4.0, https://commons.wikimedia.org/w/index.php?curid=64484791

Statistics within urban slums indicate that areas without adequate wastewater control quickly become disease hotspots. One survey in Dhaka, for instance, estimated an alarming number: approximately 16,276 instances of disease each year associated with dirty surfaces and floodwaters. Children, for the most part, wind up suffering greatly from gastrointestinal diseases, stealing healthy years from them. This leaves a stark image: immediate, directed action is called for to reduce microbial exposure, making this an urgent appeal to urban health policy (Islam, 2025). Shoddy infrastructure merely exacerbates the situation in overcrowded, under-equipped slums. Throughout the world, you continue to find this same pattern—a definite correlation between challenging sanitation and elevated health threats. In Bangladesh's Khulna, approximately 70% of the slums surveyed had risk scores significantly higher than what most would consider acceptable. Both officially controlled and informal settlements appear to have this dismal destiny, indicating that these are not isolated issues but a result of overarching, systemic failures in city planning and skewed resource allocation. It appears that addressing these requires a hybrid solution: increasing sanitation infrastructure, enhancing public health awareness, and implementing pragmatic measures to stay ahead of these dangers (Islam et al., 2025). Poor sanitation not only leads to the immediate health crises, it can jeopardize long-term community development. Diseases spread through water, bred from bad sanitation, do not only damage individual health; they also destroy community progress by draining productivity, burdening over-taxed healthcare systems, and generally reducing the quality of life. To summarize, if we're going to have sustainable development, better sanitation must be part of a broader, interconnected solution. Policymakers must understand that investing in integrated, all-encompassing sanitation programs that lower exposure, facilitate ease of health risks, and enhance community resilience is a smart, forward-looking action. In the process, societies not only tackle local health issues, but also lay the foundation for wider global development and SDGs (Islam & Kabir, 2025).

12.3.3. Gender Disparities in Sanitation Access

Most global efforts focus on alleviating sanitation challenges, yet research continues to highlight that not all people are equally impacted; marginalized populations (particularly women and girls) encounter special challenges that continue in most areas. A lack of access to basic hygiene further entrenches both health issues and social inequalities. Women, for instance, consistently get into trouble due to locational restrictions, safety concerns, and cultural reasons that at times restrict their usage of accessible facilities. In general terms, addressing those challenges involves seeing obstacles associated not just with gender but with ethnicity and income as well. Implementing inclusive, gender-sensitive approaches could unlock access while empowering women and enhancing their general health and participation in public life (Sultana et al., 2025). Evidence indicates an evident link between not having adequate sanitation and the educational reversals that many girls experience in low- and middle-income countries (LMICs). In most schools, the lack of functioning and safe menstrual hygiene management (MHM) facilities means girls miss school, a gap that only increases the gender gap, and primarily in areas with limited resources. In most instances, these sanitation problems significantly influence learning outcomes, which means policies must shift rapidly. Although some promising interventions are already underway to address these education- and gender-specific barriers in sanitation and education, very significant gaps exist. Stronger evidence is required to explore what works best in settings that support girls, especially in rural or marginalized settings

(Psaki et al., 2022). The settings in refugee camps throw an added dimension to these sanitation issues, pointing toward a pressing need for tailor-made solutions that deal with gender gaps. In settings such as the Rohingya camps in Cox's Bazar, the combination of displacement, cultural norms, and scarce resources paints a complicated picture, one in which women and girls themselves are often doubly affected by deficiency in safe and dignified sanitation. At other times, the complex obstacles all at once can feel almost impossibly tangled up to study, yet they must still be identified and addressed. Developing targeted policies that focus on these vulnerable groups, even though they are applied unevenly at times—may lead the way toward improved sanitation outcomes and, in the end, a more equitable social balance (Sultana et al., 2025).

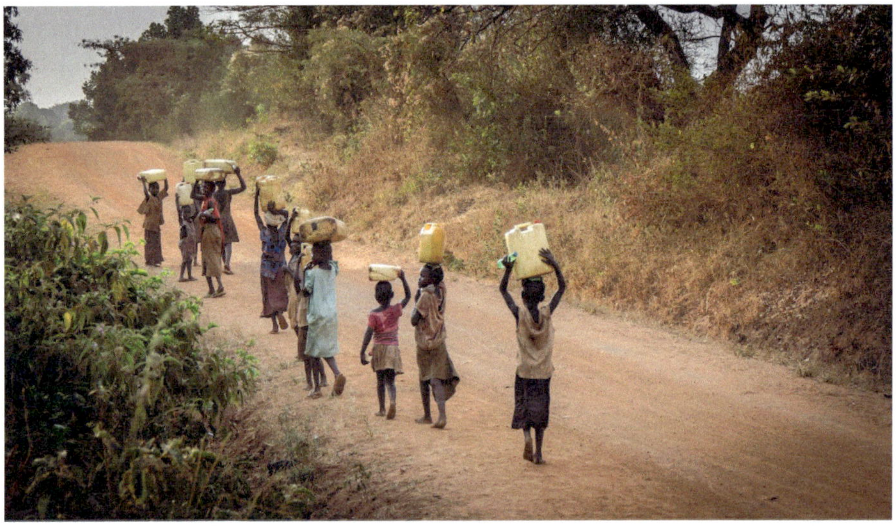

Source: Ackley, J. (2018). *Group of People Walking on the Road Carrying Containers.* Unsplash. https://iwa-network.org/wp-content/uploads/2023/03/jeff-ackley-YwDo_HwORXs-unsplash.jpg.

12.4. International Organizations and Their Roles

International institutions play a massive role in how water and sanitation are dealt with worldwide. They assemble resources and expertise—consider the United Nations or the World Health Organization, and establish quick-fix solutions as well as long-term plans. At times, these organizations get countries together on the fly to address issues such as water shortages and pollution. It is not just technical fixes either; usually, there is a strong push for equitable access to water and linking social justice directly into environmental stewardship. Overall, these organizations allow countries to share experiences and best practices, usually enhancing policymaking around water management and building communities that are resilient to future hurdles (Intergovernmental Panel on Climate Change, 2023). Apart from providing advice, these organizations tend to initiate funding initiatives worldwide. In many instances, by joining hands with both governmental and nongovernmental organizations, they rally the funds necessary to modernize infrastructure and implement new technologies in poorer areas. At times, innovative concepts, such as decentralized sanitation or water initiatives that suit local demands, are given attention. They also maintain a watchful eye on accountability, where money can be traced and outcomes can be measured. When investments pay dividends that are noticeable, trust is built among the stakeholders and local communities, confirming the worth of their diversified approach (Yoshikawa et al., 2020). Cooperation appears to be at the center of what these organizations are about. Just think of how the United Nations SDGs integrate water and sanitation into broader social and economic goals. By combining efforts from various sectors, the various stakeholders can then address better where health and the environment intersect. These institutions oftentimes end up being unofficial centers through which ideas get exchanged and capacity is developed, equipping nations with effective strategies for their water management. This collaborative work—in no way necessarily always well-oiled, but certainly effective—pays itself off when hard-hitting crises such as climate change, economic shocks, or health emergencies strike. Oftentimes, these global actors inform policy that is both responsive and effective (Intergovernmental Panel on Climate Change, 2023).

12.4.1. The United Nations and Its Initiatives

Water and sanitation issues globally are severe, and the UN has leapt in with a wide, if not always neatly tidy, system that connects to SDG 6—basically guaranteeing everyone consistent water access along with durable sanitation. Rather than traveling along the typical path, the UN solution blends new concepts such as water management and nature-based solutions; these strategies, based both on new technology and local government expertise, demonstrate that providing water isn't merely a matter of filling basic needs but also generating economic development and safeguarding our nature (Figure 12.8). Local communities receive some attention as well—by engaging regular people in policy-making, the intention is to increase accountability and overall policy effect (Takhumova et al., 2025). Money, it seems, is a large part of this equation. In much of the world with scarce resources, there simply isn't enough funding, so government budgets and infrastructure suffer. The UN has supported seeking out diversified funding sources—consider public-private partnerships combined with global assistance—to bolster local systems. Research on rural communities even suggests that when formal channels falter, informal community means take over and maintain operations. It comes as no surprise, therefore, that these informal routes prove essential in keeping services running, demonstrating unequivocally that a responsive approach to resource management can truly enhance service delivery, while also facilitating better government systems that are stronger, more sustainable (Landa et al., 2025).

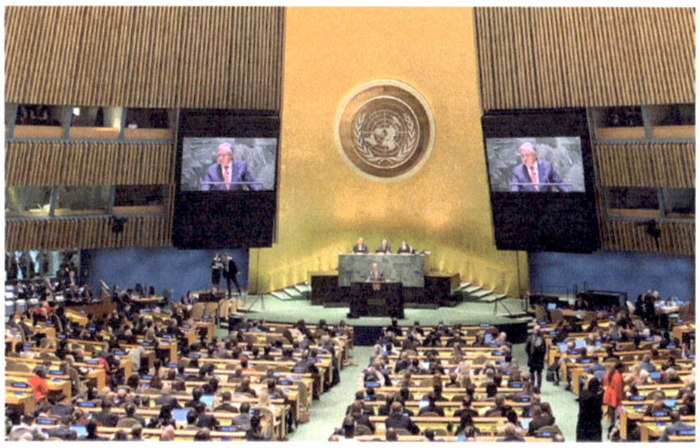

Figure 12.8. Ensuring climate-resilient water and sanitation in the UN.

Source: World Health Organization. (2018). *News: Protocol on Water and Health is a Global Example of Ensuring Climate-Resilient Water And Sanitation for All.*

After it is all said and done, the UN's approach to addressing water and sanitation problems interweaves a lot of various strategies in ways sometimes a little scattered. Working the twists and turns of international development appears always to circle back to putting local capacities and people's voices at the table, even if sometimes those most attuned to local requirements have too little voice in the final outcome. An attempt to remedy that is to create forums wherein local organizations can fully participate. Making that possible is regarded as central to improving efficiency as well as promoting fairness. Mixing formal systems with informal resource flow may well prove to be the recipe for achieving access to water and sanitation services for all, sooner rather than later (Landa et al., 2025; Takhumova et al., 2025).

12.4.2. Non-Governmental Organizations (NGOs) and Their Contributions

International water and sanitation problems have long been a complex arena, and NGOs have moved in as remarkably adaptive players. NGOs introduce their own type of grassroots local knowledge that, in most instances, shines more brightly than traditional government efforts. They include small grassroots projects to work on the global level, frequently filling the gap between cut-off communities and policymakers. Operating up close and personal on the ground, they gather actual facts, advocate for changes that serve local requirements, and even—if you look at reports such as GLAAS 2017—reorganize the way nations address financing matters surrounding water, sanitation, and hygiene (WASH) (WSP, 2011; WHO, 2015). NGOs are also indispensable in mobilizing resources and making various groups cooperate. Overall, they can enhance the distribution of aid when conventional means bias the wealthier regions against the poorer ones. In a not too uncommon situation, governments spend money in the regions they should probably prioritize over poorer communities, which suffer as a result (WSP, 2011; WHO, 2015). By keeping inclusivity at the forefront, such organizations ensure resources and investments reach those who need them most. Sometimes, they even break new ground with new funding arrangements that seek a more equitable distribution of support toward safe water and improved sanitation. Furthermore, the community engagement and advocacy work conducted by NGOs are essential for sustainable change. They endeavor to increase awareness regarding the significance of a pure water supply and proper sanitation facilities—frequently reminding residents of health hazards associated with abandonment. Such grassroots education, even when at times it appears repetitious, empowers citizens to demand increased accountability from governments and participate in important decisions regarding their lives. Accounts indicate that community ownership can influence national policies, and full NGO programs typically create an instant response with scope for long-term sustainable change. All of these serve to do a great deal to reach world goals for universal access to clean water and sanitation (WSP, 2011; WHO, 2015).

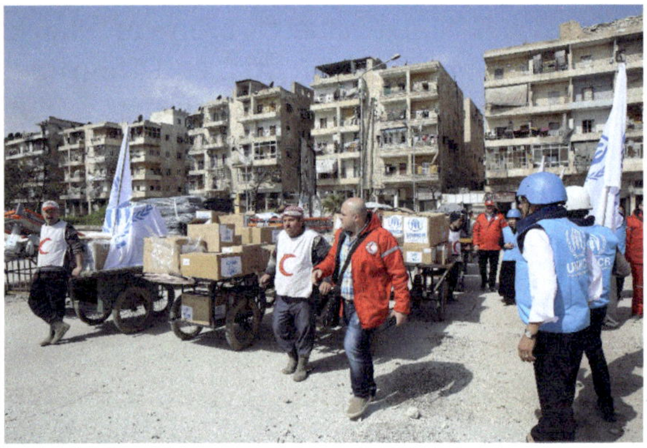

Source: United Nations High Commissioner for Refugees. (n.d.). *UNHCR Refugee Camp.*

Source: https://www.unhcr.org/sites/default/files/legacy-images/56e93ee84.jpg.

12.4.3. The Role of Local Governments in Implementing Policies

Local authorities are very important now, particularly in our increasingly interconnected world. They are centered in the communities themselves, and they catch the genuine, everyday nuances of people. This proximity allows them to close that gap between far-away policymaking and the gritty details of everyday life. Frequently, they craft plans to fit local cultural attitudes, social patterns, and even economic idiosyncrasies—a nimbleness not always available at higher levels. For instance, numerous local authorities spearhead community outreach and conduct education campaigns that reinforce basic hygiene practices and promote water usage that endures. In most situations, even if central backing falters, this local-level intervention assists in achieving overall standards as well as cultivating a sense of responsibility and concern for public resources. The convergence of water, sanitation, and nutrition concepts truly reveals how essential local contribution is to public health. Different case studies show that when municipalities collaborate to address different aspects simultaneously, they succeed in developing ways that work. Some town-scale initiatives, for example, combine water and sanitation improvements with nutrition education, and the health gains for the community can be dramatic. In general, the literature indicates that addressing these problems concurrently can reduce poverty and reduce disease rates—reiterating that local government is integral in implementing such complex policies. In this context, coordination between local government and NGOs, community associations, and foreign partners becomes critical to the stretching of resources and for making projects genuinely effective (WSP, 2011; WHO, 2015). Nevertheless, despite their such significance, local governments frequently encounter challenges such as limited resources, irregular training, and inadequate support from above. It is this phenomenon that makes it virtually necessary to invest in capacity building and resource mobilization. Improved training can provide local authorities with the type of expertise required to manage water and sanitation duties effectively. Similarly, collaborating with international organizations can both provide finances and that valuable technical know-how required to overcome infrastructural and logistical hurdles. When national and international benefactors invest in local institutions, such institutions can more effectively serve local populations while implementing global WSPs, often even avoiding anticipated hurdles. In the end, an effectively supported local government can be a strong change agent, advancing core public health objectives and securing equitable access to necessary services (Mahmud & Mbuya, 2016).

12.5. Innovative Solutions and Technologies

Global water and sanitation policies are being turned on their head with new technology and innovative concepts that are taking on real community issues head-on. Market-based strategies, more than ever, are appearing essential for driving sustainable sanitation initiatives to a larger scale. When you consider initiatives such as the Unclogging the Blockages conference, there's a stark reminder that these market-led strategies break through the traditional barriers to sanitation access and quality. This new approach weaves together components of housing, energy, business, health, and education that allow various players to collaborate alongside each other in a manner that makes services efficient and accessible to the people (Narracott et al., 2014). Technology also has its role. Live data and intelligent information systems can now allow closer monitoring of water projects, frequently ensuring that resources are used to their full potential. Broadly speaking, this enthusiasm for technology-led monitoring corresponds to recent reports emphasizing the need to develop capacity in water management as part of a green economy. Several case studies even demonstrate how applied tech solutions can establish water supply and sanitation systems that can adapt to evolving needs, a type of resilience that gets communities ready not just for the problems of today but also for the unknowns of tomorrow (Peemans et al., 2012). Strengthening the capacity of institutions with new program concepts is another cornerstone of the solution. During the Unclogging the Blockages conference, various specialists emphasized that collaboration—sharing expertise and sharing resources, is the future. Through cooperation in arrangements such as a Global Sanitation Financing Alliance, institutions can access new financial arrangements that ignite bottom-line entrepreneurial initiatives in sanitation. Not only does this type of cooperation support local businesses to flourish, but it also initiates research that gets down to the nitty-gritty of market realities. In short, developing an ecosystem that relies on innovative tech innovations can enhance the overall effect of global water and sanitation policies, raising the quality of life for communities all over the world (Narracott et al., 2014).

12.5.1. Advances in Water Purification Technologies

Water sources come under tremendous pressure today—the population surging and industries expanding relentlessly compress our finite freshwater resources. It's rather obvious we must have new ways of purifying water. Recently, technological leaps turned things around: techniques such as membrane filtration, advanced oxidation, and even allowing nature to assist through bioremediation are now dominating the process of water treatment and reuse. For example, membrane filters not only capture large particles; they operate at the molecular level itself to catch pollutants that previously escaped. This innovation is converting rejected water into a usable commodity, pushing us toward more sustainable management strategies and redefining water and sanitation policies worldwide (Singh et al., 2023). Recent research, overall, reminds us just how important it is to keep an eye on wastewater treatment in the long term. Treating wastewater prevents not just pollutants but even annoying pathogens from making their way into our water, keeping it safe for us to drink. Some newer systems even trap bio-methane and produce nutrient-rich byproducts, helping to boost agricultural production. A closer examination of several reviews of studies reveals that enhanced treatment methods can alleviate the pressure on natural water resources and at the same time unlock renewable energy potential and sustain local economies.

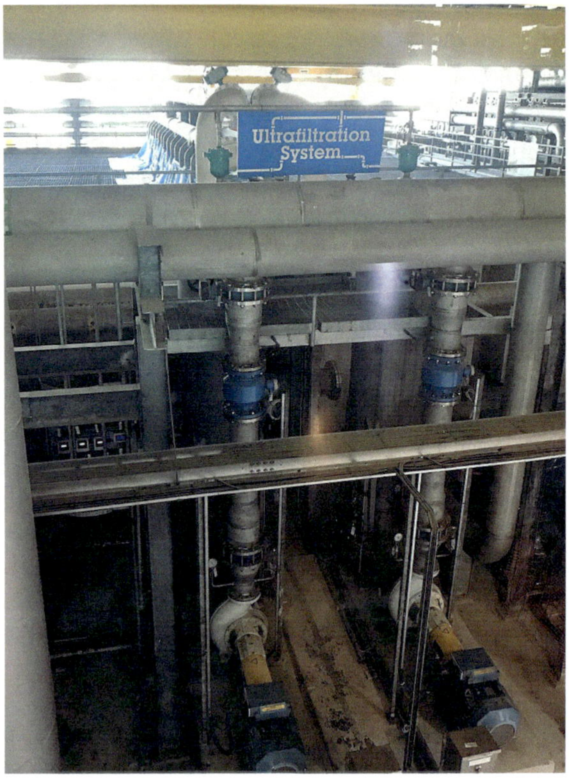

Figure 12.9. Illustration of advanced water purification.

Source: By Z22 - Own work, CC BY-SA 4.0, https://commons.wikimedia.org/w/index.php?curid=112506294

For most instances, the combination of technological innovation with reasonable regulation seems to be the formula to constructing resilient and sustainable water infrastructure (JASíguez de Miguel, 2023). Leaping onto the circular economy wagon for water cleaning creates a wider vision of sustainability. Advances today are not just about cleaving water to crystal clarity—but about recycling it, which mitigates water scarcity issues. Consider bioremediation as an example: employing living things to degrade pollutants provides a natural, efficient cleanup solution that aligns perfectly with sustainability objectives (Figure 12.9). When these technologies combine with robust policy initiatives, they are capable of creating a type of synergy that supports more intelligent water management strategies. Even research suggests that interactivity between stakeholders is the solution to overcoming concerns such as aging infrastructure and limited budgets. Mostly, the combination of technology, reasonable rules, and public participation appears to be the best way toward water and sanitation targets that are both equitable and sustainable (Singh et al., 2023).

12.5.2. Sustainable Sanitation Solutions

Policy and technology tend to blend in ways that increase our potential for sustainable sanitation in international water management. New solutions, such as segmenting wastewater treatment into smaller, decentralized systems and discovering how to recover valuable resources—demonstrate that technology can reduce harm to the environment while enhancing services. Consider anaerobic digestion, for instance; it treats wastewater while simultaneously producing biogas, providing a sort of double dividend in sanitation and energy generation. Most countries, by and large, are attempting to achieve UN SDG 6 by incorporating these new technologies into their domestic policy. Ultimately, combining technological sparks with practical policy can just construct a functional model that serves today's resource needs and improves health and the general well-being of communities (Takhumova et al., 2025). Reviewing the historical background of WASH, it happens that learning about past legacies really does matter for defining what is next. There's been a strong emphasis on technology, extending services to all, and relying on individuals to take up responsibilities, which means that there must be a turn toward sustainability. Picking apart what did and didn't work in past attempts, policymakers can sometimes find buried ideas and call for 'smarter' practices that are more equitable in the long run. A combination of perspectives, ranging from those residing in poorer areas to experienced technocrats—adds depth to the policymaking process, tending to make sanitation programs more effective and pertinent. When local populations are involved, solutions coming out of it are likely both culturally appropriate and economically feasible, fostering a sense of ownership conducive to long-term sustainable objectives (Sara de Wit et al., 2024).

Having sustainable sanitation up and operational isn't without its challenging socio-political and economic challenges, which tend to hinder progress in many cases. Budget constraints and unstable infrastructure continue to be issues, particularly where sanitation choices are in dire need. One handy solution could be to continue funding innovative funding solutions and create collaboration between the private and public sectors to construct stronger sanitation systems. It's also important to address entrenched disparities in sanitation access if equitable public health outcomes are to be achieved. Policymakers simply must confront the unpalatable reality that structural gaps do exist—gaps that serve to exacerbate vulnerabilities. After we embrace the fact that these challenges are multidimensional and sometimes complex, we can begin designing interventions that stretch beyond technological Band-Aids to tackle the economic and social layers of sanitation to pave an inclusive way toward improved public health and environmental stewardship (Takhumova et al., 2025).

12.5.3. Community-Based Water Management (CBWM) Practices

Local communities in control of water management have proved to be a game-changer in addressing water scarcity and sanitation issues across the globe (Figure 12.10). When the people own the water resources, somehow there is a greater sense of accountability and it motivates a steadier, sustainable utilization, even though the conditions are, most of the time, quite tough. Typically, you find that communities rely on traditional local governance practices to adapt solutions that meet their specific cultural and environmental requirements, a fact supported by the USAID Field Guide, which points out that such community efforts have a tendency to unite people and enhance long-term success (WSP, 2011; WHO, 2015). Yet, simultaneously, you can't help but notice how such community efforts blend with public health approaches. Consider southern Africa, for instance; in that area, water, sanitation and health issues just about come together by chance, underlining the necessity of policy approaches that go hand-in-hand. A field-level rapid assessment in the region typically indicates that the integration of HIV efforts with WASH interventions builds natural synergies. These intersections not only enhance access to water but also tackle broader health concerns, resulting in an increase in resilience and overall improved quality of life (WSP, 2011; WHO, 2015). Naturally, it is not all plain sailing to be a leader in community-based water management (CBWM). Challenges such as decaying infrastructure, limited financial resources, and disparate community engagement can sometimes throw a wrench into the machinery. Nevertheless, there are success stories where collaboration between local governments, NGOs, and residents have, step by step, closed these gaps. Knowledge sharing, capacity building, and ongoing learning are at the heart of the process; with an adaptive strategy embracing feedback (even if not always delivered perfectly), communities gradually work to refine their strategies in order to keep pace with constantly shifting environmental and socio-economic circumstances.

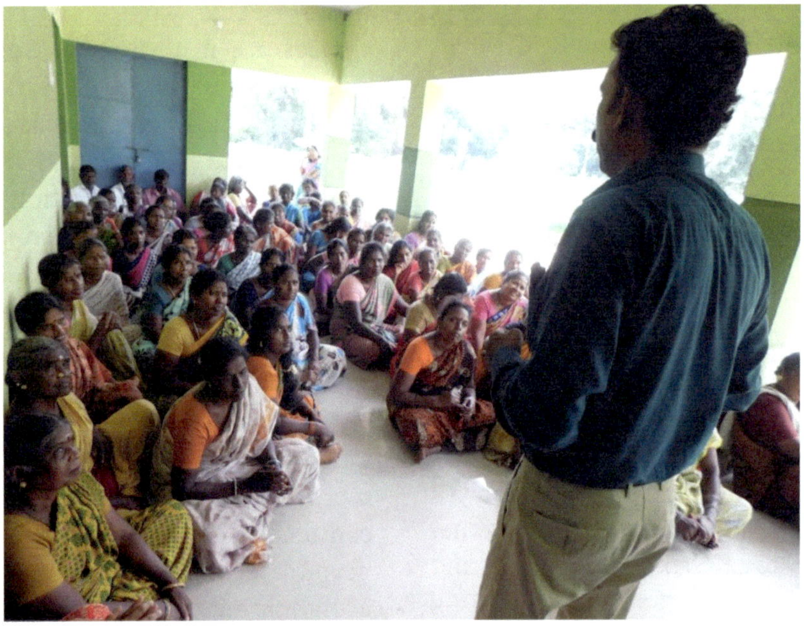

Figure 12.10. Community-engagement-in-water-management.

Source: ADI International. (2023). *Community Engagement in Water Management.*

12.6. Policy Recommendations

Sanitation and water concerns challenge us to think anew, requiring innovative, new-in-their-fields recommendations that take us in the direction of sustainability. In numerous instances, market-driven solutions have appeared as a primary step to get sanitation initiatives underway. Learnings from the Unclogging the Blockages conference even identified that if you operate sanitation as a business, you can trigger investment and fresh, outside-the-box tech. This concept not only enhances solutions but also creates unlikely synergies across industries such as housing, energy, and healthcare. When money is open to investment—both for firms and families—a configuration like the Global Sanitation Financing Alliance (Narracott et al., 2014) could heighten sanitation programming while supporting necessary on-the-ground tech innovation. Getting various sectors to collaborate is almost a requirement when addressing the complex combination of water and sanitation issues. Water, food, and nutrition tend to intertwine into each other, making it difficult to make policies work. At other times, concentrating too much on one objective, such as the battle against zero hunger in SDG 2—may inadvertently retard the achievement of access to clean water for SDG 6. In general, it is worth it when nutrition groups and those in charge of managing water resources talk more frequently with each other, usually discovering small successes that advance all. In the absence of such coordination, there's a very real potential that shortages of resources will cumulatively harm and undermine fundamental rights to food as well as water (Committee UNSS on Nutrition, 2020). Ahead of us, we must also confront the impending challenges of climate change and increasing competition for resources. Strong policies must be nimble—capable of adapting as conditions change in the environment and as areas face varying water availability. Large initiatives, such as the UN Decade of Action on Nutrition and the International Decade for Action on Water for Sustainable Development, are pushing us to look more carefully at our collective objectives. With more powerful, sometimes surprising, alliances, stakeholders may very well develop policies that integrate initiatives across several disciplines. Ultimately, it all really comes down to a combination of real collaboration and creative thinking that can revolutionize water and sanitation infrastructure for generations to come (Committee UNSS on Nutrition, 2020).

12.6.1. Strategies for Improving Global Water Access

Water is that fundamental ingredient driving sustainable development, it touches our well-being, powers our economy, and even influences social equity. In some cases, the solution is to modify the way things are done, such as giving a bit of an update to governance in a way that services run more smoothly. Recent research, particularly focusing on some African countries, indicates that having good, firm rules makes a difference. It so happens that building stronger legal systems—ensuring property rights hold and corruption is caught early, is a game changer, as rampant corruption tends to deter investment in water infrastructure. For the most part, when nations direct their efforts toward these governance actions, they establish a more equitable system, one which facilitates consistent water management and eventually improves public health within communities that are in most need (Cesar et al., 2010) (Figure 12.11). Apart from refurbishing governance, one additional piece of the equation is pumping more funds into WASH projects—what people refer to as WASH. The GLAAS 2017 report, for instance, points out that attracting additional resources from public and private sectors is quite essential if we are to access the most vulnerable. Through the development of financing mechanisms that address local water challenges directly, the officials can support projects that truly reflect the needs of the people. And if you integrate WASH funding into larger economic strategies, you end up with a more sustainable system as a whole. Not only does this create the infrastructure needed, but it also increases capacity building, ensuring water services work efficiently in the long term (WSP, 2011; WHO, 2015). Education, especially when it is empowering women and girls, ends up being another giant driver of water access improvement. There's loads of evidence that smarter schooling is associated with smarter water management, when girls are educated, communities tend to use water more sustainably and have improved sanitation results. Education investment generates a generation that's equipped to participate in governance, raise their voice for their communities, and devise new solutions to water problems. Even small steps, such as educating water conservation and hygiene to students in schools, can change the way communities manage water on a daily basis over time. Essentially, combining education with water access plans not only raises tomorrow's leaders but also forms the bases for long-term, sustainable development, a component that completes the puzzle of making water access a reality globally (Cesar et al., 2010).

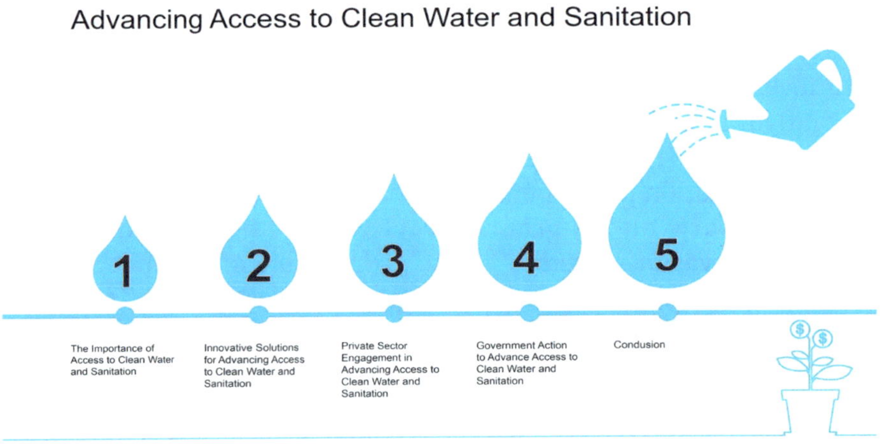

Figure 12.11. Advancing-access-to-clean-water-and-sanitation.

Source: FasterCapital. (n.d.). *Healthy Planet: The UN Global Compact's Health Agenda – Advancing Access to Clean Water and Sanitation.*

https://fastercapital.co/i/Healthy-Planet--The-UN-Global-Compact-s-Health-Agenda--Advancing-Access-to-Clean-Water-and-Sanitation.webp.

12.6.2. Enhancing Sanitation Infrastructure in Developing Countries

Public health and sanitation in most developing countries truly go together, even if sometimes it may be easy to overlook exactly how closely interdependent they are. When good facilities are not accessible, waterborne diseases have a free ride, and they tend to affect marginalized communities all the more. In other places, the absence of even the most basic infrastructure simply provides an easier means for infections to move from person to person, which further widens health disparities. Many experts now contend that constructing more toilets and water infrastructure isn't sufficient; educating individuals about proper hygiene is equally vital. Most often, pairing hands-on building with on-the-ground education ensures that each dollar spent truly enhances public health. At other times, this involves conducting campaigns in parallel with construction projects so that individuals, particularly women and girls, can have greater control over their own hygiene and sanitation (Wang et al., 2024). It is also important to design sanitation solutions that suit the daily demands of vulnerable individuals. Wherever they've been constructed, the systems that have been developed weren't developed with a local voice, so they usually end up conflicting with cultural practices or individual preferences. Having locals engaged with a more people-centered design process can result in facilities that aren't only practical but also culturally significant. This is done repeatedly throughout various studies and has the effect of increasing how widely these services are utilized. For instance, a study in Mozambique found that involving young women in developing sanitation plans helped to solve their particular problems and enhance their overall well-being (Wang et al., 2024). All of this contributes to building local pride and ensuring that these programs remain in place for the long term. And then there is the entire question of climate issues combined with sanitation. In most developing regions, intense weather occurrences such as heavy rains and floods exert additional pressure on already weak water systems. Upgrading these arrangements entails developing adaptable designs that can cope with the surprises of nature while still ensuring that sanitation is available for all. In most cases, policymakers must integrate climate adaptation concepts into sanitation upgrades, it's not a matter of having more facilities, but ensuring that they are resilient enough to withstand harsh environments (Figure 12.12). For example, decentralized systems could be a wise replacement for outdated methods that simply can't withstand intense weather. By addressing these intertwined issues with solutions that reconcile sanitation requirements and climate adaptability, communities can move toward a more equitable, healthier future, one that reduces the impact of both poor sanitation and a changing climate.

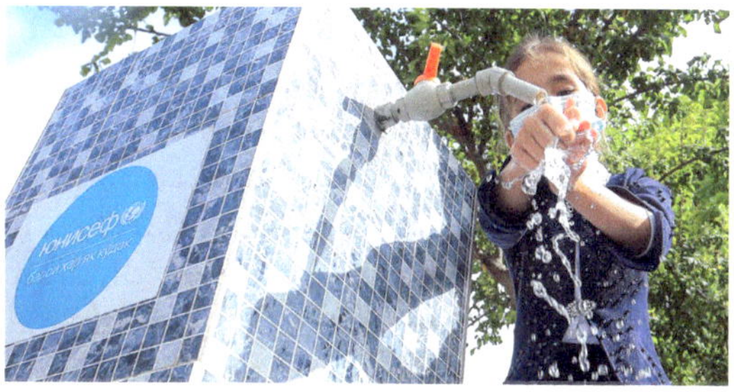

Figure 12.12. Developing sustainable water and sanitation in Central Asia's rural areas.

Source: Asian Development Bank. (n.d.). *WASH Girl*. Development Asia. https://development.asia/sites/default/files/styles/1200x600/public/summary/washgirl.jpg?itok=iTdQGu1v.

12.6.3. Promoting Public Awareness and Education on Water Issues

Water issues provide the setting for change, and everything begins with when people start to discuss them. Simple and easy-to-understand messages set off a fire that engages people at the local community level, oftentimes persuading neighbors to do their fair share of duty. School education programs, for instance, integrate instructions on water shortages, pollution, and handling so that normal citizens can obtain what's really involved. Often, when educators integrate these concepts into daily learning, citizens are more prepared to defend intelligent, sustainable choices. Some case studies (WSP, 2011; WHO, 2015) suggest employing a combination of methods—albeit not necessarily neat, is an effective way to increase these initiatives, with the result that when various communities collaborate, they all end up looking at the larger picture. Water in public spaces is something that really speaks to what policies ultimately have on our lives. From neighborhood collectings to United Nations-hosted sessions, there's an emerging sense of people freely discussing sustainable development and the care of resources. Sometimes the discussions are less structured and other times slightly rough around the edges, as people share hopes and fears for water quality and access. For the most part, allowing individuals to speak their minds not only allows them a voice but also bases policies on real life so that decisions strike close to home (WSP, 2011; WHO, 2015). Today, our online world opens up some rather distinctive avenues for sharing news about water problems. Social media alerts, interactive sites, and virtual chats dissolve the traditional geographical boundaries, allowing the stories and actions to move spontaneously and authentically. There is a kind of digital heartbeat here that easily allows communities to monitor water use and become inventive about saving it. While technology is no silver bullet, as several reports (WSP, 2011; WHO, 2015) state, combining web tools with face-to-face learning is essential to fulfilling SDGs—demonstrating that a touch of digital spark, combined with authentic local action, can go a long way.

SUMMARY

International water and sanitation policies really accumulate levels of difficulties. A combination of circumstances necessitates our having a hands-on, multi-faceted strategy to minimize those health risks that arise when WASH is in deficit. A high disease burden attributed to substandard facilities illustrates just how necessary enforceable regulations are, even when it comes to such circumstances as antimicrobial resistance (AMR). Other nations have already implemented National Action Plans to improve their WASH systems, but with no legal clout, momentum can come to a halt. Policymakers, in the majority of instances, must really understand the way that the rules operate if they're going to implement changes that don't just raise public health but also narrow the economic disparities underscored in international research (Weets et al., 2024). Looking to the future, scaling up global water and sanitation efforts means digging through the social and economic strata that determine WASH access. The urban/rural split, for instance, exposes an inefficient system that plain and simply cries out for intelligent, targeted action. Mainland China's journey over the last 20 years is a prime example—impressive achievements coupled with continued challenges, reminding us that persistent, sustainable funding is essential for defending the most vulnerable (Li et al., 2024). Once these imbalances are clearly seen, policymakers can hopefully begin putting money to work in a more unequal, but nuanced, fashion, working toward Fairness+Efficiency, instead of Efficiency-At- Fairness. In the context of a future-proof strategy in this area, the solution is in countries collaborating, harmonizing their regulatory playbooks, and relying on good research to determine what really works. Continuous work to chart out WASH policies serves as a building block for identifying strategies that cut down on health hazards associated with insufficient sanitation and water quality. With leaders striving to close policy gaps in various parts of the globe, maintaining a watch on adaptability and responsiveness will be truly crucial (Weets et al., 2024). Ultimately, only by collaborating and cooperating can nations truly strive for global access to safe water and sanitation, clearing the way for subsequent SDGs that form the foundation of global health and happiness.

Water and sanitation problems have been on everyone's radar recently, particularly in areas where resources are limited. Approximately 38% of healthcare facilities in these areas don't even have the fundamentals concerning WASH, which in most instances means an actual threat to public health. It's as if these lapses cry out for a rapid, across-the-board solution. Large players such as the World Health Organization, UNICEF, and governments must convene on an agenda that attacks these gaps directly. Investment in WASH infrastructure is not simply a matter of upgrading facilities, it's about bringing clean water and proper sanitation to all people, a fundamental right upon which modern health policy relies (WSP, 2011; WHO, 2015). On the financial side, microfinance has also recently appeared as a potential solution to enhance water and sanitation services. The Bill & Melinda Gates Foundation report broadly identifies microfinance as an approach to access previously untapped investment prospects in water. By identifying the appropriate opportunities for assistance, stakeholders can assist such service models to develop sustainably (Dondeynaz et al., 2010). This concept not only initiates some local economic development but also enables communities to become self-sufficient in addressing their water and sanitation requirements, with a mention of SDG 6 seeking universal access. In short, microfinance is more than a fiscal extra, it's an essential ingredient in a broader policy blend (Mehta, 2008). The connection between water, sanitation, and health outcomes cannot be argued. Come up short on these basics and infectious diseases can propagate more readily—striking children and the elderly especially hard. Targeted, community-based measures appear to be necessary to level these inequalities. Water and sanitation policies, which are geared toward enhancing health, must listen to the specific requirements of each community instead of operating from some generic checklist. This mode of thinking promotes local participation and ensures that interventions become meaningful and effective in day-to-day life. Merging investments in healthcare infrastructure with a strong emphasis on water and sanitation can reduce health inequalities and propel sustainable development (WSP, 2011; WHO, 2015).

KEY TERMS FROM THIS CHAPTER

- Aging infrastructure
- Cholera epidemics
- Disease rates
- Economic growth
- Gender-sensitive policies
- Integrated Water Resources Management
- Low- and middle-income countries (LMICs)
- Poor sanitation
- Sanitation policies
- Virtuous cycle
- Water and sanitation projects
- AI-based models
- Cultural norms
- Disease transmission
- Financing mechanisms
- Green infrastructure
- Long-term stewardship
- Menstrual hygiene management (MHM)
- Resilient water
- Sanitation requirements
- WASH systems

CLOSER LOOK

SUSTAINABLE DEVELOPMENT GOAL 6

Sustainable Development Goal 6 (SDG 6 or Global Goal 6) proclaims the necessity of securing "clean water and sanitation for all." It is one of the 17 SDGs the United Nations General Assembly has adopted to replace the previous Millennium Development Goals (MDGs). As defined by the United Nations, the overall aim is to: "Ensure availability and sustainable management of water and sanitation for all." The objective contains eight targets to be met by 2030 that span the key areas of water supply and sanitation and sustainable management of water resources. Measures of progress against the targets are to be made using 11 indicators.

The six major outcome goals to be met by 2030 are:

- Attentive universal and equitable access to safe and economical drinking water for all;
- Ensure access to safe and equal sanitation and hygiene for all and break the cycle of open defecation, giving priority to women and girls and vulnerable individuals;
- Enhance water quality, by lowering pollution, stopping dumping and reducing the release of toxic chemicals and materials, cutting in half the percentage of untreated wastewater (wastewater treatment) and doubling recycling and safe reuse worldwide;
- Significantly enhance water-use efficiency in all sectors and ensure sustainable withdrawals and supply of fresh water to mitigate water scarcity and significantly decrease the number of individuals facing water scarcity;
- Apply integrated water resources management (IWRM), at all scales, including through transboundary cooperation as necessary;
- Safeguard and recover water-related ecosystems, which include mountains, forests, wetlands, rivers, aquifers and lakes.

The two ways of translating into action are to increase global cooperation and capacity-building assistance to developing nations and to assist local participation in sustainable and participatory water and sanitation management.

Even with Official development assistance (ODA) disbursals to the water sector rising to $9 billion in 2018. the WHO and UNICEF Joint Monitoring Programme (JMP) in 2017 stated that 4.5 billion people lacked safely managed sanitation. In 2017, only 71% of the world's population used safely managed drinking water, and 2.2 billion individuals remained without safely managed drinking water. Other water-related risks connected with flooding and drought are also ongoing threats to human development and well-being.

Similar to the rest, this SDG is also intertwined with the rest of the SDGs. For instance, having access to clean water will enhance health and well-being, which results in an improvement in SDG 3; and, good health means that children will go to school, advancing SDG 4, and enhancing quality education. SDG6 is only possible if other SDGs are also met. (Ariho et al., 2024)

References

1. Ariho A, Aja L, Muhammad T and Mohammad L. Water pollution: causes, impacts and current efforts to address the issues of water pollution along river Meizimera-kihihi, Kanugu District,Uganda. [version 2; peer review: 2 approved with reservations]. *F1000Research* 2025, **13**:1298 (https://doi.org/10.12688/f1000research.155162.2) (accessed on 14 May 2025).

2. Anjum, G., & Aziz, M. (2025). Climate change and gendered vulnerability: A systematic review of women's health. *Women's Health, 21*. https://www.semanticscholar.org/paper/2a6d52d50856459296e1c91b78e6e0a7c9591db2 (accessed on 14 May 2025).

3. Andres, Luis A. & Briceno, Bertha & Chase, Claire & Echenique, Juan A., 2014. "**Sanitation and externalities : evidence from early childhood health in rural India**," Policy Research Working Paper Series 6737, The World Bank.(accessed on 14 May 2025).

4. Calvin, K., Dasgupta, D., Krinner, G., Mukherji, A., Thorne, P., Trisos, C. H., Romero, J., et al. (2023). *IPCC, 2023: Climate Change 2023: Synthesis Report. Contribution of Working Groups I, II and III to the Sixth Assessment Report of the Intergovernmental Panel on Climate Change* (H. Lee & J. Romero, Eds.). IPCC. https://doi.org/10.59327/ipcc/ar6-9789291691647.

5. Carbonell, Lucila; Hofmann, Pascale; Srikissoon, Nevana; Campos, Luiza C; Mbatha, Sandile; Lakhanpaul, Monica; Mabeer, Vishnu; ... Parikh, Priti; + view all (2022) Localisation of links between sanitation and the Sustainable Development Goals to inform municipal policy in eThekwini Municipality, South Africa. **World Development Sustainability** , 2 , Article 100038. 10.1016/j.wds.2022.100038 (accessed on 14 May 2025).

6. Celine Dondeynaz, Cesar Carmona-Moreno, Andrea Leone, Daoyi Chen (2010). *Analysing Inter-Relationships Among Water, Governance, and Human Development Variables in Developing countries–Preliminary Results on Africa for 2004*. JRC 59047 ISSN 1018-5593 ISBN-13: 978-92-79-18410-9 doi:10.2788/43519 Luxembourg: Publications Office of the European Union. https://core.ac.uk/download/38620805.pdf (accessed on 14 May 2025).

7. Carvalho, M., Martins, S., & Santos, E. (2023). *Sustainable Water Management: Understanding The Socioeconomic and Cultural Dimensions*. https://core.ac.uk/download/599418311.pdf (accessed on 14 May 2025).

8. Dagdeviren, H., & Robertson, S. A. (2009). *Access to Water in The Slums of The Developing World*. https://core.ac.uk/download/29841360.pdf (accessed on 14 May 2025).

9. de Wit, S., Luseka, E., Bradley, D., Brown, J., Bhagwan, J., Evans, B. E., Freeman, M. C., et al. (2024). Water, sanitation and hygiene (WASH): The evolution of a global health and development sector. *BMJ Global Health, 9*. https://www.semanticscholar.org/paper/acd5468d9dddc4c7cf921add7c8efcf6b4bc92c3 (accessed on 14 May 2025).

10. Nicolay, Gian L. and Fliessbach, Andreas (2012) Production of Innovations within Farmer–Researcher Associations Applying Transdisciplinary Research Principles. In: *International Conference on Research for Development (ICRD 2012). Research for Global Transformation, Theme 4: Enabling Research in Global Transformation Session 26: Integrated Development Research Approach*, NCCR North-South Dialogue, no. 44, p. 164.(accessed on 14 May 2025).

11. WWAP (World Water Assessment Programme). 2012. The United Nations World Water Development Report 4: Managing Water under Uncertainty and Risk. Paris, UNESCO. The United Nations World Water Development Report 4: Managing Water under Uncertainty

and Risk (Vol. 1),Knowledge Base (Vol. 2) and Facing the Challenges (Vol. 3). (accessed on 14 May 2025).

12. Gumbo, B., Indij, D., Coates, D., Lentini, E., Sewilam, H., Liebe, J., Bernaudat, L., et al. (2012). *Water in the Green Economy: Capacity Development Aspects*. https://core.ac.uk/download/71360162.pdf (accessed on 14 May 2025).
13. Intergovernmental Panel on Climate Change. (2023). *Climate Change 2022–Impacts, Adaptation and Vulnerability*. https://doi.org/10.1017/9781009325844.
14. M. M. Majedul Islam; Assessing health risks and disease burden from waterborne pathogens across multiple urban exposure pathways. *Journal of Water, Sanitation and Hygiene for Development* 1 April 2025; 15 (4): 322–332. doi: https://doi.org/10.2166/washdev.2025.306 (accessed on 14 May 2025).
15. Islam, S. M. T., & Kabir, Md. A. (2025). Quantification of health risk due to poor sanitation infrastructure in slums of urban Khulna, Bangladesh. *International Journal of Environmental Health Research*, 1–19. https://doi.org/10.1080/09603123.2025.2489128 (accessed on 14 May 2025).
16. Landa S, Sanoussi EY, Mahamane E, Mahamadou KOB, Salzberg A, Anderson DM (2025) Resource allocation for environmental health services in healthcare facilities: A qualitative case study from Niger. PLOS Water 4(2): e0000330. https://doi.org/10.1371/journal.pwat.0000330 (accessed on 14 May 2025).
17. Li, S., Gong, A., Yin, Y., & Su, Q. (2024). Spatiotemporal characteristics and socioeconomic inequalities in water, sanitation, and hygiene access in China from 2000 to 2020: Analysis of data from three national censuses. *BMC Public Health, 24*. https://www.semanticscholar.org/paper/0cd614a1f66c3393ef3a5ae5cec9ce247c59b96e (accessed on 14 May 2025).
18. Lief, E., Kates, J., & Pearson, J. (2009). *U.S. global health policy: Donor funding for health in low- & middle-income countries, 2001–2007*. https://core.ac.uk/download/71348668.pdf (accessed on 14 May 2025).
19. Morse, Tracy and Lungu, Kingsley and Taulo, Steven (2010) Gap Analysis of Environmental Health Research in Malawi : Report to the National Commission of Science and Technology. National Commission for Science and Technology (Malawi), Malawi. (accessed on 14 May 2025).
20. Mahmud, Iffat, 1982- author.; Mbuya, Nkosinathi, author.; World Bank, issuing body.
21. Washington, DC : International Bank for Reconstruction and Development/The World Bank; 2016
22. Library Catalog ; MMS ID 9916637343406676; ISBN 9781464806988 (paper); NLM Unique ID 101663734 (accessed on 14 May 2025).
23. Mehta, M. (2008). *Assessing Microfinance for Water and Sanitation: Exploring Opportunities for Sustainable Scaling Up*. https://core.ac.uk/download/71345975.pdf (accessed on 14 May 2025).
24. WSP (2011). Political economy of sanitation: How can we increase investment and improve service for the poor? Operational experiences from case studies in Brazil, India, Indonesia and Senegal World Bank, Water and Sanitation Program (WSP), USA (accessed on 14 May 2025).
25. WHO Library Cataloguing (2015)-in-Publication Data Water, sanitation and hygiene in health

care facilities: status in low and middle income countries and way forward. 1.Water supply. 2.Water Quality. 3.Sanitation. 4.Hygiene. 5.Quality of care. 6.Health care facilities. 7.Developing Countries. I.World Health Organization. II.UNICEF. ISBN 978 92 4 150847 6. https://core.ac.uk/download/75783071.pdf (accessed on 14 May 2025).

26. Narracott, A., Nothomb, C., Sauer, J., & Snell, M. (2014). *Sanitation as a Business: Unclogging the Blockages*. https://core.ac.uk/download/75778737.pdf (accessed on 14 May 2025).

27. Obringer, R., Kumar, R., & Madani, K. (2024). Harnessing the power of AI for climate change impact assessment. "Harnessing the Power of AI for Climate Change Impact Assessment," United Nations University, UNU-INWEH, 2024-08-27, https://unu.edu/inweh/article/harnessing-power-ai-climate-change-impact-assessment.(accessed on 14 May 2025).

28. Psaki, S., Haberland, N., Mensch, B., Woyczynski, L. P., & Chuang, E. (2022). Policies and interventions to remove gender-related barriers to girls' school participation and learning in low- and middle-income countries: A systematic review of the evidence. *Campbell Systematic Reviews, 18*. https://www.semanticscholar.org/paper/c041dc01ca606f7fb20e87dcb7549378283d3d4b (accessed on 14 May 2025).

29. Satterthwaite, D., Archer, D., Colenbrander, S., Dodman, D., Hardoy, J., Mitlin, D., & Patel, S. (2020). Building resilience to climate change in informal settlements. *One Earth, 2*, 143–156. https://doi.org/10.1016/j.oneear.2020.02.002.

30. Silva Rodríguez de San Miguel, J. A. (2023). Wastewater treatment and reuse for sustainable water resources management: A systematic literature review. *Sustainability, 15*, Article 10940. https://doi.org/10.3390/su151410940.

31. Singh, B. J., Chakraborty, A., & Sehgal, R. (2023). A systematic review of industrial wastewater management: Evaluating challenges and enablers. *Journal of Environmental Management, 348*, Article 119230. https://doi.org/10.1016/j.jenvman.2023.119230.

32. Shekhar Singh, Manish Kumar Goyal; A review of India's water policy and implementation toward a sustainable future. *Journal of Water and Climate Change* 1 February 2025; 16 (2): 493–510. doi: https://doi.org/10.2166/wcc.2025.560 (accessed on 14 May 2025).

33. Sultana, U. B. F., & Rahman, M. M. (2025). Water, sanitation & hygiene inequalities in Rohingya camps and host communities of Cox's Bazar: An intersectional multilevel ecological model perspective. *Social Science Review*. https://www.semanticscholar.org/paper/216c812a90b0a3354ea4372e2ab09ffc2464d3d8 (accessed on 14 May 2025).

34. Takhumova, O., & Goncharova, M. (2025). Innovative approaches to water resource management in achieving sustainable development goals. *E3S Web of Conferences*. Volume 614, 2025

35. International Conference on Agritech and Water Management (ICAW 2024). DOI https://doi.org/10.1051/e3sconf/202561404019 (accessed on 14 May 2025).

36. Thibodeau, Mary, "Decolonizing WASH Practices Between National Policies & International Standards: A Case Study in Tanzania" (2023). *Capstone Collection*. 3289. https://digitalcollections.sit.edu/capstones/3289(accessed on 14 May 2025).

37. United Nations System Standing Committee on Nutrition. (2020). *Water and nutrition: Harmonizing actions for the United Nations Decade of Action on Nutrition and the United Nations Water Action Decade*. https://core.ac.uk/download/288633623.pdf (accessed on 14 May 2025).

38. Walimah, E., Andayani, H. F., Sonjati, E., Siagian, I. O., & Silapurna, E. L. (2024). Mitigating the impact of climate change on public health: Strategies for resilience. *Global International Journal of Innovative Research*. 2. 2231-2244. 10.59613/global.v2i9.308. accessed on 14 May 2025).

39. Wang, C., Nitto, R., Kuroki, T., Ban, Y., Nakai, M., Shimizu, J., Ashikaga, T., Warisawa, S. (2024). Constructing a Transformer-based Model to Infer Daytime Productivity from Biometric Information During Sleep. In: Tareq Ahram, Waldemar Karwowski, Darko Etinger and Tea Mijač (eds) Human Systems Engineering and Design (IHSED2024): Future Trends and Applications. AHFE (2024) International Conference. AHFE Open Access, vol -2. AHFE International, USA.

40. Weets, C. M., & Katz, R. (2024). Global approaches to tackling antimicrobial resistance: A comprehensive analysis of water, sanitation and hygiene policies. *BMJ Global Health, 9*. https://www.semanticscholar.org/paper/16b183bef74c48e99c1721b3610dc82b64abc31e (accessed on 14 May 2025).

41. Yoshikawa, H., Wuermli, A. J., Britto, P. R., Dreyer, B. P., Leckman, J. F., Lye, S. J., Ponguta, L. A., et al. (2020). Effects of the global coronavirus disease-2019 pandemic on early childhood development: Short- and long-term risks and mitigating program and policy actions. *The Journal of Pediatrics, 223*, 188–193. https://doi.org/10.1016/j.jpeds.2020.05.020.

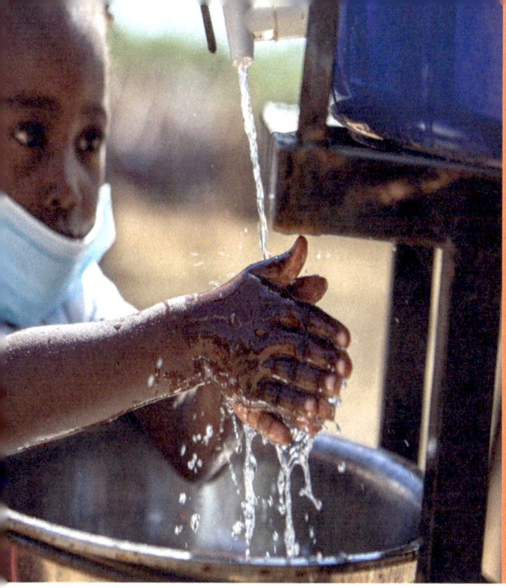

Chapter 13

WATER-RELATED HEALTH INTERVENTIONS AND PROGRAMS

Contents

Introduction

Pure water and good sanitation are not luxuries—their absence is the foundation of unhealthy communities, particularly where waterborne disease is a common risk. Recently, there has been evidence to suggest that increasing water, sanitation, and hygiene services (WASH) significantly reduces avoidable disease. Nigeria, for instance, presents a confusing image: though sometimes regarded as one of Africa's richer countries in terms of some indicators, much of its population continues to suffer from suboptimal health statistics as a result of endemic systemic deficiencies. Approximately 40% of Nigerians remain impoverished, facing extreme threats that only increase with a below-par water supply and less-than-optimal sanitation arrangements. Strong WASH programs, therefore, address immediate hygiene requirements as well as trigger long-term health education and community engagement (Abubakar et al., 2022). NGOs have truly filled gaps in areas where resources are lacking ,, in many cases serving as a link between government initiatives and community. They don't merely direct funds and technical expertise; they mobilize people in favor of health issues regarding clean water and improved sanitation. At other times, it's not a matter of just distributing pamphlets; these organizations work closely with people so that health messages have the proper local tone and really make an impact. Recent research even indicates that when NGOs tailor their methods to meet community details, they assist in breaking down myths surrounding waterborne diseases, a key step in areas that are faced with both infrastructure and knowledge deficiencies (Adebisi et al., 2021). Tracking these programs is important—without careful monitoring, it's difficult to see what does and doesn't work, or what needs revision. A good evaluation structure does more than highlight short-term gains; it also ensures that programs are sustainable enough to have genuine impacts. Information-driven analysis allows decision-makers to make adjustments to resource deployment and think more wisely about the next step. The difficulties encountered during the time of COVID-19 highlighted how important solid health surveillance is, and how well-coordinated WASH interventions do indeed contribute to making a more resilient public health system. Overall, acquiring a general, if occasionally imperfect, picture of robustly how WASH programs, NGO activities, and health education fit together is central to achieving sustainable public health gains (Abubakar et al., 2022).

Definition of Water-Related Health Interventions

Public health is not all about everyday services, it is usually divided into straightforward care and water-oriented interventions, if you like. These water interventions address the dynamic, though unglamorous, interactions between water, sanitation, hygiene, and health outcomes (Figure 13.1). They experiment with combinations of ideas: increasing access to safe drinking water, installing improved sanitation facilities, and encouraging regular hygiene practices in order to drive down waterborne diseases. In much of low- and middle-income settings, where poor WASH services contribute to expanding health disparities, such interventions are truly important. In general, such interventions not only reduce disease and mortality but also bring the community on board in making health choices, helping improve overall wellbeing and even enhance health system capacity (Abubakar et al., 2022). Look a bit closer and you'll see that water-related health actions aren't all about infrastructure; education and community mobilization play their part too. Health education campaigns, for instance, have come to the forefront in making folks aware of basic hygiene, such as simple lessons on handwashing or even proper menstrual hygiene management (MHM). These programs seek to give communities the day-to-day expertise they require, which in turn lowers diseases associated with poor water quality and unsanitary conditions. Interventions such as MHM in 10 integrate in-class instruction with actual infrastructure development, clearly making the school life of menstruating girls more tolerable and helping to fulfill years of neglected health requirements (Sommer et al., 2021). It's an uneasy, at times uneven blend, but one which creates stronger, more health-informed communities. Monitoring and evaluation become the humble heroes of this endeavor. Routine checks and evaluations provide essential information that informs policy adjustments and program realignments. Quite often, these evaluation systems indicate what's effective and, perhaps just as valuable, what's missing in places where services must be strengthened. They ensure interventions are informed by sound, ground-level data. By rooting out these conclusions, governments, NGOs, and even neighborhood leaders can make strategies more responsive to local needs, advocating for more equitable health outcomes. Thus, constant surveillance drives a round of sustainability and accountability that informs global objectives such as universal health coverage and general social equality (Abubakar et al., 2022).

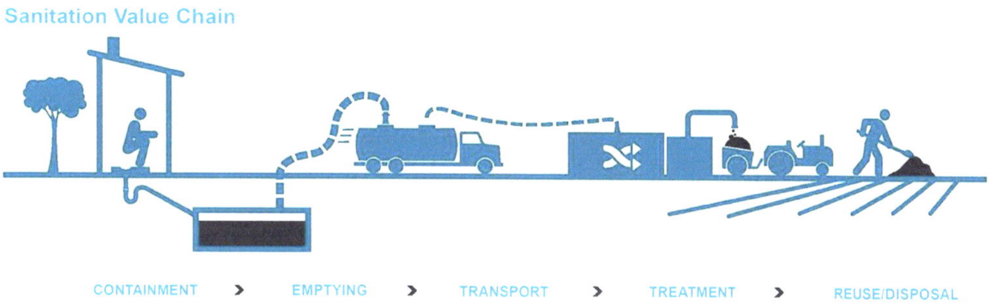

Figure 13.1. Effects of water and sanitation interventions on health.

Source: https://en.wikipedia.org/wiki/File:Sanitation_Value_Chain.jpg

Importance of WASH (Water, Sanitation, and Hygiene) Programs

Public well-being and health are motivated by a combination of social determinants and emerging developments, and that obviously guides us toward the necessity of effective WASH programs. Communities have equitable access to safe water, acceptable sanitation, and effective hygiene education, which in turn keeps preventable disease at bay and improves overall health. Consider Nigeria, for example; there, are unbalanced conditions so that WASH initiatives not only address the resultant short-term health concerns but also deal with broader economic and social issues that accompany waterborne diseases. Basic hygiene habits, if effectively promoted, tend to reduce rates of disease and death, particularly among vulnerable individuals such as children and pregnant women. In most instances, empowering local communities through such programs sets the ground for better living and public care indicators (Nielsen et al., 2022). NGOs, however, have a fairly crucial role to play in ensuring these programs function. They normally serve as the link between government organizations and the local community, tapping local expertise while establishing partnerships that count. Often, you'll see these organizations training community members in basic sanitation practices and encouraging behavior shifts that lift overall public health standards (Figure 13.2). They also get involved in capacity-building efforts, which, generally speaking, help local leaders manage water and sanitation resources more effectively. This kind of collaboration boosts community engagement and helps keep the programs going strong, a crucial need in underserved areas (Nielsen et al., 2022). Monitoring and evaluation in regular checks are important to make these efforts effective. Regular reviews provide useful feedback, sometimes even highlighting impediments to access that require urgent adjustments in strategy. Operating with good data ensures interventions remain adaptable enough to respond to changing needs, and in most instances, this helps ensure that the resources are spent wisely. Briefly, when programs are closely tracked and tuned as necessary, they become critical instruments in combating inequality and fostering sustainable health equity (Abubakar et al., 2022).

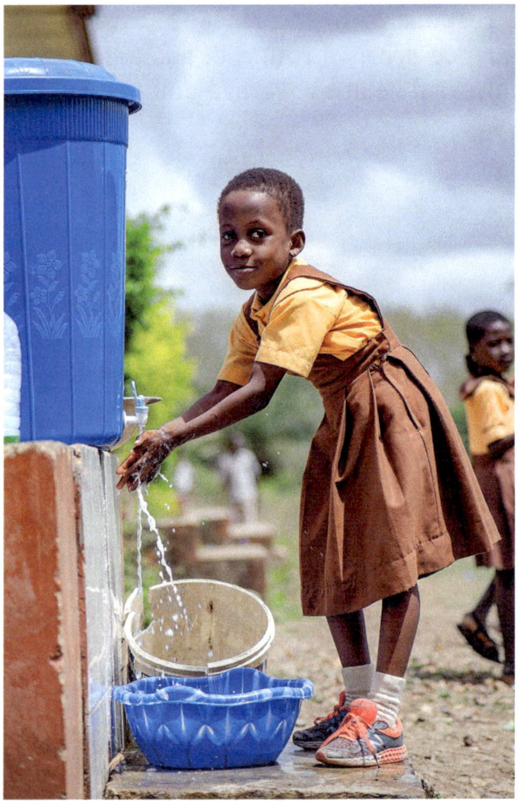

Figure 13.2. A schoolgirl using a Veronica Bucket in Ghana for washing her hands.

Source: Wikimedia Commons. (2021). *Pupil Washes Hands During COVID-19 Pandemic in Ghana.*

13.1. Understanding WASH Programs

Public engagement and alterations to the way individuals act are just at the center of reforming public health with WASH initiatives. Rather than implementing the standard, general fixes, the majority of projects start by listening to what every community is all about – catching daily routines, customs, and social idiosyncrasies. They begin by determining just who they're working with and then customize their approach so individuals feel the program is addressing them. This type of bottom-up strategy sets up habits that can endure for a lifetime and lead to healthy behaviors every day, keeping waterborne diseases in check. Case studies – even from projects in other regions of Asia and Africa (The Water and Sanitation Program, 2011; WaterAid Australia, 2011) – continue to indicate that understanding needs at the community level is simply a key to success. Look, if you take a peek at Southeast Asia you'll see some quite innovative means of implementing WASH." In Vietnam, for instance, the team went deep into domestic behavior patterns and rather than attempting to force outside solutions, they homed in on comprehending traditions and motivations that are local in nature.

The outcome? An approach that seamlessly integrates handwashing into daily routines. In Indonesia, there's a similar feel where initiatives collaborate with private partners to increase reach and softly reinforce positive habits. These types of collaborative endeavors truly demonstrate that combining local flavor with a dash of external assistance really can make a lasting impact on community health (The Water and Sanitation Program, 2011; WaterAid Australia, 2011).

Apart from initiating things, the entire WASH program story also depends on monitoring progress along the way. Regular tracking and continuous monitoring allow teams to visualize the practical effects these projects have in real life, and they are fast to alter based on new on-the-ground input. Most often, this is not simply about tracking increases in hygiene—but also about keeping community voices involved, which creates accountability. With regular checkups and a dose of good health education, the programs go on to refine their strategies and make every resource count, demonstrating that ongoing learning and adjustment is an integral component of long-term achievement (Figure 13.3).

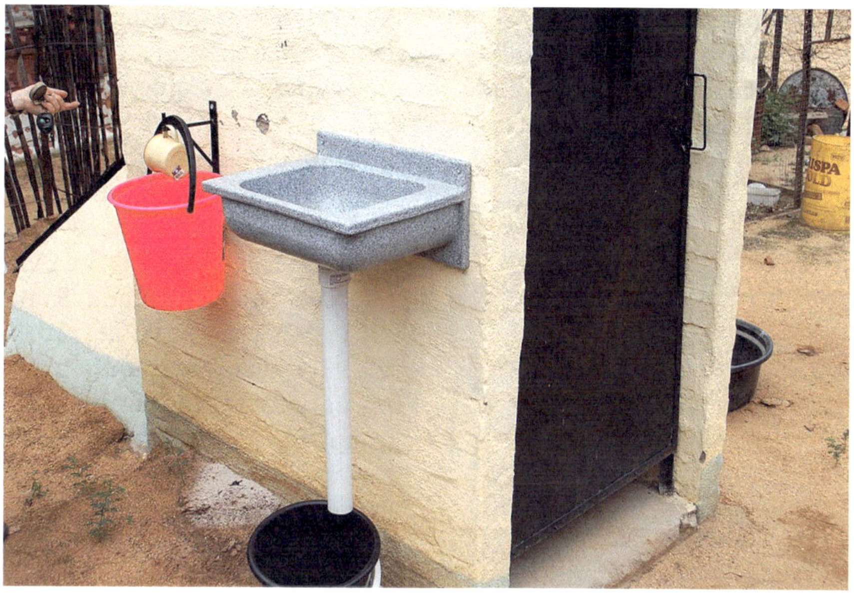

Figure 13.3. Simple handwashing facilities were attached to each toilet.

Source: SuSanA Secretariat. (2011). *Handwashing*. Wikimedia Commons.

13.1.1. Components of WASH Programs

Most communities have achieved some progress but still falter at establishing effective WASH programs. Clean water is not only a nicety, it's necessary to prevent waterborne diseases. For instance, successful household chlorination activities in some rural and disadvantaged communities have rendered drinking water microbiologically safer. Nevertheless, water quality problems, such as unanticipated turbidity or additional dissolved organic matter, can disrupt the effectiveness of such treatments. Occasionally it is useful to adjust the strategy for the local environment, considering factors such as product quality and what consumers like (Nielsen et al., 2022). Generally, getting a solid water supply right is central to driving forward wider public health objectives. Sanitation, too, holds a major sway over public health, especially when we're talking about cutting down on gastrointestinal and respiratory diseases. The stark reality is that many people, particularly women and children, still lack proper sanitation facilities, leading to millions of preventable deaths every year. A good sanitation system doesn't just lower disease rates; it also boosts dignity and safety. In general, closing the sanitation gap fits with goals such as SDG 6, which mandates universal access to safely managed facilities by 2030, and benefits even poverty alleviation (SDG 1) and education advancements (SDG 4) to some extent. Integrating holistic sanitation interventions into WASH interventions is, for many, a requirement to improve the overall standard of living (Chirgwin et al., 2021). Health education caps these initiatives by leading communities to adopt healthy hygiene practices. It's not only a matter of frequent handwashing; it's also about safe water storage and intelligent sanitation, which in unison can significantly reduce health problems associated with unhygienic WASH conditions (Figure 13.4). These education campaigns tend to require tuning into the local culture and adaptation to the particular needs of the community—sometimes employing interactive workshops and local opinion leaders to initiate deep-seated changes in behavior. Monitoring these activities can be slightly spotty at times, but it's vital for gauging their effectiveness and adjusting strategies accordingly. Together with the rest of WASH, health education contributes to building stronger communities capable of maintaining good health outcomes in the long term (Nielsen et al., 2022).

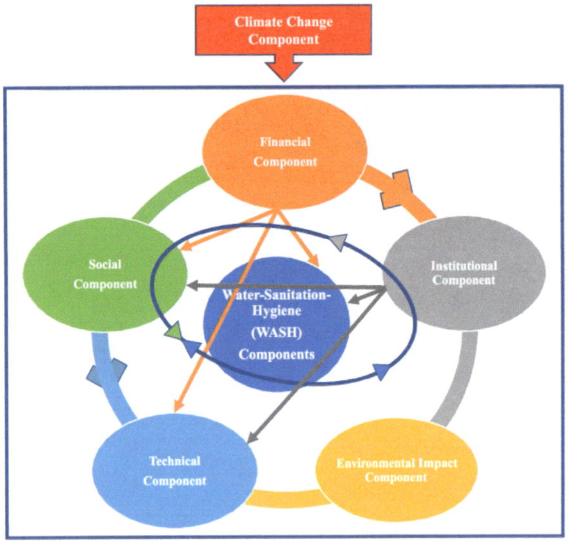

Figure 13.4. Components of integrated WASH assessment tool and their interactions.

Source: Daniel, D. (2024). *Components of integrated WASH Assessment Tool and Their Interactions*. In C. Z. Win, D. Daniel, N. M. U. Dwipayanti, & W. Jawjit, *Development of Integrated Assessment Tool For Water, Sanitation and Hygiene (WASH) Services in Non-Household Settings Under Climate Change Context. Heliyon*, 10(Suppl. 1), e37645. https://doi.org/10.1016/j.heliyon.2024.e37645.

13.1.2. Global Impact of WASH Initiatives

Water, sanitation, and hygiene (WASH) initiatives rely on a combination of circumstances that dictate their success, particularly in low-resource countries. Most programs are designed to modify daily practices, which, in most situations, reduces waterborne diseases. Consider Vietnam as an example; its initiative illustrates that addressing local habits counts before implementing any solutions. They spent observing how people conduct their daily routines and, based on those observations, developed means of changing habits toward improved health. By relying on feedback from the community and these behavioral insights, such projects slowly lift the burden of avoidable disease (The Water and Sanitation Program, 2011; WaterAid Australia, 2011). Collaboration rears its head repeatedly as another essential ingredient. In Indonesia, when government groups partnered with private firms and NGOs, they were able to take handwashing campaigns much farther than ever before—beyond small, targeted populations. Collaborating in sometimes surprising combinations, they employed existing market channels and networks to discover new avenues to reach more individuals. Such collaboration not only enhances the way resources are shared but also disseminates useful hygiene habits across the country; policies and local initiatives ultimately support each other, sort of like a positive feedback loop (The Water and Sanitation Program, 2011; WaterAid Australia, 2011). Monitoring what works is as crucial as the effort itself. A good evaluation framework allows individuals to get to the bottom of numbers on health results, how groups act, and where funds end up. That data, in the majority of instances, is important to inform wiser, data-driven changes and to make adjustments to where money and effort are directed. Case studies, particularly out in South and Southeast Asia—emphasize the necessity to know who is being served and to set conditions that encourage improved hygiene practices (Figure 13.5). Through ongoing monitoring and adjustment of programs, international health initiatives can maintain their velocity and confidently address water-based problems (The Water and Sanitation Program, 2011; WaterAid Australia, 2011).

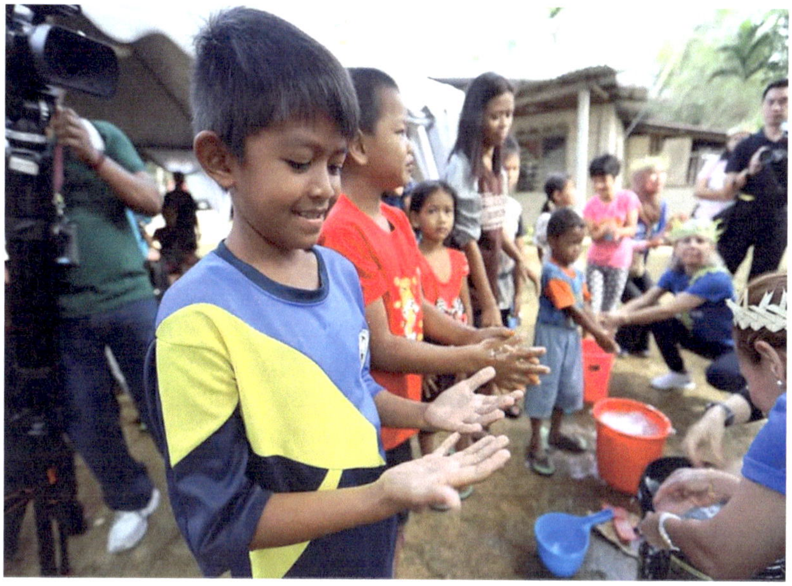

Figure 13.5. GPF Malaysia WASH program teaches children hygiene and sanitation.

Source: WASH Malaysia. (2023). *WASH Malaysia*.

https://b3244667.smushcdn.com/3244667/wp-content/uploads/2023/05/WASH-Malaysia.jpeg?lossy=0&strip=1&webp=1.

13.1.3. Case Studies of Successful WASH Implementations

Community engagement has demonstrated a remarkable effect on WASH installations. A series of case studies indicate that once individuals in the community intervene and take ownership of their water and sanitation facilities, gains appear in access to safe water and overall well-being. It appears that a little sense of responsibility – something akin to a self-regulatory check – can go quite far toward sustaining these initiatives. Studies even suggest five drivers of such good outcomes, accountability, diffusion, market forces, ownership, and, yes, even shame (Nelson et al., 2021). Essentially, relying on local resources and allowing community leaders to lead proves to be the secret to success in the long run. Being able to get a handle on how all the stakeholders function together is another necessity. Certain research indicates that roles will blur in undesirable patterns: NGOs and local authorities may either complement each other or, sometimes, tread on each other's toes. International NGOs tend to initiate such projects, but it is challenging to harmonize their grand designs with what the locals anticipate – as well as the prevailing social context – at times nullifying the purpose of the project. Overall, a closer examination of local politics and initial, informal conversations with locals appear to set the stage for results that suit the culture (Malik et al., 2019). This chaotic but authentic combination of elements can ultimately enhance a project's overall effect. Health education puts yet another spin on the tale. When sanitation and water projects are combined with a dose of health instruction, communities apparently get the message about the need for good hygiene, which subsequently approves of improved public health results. Tracking can't simply begin with the numbers on infrastructure, it must monitor when and how attitudes shift, too. By combining hands-on solutions with constant learning (and yes, occasionally with a bit of mess in the process), WASH programs create a more comprehensive system of public health, connecting practical solutions with daily learning (Malik et al., 2019).

13.2. Role of Non-Governmental Organizations (NGOs)

Water health projects rely heavily on nonprofits. NGOs fill the gap where government initiatives sometimes fall short, particularly in less visited communities. They initiate grassroots-level projects and also coordinate resources and expertise in WASH. In most instances, these organizations modify programs so they are molded according to local culture and requirements. They can switch approaches in an instant when public opinion comes flooding in, ensuring the efforts make a real difference.

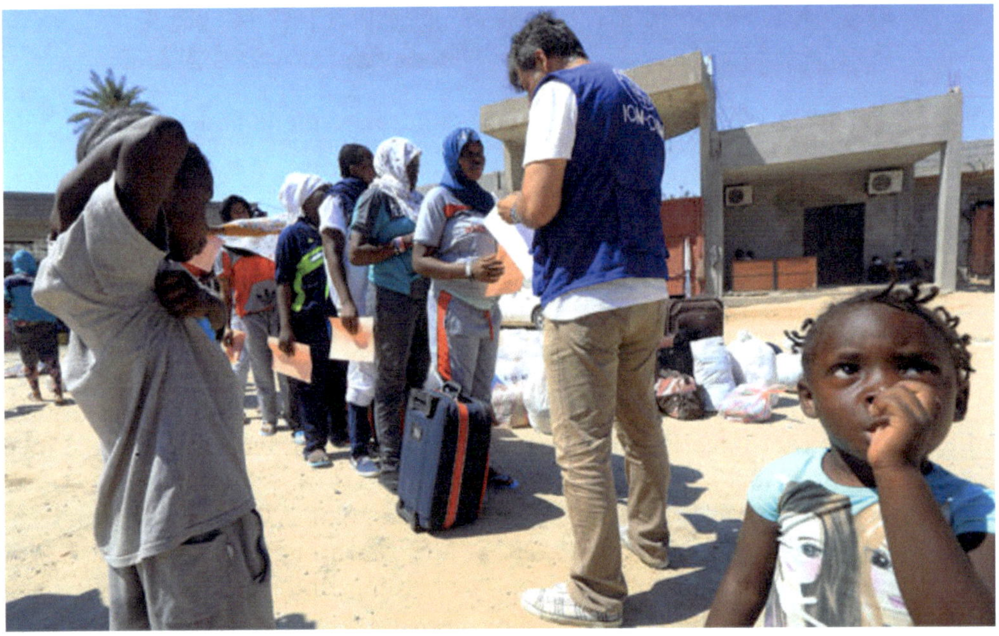

Source: WASH Malaysia. (2023). *WASH Malaysia*.https://www.arabnews.com/sites/default/files/styles/n_670_395/public/2017/08/17/972891-1772188992.jpg?itok=5mQ3uRWh.

All this translates to them often being the driving force for real-world, creative health solutions that address local circumstances. NGOs do not only stop at establishing projects—but also spearhead education campaigns that increase awareness regarding health issues due to water. By speaking plainly about the value of simple sanitation and hygiene, they empower people to take charge of their own health. Good communication is absolutely essential; it sets the foundation for a healthier life in these respects. You can observe it in some case studies in South and Southeast Asia, where targeted educational activities have brought significant changes in behavior, as communities adopted better hygiene habits. NGOs not only raise awareness but also create a culture that pushes all individuals toward healthier practices, laying the groundwork for better water quality

(The Water and Sanitation Program, 2011; WaterAid Australia, 2011). Additionally, these agencies remain vigilant about their efforts by monitoring and evaluating them—a process that many miss. Their assessments ensure that all WASH interventions are quantified in impact and effectiveness. They gather valuable data that informs not just local projects but also frames overarching public health policy. This strategy—depicted in rich reports on water, sanitation, and nutrition, is useful in unraveling the intricacies of the challenges facing communities (Mahmud & Mbuya, 2016). By flaunting the successes, these organizations build an increasing repository of success stories that create more advocacy in terms of government and international donor support. Briefly, their constant combination of checking, listening, and adapting becomes crucial in creating a long-term impact in public health.

13.2.1. Overview of Key NGOs Involved in Water-Related Health

NGOs and water health issues thoroughly blend with each other in ways that determine the way communities remain healthy. WaterAid, the International Committee of the Red Cross, and a few others go directly into action by enhancing clean water availability and sanitation facilities. They implement large-scale WASH programs that introduce new approaches to local communities. Consider WaterAid—whether or not they insist on knowing the individuals they help, so community requirements take precedence. This type of hands-on, lesson-learned strategy typically creates a road to long-term change and improved hygiene habits (The Water and Sanitation Program, 2011; WaterAid Australia, 2011).

By mobilizing resources as well as local expertise, these organizations provide not just short-term solutions but also address long-term solutions for those who are most vulnerable. Confronting serious health challenges, numerous NGOs now concentrate on the relationship between water quality and nutrition, combining multiple approaches to increase public health. Organizations such as UNICEF and Save the Children combine WASH projects with nutrition initiatives in ways that naturally happen in regions where undernutrition, usually exacerbated by poor water and sanitation, is rampant. An extensive study on the WASH-nutrition link even illustrates that improved water and sanitation can drastically reduce undernutrition. In most situations, the findings of this research, particularly in countries such as Bangladesh where NGOs observe positive gains firsthand, highlight why the combination of clean water initiatives and nutrition assistance is so critical (Mahmud & Mbuya, 2016). Overall, these combined actions are central to health initiatives addressing both the immediate problems and the more embedded, persistent issues. Health education also plays a large role in how well these water-related initiatives succeed. Organizations like Oxfam and CARE construct programs that engage communities and increase awareness; they want individuals to realize just how much good hygiene and proper sanitation matter. These projects, which also involve teachings on intelligent water management and subtle behavior changes, strive to reduce the transmission of waterborne diseases. This emphasis on instruction relates back to previous experiences demonstrating how encouraging individuals to stay clean really pays dividends, even if it necessitates a little bit of extra repetition along the way. Ultimately, these training activities solidify the returns on WASH interventions, so people continue practicing healthy habits to protect against disease associated with poor water quality, and thereby establish overall public health resiliency (The Water and Sanitation Program, 2011; WaterAid Australia, 2011).

13.2.2. Strategies Employed by NGOs in Water Interventions

NGOs shake things up when it comes to managing water issues. NGOs tend to involve local people from the very beginning, and they ask them to contribute to designing and implementing WASH programs (Figure 13.6). This participatory approach makes the programs feel like they're truly owned by the community and are what the people require , something that continues to resurface as you observe such interventions. By talking with locals and collecting their opinions, NGOs develop solutions that accommodate local traditions, which in most cases causes the projects to survive longer. It's a nice progression: the more people participate, the more they learn about why clean water and proper hygiene are important, and the resulting education only makes the positive effects even more powerful. Good monitoring and evaluation also have a critical, but sometimes forgotten, role. Most NGOs depend on a combination of pre- and post-project surveys, informal focus groups, and even participatory reviews to observe what's changing in community attitudes and practices toward water and sanitation. Evidence from Bangladesh and other settings tends to suggest that improved water and sanitation conditions can alleviate undernutrition. More often than not, the constant stream of information allows organizations to adjust their approach as issues arise, ensuring that each action—no matter how small—contributes to more robust, more resilient communities. Education also comes into play as a force to be reckoned with. Health initiatives are established not only to educate but to generate true awareness of how water purity, sanitation, and general health are interlinked. When such campaigns are directed at an assortment of various groups, the message is more likely to resonate with them and slowly increase the community's understanding of practicing good hygiene. Points taken from places in South and Southeast Asia and Africa, in general, remind us that one needs to understand who their audience is and how one can find those golden opportunities to guide behavior in a positive direction. By incorporating these educational programs into WASH programs, NGOs demonstrate that addressing water issues is not merely a matter of infrastructure, it's creating an entire environment in which public health can flourish.

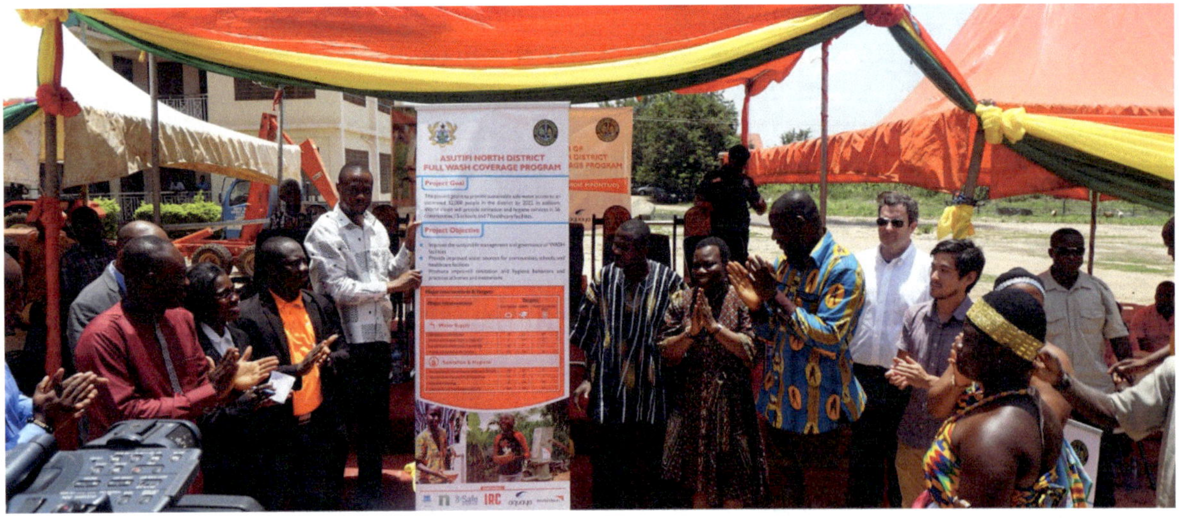

Figure 13.6. Local NGOs to support WASH master plan in Ghana.

Source: Dutch Water Sector (2021). *IRC Asutifi Programme Launch.*

13.2.3. Challenges Faced by NGOs in Implementing Programs

Water and health projects are confronted with a multitude of issues, and NGOs appear to be stuck in a whirlpool of struggles. A significant impediment is the scarcity of resources, which more often than not translates to them being unable to provide consistent, quality services where safe WASH is most important. Political instability and poverty, particularly within sections of Sub-Saharan Africa, fuel the fire, leaving citizens at greater risk of cholera and other water-borne diseases. Inadequate infrastructure only makes things more complicated, further complicating it to deliver assistance where it is required. And then, when emergencies arrive, such as a cholera epidemic, the meager supplies can get stretched almost to breaking point, a condition documented in research on health inequities and intervention effectiveness (Siamalube et al., 2025). Having to work within a complex political and regulatory terrain is another thorn for such organizations. Weak governance in most areas drives NGOs into the quicksand of bureaucracies—adversarial relations with red tape, minimal cooperation from local authorities, and even hostility from governments desperate to preserve sovereignty. Coordination tends to disintegrate among stakeholders, meaning that attempts to improve health outcomes around water end up scattered, and not focused. Political environments can turn on a dime, making long-term plans logistical nightmares; such is the grim reality highlighted in a number of governance and health service delivery evaluations (Abubakar et al., 2022). And then, of course, there is the cultural and social aspect, which brings an added measure of complexity. Some communities resist external intervention, largely out of mistrust or simply because they have different opinions regarding health practices. Gender roles also contribute, especially in regions where girls and women bear the brunt of caregiving. In the end, however, WASH programs' success hinges on knowing what a community values and requires, it's about communication and honest involvement rather than just checking boxes. While programs ignore these cultural subtleties, they jeopardize alienating exactly those individuals they hope to assist, further undermining efforts to reduce waterborne diseases and increase overall health. The answer, therefore, is embracing sensitive strategies that foster actual trust with regional stakeholders (Siamalube et al., 2025).

13.3. Health Education Campaigns

Health education concepts thrown into water-related health initiatives can kick off community awareness and slowly modify behavior (Figure 13.7). When information dissemination is the only objective, such programs assist people in perceiving why proper clean water, sanitation, and daily hygiene are so important. Many times, messages integrate with indigenous culture in a way that individuals feel invested in improving public health. There is even some research that indicates when communities are involved in such campaigns, they remember and act upon the ideas more, ultimately enhancing better well-being. This combination of knowing and doing is particularly significant in locations such as Nigeria, where disparities between cities and rural areas reveal how disproportionate access to clean water and sanitation can be (Abubakar et al., 2022). Health education initiatives are not all about small changes in behavior either; they can trigger dramatic reforms in public health infrastructure. Often, these campaigns partner with NGOs to spearhead local initiatives that do more than promote clean habits – they advocate for long-term access to clean water as well. When these initiatives work in concert, they not only concentrate on a single aspect of the problem but address more general social issues, striving toward equity in all communities. For instance, events taking place in schools or in community centers can enhance awareness of waterborne problems and hygiene, even prompting policy shifts toward improved WASH facilities at times (Sommer et al., 2021).

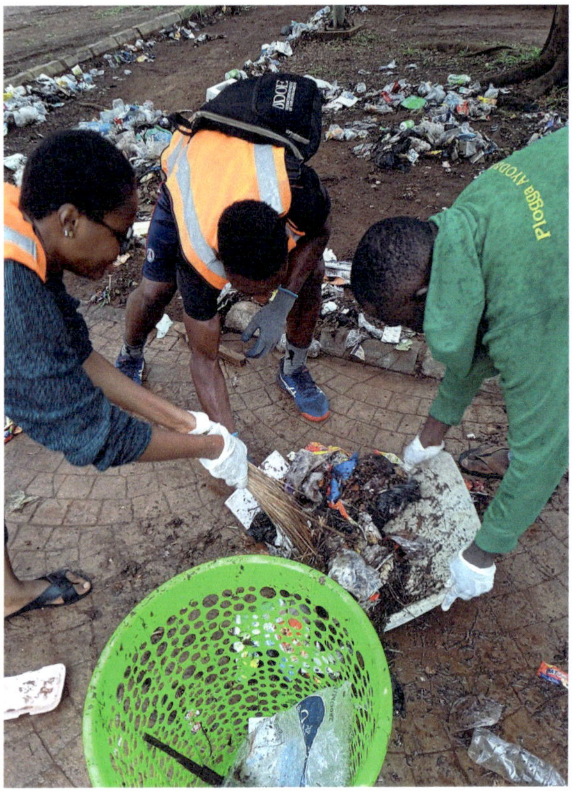

Figure 13.7. Community education campaigns for the prevention of diseases.

Source: By SusuGeo - Own work, CC BY-SA 4.0, https://commons.wikimedia.org/w/index.php?curid=151832393

It really depends on how adaptable these projects are able to be in terms of responding to what individuals genuinely require on the ground. Monitoring progress through frequent checks is another important aspect of making these health initiatives succeed, even if the process isn't always flawless. By keeping a close eye on how well educational concepts are catching on, stakeholders can identify where there are still gaps and adjust their strategy accordingly. This constant, sometimes imperfect, feedback loop not only reinforces what's working but also directs resources where they're needed most. Strong evaluation strategies put a spotlight on behavior change shifts that bring about concrete health gains, driving future planning. In water projects, ongoing monitoring guarantees that at-risk populations are not left behind, addressing issues with access to safe water and adequate sanitation (Abubakar et al., 2022). Ultimately, combining community education, NGO partnership, and regular evaluations creates a fairly solid platform for advancing public health.

13.3.1. Importance of Health Education in Water-Related Health

Clean water and proper sanitation aren't just logistical issues, they strike at the very core of public health. In most cases, access to clean water challenges individuals to re-examine their daily routines, demanding better choices and evasive behavior changes. Health education programs, therefore, become a primary vehicle for disseminating information on the risks of waterborne disease and why cleaning up counts. Through sharing practical information, these projects empower communities to adapt the way they consume water and deal with sanitation on a daily basis. Organizations such as NGOs and government institutions, collaboratively (at times in creative ways), assist in reaching people at the fringes, giving all individuals an opportunity for improved health. For many, learning big about water safety ultimately closes health disparities created through inadequate access, paving the way for long-term community wellness. Health classes focused on water problems can modify day-to-day activities, which is quite significant. Consider simple things such as handwashing with soap, keeping drinking water safe, or using proper sanitation facilities—each one helps reduce the spread of infections. Campaigns based on these concepts, frequently conducted by organizations that specialize in

WASH, increase not only awareness but also a sort of public health consciousness. These programs combine what individuals know with what they do, so that education on water safety flows by proxy into daily habits. This type of program demonstrates, quite obviously, the strength of health education in bringing about lasting, sustainable change. Monitoring and refining these education programs only makes their effectiveness more apparent. In the majority of instances, frequent assessment and public input ensure that both the good points and the weak areas of various approaches, are identified, and subsequently decision-makers are able to modify approaches based on actual facts. The relentless process, though at times a little bit challenging, is such that learning resources are constantly redone to fit what people really require. Combined with constant local involvement, it supports the broader public health efforts associated with water concerns. And, perhaps remarkably, discussions regarding menstrual equity and reproductive health make it clear that sometimes these initiatives must tackle some very particular concerns that disproportionately impact women and the most vulnerable communities. Ultimately, effective health education is a fundamental component of an integrated strategy meant to improve public health through wiser water-based interventions.

13.3.2. Methods of Delivering Health Education

Good health education isn't a tidy afterthought, it alters how communities approach water safety and sanitation (Figure 13.8). The community members become engaged in hands-on workshops where talking about sanitation and hygiene becomes something you do, rather than something you hear. Community leaders and local NGOs get involved naturally, filling in that gap between textbook science and the people's everyday habits.

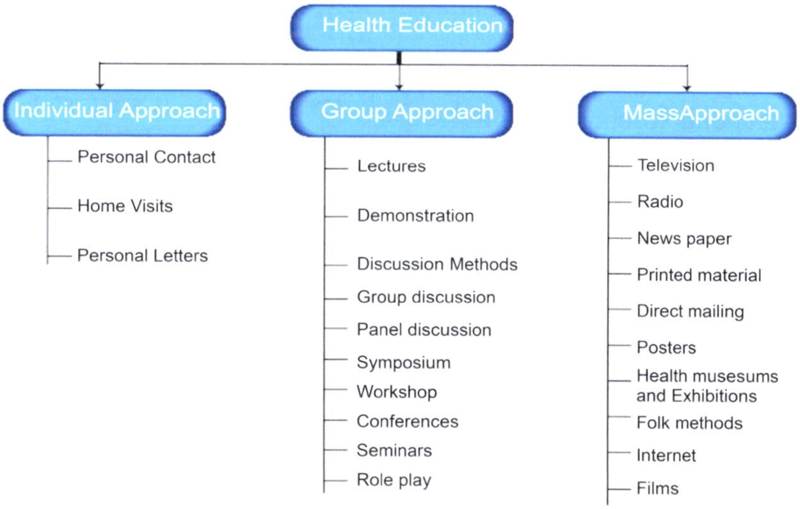

Figure 13.8. Health education.

Source: Gyan Sanchay. (2022). *Health Education Methods.*

It's most often in local languages and with materials that just resonate with people, so the message takes. Workshops blend interactive dialogue with hands-on demos, making it all feel easy while still conveying the major points. And then there's the entire media aspect of it.

Health messages regarding WASH appear on posters, are passed around on social media, or spoken of over the radio, particularly in waves where technology is limited. Radio shows, for instance, are a wonder in rural regions, reaching individuals who don't read that well, and the storytelling there is what makes the lessons resonate emotionally. Now and again community feedback in the form of surveys or local debates gets through some extra nuance, pushing these campaigns to gradually get even better over time. Keeping track of what works, and doesn't, is part of this complicated equation. By visiting different health education projects, organizations can identify what works best and where they are lacking; this is especially the case in challenging settings such as conflict zones where loopholes in water and hygiene programs appear evidently (Als et al., 2020). Most often, pilot projects, such as those where hygiene promotion is integrated with vaccination campaigns (Velleman et al., 2013), are test runs prior to when ideas are implemented at a larger level. Such continuous, in-the-field review assists teams in refining strategies so that they are better able to respond to changing needs and desires of their communities.

13.3.3. Evaluation of the Effectiveness of Health Education Campaigns

Assessing health education campaigns is crucial in determining whether or not they modify the behavior of individuals and improve overall health. Rather than adhering to a tidy checklist, one may observe how people interact, retain information, and slowly modify their behaviors over time. Frequently a great campaign employs culturally attuned messages packed in with real community participation to induce the content to resonate with different groups in different ways. Overall, the more messages resonate with the local culture, the greater the chance people will adopt healthy habits that, by extension, reduce waterborne diseases. Routine monitoring using transparent metrics allows organizations to refine their strategies, which in most instances also makes a compelling case for continued funding and support (Critchley et al., 2020).

A good monitoring system for tracking and following up on these endeavors frequently produces surprises regarding the long-term returns from health education. It can combine both numbers-based (quantitative) measures and personal (qualitative) understanding, such as observing how well ideas catch on over months or years, and whether or not behavior change lasts. Feedback loops, when applied, even enable on-the-fly adjustments during a campaign's execution, ensuring the content remains current and useful.

At other times, combining various approaches—perhaps surveys with informal interviews—offers more nuanced information about the way people act and become involved with health information. The conclusions don't just refine what is happening today but also inform how things are formed in future projects, initiating a process of perpetual improvement (Farrand et al., 2019). Collaborating with a diverse set of players is another essential part when it comes to assessing health education projects. Collaborating together, whether with government agencies, NGOs, or local civic leaders, tends to increase trust and exposure in unusual ways.

Those types of collaborations assist in overcoming daily challenges, making sure that the educational content reaches channels people already have faith in, even if things get a little complex along the way at times. In most instances, arm-in-arm with neighborhood influencers or community organizations can add momentum to a campaign, creating a feeling of local stewardship over health decisions. Co-shared responsibility for evaluation fosters greater organic transparency and accountability, opening the door to sustainable enhancement in public health initiatives (Critchley et al., 2020).

13.4. Monitoring and Evaluation in Public Health

Water health initiatives rely heavily on effective monitoring and evaluation systems that enable individuals to see the effects of what is being achieved. In WASH programs, that is, WASH, M&E is not merely about data crunching; it is a snapshot of what does and does not work, informing funders and communities where they are (Figure 13.9). For instance, a good M&E system will not just verify whether access to clean water is increasing but also record changes in waterborne disease and general community health. At other times, local NGOs and public health professionals conduct these reviews, allowing actual data to inform alterations without relying on intuition; this means interventions last longer and even attract additional support when gaps are identified. Overall, data collection and winnowing out is the beginning of learning and adjusting public health practice, even if it's a little rough around the edges.

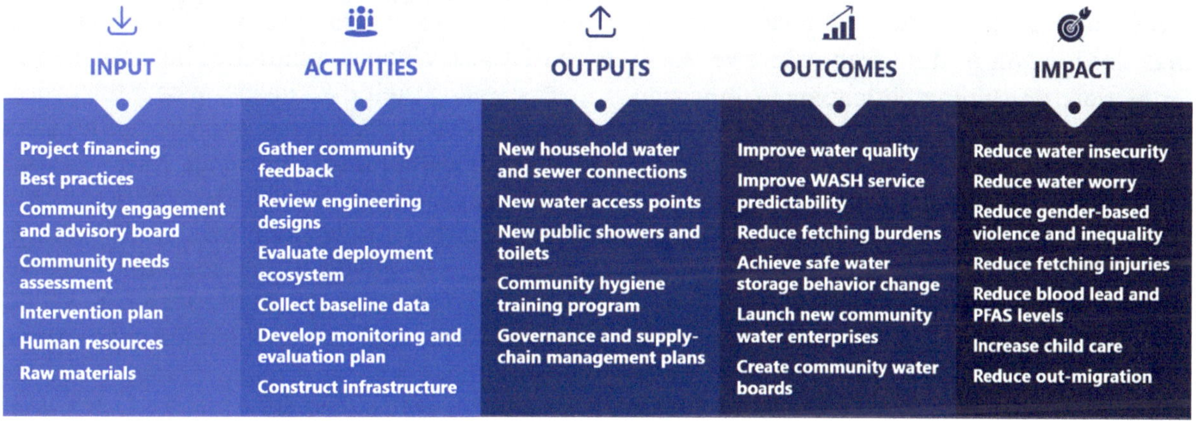

Figure 13.9. Hypothetical logic model of a WASH intervention with examples of human-centered impacts beyond microbiological indicators.

Source: Cumming, O., et al. (2023). *Measuring Transformative WASH: A New Paradigm for Evaluating Water, Sanitation, and Hygiene Interventions*. WIREs Water, 10(1), e1674. https://doi.org/10.1002/wat2.1674.

Local participation in these appraisals is absolutely essential—nearly without fail. Getting local people into the process isn't done as a tokenistic exercise; it ensures interventions address local priorities and honor cultural idiosyncrasies. When locals assist in monitoring how programs are functioning, they not only feel a sense of ownership but also increase the possibility of sustained change in water usage, sanitation practices, and hygiene education. Community-based assessments tend to elicit those nuanced social dynamics plain numbers may overlook, making sense of why people act as they do. This experiential learning can empower all participants and, candidly, create more responsible and adaptable health programs. And when feedback is coming in continuously, it's simple to modify programs at the moment as the community needs change. And then there's technology—a true game-changer today. Technology such as mobile health applications and intelligent data analytics can bring M&E in public health to the next level with its capacity to record and dissect data in real-time, especially important when dealing with water-related concerns. Where conventional monitoring strategies may not be effective, technology provides new avenues of monitoring data in different areas and even between differing socio-economic categories. This technology-led change not only causes programs to be more effective but also aligns seamlessly with larger objectives such as advancing gender equity and enhancing health literacy. In all but a few instances, combining technological innovation with a community-oriented approach provides a more complete, richer description of how truly effective these interventions are, ultimately leading to improved health outcomes across the board.

13.4.1. Importance of Monitoring and Evaluation in WASH Programs

WASH efforts rely heavily on solid monitoring and evaluation, they're sort of the secret ingredient driving actual progress. Data collection and analysis indicate where it's working and where it's not, which in most instances assists decision-makers in keeping projects aligned with public health objectives. An effective M&E system can reveal areas of service shortages so resources can be directed more effectively. Consider the Conrad N. Hilton Foundation, for instance; more than 20 years of continuous attention to safe water access have taught them valuable lessons regarding the importance of robust partnerships and enduring, supportive engagement in WASH efforts (Nagpal, 2012). Without a regular routine of evaluation, the overall impact tapers off and it's much more difficult to push forward on improvement in community health. A well-designed M&E system does more than simply count impacts, it also establishes accountability across all parties, from local NGOs to government agencies. In most instances, regular checks of outcomes maintain everyone on schedule and dedicated to their objectives. This concept aligns with USAID's attempt to improve water quality and sanitation throughout numerous regions, as indicated within their 2013–2018 Water and Development Strategy (The Water and Sanitation Program, 2011; WaterAid Australia, 2011). Effective monitoring mechanisms serve to spotlight success as well as challenges, thereby increasing transparency and establishing trust in stakeholder engagement demands. Also, the inherent feedback loop of consistent assessment can prod program adjustments so that health education campaigns truly resonate with a diverse set of communities. Ultimately, maintaining that ever-present cycle of monitoring and evaluation is crucial to the long-term viability of WASH initiatives. When communities become involved in assessing their own needs, even if the process is somewhat disorganized, it promotes an actual sense of ownership over local water supplies and sanitation infrastructure. With good M&E, people better know their own health and are more able to advocate for necessary changes. This sort of participatory approach, by and large, aligns with worldwide efforts to support self-reliance and resilience among poor and vulnerable groups. Overall, a targeted assessment not only heightens program performance but also intensifies community involvement, which is essential for sustainable public health impact.

13.4.2. Tools and Methodologies for Effective Evaluation

Water health projects appear to rely on the quality of our verification of what they do and how they do it. Too often, researchers blend hard data, such as water quality measures and overall health results, with local residents' personal input and community voices. This type of methodology, in many instances, isn't merely a matter of the numbers; it also catches on to those fine details of day-to-day application that conventional techniques may overlook. At times, techniques pilfered from, for example, early childhood development are adapted to guard over health interventions, identifying those critical junctures where intervention may need adjustment. And remember, leveraging technology such as mobile data collection can bring immediate feedback, allowing teams to make real-time adjustments to keep progress rolling (Kosenchuk & Tarnavska, 2024). Outcome measurement tools also figure prominently in how WASH programs are measured. It's not just about tallying instances of disease prevention but also observing community participation and changes in the way people use water. For example, longitudinal studies comparing populations with improved sanitation and populations without can support evidence for impact. Based on concepts in environmental education—eco-literacy and even naturalistic intelligence, some argue, can softly turn around community perception of water conservation and sanitation. By establishing clear targets and measuring actual indicators, health agencies have a better sense of how these programs translate into healthier communities, ultimately resulting in wiser resource utilization and data-driven policy-making decisions (Setyaningsih et al., 2024). Involving local communities, NGOs, and government agencies in the assessment process provides a level of ownership and responsibility that truly pays off in the long run. When members of the community contribute to defining and administering how these programs will be measured, the data will more likely be richer and more representative of actual life situations. This interactive process ultimately closes the gap between strictly technical evaluations and the day-to-day realities of residents, resulting in programs that are both culturally appropriate and effective. Having workshops or casual focus groups can also generate useful debate, combining qualitative findings with the raw numbers, and providing a richer understanding of how water-and-health interventions could be refined to benefit everyone more (Kosenchuk & Tarnavska, 2024).

13.4.3. Case Studies Highlighting Successful Monitoring Practices

Monitoring has an enormous role in demonstrating the performance of water health programs, particularly in WASH programs. A USAID/Ethiopia, for instance, assessment looks closer at the Millennium Water Alliances (MWA) activities in 28 districts (Figure 13.10). The report indicates that even as water access and sanitation experienced perceptible improvements, a short planning time frame frequently disrupted long-term behavior changes in communities. More often than not, this would be achieved by transitioning to longer-term strategies so these changes truly take hold. There's also an unmistakable message about increasing investment in research and development and aligning methods with what people broadly acknowledge as best practices. Overall, this case is a reminder that measuring isn't merely about tallying outcomes, it's about monitoring outcomes over time to ensure health gains stick (Aregai et al., 2008). Combining various approaches to development also appears to be important for advancing effective health interventions. According to a report based on 17 countries' case studies, where primary care, clean water, and adequate nutrition are combined, overall program impact skyrockets. What researchers find is that multi-element strategies tend to bind communities together while enhancing overall health in a balanced manner. Most experts believe that these mix-and-match strategies address the complex interdependencies of disease and poverty more effectively than stand-alone efforts could. Integrated programming such as this requires monitoring systems to watch how various components of a program relate to one another and how stakeholders receive an accurate picture of both individual and combined impact. If you examine all of these case studies, the evidence truly supports integrated programming in public health (The Water and Sanitation Program, 2011; WaterAid Australia, 2011). Constructing good monitoring and evaluation systems is also important in understanding what these WASH programs translate to in real life. Several case studies highlight that utilizing customized metrics, one that suits the particular challenge and context of each community—results in data that are actionable. When monitoring practices are aligned with the local context, the insights that emerge can be far more useful. For example, a lot of successful projects included community feedback mechanisms to test the acceptance of health messages socially; these findings then informed ongoing education campaigns. This adaptive, flexible style not only makes programs more effective but allows individuals to feel more invested in the process. Finally, maintaining an ongoing, responsive evaluation process is necessary for sincerely sustainable water-related health gains (Aregai et al., 2008; The Water and Sanitation Program, 2011; WaterAid Australia, 2011).

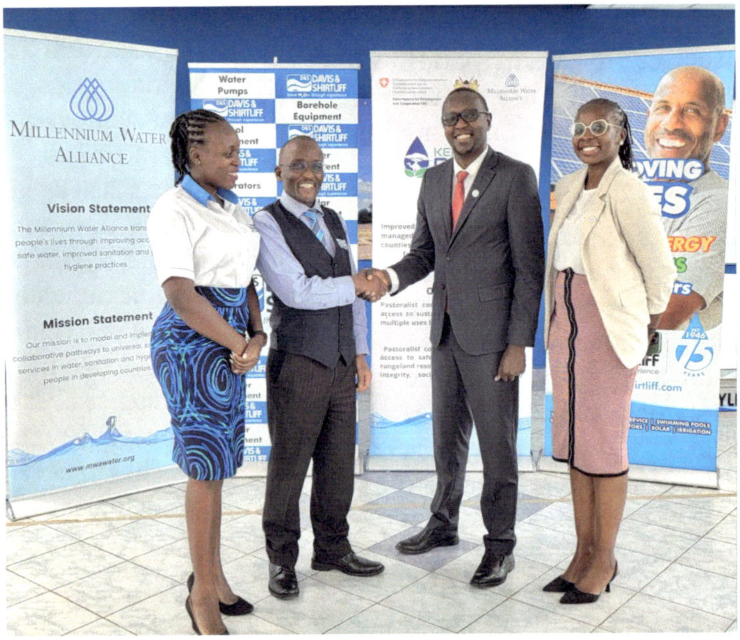

Figure 13.10. Millennium Water Alliances (MWA).

Source: https://pbs.twimg.com/media/F3KOFm1agAAPz8s.jpg.

13.5. Community Involvement and Engagement

Community engagement truly shines when addressing waterborne health problems. Local associations, government departments, and NGOs tend to come together in a manner that provides a huge impetus to WASH initiatives—that's WASH in plain language. At times such agencies serve as vital conduits, mobilizing resources and raising awareness of risks associated with inadequate facilities. You can witness it in action in areas such as the Kallakurichi District of Tamil Nadu; schools there have experienced noticeable improvement in student health and overall performance after the community became involved. For the most part, addressing local needs directly translates to strategies that stick and contribute toward enhancing day-to-day hygiene practices (Anushya & Subramaniyan, 2024). Combining health education campaigns with a community approach can truly make all the difference. If people assist in planning and implementing these campaigns, the messages, of course, become more relatable and accessible—health information just seems better understood. Research tends to indicate that when locals are involved in creating their own health messages, those messages resonate more strongly with everyone else. For instance, efforts in collaboration with organizations such as UNICEF have established that incorporating community input into hygiene promotion can enhance adherence to healthy behaviors. Such dynamic interactions establish trust and lead to communities being responsible for their own health, which is quite remarkable in general (Murphy, 2009). Sustained success for WASH programs depends heavily on maintaining community involvement, despite this component being neglected at times. NGOs have to deal with challenges such as limited finances and bureaucratic barriers, which highlights the significance of solid, grassroots networks. These networks tend to offer consistent feedback that assists in refining water and sanitation activities. When government authorities, NGOs, and locals collaborate, what is required is a multi-layered strategy to reduce barriers. Further, when people begin to claim a program as their own, they remain committed for longer, this ownership is, in most instances, paramount to maintaining health interventions effective and sustainable (Anushya & Subramaniyan, 2024).

13.5.1. Role of Community Participation in WASH Programs

Community engagement is really at the center of WASH initiatives, those initiatives working on WASH. When locals get involved right from the start, they feel a sense of ownership that persists, taking care of water and sanitation resources in a lasting manner. For instance, the MWA initiatives in Ethiopia demonstrate how combining local expertise with international concepts can truly disrupt. Engaging the community does not only enhance the access to safe water and good sanitation, but it also shares healthier hygiene practices. Short-term thinking often tends to hold things back, according to some assessments, which usually implies continued, grassroots action (Aregai et al., 2008). And, too, when individuals are involved in decision-making, it provokes behavioral changes that are quite important to public health in these programs. Local residents involved in the process are more likely to implement practices that enhance sanitation and hygiene in general (and, honestly, that's a win-win). This type of participation even extends to health education, increasing day-to-day awareness about why mindful water use and sanitation are important. In Bangladesh, a study indicates a strong link between solid WASH behaviors and improved nutrition outcomes and suggests that scaling up in these programs can impact public health issues at large (Mahmud & Mbuya, 2016).

Collaborating, communities devise means to manage their own particular issues, keeping WASH activities both culturally attuned and effective. Adding community perspectives to the mix also raises the stakes with regard to monitoring and fine-tuning WASH projects. Training local people to assist in collecting and checking data not only accesses knowledge that may otherwise go unnoticed but also flags areas where things require tweaking. This approach empowers those on the ground while allowing managers to be adaptable—shifting gears when necessary. Looking over the MWA projects, it seems that developing local capacity—be it through on-the-job training or improved resource backing, can foster collaborative partnerships between community groups, NGOs, and government agencies. Ultimately, it's not merely about presence; true community engagement is what propels sustained health outcomes improvement through WASH programs (Aregai et al., 2008).

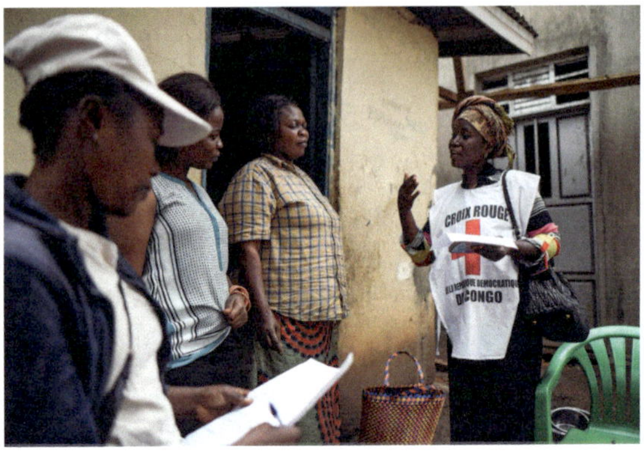

Source: Butler, C. (2023). *Community Engagement and Accountability Activities in DR Congo*. Prepare Center.

13.5.2. Strategies for Enhancing Community Engagement

Community involvement in water health initiatives begins with creating real connections between various groups. Collaborating with locals, NGOs, and even government stakeholders harnesses the know-how and capacities that make WASH projects succeed. Consider NGOs and CSOs–they're the ones energizing community backing and spreading the word on clean water and quality sanitation in homes and schools. In Tamil Nadu's Kallakurichi District, local NGOs have demonstrated in a very concrete fashion how local participation can catalyze shifts in WASH facilities, improving health benefits and even pushing up school enrollment (Anushya & Subramaniyan, 2024). This whole-hog intervention not only suits local priorities but also lingers on, making individuals feel as if they own the transformation. Health education initiatives also provide a strong impetus to the way communities mobilize. When people are made aware of the importance of hygiene, availability of clean water, and sanitation, they come to realize the danger of badly maintained facilities and, in most instances, demand better amenities in their own communities. At the Paths Forward for the Global WASH Sector conference, individuals spouted about the necessity for innovative measures to raise awareness and put the problems in front of more eyes (The Water and Sanitation Program, 2011; WaterAid Australia, 2011). Participatory workshops, youth-attracting programs, and even active social media discussions all blend to create a sort of open discussion — one that tends to attract community support for WASH initiatives. All the while, monitoring progress makes a huge difference too. When the community pitches in to assist with evaluations, it lays the foundation for candid commentary and trust-building, even when it reveals inconvenient glitches along the way. Community-driven reviews not only identify what works and what doesn't but also permit rapid adjustments when something goes wrong. Insights gained in these sessions ensure that existing plans are bettered and even lay the groundwork for upcoming projects. Several speeches have indicated that to maintain WASH programs on course, an on-going check-and-adjust process is necessary (The Water and Sanitation Program, 2011; WaterAid Australia, 2011). Finally, intermingling teamwork, education, and a bit of reality-checking is the key to making water-related health initiatives endure.

13.5.3. Impact of Community Involvement on Program Success

Community engagement is a major factor in helping water-health projects succeed. When the locals join in, there's an actual sense that the improvements are their own, and the strategies can organically integrate into the special way each community lives and thinks. Usually, when individuals feel personally engaged, the new routines stick much longer, producing outcomes that take hold over time. Use the Conrad N. Hilton Foundation's activities in West Africa as a case in point, it's there that building smart partnerships really maximizes the use of WASH money, as local people's input informs what the projects can do and how they're managed (Nagpal, 2012). In most instances, these community-led approaches not only maximize participation but lead to a form of continuous improvement cycle that continually streamlines outcomes. Local involvement also has a tendency to increase cooperation and trust among all stakeholders involved, particularly when designing educational campaigns about health and sanitation.

It may be self-evident, but when there are government agencies and NGOs chasing wide health objectives, the grassroots wisdom of community voices frequently alters the way these initiatives are perceived, sometimes in unexpected manners. A report usually states that the combination of various ideas for development – particularly in areas that strike at the very center of public health such as clean water and nutrition – can raise program success (The Water and Sanitation Program, 2011; WaterAid Australia, 2011).

By combining local know-how with professional designs, projects stand a better chance of addressing the actual underlying issues, cutting down on such problems as waterborne diseases and poor sanitation procedures. There's also the recurring issue of having community members stay vigilant and provide feedback on health projects.

Their constant input, informed by day-to-day experiences, makes the entire process much more open and accountable. This sort of feedback loop not only provides individuals with voice but also stimulates adaptable management approaches—something that's fairly vital for responsive public health practice. With everyone discussing freely, it's easier to identify both successes and glitches in the moment, making it easy to quell them if necessary. Ultimately, incorporating local views into the way programs are evaluated serves to build trust and makes these health programs both contextual and effective in the long term.

13.6. Policy and Governance

Water health interventions take a variety of forms and require pragmatic policies and efficient regulation. WASH programs—that combination of WASH—require clear guidance to function optimally. In certain cases, there is local government distribution of resources and collaboration of a combination of NGOs and public agencies, so a type of hands-on government becomes necessary. One must avoid duplicating efforts and, bluntly, ensure that everything meshes. Clear governance creates accountability and citizen trust, which then increases community engagement and assists individuals in remaining with sustainable changes, particularly where resources are limited. Examining ongoing projects demonstrates how policy influences everyday success. For instance, assessments of MWA in a number of districts showed enhanced water and sanitation access, although short-term agendas occasionally stifle sustainable change. Generally, the reviewers indicate that planning for the long term and applying strong indicators is central; one set of assessments had this explicitly highlighted (Aregai et al., 2008). Merging these findings into policy is not only likely to improve WASH activities but also link them more closely with broader health and education policies, forming a usable and cohesive strategy. At the center of every effective WASH initiative is the combination of governance and community participation, particularly through health education campaigns. These campaigns are daily avenues for conveying the significance of safe water, solid sanitation, and consistent hygiene practices: even if the underlying messages do end up being presented in different ways throughout the community. Evidence indicates that intelligent, at times less tense communication can assist populations in becoming effectively informed and result in enhanced health results in areas where undernourishment is prevalent due to low-quality WASH conditions. A systematic review highlighted a considerable gap between sanitation and nutrition, and it was shown that focused policies can contribute to tangible change (Mahmud & Mbuya, 2016). Where water and nutrition targets come together, governments are able to encourage a model that blends health education, infrastructure improvements, and people empowerment, all of which enhance a stronger public health system.

13.6.1. Overview of Policies Affecting Water-Related Health Interventions

Health impacts in populations tend to rest on the combination of water programs and health policy. You see that when countries highlight WASH, it gets better for people who are most vulnerable to waterborne disease. There's loads of research, even research that indicates more access to water reduces nutrition issues in populations where poverty is such that basic needs just aren't provided (Mahmud & Mbuya, 2016).

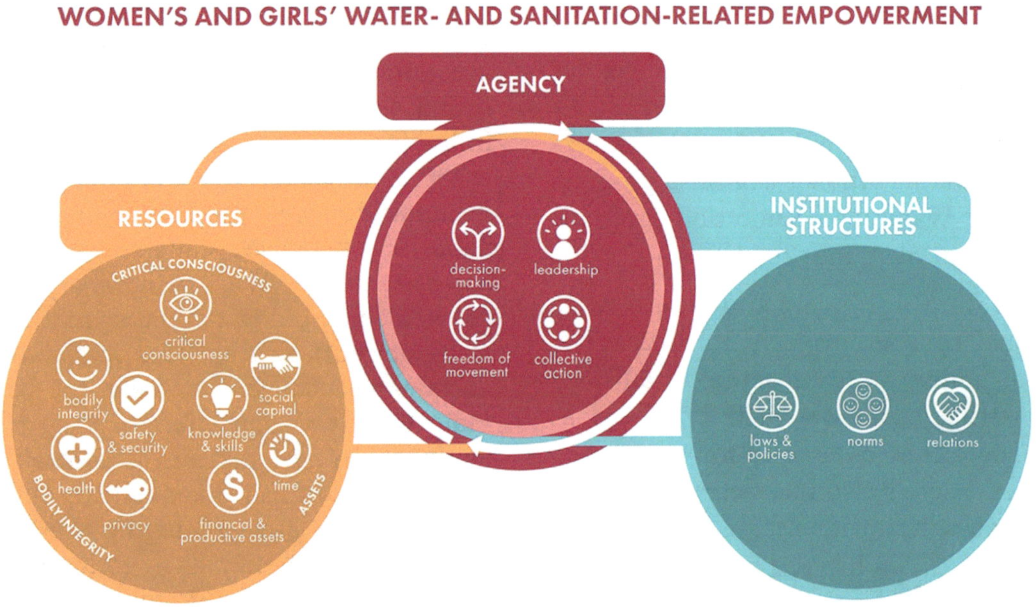

Figure 13.11. Relationship between the domains and sub-domains of women's and girls' water and sanitation-related empowerment.

Source: Doma, R., et al. (2023). *An Exploration of Sanitation-Related Decision-Making, Leadership, Collective Action, and Freedom of Movement Among Women in Urban Tiruchirappalli, India. Frontiers in Water, 5*, Article 1048772. https://doi.org/10.3389/frwa.2023.1048772.

It would appear that creating policies to support these water initiatives is truly important to maintaining communities intact and their health viable. When crises occur and individuals become displaced, the combination of water policies becomes increasingly complicated. Attaining care in these instances is not easy; there tend to be significant access barriers that complicate relief efforts (Santos et al., 2024). Leaders thus struggle to balance immediate humanitarian response with the compulsion to establish medium- and long-term water and sanitation arrangements. Balancing fast fixes with durable infrastructure could quite possibly improve how WASH programs function, so that displaced communities receive not just emergency care but assured access to vital services as well. It is also important to verify if these water-health policies perform and adjust as needs evolve. By monitoring the performance of WASH projects, stakeholders can collect the type of data that informs and refines policies in the process. This regular review is not simply about statistics, it indicates where water management intersects with public health in a more comprehensive way and even illustrates where these service gaps manifest across various groups. Briefly, through continually refining policies and leveraging a well-crafted monitoring system, communities can accumulate resilience to future health threats, even if the process isn't necessarily tidy and neat (Figure 13.11).

13.6.2. Role of Government in Supporting WASH Initiatives

Encouraging long-term public health ultimately depends on the extent to which governments become actively engaged in WASH initiatives. They begin by investing and establishing pragmatic guidelines—initiatives that can improve program success in the most unlikely ways. These organizations often serve to bridge, bringing together NGOs and local groups even when interests are fragmented. Collaboration of this sort is quite central in dealing with the numerous layers of health challenges relating to water. In most instances, their leadership is not only ensuring money comes through but also about basing projects within realities on the ground. An example is the West Africa Water Initiative, where partnerships appear to double both financial incentives and human energy (Nagpal, 2012). Beyond just funding and coordination, there's also a big role for governments in raising awareness and promoting proper hygiene practices. You'll find that comprehensive health education campaigns often sprout from government actions that are meant to clear up common misconceptions about water and sanitation. When agencies dish out clear, sometimes plainspoken, evidence-based info, community engagement naturally follows and gradually ushers in some healthy behavior changes. It's often the tracking of these initiatives, though, that introduces changes as fresh data and feedback come in, fostering that trust and accountability in WASH projects (The Water and Sanitation Program, 2011; WaterAid Australia, 2011). Policymaking introduces yet one more layer to this equation. Governments can enact legislation intended to provide a level playing field for access to water and sanitation for all, particularly those most vulnerable. By establishing long-term structures and supporting investments in key infrastructure, these agencies create the kind of ecosystem where WASH efforts succeed. And then there's when policies also prod the private sector to think out of the box, and it all comes together in synergistic ways. All things considered, when governments intervene in such areas as regulation, distribution of resources, and policy-making, they set the stage for a healthier populace, demonstrating the extent to which good governance works its way into better public health outcomes.

13.6.3. Importance of Multi-Sectoral Collaboration

Water-related health issues aren't a single-note issue, they challenge us to think beyond the normal confines. Rather than attempting to address things in isolation, health, environmental and educational groups must come together. Consider WASH programs, for instance; these are an actual pillar of public health. When different sectors chip in with their own strengths and resources, they can whip up strategies that tackle the many layers of these issues. In most instances, this type of collaboration not only streamlines service provision but also boosts health outcomes, mirroring paradigms that take care of human, animal, plant and environmental threats – just like in the One Health Joint Plan of Action rolled out by a number of prominent bodies. Another aspect of the equation addresses deeply ingrained social factors such as the stigma of menstrual health. Public policies are essential, but they usually have a hard time dismantling the norms that sustain shame and stigma. It's necessary to see, more broadly, that an array of determinants influences the way individuals perceive and manage menstruation in larger health initiatives. When health, education and gender advocacy work come together, a more holistic approach naturally emerges, one that doesn't merely pursue tangible health outcomes but also pushes the attitudes of society to shift. Well-planned education campaigns, for instance, have the potential to empower individuals with both the information and self-assurance necessary to speak openly about menstrual health and to eliminate barriers that prevent girls and women from accessing necessary health services (Mary et al., 2022). And then there's the entire matter of ensuring these partnerships really deliver through effective monitoring and evaluation. Implementing mechanisms to monitor progress not only holds everyone accountable but also stimulates continuous learning, even if the process can sometimes be a little haphazard. Stakeholders from all sectors must evaluate program outcomes, relying on data to determine what's working and where a small adjustment might be required, so they can adjust as health issues change. Combining evidence-based practice with direct policy intervention constructs health programs that, in turn, augment broader public health objectives. Overall, this sort of concerted, cross-sector approach is the most important component of constructing resilient and sustainable health interventions, igniting positive developments that extend far beyond the limits of any single effort.

SUMMARY

Good health relies on clean water, safe sanitation, and adequate hygiene. When those fundamentals fail, severe disease, and even death—may ensue, particularly in the already vulnerable. It is not simply a matter of constructing new facilities; engaging local people can make all the difference. In most instances, research has indicated that communities owning their own WASH initiatives have longer-lasting and more effective programs (Abubakar et al., 2022). NGOs, through initiating local ownership and exchanging useful health advice, contribute to stronger public health systems even though the progress at times seems somewhat uneven. Health education continues to gear up, and that is significant. Consider big crises such as the COVID-19 pandemic; simple, easy-to-understand explanations of risk truly come into play at those times. A number of African countries, for instance, illustrate how small changes to messages to resonate with local cultural differences create quicker, more effective responses. People tend to see that when the voice of a community is blended in with professional guidance, issues such as mistrust and disinformation are addressed more head-on (Adebisi et al., 2021). Generally speaking, crafting these messages in a tailored manner, sometimes restating key ideas in fresh terms, seems to plug holes left by more generic campaigns. Overall, addressing waterborne health problems is not a one-trick pony. Lasting public health progress arises from combining sound WASH enhancements with genuine community participation and ongoing data-informed check-ins. When government offices, NGOs, and ordinary community members all contribute, the opportunity for equitable, sustained progress increases. If we continue to concentrate on both physical infrastructure and social aspects of health, we're making vital strides toward bridging disparities and constructing healthier futures (Abubakar et al., 2022).

Water, sanitation, and nutrition are coming into their own as public health protagonists. Individuals are realizing that when communities have improved access to WASH, issues such as undernutrition ease up, with overall health improving. An examination of a range of research, one even highlighting achievements in Bangladesh (Mahmud & Mbuya, 2016)—demonstrates that where water and sanitation interventions reduce waterborne diseases, the most at-risk, including children and pregnant women, receive a welcome respite. In most instances, integrating WASH with nutrition approaches allows health interventions address issues from so many facets, sometimes from unanticipated directions. NGOs also have a major role to play in making WASH programs available, particularly in areas left behind. Most NGOs partner with local organizations to implement services that truly align with what each community requires, enhancing the chances of participation and sustainability. For instance, a fast-track study conducted in Southern Africa that examined WASH and HIV interlinkages mapped out how important it is for various health sectors to collaborate in Lesotho and Mozambique (The Water and Sanitation Program, 2011; WaterAid Australia, 2011). Such organizations typically conduct education campaigns that not only teach but also inspire individuals to adopt better sanitation practices, incrementally creating a true culture of health, one that extends far beyond mere service delivery. Lastly, paying close attention to how water-related interventions are working is something that simply can't be ignored. Ongoing monitoring—sometimes with a few small adjustments to the system—keeps WASH projects on track and responding to emerging public health trends. These repeated checks enable decision-makers to identify gaps in service delivery early, and such forward planning enhances both transparency and accountability. And, additionally, by employing data, public health individuals are able to refine their approaches to better address health emergencies related to water and sanitation. So, when you combine WASH interventions, engaged NGOs, committed health education, and robust evaluation procedures, what you end up with is an expansive approach that propels public health results in the positive direction.

KEY TERMS FROM THIS CHAPTER

- Educational programs
- Good hygiene
- Health education
- Health statistics
- Nutrition initiatives
- Public health consciousness
- Sanitation resources
- Undernutrition
- WASH services
- Water-based problems
- General social equality
- Ground-level data
- Health service
- Health surveillance
- Poverty alleviation
- Sanitation infrastructure
- Stigma
- WASH conditions
- Water health interventions
- Well-planned education campaigns

CLOSER LOOK

CATEGORIES OF DRINKING WATER INTERVENTIONS

Water interventions for drinking can be generally divided into source water protection, point-of-entry treatment, and point-of-use treatment. Source water protection involves the prevention of contamination at the source, point-of-entry treatment deals with water before entry into a household or community, and point-of-use methods are implemented at the end-user level.

1. Source-Based Interventions

- These seek to safeguard or enhance water at source (e.g., springs, wells, surface water).
- Examples: Spring capping, borehole drilling, protected wells, piped water systems.
- Effectiveness: Often successful long term but needs infrastructure, upkeep, and community involvement.

2. Point-of-Use (POU) Interventions

- These treat water at the domestic level.
- Examples: Chlorination, ceramic filters, solar disinfection (SODIS), boiling, bio sand filters.
- Effectiveness: Has been shown to decrease diarrheal disease by 40–50% when used regularly, but adoption and continued use are inconsistent.

3. Distribution and Storage Interventions

- Focus on how water is stored and transported after collection.
- Examples: Safe water containers, narrow-mouthed storage jugs.
- Effectiveness: Helpful in reducing contamination post-collection, especially when combined with hygiene education.

4. Behavioral Interventions

- Educating communities on safe water handling, storage, and sanitation practices.
- Effectiveness: Mixed results; behavior change is difficult to sustain without ongoing support and community buy-in.

5. Integrated WASH (Water, Sanitation, and Hygiene) Programs

- Combine water interventions with sanitation and hygiene promotion.
- Effectiveness: Tend to have the most substantial impact on health outcomes, particularly diarrheal disease, child growth, and school attendance.

References

1. Nelson, S., Drabarek, D., Jenkins, A., Negin, J., & Abimbola, S. (2021). How community participation in water and sanitation interventions impacts human health, WASH infrastructure and service longevity in low-income and middle-income countries: a realist review. *BMJ open*, *11*(12), e053320. https://doi.org/10.1136/bmjopen-2021-053320 (accessed on 14 May 2025).
2. Abubakar, I., Dalglish, S. L., Angell, B., Sanuade, O. A., Abímbọ́lá, Ṣ., Adamu, A. L., Adetifa, I., et al. (2022). The Lancet Nigeria Commission: Investing in health and the future of the nation. *The Lancet, 399*, 1155–1200. https://doi.org/10.1016/s0140-6736(21)02488-0.
3. Adebisi, Y. A., Rabe, A. P. J., & Lucero-Prisno, D. E. (2021). Risk communication and community engagement strategies for COVID-19 in 13 African countries. *Health Promotion Perspectives, 11*, 137–147. https://doi.org/10.34172/hpp.2021.18.
4. Als, D., Meteke, S., Stefopulos, M., Gaffey, M. F., Kamali, M., Munyuzangabo, M., Shah, S., Jain, R. P., Radhakrishnan, A., Siddiqui, F. J., Ataullahjan, A., & Bhutta, Z. A. (2020). Delivering water, sanitation and hygiene interventions to women and children in conflict settings: a systematic review. *BMJ global health*, *5*(Suppl 1), e002064. https://doi.org/10.1136/bmjgh-2019-002064 (accessed on 14 May 2025).
5. Anushya, S., & Subramaniyan, D. J. (2024). Role of NGOs and Civil Society Organizations in Enhancing WASH Facilities in Government Schools: Lessons from Kallakurichi District, Tamil Nadu. *South Eastern European Journal of Public Health*, 1034–1046. https://doi.org/10.70135/seejph.vi.3167(accessed on 14 May 2025).
6. Aregai, B., & Dinku, S. (2008). *External Program Evaluation: Water, Sanitation and Hygiene (WASH) Program in Ethiopia*. https://core.ac.uk/download/71360955.pdf (accessed on 14 May 2025).
7. Chirgwin, H., Cairncross, S., Zehra, D., & Waddington, H. (2021). Interventions promoting uptake of water, sanitation and hygiene (WASH) technologies in low- and middle-income countries: An evidence and gap map of effectiveness studies. *Campbell Systematic Reviews, 17*. https://doi.org/10.1002/cl2.1194.
8. Critchley, H., Babayev, E., Bulun, S. E., Clark, S., Garcia-Grau, I., Gregersen, P. K., Kilcoyne, A., et al. (2020). Menstruation: Science and society. *American Journal of Obstetrics and Gynecology, 223*, 624–664. https://doi.org/10.1016/j.ajog.2020.06.004.
9. Farrand, C., MacGregor, G. A., Campbell, N. R. C., & Webster, J. (2019). Potential use of salt substitutes to reduce blood pressure. *Journal of Clinical Hypertension, 21*, 350–354. https://doi.org/10.1111/jch.13482.
10. Yael Velleman, Katie Greenland, Om Prasad Gautam; An opportunity not to be missed – immunisation as an entry point for hygiene promotion and diarrhoeal disease reduction in Nepal. *Journal of Water, Sanitation and Hygiene for Development* 1 September 2013; 3 (3): 459–466. doi: https://doi.org/10.2166/washdev.2013.085 (accessed on 14 May 2025).
11. Kosenchuk, O. ., & Tarnavska, N. . (2024). Mental Health in Education for Crisis-affected Preschool Children: Multilevel Monitoring. *Mental Health: Global Challenges Journal*, *7*(1), 95–117. https://doi.org/10.56508/mhgcj.v7i1.235 (accessed on 14 May 2025).
12. Mahmud, Iffat, 1982- author.; Mbuya, Nkosinathi, author.; World Bank, issuing body.

13. Washington, DC : International Bank for Reconstruction and Development/The World Bank; 2016

14. Library Catalog ; MMS ID 9916637343406676; ISBN 9781464806988 (paper); NLM Unique ID 101663734(accessed on 14 May 2025).

15. Malik, A. J. (2019). *The Social Construction of Sanitation Technologies: An Analysis of The Technology Selection and Implementation Process in District Mansehra, Pakistan*. https://core.ac.uk/download/197481127.pdf (accessed on 14 May 2025).

16. Murphy, D. F. (2009). *Study on the UNICEF-UNILEVER Partnership for Hygiene Promotion in Primary Schools in Nigeria: Final Report. Study on the UNICEF-UNILEVER Partnership for Hygiene Promotion in Primary Schools in Nigeria: final report.* UNICEF Nigeria, Abuja, Nigeria. (accessed on 14 May 2025).

17. The Water and Sanitation Program (2011). *Handwashing with Soap—Two Paths to National-Scale Programs: Lessons from the Field: Vietnam and Indonesia*. This document was written by Penelope Dutton with contributions from Isabel Blackett, Nga Kim Nguyen, Ida Rafiqah, Wendy Sarasdyani, Minh Hien Nguyen, Amy Lynn Grossman and Almud Weitz. It was peer reviewed by Nathaniel Paynter and Jacqueline Devine. https://core.ac.uk/download/75783149.pdf (accessed on 14 May 2025).

18. WaterAid Australia, International WaterCentre, IRC International Water and Sanitation Centre. (2011). Promoting good hygiene practices: Key elements and practical lessons.(accessed on 14 May 2025).

19. Nagpal, T. (2012). *Providing Access to Safe Water: Lessons Learned from Two Decades of Philanthropic Investment in The Rural Poor*. https://www.wvi.org/publication/providing-access-safe-water-lessons-learned-two-decades-philanthropic-investment-rural (accessed on 14 May 2025).

20. Olson, M. M., Alhelou, N., Kavattur, P. S., Rountree, L., & Winkler, I. T. (2022). The persistent power of stigma: A critical review of policy initiatives to break the menstrual silence and advance menstrual literacy. *PLOS Global Public Health, 2*, e0000070. https://doi.org/10.1371/journal.pgph.0000070.

21. Pedrosa, A. L., Bitencourt, L., Fróes, A. C. F., Cazumbá, M. L. B., Campos, R. G. B., de Brito, S. B. C. S., & Simões e Silva, A. C. (2020). Emotional, behavioral, and psychological impact of the COVID-19 pandemic. *Frontiers in Psychology, 11*. https://doi.org/10.3389/fpsyg.2020.566212.

22. Ross, R., Chaput, J. P., Giangregorio, L., Janssen, I., Saunders, T. J., Kho, M. E., Poitras, V. J., et al. (2020). Canadian 24-hour movement guidelines for adults aged 18–64 years and adults aged 65 years or older: An integration of physical activity, sedentary behaviour, and sleep. *Applied Physiology, Nutrition, and Metabolism, 45*(S57–S102). https://doi.org/10.1139/apnm-2020-0467.

23. Santos, M. S. C. (2024). *Emergency Healthcare Response in Settings of Forcibly Displaced People: A Review*. https://core.ac.uk/download/639872725.pdf (accessed on 14 May 2025).

24. Setyaningsih, D., Handasah, R. R., Mamma, A. T., Krobo, A., Olua, E., & Iryouw, V. (2024). Fostering Eco-literacy and Naturalistic Intelligence through Environmentally Based Education in Coastal Preschool . *JPUD - Jurnal Pendidikan Usia Dini, 18*(1), 251–269. https://doi.org/10.21009/JPUD.181.18 (accessed on 14 May 2025).

25. Siamalube, B., & Ehinmitan, E. (2025). Unmasking the neglected cholera outbreaks in Sub-Saharan Africa. *International Journal of Public Health, 69*. https://doi.org/10.3389/ijph.2024.1607990.

26. Sommer, M., Caruso, B. A., Torondel, B., Warren, E. C., Yamakoshi, B., Haver, J., Long, J. L., et al. (2021). Menstrual hygiene management in schools: Midway progress update on the "MHM in Ten" 2014–2024 global agenda. *Health Research Policy and Systems, 19*. https://doi.org/10.1186/s12961-020-00669-8.

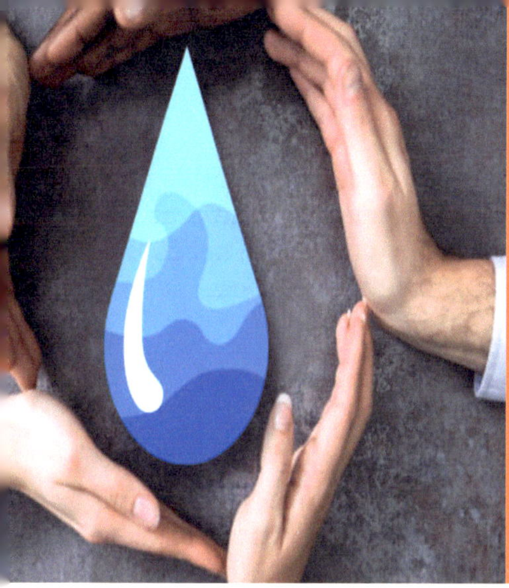

Chapter 14

COMMUNITY-BASED WATER MANAGEMENT AND SUSTAINABILITY

Contents

Introduction

The modern world is faced with a number of water management issues with rapid urbanization, increasing population, and climate change as the most pressing among them. Such pressures call for innovative and sustainable approaches to achieve equal access to clean water, especially in community environments. The idea of community-based water management (CBWM) has been a groundbreaking approach that can help support the participation of local communities in their water management. By engaging local knowledge and resources, the strategy brings sense and ownership at the community level, thus resulting in more sustainable action. Integrating community action with overall Sustainable Development Goals (SDGs) maximizes their reach, especially in settings where conventional management methods have not been able to address the needs of inhabitants. The understanding of the interlinkages of water resource management and community sustainability is critical in addressing current environmental and socio-economic issues. Effective CBWM programs are impressive in the manner they effectively address local requirements as well as environmental conservation. Cooperative models, for instance, have proven to greatly enhance livelihoods while at the same time resolving ecological issues. A good example is the Simbuco Aqua-Marine Multi-Purpose Cooperative (SAMMPC), which not only focused on economic sustainability but also served social inclusivity by enhancing women's involvement in aquaculture and strengthening community unity. The cooperatives' alignment with several SDGs, such as SDG 14 (Life Below Water) and SDG 5 (Gender Equality), demonstrates how concerted efforts can trigger revolutionary change among communities. But with challenges like resource depletion and environmental degradation manifesting the intricacies in balancing development with ecological sustainability, meeting these challenges demands addressing them with a multi-faceted system considering input and participation of multiple stakeholders in the water management process. The success of CBWM is through stakeholder participation, and this is a key factor in promoting project sustainability. This aspect was particularly emphasized in a study carried out in Mavoko Constituency, where social participation and participation were key factors that enhanced the likelihood of maintaining water projects. Through involvement in decision-making by different segments of society, including marginal groups, the projects are likely to be successful. Good planning is also a staple of these participatory approaches, illustrating how the combined strategic effort of local stakeholders can have great dividends. Generally, community engagement, effective stakeholder engagement, and planning are key for long-term success in water management. Addressing challenges and community resilience offer the foundation upon which sustainable water management practices are harmonized both with local needs and international sustainability programs.

Definition of Community-Based Water Management (CBWM)

Community-based water management (CBWM) includes different participatory methods, enabling local communities to own and manage their water resources. Stakeholder involvement is the focus of CBWM, accepting that social, economic, and environmental factors are part of the complex interaction in water management. Combining traditional water management practices with indigenous knowledge, CBWM fosters ownership among the people involved, which ultimately enhances sustainability. This approach aligns with the principles of Integrated Water Resources Management (IWRM), which fosters an inclusive approach that brings together various water-related activities and actors (Heath et al., 2010). By adopting such integration, communities can maintain their respective needs and develop customized solutions and thus improving water quality and quantity, social equity and resilience to climate change. Decentralization of local institutions is one of the characterizing components of CBWM; it focuses on empowering the community to use its water resources in the best possible way. Decentralization facilitates faster decision-making and response to local conditions. The stakeholders in society have a tendency to self-organize into water user associations or cooperatives, which leads to collective practice that reinforces social relations. Second, the system provides accountability and transparency since the local stakeholders participate directly in practicing water management. These governance models can be applied so as to result in better management of water conflicts because the conflict is settled within the local community context as opposed to being settled by third-party regulating authorities

(BSR et al., 2006). Therefore, CBWM not only deals with the issue of water scarcity but also encourages community integration, which is an important aspect of sustainability over time. Implementation of CBWM is slowed down by insufficient financial means, technical ineptness, and differences in levels of support from the government. Communities and local governments may be hampered by out-of-date infrastructure or insufficient training, which could render them incapable of effectively operating water systems. Opposition might also come from local governments or other external groups who are inclined toward central control of water resources. Despite these difficulties, successful programs show that through increased participation, education, and funding, communities can overcome to successfully manage their water resources. Through these challenges and past successes, CBWM has the potential to develop as a strong model for sustainable water management that is consonant with larger aims of environmental protection and social justice (Heath et al., 2010).

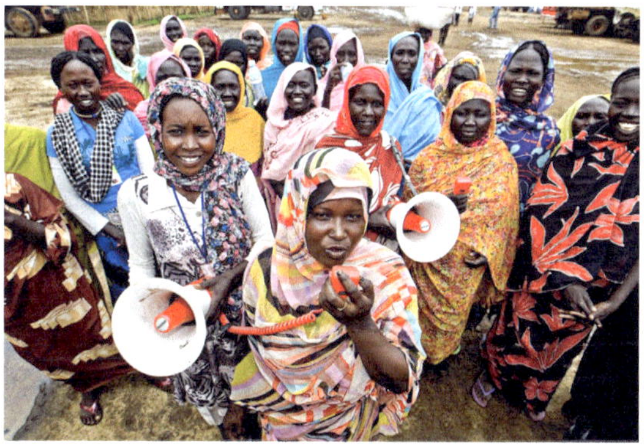

Source: Ferguson, J. (n.d.). *Photograph of women advocating for rights in South Sudan.* Oxfam Novib. https://www.oxfamwash.org/images/f/9/3/4/d/f934d4019e8d486228ee06f7b858582680244a9a-oxfam-novib-zuid-sudan-vrouwenrechten-56071-john-ferguson-oxfam.jpg.

Importance of Sustainability in Water Management

The urgency of building local participation in water management highlights the deep significance of sustainability for community resilience and environmental health. Where possible, traditional knowledge remains vital to effective water resource management, permitting communities to establish sustainable practices adapted to their local conditions. At the local-level scale, in addition to providing optimized use of resources, it enables the owners of the local residents' water systems. With the integration of sustainable principles, communities can mitigate challenges such as climate change, bad infrastructure, and loopholes in policies that threaten their water source. Such integration is vital in the achievement of SDGs, in this case, SDG 6, ensuring availability and sustainable management of water for all, emphasizing the indispensable role of local communities in addressing the pressing needs of global water issues (Ash-Shiddiqie, 2025). Moreover, sustainable water management enhances economic development at the same time as it maintains ecosystems. Approaches like community-based tourism, which integrates local practice and knowledge, illustrate how economic benefits can be generated from sustainable water management. For instance, places like Subak Teba Majelangu in Bali illustrate how native irrigation techniques provide essential water while also supporting eco-tourism and agriculture and thus contributing to the livelihoods of the locals. Such a two-pronged approach reflects the spirit of sustainability, wherein economic growth is harmonized with the conservation of the environment. A focus on equitable distribution of benefits guarantees that the economic gains arising from water management enhance community institutions rather than undermining them. As illustrated, good water governance has to be mindful of economic sustainability in addition to environmental targets, building an integrated framework for community development and resource conservation (Yastini et al., 2024). In tackling the many issues of water scarcity and water management, the need for sustainability is even more critical. Ecological threats such as water quality pollution and over-pumping require adaptation mechanisms that hinge on sustainable strategies. CBWM initiatives are significant forums for such issues to be addressed, paving the way for solutions that find their inception at a grassroots level for grasping ecological development processes. Strategic flexibility is therefore critical in the uncertainty provided by climate change where traditional strategies would not work. Further, they can offer spaces for lobbying as much as for policies so that voices emanating from grassroots sources influence guidelines in governance within a regional context. Finally, the call for water management toward sustainability not only resonates with environmental ends but also supports community resilience against impending adversity, promoting proactive stewardship of precious water resources (Ash-Shiddiqie, 2025).

14.1. Principles of Community-Based Water Management (CBWM)

The growing realization of the need for involvement in water management has rendered CBWM principles more relevant (Figure 14.1). Local communities possess their own close knowledge of their own water resources and the problems that come with them, enabling them to come up with solutions that are appropriate to their own specific situations. By promoting local ownership and accountability, these values invite stakeholders to take active participation in the planning and implementation process, thus promoting sustainability. Effective participation in communities does not merely allow room for improved management processes but also empowers the people to be able to convey their desires and needs. As communities continue to manage water resources, they can rely on local traditions and practices to inform their methods, thus their methods become more culturally adapted and sustainable. Finally, the incorporation of local knowledge into water management activities places the focus on participatory systems that empower community voices and whose participation in decision-making becomes necessary. Collaboration has the leading position in the realm of CBWM since it can coordinate collective action for a variety of actors. Appreciating the compound character of water resources, practitioners build multistakeholder alliances that go beyond customary governance systems. Multistakeholder alliances allow for interaction across different stakeholders, such as government bodies, local communities, NGOs, and private interests, to enhance shared responsibility for the sustainable management of water resources. To this end, it is crucial to create institutionalized systems of governance that will assist in mediating conflicting interests and promoting fair access to water. However, as (Cokburn et al., 2019) have been seen to stress, it is on the identification of contextual issues influencing stakeholder relationships that the success of such collaborative practices is based, including the social, political, and historical dynamics. In bringing these factors together in collaborative systems, CBWM is stronger and fairer. Without resolving the systemic issues that tend to suppress progress, water management will not be sustainable. Financial, infrastructure, and political challenges may stall community efforts, and this necessitates an enabling system. The participation of institutional investors and private institutions can be a turning point, as noted in (United Nations Global Compact, 2015a), by uniting their capacity and expertise with community development. New funding models and investment strategies can allow communities to implement their water management approaches. Also important is to appreciate the social-ecological interplay inherent in water systems, which necessitates adaptive management approaches that can adapt to evolving conditions over time. Adopting a holistic appreciation of water as integral to complex ecosystems supports resilience and sustainability, ultimately culminating in effective community-based projects that can be replicable and scalable in various contexts.

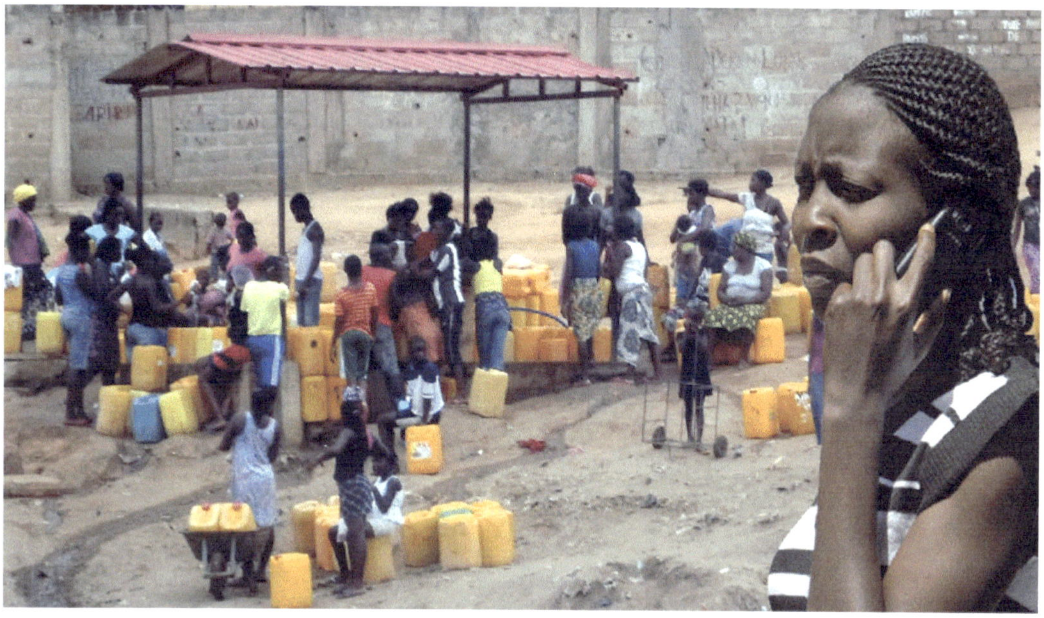

Figure 14.1. Community water management using the mobile-phone-based Vera Agua monitoring system.

Source: Cain, A. (2018). *Community Water Management Using the Mobile-Phone-Based Veraagua Monitoring System.* In *Informal Water Markets and Community Management in Peri-Urban Luanda, Angola. Water International, 43*(2), 248–263. https://doi.org/10.1080/02508060.2018.1447911.

14.1.1. Local Participation and Empowerment

The complex interdependence of empowerment and participation is at the core of effective CBWM programs. The involvement of local people not only ensures ownership but also ensures project sustainability. Ownership tends to produce creative and place-specific solutions to issues in the locale, as evidenced by the adoption of the Sufficiency Economy Philosophy (SEP) in Thailand. Through emphasizing self-sufficiency and communal effort, programs operating on this ideology are a platform where the community members come together to craft adaptation mechanisms for effective management of water resources. Local engagement not only serves to handle water management problems immediately but also develops resilience for the long term against climatic pressures, hence supporting environmental sustainability and economic security (Tanpipat et al., 2024). Apart from promoting innovation, local engagement is also important for the purpose of making sure that various community voices are represented and catered to in decision-making. Water borehole projects in Mavoko Constituency directly point out that stakeholder involvement plays an important role in supporting the sustainability of community-led initiatives. The research showed that active social inclusion raised chances for sustainability by an impressive 5.6 times and that successful planning results also heavily depended on the participation of stakeholders. This underscores the imperative of practitioners to integrate holistic means that facilitate equal participation by various groups of communities, especially the marginalized women and youth. This diversified participation enhances the capacity of local actors to make effective contributions to water management, shaping initiatives responding to community needs and priorities (Machuma et al., 2024). Besides, the empowerment of local communities is not only participation but also includes the capacity-building processes that enable individuals to actively shape and sustain development initiatives. Through training, resources, and education in water management practices, people can learn skills to sustain and manage their water resources. This empowerment is significant in building a sense of responsibility and agency, which allows communities to manage external adversity, including that arising from climatic variability and resource scarcity. Community-led efforts in this instance serve as experimentation laboratories, whereby locals experiment and refine measures most suited to their own situations (Figure 14.2). Therefore, the function of local empowerment and participation in CBWM is not just essential; it is revolutionary, providing avenues for sustainable development and resilience (Machuma et al., 2024; Tanpipat et al., 2024).

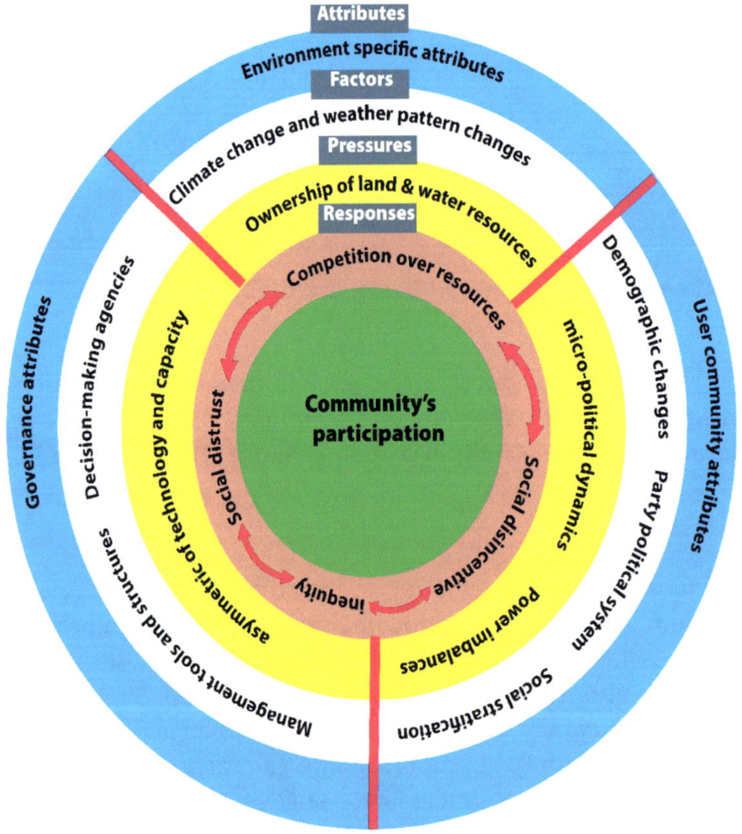

Figure 14.2. A conceptual framework for analyzing the impacting factors of community participation.

Source: Sultana, F., & Thompson, J. (2022). *Barriers in Participative Water Governance: A Critical Analysis of Community Water Management in South Asia. Water, 14*(5), 762. https://doi.org/10.3390/w14050762.

14.1.2. Integrated Resource Management (IRM)

Within modern discourse relating to sustainability, the theory of integrated resource management (IRM) is a critical paradigm that combines multiple resources to produce maximum results (Figure 14.3). The theory focuses on the holistic interrelatedness of environmental, economic, and social factors. IRM aims to simplify processes that regulate resource allocation, especially in water management, by unifying the stakeholders within the community. The move toward CBWM programs—central to sustainable approaches—tends to draw from the philosophy of IRM since it builds local capacity and strengthens the user base through participatory management. Such involvement not only increases community ownership but also promotes enhanced coping with changes in climate and resource availability, consistent with the recommendations of the IPCC, which emphasize the implications of coordinated approaches in developing solutions to enduring environmental issues (Intergovernmental Panel on Climate Change, 2023).

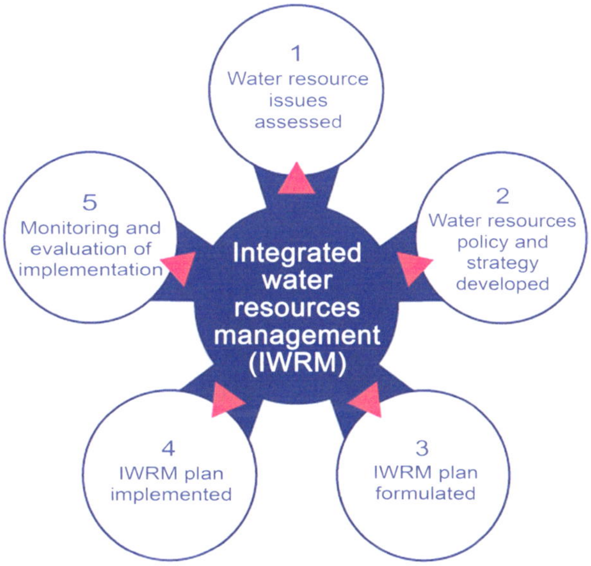

Figure 14.3. Integrated water resource management (IWRM).

Source: Springer Nature. (n.d.). *[Figure 1: Water Quality Monitoring System Schematic]*. In *Water Quality Monitoring and Management: A Global Perspective* (pp. 1–10). https://doi.org/10.1007/978-3-031-62079-9_18.

The benefits of IRM are vast, particularly in addressing the complex demands of local societies in the wake of climate change. Through the incorporation of economic and social considerations into environmental decision-making, IRM creates a sense of shared responsibility that encourages stewardship by local communities. Communities adopting this paradigm can avoid risks from resource deficits and thus build resilience. The economic advantages of renewable resources utilization, as presented in recent literature, show efficiency-technology synergy. Such coordination does not just ensure optimal use of resources but also aligns with climate agendas, thereby significantly reducing greenhouse emissions (Gielen et al., 2019). Hence, the values underlying IRM show how much sustainability can be enabled through localized and community-based systems. Although there are conceivable advantages to the implementation of IRM, its practice has substantial constraints that undermine achievement in community water programs. Interest conflict among the stakeholders, official resistance, and poor data limit integration. In some cases, communities may experience difficulty integrating due to the dilution of group participation when organizational structures are in hierarchical form. In addition, noteworthy differences in resources and capacity can act as hindrances to equal participation. To counter such issues, promoting open channels of communication and putting participatory mechanisms in place are indispensable moves. Through such mechanisms, communities are in a position to make sure different perspectives are considered, improving the effectiveness of their water management regime. By comprehending and reacting to such challenges, communities are in a better position to align their activities toward the overall goals of sustainability, enhancing the resilience of their economies and ecosystems.

14.1.3. Adaptive Management Strategies

Adaptive management practices are central to the development and success of CBWM programs. Through an iterative learning process, these practices enable communities to put policies into place that can be refined using real-time data and results. This method produces resilient water management systems capable of responding well to changing environmental circumstances and shifts in water availability. Through repeated testing and assessment, stakeholders are able to determine which practices work best, and thus maximize the general efficiency of water use while conserving as much as possible. The involvement of stakeholders, prioritized in adaptive management, also promotes local ownership of water resources, evoking a sense of responsibility and commitment to sustainable utilization within a society (George et al., 2019). With the complexities of climate change and population pressure unraveling vital challenges for water resources, adaptive management acts as a tool for setting resilient structures to withstand external pressures. Through scientific research, indigenous knowledge, and engaging stakeholders, all dimensions of water management about ecological, social, and economic factors are addressed by these strategies. An integrated approach is required to develop sustained solutions that are context-specific as well as dynamic in nature to respond to uncertainties of the future. Moreover, adaptive management enhances the ability of communities to collaborate effectively with multiple actors—governmental agencies via NGOs, starting interdisciplinary cooperation that can access more resources and experience (Andoni et al., 2018). Efficient application of adaptive management depends on constant monitoring of the health of ecosystems and the requirements of communities. This involves integrating technology, such as data-collecting tools and models, to inform parties about water quality and availability. Periodic assessment allows for early detection of issues as they begin to emerge, allowing communities to adjust their management in advance. Adaptive management also offers an opportunity for capacity development and training of the community so that the locals are well-equipped to deal with upcoming challenges. By putting the community at the center of the management, adaptive strategies not only improve the sustainability of water resources but also empower individuals to become active agents of managing their own stewardship (George et al., 2019).

14.2. Benefits of Community-Based Water Management (CBWM)

CBWM has become a revolutionary practice, particularly in those areas with severe socioeconomic challenges. By involving the participation of locals, CBWM makes it possible for communities to take charge of their water sources, thus having higher ownership of such vital resources. This form of local governance not only promotes sustainable action but also raises resilience to environmental change. For instance, initiatives like the Simbuco Aqua-Marine Multi-Purpose Cooperative (SAMMPC) show how community participation can enhance economic growth and environmental sustainability in alignment with Sustainable Development Goals (SDGs). The cooperative improved members' livelihood and social harmony, reflecting CBWMs double attention to economic and social effects (Pamesa et al., 2025).

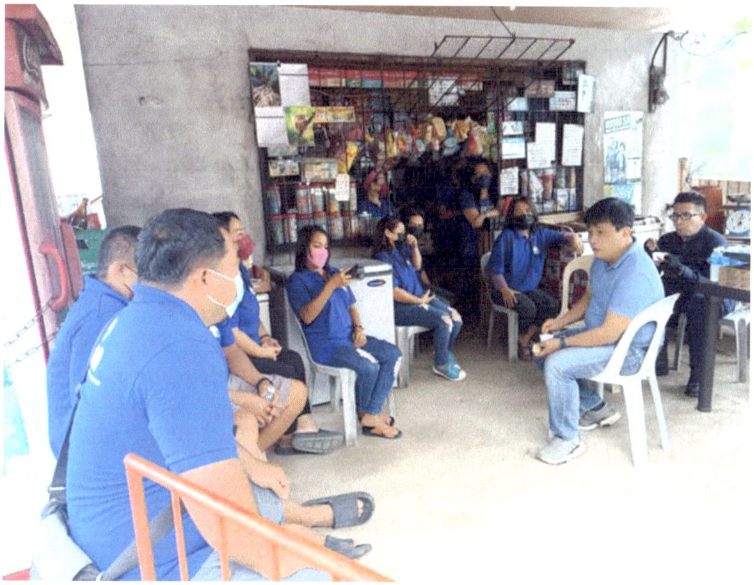

Source: https://scontent.fdel11-4.fna.fbcdn.net/v/t39.30808-6/476524999_3645704919053368_3567199205387968696_n.jpg?stp=dst-jpg_s600x600_tt6&_nc_cat=105&ccb=1-7&_nc_sid=833d8c&_nc_ohc=syKI-U91wQcQ7kNvwF42sqm&_nc_oc=AdnOq0YhF7lrg-TzyyktpEKIumoovfGL0oO5tdQ98iMlIpW25fd3Yo-nLB1Aq_d8ZI_Sh7xVmv5DbINIt0QioQJ2&_nc_zt=23&_nc_ht=scontent.fdel11-4.fna&_nc_gid=Vja8S4fipP1DHviWWMyivg&oh=00_AfEoeG2gNeRlUzMWCPnL-mFW6-0wzkTjWcW4e6AVM9FZLw&oe=680FF9DB.

Such programs demonstrate how local involvement can effectively address local issues while promoting collective sustainability projects. Its other important advantage is in its ability to facilitate inclusive participation, especially for marginalized groups. By providing empowering platforms for women and disadvantaged groups, CBWM supports social equality and promotes gender equality. Empirical research shows that working together in community-based water programs can lead to diversified income sources and higher resource access, and therefore community well-being (Pamesa et al., 2025). Inclusivity not only strengthens the ties in a community but also enables different voices to be heard in the process of decision-making. By engaging these groups directly in the management of water resources, typically more targeted and tangible solutions to local issues are obtained. Through prioritizing inclusivity, CBWM ensures more active participation by communities, ensuring that the benefits of sustainable water management trickle down to all segments of society. In turn, CBWM supports flexibility and adaptation toward climate change, particularly in the city where scarcity of water becomes a usual case. As cities try to cope with the effects of accelerated population increase and environmental transformation, proper water management is a priority. Community-based initiatives can harness local knowledge and practices to build innovative solutions that are adapted to unique environmental conditions. For example, incorporating green infrastructure into city CBWM projects can improve water management, biodiversity, and ecological well-being. These multifaceted approaches not only reduce the negative impacts of urbanization but also promote long-term sustainability by engaging various stakeholders, including government agencies, local enterprises, and citizens. With concerted effort, CBWM is a realistic model to manage the multifaceted challenges posed by climate change, both preserving access to water and quality for future generations.

14.2.1. Enhanced Local Knowledge and Expertise

Involving community members in water management projects harnesses local knowledge critical to the sustainability and success of the projects. When residents are involved personally in decision-making, they give invaluable information about their environment, culture, and previous experience with water sources. This localized knowledge facilitates the finding of context-specific challenges that might be hidden from outside experts. For instance, adapting to seasonal cycles and bouts of drought requires intelligence that is only known to local users. Through the use of such knowledge, CBWM encourages adaptive approaches responsive to the specific needs and situations of each locality for increasing resilience to environmental change. In addition, local knowledge encourages ownership and responsibility among the people, essential factors for sustainable water management. The communal investment in water infrastructure creates a culture of stewardship, with the community members encouraged to protect and maintain water resources. Evidence asserts that sustainable projects are more likely to flourish where indigenous peoples are not only passive recipients but active participants in the management process. This framework is radically different from top-down approaches that are unconcerned with local realities, potentially leading to poor resource management and disapproval by the locals. Greater local knowledge is a cornerstone in gaining transparency and trust—two requisites for sustained commitment to water management strategies. Finally, local and external collaborations can also be used to build the knowledge base that captures water management. Having governmental institutions, NGOs, and academic institutions on the board can cause a value-enhancing sharing of information in an interdisciplinary manner through a synergistic collaboration. That enhances the projects' efficacy at a higher degree through holistic approaches to water management. For instance, combining existing technologies, discussed in scholarly works critiquing blockchain solutions, with traditional approaches can optimize the management of water resources by ensuring adequate accessibility and transparency. Interdisciplinary collaboration plays a central role in the transition to sustainable water systems that are adaptive to community needs and environmental health, hence catering to broader objectives associated with sustainability and public health (Andoni et al., 2018; Margaret et al., 2018).

14.2.2. Improved Water Quality and Availability

Strategic enhancement of water quality and accessibility is a key component for sustainable community development. The mining industry, particularly in nations like Mongolia's Gobi

Desert, is an excellent case study of the necessity to consider water quality and accessibility concerns. Stakeholder engagement, both community and mining organization, has become a basic principle of IWRM. Empirical research in this area indicates that measures such as participatory water monitoring and autonomous water auditing enhance water management outcomes significantly. Community involvement in these initiatives not only increases transparency but also fosters a general feeling of responsibility, hence ensuring that different interests are brought into equilibrium in the interest of fostering sustainability. Therefore, improving water quality entails synthesizing the views of the people in decision-making, which can promote effective practice that emphasizes both economic effectiveness and environmental sustainability (Purevjav et al., 2025). Another effective endeavor aimed at enhancing water quality is integrating service-learning projects into school curricula. A good example is from The Hong Kong Polytechnic University, where students undertook a project tackling water quality in disadvantaged communities. This practical experience provided opportunities for students to translate what they had learned in class into actual practice by setting up water filtration systems that directly impacted nearby communities. Such an educational model not only enables students to learn practically but also makes them active citizens with sensitivity toward underprivileged communities. By connecting academic study with concrete community returns, such projects highlight the double returns of educational community projects: they achieve not only better water quality but also instill social responsibility in future leaders (Wong et al., 2025). Enhancing water quality and access by means of community-organized projects reflects a paradigm shift toward more sustainable methods. These programs tend to embrace both indigenous knowledge and scientific approaches to formulate holistic solutions that are suited to context-specific environments. For example, the design of herder's well improvement initiatives in Mongolia is a case where community-based approaches can adequately address local water issues. Through the integration of community stakeholders into the planning and implementation of the project, inherent limitations are addressed more ably (Figure 14.4). Stakeholder cooperation assures not just practical solutions but proper alignment with culture at the local level. By embracing a holistic, stakeholder-driven process for water management, stakeholders may ensure sustainable increases in water quality and quantity in the long-term and therefore toward greater sustainability ends (Purevjav et al., 2025).

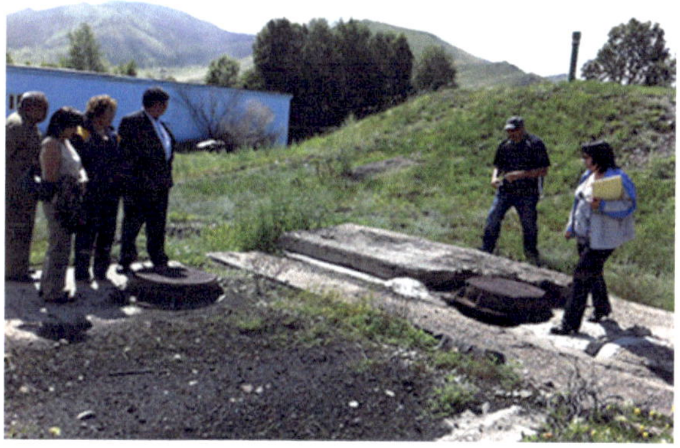

Figure 14.4. Implementing water safety plans.

Source: World Health Organization. (n.d.). *Water Safety Plans.* https://www.who.int/images/default-source/wpro/countries/mongolia/news/water-safety-plans-1.jpg?sfvrsn=a6c59f0_2.

14.2.3. Strengthened Community Resilience and Social Cohesion

Community-based water management tends to function as a key tool for building social cohesion and resilience among communities (Figure 14.5). By convening diverse stakeholders, these programs empower citizens to actively engage in making decisions about local resources.

An example is the Simbuco Aqua-Marine Multi-Purpose Cooperative (SAMMPC), which illustrates how cooperative structures can build stronger social relationships among members and enable collective action to confront common challenges. As members become involved in aquaculture, they not only enhance diversified income but also forge resilient networks, thus enhancing the social fabric of community existence. The inclusivity that is facilitated by such cooperatives especially enhances women's participation, going in line with the SDGs and even supporting their resilience to economic and environmental shocks (Pamesa et al., 2025). In measuring resilience at the community level, it is clear that social cohesion serves to cushion against adversity. For instance, Malian agricultural cooperatives provide members with valuable resources and support systems that are especially important during difficult periods like droughts and floods. By facilitating higher farm production and ensuring access to sustainable water, these cooperatives are central to food security and well-being. The sharing of resources, information, and emotional support among the members generates a state in which group problem-solving can flourish. Hence, the formation of cooperative networks not only addresses short-term issues but also fosters long-term resilience by establishing a denser community, which can function as a collective during times of crisis (Mumararungu et al., 2024). Moreover, the dynamics of inclusion have a central function in closing the loop of community resilience and social cohesion. Though there are several advantages of cooperative arrangements, unequal accessibility to members and non-members could lead to perceptions of exclusion. Effective cooperative undertakings will have to stress inclusivity and engage non-members actively, therefore avoiding fragmentation which undermines social cohesion. Cooperative participation in water management schemes, for instance, is able to enhance knowledge regarding cooperative benefits and confidence among all members of the residential community. As illustrated through most case studies, cooperatives' ability to serve as instruments of open decision-making and conflict resolution highlights their potential to ensure social harmony. Lastly, resilient resilience through cooperative membership collaboration not only addresses the immediate issue but also fosters a stronger and empowered society (Mumararungu et al., 2024).

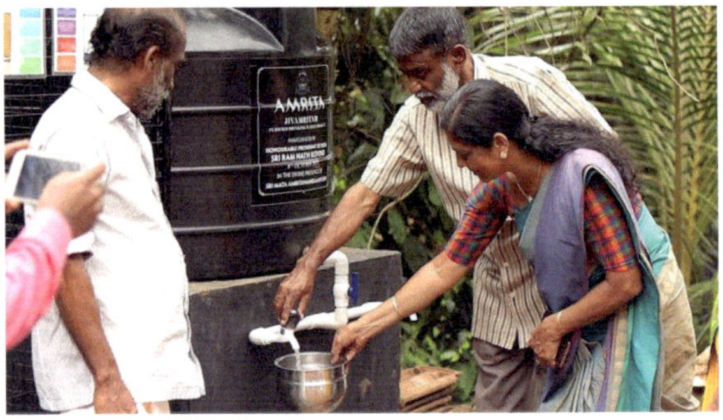

Figure 14.5. A community-based purified drinking water solution.

Source: Global Water Partnership. (n.d.). *Jivamritam*. https://www.gwp.org/globalassets/global/water-changemaker-awards/submitted-form-media/images/added-images/final/jivamritam.jpg.

14.3. Challenges in Community-Based Water Management (CBWM)

In attempts at implementing CBWM systems, there are a number of complexities that hinder efficient sustainability. One of them is coordination and participation by a variety of stakeholders, typically resulting in conflicting interests and management practices. Conflicting priorities among the private sector, the government, and the local communities can create tensions and inefficiencies. Poor cohesive regulatory frameworks can also make it difficult to distribute water resources and struggle with conflict resolution, interfering with the collective action required to maintain practices. Fragmentation is often articulated through asymmetrical access to water resources, making socio-economic inequality worse among groups. Solving these issues of governance will demand collaborative frameworks that will ensure dialogue and consensus-building among all stakeholders to promote shared responsibility in managing water. In addition, funding issues pose huge obstacles to effective community-led water projects. Most communities do not have the required capital to invest in the construction, upkeep, and improvement of water management systems and technologies. This lack of funds can prevent routine maintenance, which causes the early deterioration of vital systems. Capacity-building through investment in money as well as human capital is important for successful water management. Many of the local stakeholders can also be lacking in the technical capabilities to practice sustainability, and this amplifies the financial issues. Initiatives to establish financial resilience, like micro-financing or collaboration with NGOs—must be created to empower communities to manage their water resources sustainably. It is crucial to ensure the economic sustainability of such projects in order to be able to deliver effective and efficient water management solutions. Lastly, environmental changes, including climate variation and pollution, are a grave challenge to CBWM. With water supplies increasingly uncertain due to unstable weather patterns, communities are typically not in a position to react in a timely manner to these changes. Extreme weather patterns such as floods and droughts have the potential to strain already limited resources and complicate water delivery. Furthermore, agricultural runoff and industrial effluent pollution pose threats to water supply quality, necessitating quick action. Water quality monitoring systems and responses to pollution incidents may be lacking within communities. The given scenario reflects the need for consolidating technology and scientific data into community-based management Systems to allow local institutions to respond effectively to environmental change and safeguard water resources for future generations.

14.3.1. Conflicts Over Water Rights and Usage

Water, a finite and essential resource, is often the target of disagreements among different interested parties, including agricultural communities, urban areas, and businesses. The disagreements arise from competing demands, particularly as population growth and climatic change place additional pressures on existing water resources. Long-established water entitlements are typically incompatible with prevailing standards of use in most places, and tensions arising can erode social cohesion and sustainability initiatives. CBWM aims to address such challenges with the advancement of cooperative models of governance that embrace local engagement and responsive practice. Through the engagement of diverse stakeholders in decision-making, such initiatives seek to balance interests and secure a more equitable distribution of resources, eliminating or reducing the possibility of conflict. Resolving the complexities of water rights is most critical, as not doing so can jeopardize both the sustainability of community management systems and overall sustainability objectives (Calvin et al., 2023). Legal frameworks often complicate negotiating water rights, typically because such laws can be ill-suited to handle local complexity. Historical entitlements often undermine attempts to create equitable and equitable water distribution, and it is challenging for communities to come to agreements. Legal compliance can also foster resentment, resulting in more conflicts between communities, particularly when perceived injustices continue. Under climate change, where resource availability is variable, it is important that community-based systems be flexible. Such systems must not only adopt fair water-sharing principles but also have ongoing discussions to revisit rights and obligations based on varying environmental conditions. This integrated governance mechanism enables communities to develop resilience while avoiding possible disputes regarding water rights and use thereby improving the sustainability of local water resources (Wang et al., 2022). In addition, effective CBWM projects tend to incorporate educational elements to develop knowledge regarding water rights and use among all stakeholders. These programs make people aware of the need for sustainable approaches and the socio-economic effects of water conflicts (Figure 14.6). By empowering people in the community with information on their rights and duties, the programs can enforce inclusiveness and create a sense of shared ownership of local water sources. Greater awareness tends to make people more closely bonded and willing to resolve conflicts peacefully. In addition, the connection of local water management with environmental policies and frameworks makes it possible for integrated strategies to respond to cross-jurisdictional problems. This way, the encouragement of collaborative mechanisms not only helps to minimize water rights conflicts but also supports the argument for sustainable water use within society (Calvin et al., 2023).

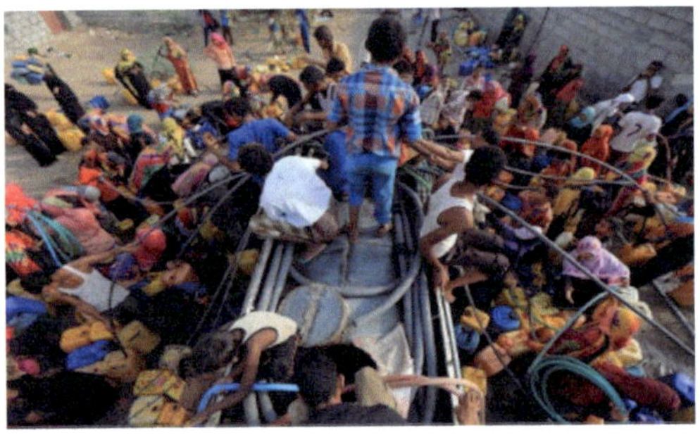

Figure 14.6. Illustration of water conflicts.

Source: Atlantic Council. (2017). *20170912_WaterScarcity*. https://www.atlanticcouncil.org/wp-content/uploads/2017/09/20170912_WaterScarcity.jpg.

14.3.2. Limited Financial Resources and Funding

The availability of adequate financial resources for CBWM programs is a significant challenge that can divert development momentum toward sustainability. Most communities, particularly those in the developing regions, have harsh funding capacity constraints that directly influence their ability to provide effective water management solutions. The financial squeeze will normally result in inadequate infrastructure, lacking proper training for local personnel, and poor maintenance of the available water infrastructure. Without such sustainable funding models, even the most creative programs risk becoming unsustainable in the long run as community members can easily put water matters ahead of other needs such as health and education. It is thus important to understand the subtleties involved in funding relationships so that there can be success and sustainability of CBWM programs. Furthermore, marginalized sections of society and women tend to be disproportionately affected when economic resources in water management systems are limited. This inequality is exacerbated because access to clean water has a strong impact on different aspects of life, including economic stability, education, and health. As indicated in (United Nations Global Compact Report, 2015b), when women are empowered through access to water and sanitation, it not only enhances the quality of life but also builds resilience in the community. In this context, developing equitable and inclusive funding strategies is essential. When funding is given in such a way that it targets these marginalized groups, the benefits are far-reaching, not only increasing the accessibility of water but also enhancing gender equity and social harmony in communities. Partnerships for funding and investment are key in filling financial gaps in CBWM. As seen in (United Nations Global Compact Report), the participation of institutional investors, firms, and foundations in the financing environment can improve the sustainability of water projects. The partnership can bring in the needed capital while promoting innovative options that suit local conditions. By enabling a cross-sector dialogue, the partnerships can tap into a wide range of views and resources, which can result in more durable water management systems. However, it is critical to make sure that the goals of such collaborations support community requirements and sustainability aims. Involving community stakeholders in decision-making guarantees that financial action not only mitigates current requirements but also makes full contributions to long-term sustainability in community development and water management.

14.3.3. Institutional Barriers and Governance Issues

Successful CBWM must involve a coherent governance framework that is oftentimes disenabled by institutional obstacles. Throughout most regions, these obstacles are seen in the form of fractured authority and the absence of coordination across water resource agencies. This form of fragmentation may result in inefficiencies by generating power disparities that advantage specific stakeholders at the expense of others. The research presenting Laikipia County shows that even with the advantages of community-based resource management (CBRM), the efficacy of such projects is often undermined by a lack of policy support and institutional weaknesses. Improving these governance lapses is important to establish an enabling environment where local efforts will flourish and where local stakeholders can safely navigate the intricacies of resource management (Keter & Mbali, 2025). Also, governance problems tend to worsen the problem of financing and resource allocation in community programs. Insufficient financial resources may hold back creative strategies in water management, which creates a cycle of reliance on insufficient financing. That constraint is experienced in Mvomero District, where community initiatives have been promising to improve water quality and household livelihoods through proactive participation and monitoring. Nevertheless, difficulties with water expenses and water-finding time still persist, mainly owing to inadequate investment in water infrastructure and capacity building (Mgonja & Massawe, 2024).

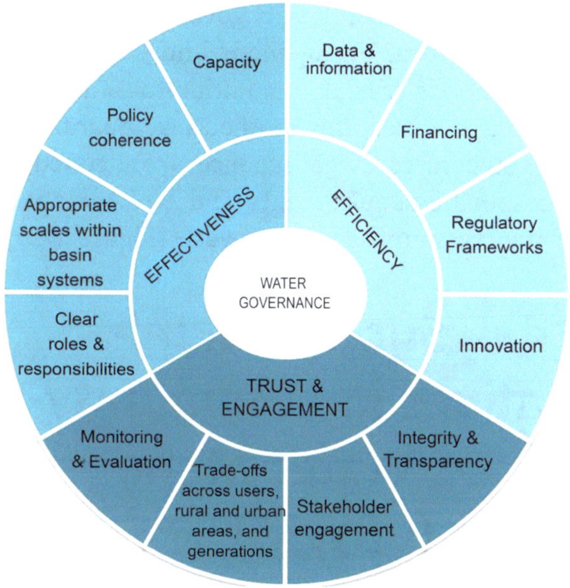

Figure 14.7. Water governance.

Source: Organization for Economic Co-operation and Development (OECD). (2015). *OECD Principles on Water Governance.* In *Water Governance in Cities: Current Trends and Future Challenges*. MDPI. https://doi.org/10.3390/w11030500.

Such fiscal challenges can potentially undermine community work, and therefore systematic reforms of governance are needed to achieve that finances need to be directed toward the goals of sustainable water governance. Moreover, the integration of local knowledge and practices into official governance remains a significant issue. Institutional concerns overlook indigenous knowledge, which could inform more sustainable local-level practices. Community empowerment to participate in governance has the potential to enhance adaptive management so that resilience to environmental changes can be enhanced. The Laikipia County case emphasizes that CBRM may strengthen social capital and local governance, though institutional challenges discourage the utilization of its full potential (Keter & Mbali, 2025). Therefore, promoting a democratic governance system based on local engagement and stakeholder interaction is crucial. In addition to reinforcing local capabilities, this method also guarantees that structures of governance are attuned to the specific requirements and circumstances of the communities they govern (Figure 14.7).

14.4. Successful Initiatives in Community-Based Water Management (CBWM)

The development of CBWM models has provided creative solutions for securing sustainable water supplies, as indicated by projects such as Costa Rica's ASADAS. These grassroots organizations exist in rural settings where there is limited clean drinking water because there are no government or private utilities. ASADAS illustrates the effectiveness of bottom-up, polycentric governance that increases water security as well as supports democratic management of resources. Yet, the troubles that confront ASADAS—financial sustainability and upkeep of infrastructure—highlight the intricacies of such projects. Around half of these organizations exhibit high performance, but numerous face water quality as well as long-term leadership problems. The resolution of these issues will help ensure the maximum potential of groundwater management through community intervention since they summarize the synergy between the local ruling and the sustainable consumption of water resources (Madrigal-Ballestero et al., 2025). Likewise, another effective project in CBWM is observed in Laikipia County where indigenous and modern-day practices are combined to promote climate security. The project promotes the active participation of local stakeholders in the management of resources, which strengthens adaptive capacity toward environmental change. Under the theory of Common-Pool Resources, it is evident that CBRM not only generates social capital but also enhances local governance institutions. Additionally, diversification of economic opportunities further consolidates the community's dependence on water resources. Nevertheless, these challenges revealed, such as resource limitation and inadequate access to climate information, need to be critically overcome to provide these initiatives with sustainability and efficacy. Strengthening CBRMs potential by breaking these bottlenecks may provide revolutionary advantages to the region (Keter & Mbali, 2025). ASADAS and Laikipia County's experiences are testimony to key lessons in the area of CBWM. Local community participation is key to addressing the specificity of social-ecological dynamics around water resources. Effective programs demonstrate that when communities can take control of their own water management, they are more likely to create innovative solutions based on their particular circumstances. Ongoing support from outside groups—be it funding, technical assistance, or policy support, is nevertheless crucial for these community-based organizations to be successful. By giving community involvement and finding ways to manage challenges top priority, it is possible to build adaptive water management systems that not only make resources available for present populations but also maintain them for the future. This integrated strategy is an important step toward sustainable water management in different settings (Keter & Mbali, 2025; Madrigal-Ballestero et al., 2025).

14.4.1. Rainwater Harvesting in Rural Communities

The balance between community participation and effective water management becomes a theme of focus in the experience of successful schemes in rural localities. Community activities that target rainwater harvesting have proved pivotal in addressing both short-term requirements and long-term issues of sustainability in the majority of regions, especially those with longstanding water shortages. The concept of rainwater harvesting not only reduces dependence on unreliable water sources but also instills a sense of ownership among individuals. A case study of rural practices shows that interventions like artificial lakes, often sponsored by local governments, allow communities to collect and utilize rainwater cost-effectively, thereby enhancing resource availability and drought resilience (Vadikar, 2024). A more detailed observation of case studies confirms diversified benefits through rainwater harvesting activities among rural communities (Figure 14.8). In regions such as Dang, Gujarat, regional populations have witnessed considerable improvements in water supplies and quality through conscientious community involvement. The participatory practice has brought cost savings and revenue gains, which further strengthen the community to engage in solving water-related problems as a collective whole. The success of such efforts rides largely on the collaborative approaches used, which are important for sustainability since they advance social connections while at the same time enhancing livelihoods. This is not without threats, though, as resource limitations and possible resource conflicts due to rights to water can hinder success (Vadikar, 2024). As demonstrated in regional and cross-national studies, community-based water management programs can greatly improve socio-economic status. The Fuatilia Maji project in Tanzania is a prime example of how community protection and monitoring of local water sources result in improved water quality, ultimately increasing household income and health. Such participation of community efforts in water management enables a more integrated framework to manage water resources, which also implies local participation can bring about not just better environmental quality but also enhanced livelihoods. However, recurring issues, including high expenses and time devoted to collecting water, underscore the necessity of ongoing investments in infrastructure and community training to ensure that rainwater harvesting continues to be a sustainable solution for water-scarce areas.

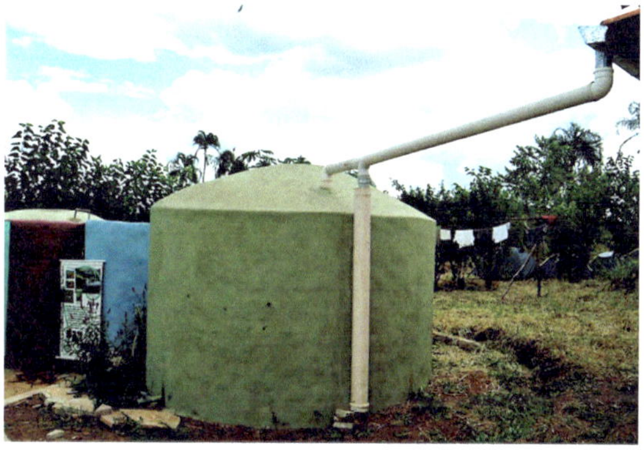

Figure 14.8. Illustration of rainwater harvesting in rural area.

Source: Dolman, M., & Lundquist, J. (2008). *Surface Tank Made Out of Ferro-Cement for the Storage Of Collected Rainwater*. Sustainable Sanitation and Water Management (SSWM).

14.4.2. Watershed Management in Urban Areas

Urban settings are confronted with special challenges regarding watershed management, especially as population grows and impervious areas increase (Figure 14.9). Modification of natural stream flow can result in many issues, including more flooding, degradation of water quality, and loss of aquatic ecosystems. Watershed management in such environments requires the incorporation of community-based practices to allow local stakeholders to participate effectively in decision-making. Through the promotion of public engagement, urban planners are able to tailor responses more finely to local conditions and enhance resilience to climate change impacts. For example, innovative green infrastructure technologies like rain gardens and pervious pavements reduce runoff but also promote biodiversity, demonstrating the potential for urban watershed management to contribute to wider sustainability objectives (Intergovernmental Panel on Climate Change, 2023). In addition, the complexity of urban watersheds is usually compounded by socio-economic disparities that express themselves in unequal access to clean water and green areas. Community participation and the integration of marginalized voices in planning efforts are needed to address these disparities. Community-based management techniques can most effectively mobilize social capital so that residents can work together on projects restoring and conserving local water resources. These partnerships tend to promote better environmental education, increasing awareness of the interdependence of human health and ecological health. Successful projects, such as neighborhood clean-up days and tree planting activities, can not only increase habitat restoration but also foster a sense of ownership by community members, supporting sustainable behavior in urban watersheds (Whitmee et al., 2015). Lastly, assessing the effectiveness of watershed management approaches requires integrated monitoring and adaptive management systems. Urban environments tend to have incomplete data on water quality, flow regimes, and ecological conditions, making it difficult to assess the effect of management interventions. Effective partnerships between local governments, universities, and non-profit organizations can enable the collecting of relevant data to support continuous strategy refinement. This adaptive strategy is supportive of the principles of sustainability because it acknowledges the dynamic character of urban ecosystems and the importance of ongoing evolution in water management practices. Overall, leveraging community engagement and data-based decision-making can lead toward more resilient watersheds in urban areas, which can support both human populations and biodiversity as urban environments continue to transform (Intergovernmental Panel on Climate Change, 2023).

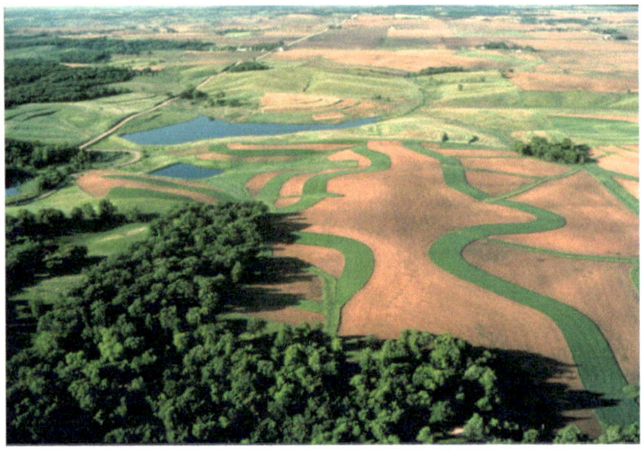

Figure 14.9. Watershed planning process.

Source: By Natural Resources Conservation Service (NRCS) - U.S. Department of Agriculture, Natural Resources Conservation Service – From National Conservation Practice Standards: "Contour Buffer Strips; Practice Introduction." Practice code 332., Public Domain, https://commons.wikimedia.org/w/index.php?curid=6262137

14.4.3. Community-Led Irrigation Systems

Successful water management has become prominent as an important strategy for countering the increasing pressures on water resources, especially in agricultural production. Community-managed irrigation systems are a good example of this, highlighting how localized management can promote water use efficiency and sustainability (Figure 14.10). By utilizing local knowledge combined with modern practices, these systems create a participatory setting where community members are actively involved in decision-making. The incorporation of local traditions and environmental concerns enables such systems not just to maximize water distribution but also to enhance social relationships among the farmers themselves. The more ownership communities have over natural resources, the more likely they are to spend time and money on the upkeep of such systems, generating a sustainable production and conservation cycle. The establishment of community-managed irrigation systems usually faces serious challenges, mainly in terms of governance and resource distribution. As farmers deal with communal water resources, there may be conflicts arising from varied agricultural requirements and preferences. Successful experiences within this arena show that clear communication mechanisms and conflict resolution procedures are fundamental in fostering cooperation and fairness among communities. Moreover, technical training access and equipment enable members of the community to adopt innovative irrigation methods that can increase productivity while preserving the environment. These difficulties, however, can be resolved through dynamic solutions that enhance resilience by facilitating adaptive learning and participatory approaches to water management. The history of these communities highlights the value of inclusiveness and collective responsibility in effectively managing essential water resources. Additionally, the scalability and flexibility of community-managed irrigation systems are worthy of further examination, especially regarding their implications for wider sustainability objectives. For regions experiencing severe environmental pressure or water shortage, these systems can be examples of decentralized water management, meeting complexities emanating from big, centralized systems of governance. Technologies like developments in data handling and digital twins could aid such initiatives by giving vital information on water consumption and availability, improving decision-making processes further (Rasheed et al., 2020). On the other hand, the socio-economic significance of enhanced access to irrigation is tremendous, encompassing increased food security and climate variability resilience among communities. Relying on diverse successful case histories across the globe can make the dissemination of best practices easier, eventually leading to the successful management of water resources and enhancing community empowerment.

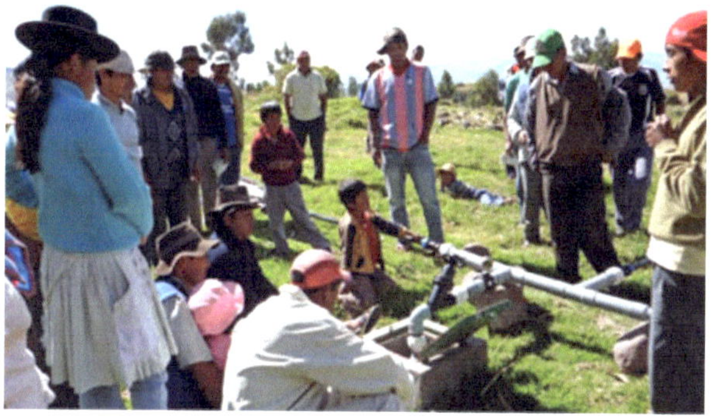

Figure 14.10. Community-led irrigation systems.

Source: World Bank. (n.d.). *Modernización de sistemas de riego en Perú.* https://www.worldbank.org/content/dam/Worldbank/Feature%20Story/lac/pe-modernizar-sistemas-de-riego-400x264px.jpg.

14.5. Role of Technology in Community-Based Water Management (CBWM)

Technological innovations are essentially reshaping the terrain of CBWM. Tools for collecting data, including geographic information systems (GIS) and remote sensing, enable local actors to track water availability and quality with a level of detail not previously possible (Figure 14.11). Such capacity increases community participation through the ability of residents to assist with data collecting and decision-making. The more informed the stakeholders are regarding their regional water supplies, the more effective they are at fighting for environmentally friendly practices and policies that allow for equitable access. In addition, the use of technology in water management systems enhances transparency, thereby enhancing trust levels among community members and local government, an essential aspect for sustainable water governance in the long run (United Nations Global Compact Report, 2015). Smart water management systems are among the cornerstones in enhancing the effective utilization of water in communities. These systems use sensors and analysis of real-time data to optimize water distribution, reduce wastage, and save costs. For instance, smart meters allow domestic and commercial consumers to track their consumption of water appropriately, prompting them to consume water responsibly. Technology also aids in leak detection, which reduces loss in the water infrastructure of cities by a significant amount. With these intelligent technologies, communities can create a more sustainable water cycle following the principles of effective use of resources and environmental stewardship. The issue remains, however, of providing such technologies to all people in the community, particularly for poor communities (Beckmann et al., 2019). Moreover, the role of social media and mobile apps in facilitating CBWM cannot be overemphasized. These resources enable real-time communication between residents and their local governments, a unified management of water resources. Citizens can report concerns like leaks or unauthorized water consumption, triggering prompt actions from regulators. This integration not only enhances accountability but also encourages citizens to engage proactively in local environmental management. Additionally, educational programs that capitalize on technology can inform people about water conservation, thus encouraging sustainable behavior in communities. Therefore, technology is a key driver of change in the development of CBWM frameworks toward more participatory and sustainable processes (United Nations Global Compact Report, 2015).

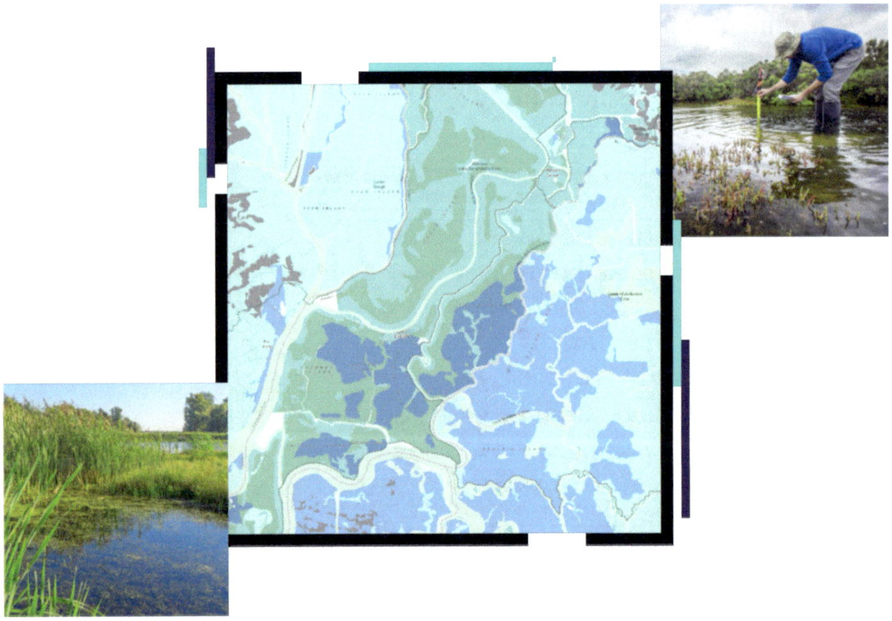

Figure 14.11. Geographic information systems (GIS) for water resources.

Source: Esri. (2021). *Water Resources Overview Banner.*

14.5.1. Use of Data Collection and Monitoring Tools

The implementation of data collection techniques in practice is essential to ensuring the proper utilization of community-based water resources. In regions like the Gobi Desert, where the availability and quality of water are issues of concern, qualitative data collection techniques such as semi-structured interviews and field observation have been highly beneficial. These methods allow researchers to maintain the different perceptions of stakeholders like local communities, government institutions, and mining companies, hence gaining a better understanding of water use trends and issues. Participatory water monitoring in this sense has emerged as a frontline method, facilitating local stakeholders' cooperation and transparency in data. The results of the aforementioned techniques are able to inform the development of tailored interventions aimed at improving the control of water to promote its sustainability in water-scarce regions that are navigating the twin horns of economic development and environmental conservation (Purevjav et al., 2025). The value added by data acquisition equipment to encourage stakeholder engagement cannot be measured. Its stakeholders' engagement in decision-making stands supreme toward making water management schemes successful in the long run. Research conducted in Mavoko Constituency has revealed that the social inclusion of people makes community projects very sustainable. Through the use of systematic tools of data collection, like questionnaires, it is possible to systematically interact with community members, representing various voices and ensuring their consideration in planning. Such studies show that increased stakeholder involvement can significantly contribute to project success, and the argument for the use of data-based strategies in community engagement is strong. The co-interdependence of data collection and stakeholder engagement enhances the need for instituting strong monitoring systems that aid in constant interaction between project implementers and beneficiaries and, through this, enhance communal investment in sustainable practices (Machuma et al., 2024). Monitoring gadgets also play an important role in evaluation processes, enabling adaptive management of water resources. Recurring data collecting provides an empirical foundation for evaluating the efficacy of multiple water management measures in the long term. Through this repeated process of data collection, analysis, and returns, communities can reveal what works and what does not, what is effective and what is not. In addition, through applying various methods of data analysis, from simple statistics to sophisticated modeling, stakeholders can develop enhanced comprehension of water processes and user interactions. The culmination of these activities not only enables the local populace to own their waters but also provides policymakers with data-driven information required for informed decision-making. Consequently, the incorporation of exhaustive data collecting and monitoring mechanisms becomes a critical element in the realization of the ambitions of sustainability and fair water management, underpinning the general principles of participatory governance and adaptive governance (Purevjav et al., 2025).

14.5.2. Implementation of Sustainable Irrigation Technologies

Agricultural innovations are more and more known to play a key role in coping with the complex challenges facing water-dependent farming communities (Figure 14.12). The use of sustainable irrigation technology has become a central component in the enhancement of water management efficiency and ensuring agricultural resilience. Through the use of systems focusing on the preservation of resources, communities are able to effectively counteract the adverse effects of climate variability and land degradation that undermine the yields of crops and food security. The technology generally uses predictive analytics and real-time data to optimize irrigation schedules for optimal efficiency, delivering water precisely where and when crops require it most. Moving to data-based practices is not only sustainable but also enables farmers to make decisions based on information that is aligned with best practices in terms of managing the environment. Supportively developing irrigation technology is particularly essential in regions where ancient forms of irrigation have proved to be inefficient or unsound for the environment. For instance, intelligent irrigation systems incorporating soil moisture sensors can help reduce wastage of water while providing optimal soil conditions for farming. These technologies can help to boost farming in developing countries, whose agricultural outputs are usually hindered by the issue of aging infrastructure and unreliable water access. With their ability to streamline water delivery and reallocate resources effectively, these technologies hold huge socioeconomic benefits such as improved farm revenues and reduced food price volatility. Successful initiatives in CBWM, combined with technological uptake, pave the way for a more equitable paradigm for agricultural growth. However, the path to mass use of sustainable irrigation technologies is littered with challenges that have to be countered collectively. Prominent roadblocks are access constraints to finances, poor infrastructure, and insufficient technical expertise among farmers. Moreover, systemic coordination between government organizations, agricultural extension systems, and local societies is critical to implementing worthwhile solutions. By fostering coalitions between stakeholders including farmers, policymakers, and scientists, communities can develop integrated frameworks that reconcile technological advancement and social equity. As seen in the study of irrigation regimes in Nigeria, these frameworks have the potential to make water governance more effective and to make technological innovations respond to local conditions, leaving local communities better placed to overcome sustainability barriers and to support food security efficiently (Adeyolanu & Okelola, 2024; Sahana et al., 2025).

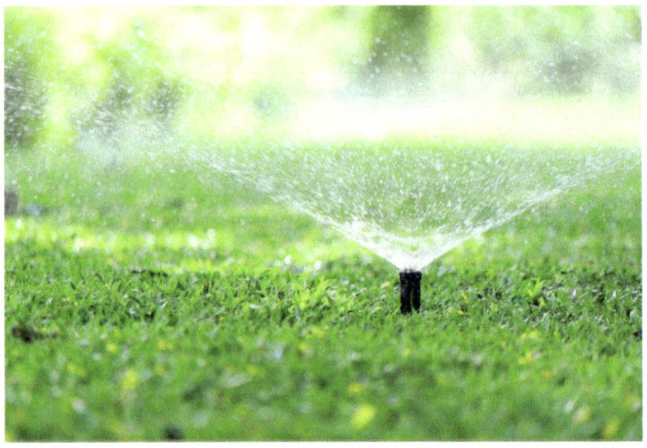

Figure 14.12. Sprinkler irrigation.

Source: Lehigh County Authority. (2021). *Sustainable Irrigation is Smart Irrigation*. Lehigh County Authority.

14.5.3. Role of Social Media in Community Engagement

Taking advantage of new technologies, especially social media, increases community participation across different fields, such as water management. By means of platforms such as Facebook, Twitter, and Instagram, the stakeholders get access to real-time comments from members of the community, fostering a more participatory approach. Besides such participation that allows the provision of necessary information with regard to water sustainability, it also inspires the local communities to participate actively in discussions and decision-making. This collective engagement is key to effective CBWM initiatives, since it produces a perceived sense of ownership on the part of the people, leading them to adopt sustainability initiatives and goals. Furthermore, social media is the platform through which success stories can be disseminated and motivate other members of the community, thus increasing their impact and prompting them to engage more in water management activities (Charlene et al., 2020). As problems relating to water quality and scarcity continue, social media's role in promoting communal responses becomes ever more central. Educational messages that highlight water crisis urgency may be rapidly propagated and tailored for specific populations to maximize the delivery of high-priority messages to those with the greatest effect. In addition, social network sites can also be used in mobilizing for clean-up or workshop activities as community events, hence creating tighter community bonds and collaborative efforts. These initiatives matter in raising environmental awareness since they not only educate volunteers but also contribute to the empowerment of local grassroots activists who are able to facilitate water sustainability activities. By exploiting the ease of social media, communities become increasingly well-positioned to organize a response to water problems, hence making them more resilient in an era characterized by precarious environmental circumstances (Margaret et al., 2018). Moreover, the effectiveness of social media in mobilizing communities is boosted by its ability to cross geographical barriers and connect different communities. This interconnectivity allows for the exchange of the best practices for the management of water elsewhere in order to learn from the successes that other regions have implemented. The exchange of ideas and material on a worldwide platform has the potential to increase overall knowledge regarding issues of water sustainability and allow communities to adapt successful initiatives in other contexts to suit their own environments. Such cross-learning builds on an integrative approach to managing water that matches the understanding of the people and needs in their environment. The interactive aspect of social media promotes constant debate so that the community members are constantly involved in the process of sustainable resource management, resulting ultimately in more adaptive and effective solutions (Charlene et al., 2020).

14.6. Policy Frameworks Supporting Community-Based Water Management (CBWM)

Adequate governance frameworks are crucial to the success of CBWM programs. In addition to affording a framework for stakeholder participation, they ensure the co-operation required to manage resources effectively. Decentralized governance shapes policies that enhance the active participation of local communities in decision-making. This integration is necessary in consolidating social capital and enhancing local governance, as seen in Laikipia County where CBWM interventions have harvested benefits such as spurring economic diversification and integrating indigenous knowledge into practices that are appropriate for local conditions (Keter & Mbali, 2025). Additionally, the capacity of communities to interact with current policy frameworks can greatly improve their adaptive capacity to environmental changes, and thus such frameworks are key to fostering sustainability. Apart from governance systems, policy frameworks supporting interdisciplinary collaboration is vital to the success of CBWM programs. These frameworks must cross sectors such as agriculture, urban planning, and the environment to facilitate an integrated strategy for water management. Breaking down silos across these sectors facilitates policies that permit the sharing of resources and information that leads to more effective general water management practices. Incorporating various viewpoints not only enhances decision-making but also enhances resilience against imminent threats such as climate change and urbanization that face water resources (Nwokediegwu et al., 2024). For example, effective urban water management has increasingly adopted stakeholder participation as a means of highlighting the value of collaborative effort in coping effectively with water problems in the rural and urban sectors. In addition, the continuous adjustment of policy environments is required to keep pace with the dynamic needs of issues confronting communities in water management. As climate change and urbanization increase, policies need to be kept responsive and flexible in relation to fresh data and community requirements. This involves not just the constant review of the success of CBWM interventions but also incorporating best management practices (BMPs) proven to work elsewhere. Through this, policy frameworks can promote innovations in water efficiency and pollution control and, in the end, empower people to sustainably manage their water resources (Nwokediegwu et al., 2024). The current discourse on CBWM stresses the need for adaptive policies that not only take into account existing issues but also look ahead to future direction, preserving long-term water security and sustainability.

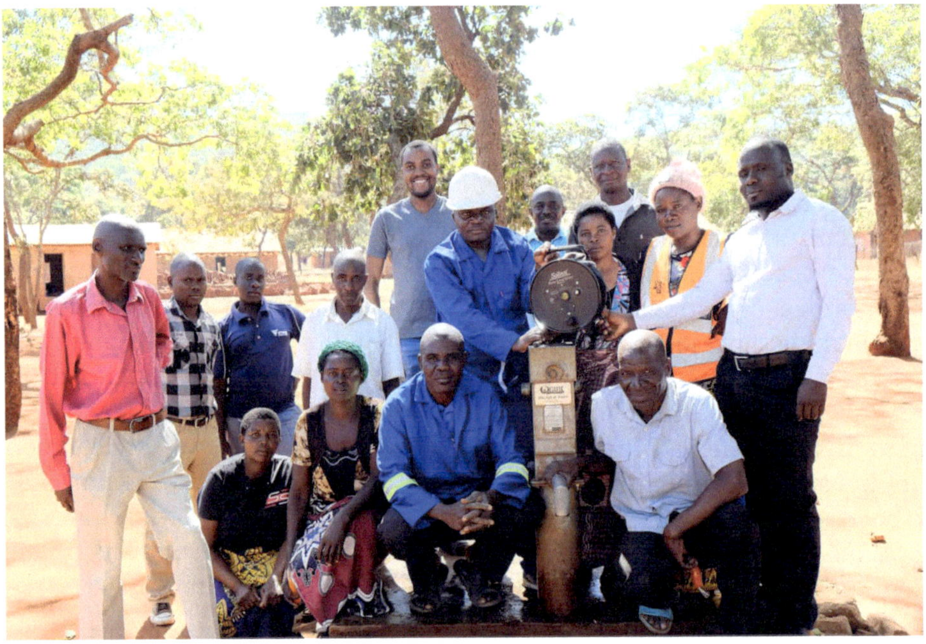

Source: Orant Charities Africa. (2021). *Community Development Project in Africa.*

14.6.1. National Policies Promoting Local Governance

The formulation and application of national policies have significant impacts on local governance, especially under CBWM. Efficient policy systems enhance the abilities of local communities to adopt sustainable practices that are sensitive to their local environmental conditions. National governments can facilitate such sensitivity through power decentralization and resource provision that allows local stakeholders to own their water resources. This empowerment statement results in higher adaptive capacity since the problems at the local level are handled better by the communities and sustainability is enhanced. Furthermore, through the integration of indigenous knowledge into such systems, national policy becomes capable of strengthening community practice and aligning it with the local ecological context and social processes and thereby leading to greater resilience against climate hazards, as already evidenced in earlier research on community-based resource management (Keter & Mbali, 2025). Secondly, the promotion of local governance at the national policy level promotes greater cooperation among actors. In promoting cooperation among government institutions, civil society, and local societies, these policies create a positive environment for mutual learning and sharing of resources. These collaborative platforms have the potential to give rise to more effective governance systems that tap into local knowledge and boost the legitimacy of decision-making. An example of this is community-led organizations such as Costa Ricas ASADAS, which are usually established where government programs are absent and offer basic services and advocate for democratic resource management. Even though such organizations come with numerous rewards like improved water security, national support is the most critical in overcoming barriers like financial viability and technical capacity (Madrigal-Ballestero et al., 2025). The crafting of a robust policy base can thus be important in reinforcing local governance and the efficiency of such community-driven initiatives. The success of CBWM also relies on overcoming the unique challenges identified by national policies. Obstacles include inadequate access to climate information, resource limitations, and institutional inefficiencies can invalidate local efforts. Policies that stress capacity building and technical assistance are critical in enabling resilient governance mechanisms. This can include training activities that prepare local leaders with the necessary skills and understanding, allowing them to better use resources. Confronting these problems head-on can strengthen civil participation and enhance the sustainability of programs that are essential to community health. As seen in productive examples such as ASADAS, merging national policies promoting local governance can open the door to creative and responsive water management practices that are both focused on meeting the needs of communities and ensuring environmental sustainability (Madrigal-Ballestero et al., 2025).

14.6.2. International Agreements and Frameworks

The sophistication of water resource management in a sustainable manner depends on the synergy between the domestic effort and larger international frameworks. The latter tend to provide legal and institutional frameworks that support community-based interventions, allowing equitable management of water. For example, the joint work of the IUCN Environmental Law Centre and The Katoomba Group has provided evidence on the legal regimes applicable to Payments for Ecosystem Services (PES) in Andean nations, showing a coordinated movement toward the institutionalization of practices supporting ecological harmony and community well-being (Figure 14.13). Through examination of current legislation and suggesting reforms that are required, such efforts work toward having a unified vision of ways in which global agreements can be used to influence domestic practices and promote sustainable water management measures that are context-specific (Greiber, 2009). Additionally, investment in nature-based solutions highlights the essence of global collaboration for solving international water issues. In one year alone, investments totaling $12.3 billion brought to focus how investors in different sectors can work together harmoniously to make watershed protection and restoration efforts provide sustainable water supplies. Such investments are not just money transactions but integral parts of a master strategic plan that incorporates sustainability with socio-economic value. With the use of innovative tools to track the success of such deals, communities are able to not only clean water but also natural disaster resilience, which shows the many advantages that can be brought by such global agreements (Bennett & Carroll, 2014). The advantages of global frameworks go beyond dollars and cents, including the structures of governance and levels of cooperation that are critical to efficient water management. The participation of various stakeholders, from governments to local citizens, provides a setting for collective responsibility and mutual accountability. These cooperations enable a better understanding of the needs of the region as well as better synchronizing them with larger environmental objectives. It is under this collaboration that successful projects are able to emerge, showcasing how global agreements are able to spur local initiatives toward sustainability. With the challenges brought about by climate change and resource constraints, the strengthening of these frameworks is essential to ensure that CBWM not only survives but also evolves to address changing conditions and needs (Greiber, 2009; Bennett & Carroll, 2014).

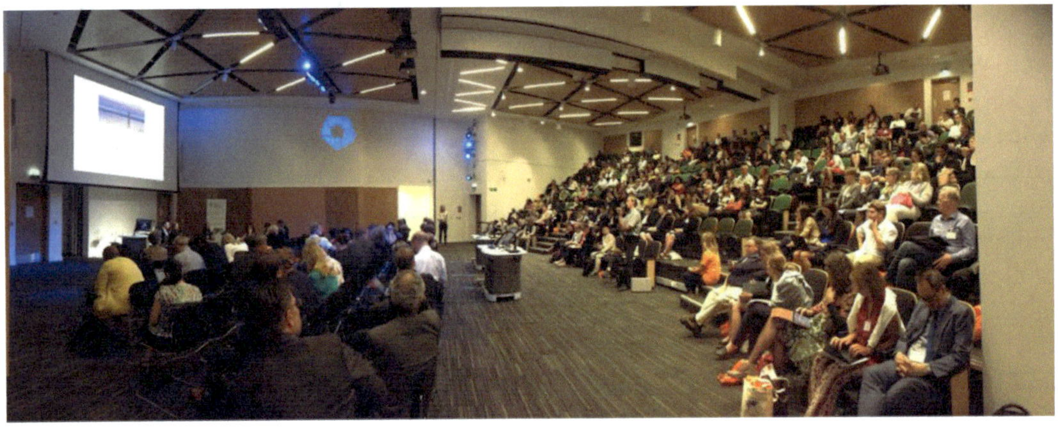

Figure 14.13. IUCN academy of environmental law colloquium.

Source: https://iucn.org/sites/default/files/content/images/2018/whatsapp_image_2018-07-04_at_4.38.59_am.jpeg.

14.6.3. Role of NGOs and Community Organizations

In modern debates regarding sustainability, the joint contribution of NGOs and community organizations comes to the forefront as a determining element in achieving efficient water management. These organizations promote community involvement, enabling local communities to become custodians of water resources. By providing educational initiatives and volunteer mobilization, these organizations instill a sense of stewardship among community members. For example, during the pandemic, the Society of Indonesian Petroleum Engineers successfully engaged stakeholders via strategic pillars that highlighted member focus and social responsibility. Not only was capacity development improved through this collaborative effort, but also notable community improvements were seen, for example, in school refurbishments that employed sustainable development practices (Santoso et al., 2024). These efforts illustrate the potential of NGOs to bring about system change by coordinating resources and efforts toward shared ecological ends. Further, the sustainability issues in cities plagued by rapid development and climate change call for creative designs typically advocated by NGOs. For instance, China's sponge city project incorporates ecological values into urban planning, encouraging water-related crisis resilience. This strategy demonstrates how community organizations can campaign for and adopt measures that combine natural and built environments. Collaborating with local governments and stakeholders, NGOs can advocate for policies that emphasize green infrastructure and community-based solutions. Through the formation of flexible frameworks, for example, the suggested ecological compensation scheme, NGOs not only improve the effectiveness of water management strategies but also ensure long-term economic viability at the same time, encouraging collective involvement (Shi et al., 2024). This is a perfect illustration of the innovative power of people-centered initiatives to address overarching environmental issues.

The NGO effect goes beyond direct project benefits; NGOs significantly influence the public image and policy around water management. Through research, information dissemination, and channeling community voices, NGOs are able to impact local and national-level decision-making. Their activism tends to underscore the need for participatory and equitable approaches to water management, which bring disadvantaged communities along. In addition, effective programs tend to be built on the formation of partnerships between private sectors, governments, and NGOs, building a multitiered strategy for managing resources. Not only does this use a broad range of expertise, but also pools them together toward a shared vision of sustainable water management. As in some successful programs, the complementary roles of NGOs and community organizations play a crucial part in building stronger and more responsive water management mechanisms that flourish against the backdrop of constant challenges.

CLOSER LOOK

Benefits of Technology in Community-Based Water Management

Technology positively impacts CBWM by boosting efficiency, lowering costs, enhancing water quality, and ensuring sustainability. It facilitates real-time monitoring, leak detection, automatic control, and enhanced decision-making, which ultimately result in more sustainable water resources and better community health.

1. Efficiency and Cost Savings:

- **Leak Detection:** Smart systems can detect and alert to leaks, minimizing water waste and reducing costs.
- **Optimized Water Usage:** Water management software and modeling tools help optimize water usage and reduce wastage.
- **Reduced Maintenance Costs:** Real-time monitoring and predictive maintenance can reduce maintenance costs by allowing for proactive repairs and replacements.

2. Improved Water Quality:

- **Real-time Monitoring:** Sensors can monitor water quality parameters like pH, temperature, and contamination, ensuring safe water delivery.
- **Early Detection of Contamination:** Real-time monitoring helps identify and address potential contamination quickly, preventing health risks.
- **Water Treatment Optimization:** Technology can optimize water treatment processes, ensuring efficient removal of pollutants.

3. Enhanced Sustainability:

- **Water Conservation:** Techniques like drip irrigation, smart irrigation systems, and soil moisture sensors help conserve water.
- **Reduced Water Waste:** By tracking water usage and identifying areas of waste, communities can reduce their overall water consumption.
- **Sustainable Infrastructure:** Smart systems can enable innovative solutions like automated water refills and optimized pump control.

4. Community Empowerment and Collaboration:

- **Increased Awareness:** Real-time data and monitoring tools can help increase community awareness about water usage and quality.
- **Improved Decision-Making:** Data-driven insights allow for better-informed decision-making about water management.
- **Capacity Building:** Training and support programs can empower local communities to manage their own water systems.

5. Improved Public Health:

- **Access to Safe Water:** Technology can help ensure access to clean and safe drinking water, improving public health outcomes.
- **Reduced Waterborne Diseases:** By monitoring water quality and addressing contamination quickly, technology can reduce the risk of waterborne diseases.
- **Improved Sanitation:** Technology can also play a role in improving sanitation systems, further enhancing public health.

SUMMARY

Upon consideration of the postulates, advantages, and limitations of CBWM, one sees that participatory models based on local involvement have much to offer in the way of sustainability. Community involvement not only creates a people's stake in resources but also more successful ecological outcomes through localization of knowledge and expertise. Such community-based activities can successfully soften competition for access to water as a means of alleviating social disparities that typically inhibit environmental conservation. Through community-based methods, it is possible for stakeholders to ensure that water management measures align with local ecosystem realities, thus supporting resilience against climate change and environmental degradation. Most importantly, the inclusion of indigenous and traditional knowledge systems in these frameworks is important, as it supports adaptive measures that are appropriate to the specifics of various regions (George et al., 2019). Nonetheless, as great as they are, CBWM initiatives are confronted with many challenges that may hinder their success. Lack of political will, inadequate funding, and poor training may undermine successful implementation and community participation. Such barriers highlight the importance of an integrated approach that not only facilitates local participation but also bridges systemic barriers. To this effect, the development of partnerships with government and non-government institutions can advance resource deployment and technical support. In addition, establishing platforms for open communication and sharing of information encourages inclusivity and encourages a space in which stakeholder opinions, including vulnerable groups, are magnified. The opportunity for community-based systems to advance sustainable water management may never be unlocked without breaking these barriers (Andoni et al., 2018). In the end, seeking sustainable water management through community engagement is a changeover that is revolutionary in terms of how resources are managed. As evidenced by effective projects around the world, creating community involvement can generate innovative solutions that crossover environmental and social objectives. By adopting a holistic approach that takes into account local contexts and ecological factors, we open the door to resilient and flexible water management practices. Additionally, coupling these efforts with larger-scale sustainability agendas, such as those prioritized by international bodies such as the UN SDGs, can guarantee long-term success. Thus, to ensure the best results from CBWM, continuous education, involvement, and encouragement of all stakeholders are critical in developing resilient and sustainable ecosystems (George et al., 2019).

The complex relationships of water management require holistic frameworks that cover both human needs and environmental sustainability. This has been compounded by issues such as climate change, which has the effect of increasing the occurrence of extreme weather conditions and material shortages. As (Gradl et al., 2012) posits, such pressures pose a daunting impediment not just to human beings but also to business organizations attempting to establish sustainable processes. Organizations rely on secure social and ecological contexts in order to succeed; yet the excessive use of common resources evokes the 'tragedy of the commons.' This issue makes community-based initiatives challenging since stakeholders may not have the interest to invest in shared sustainability objectives. Future policies should therefore prioritize cooperation among multiple actors to develop contexts that are supportive of long-term investment in water management. CBWM presents promising routes of innovation and efficacies, especially as evidenced by efforts such as 50 in10, which involves numerous stakeholders ranging from NGOs, and businesses, to governments. Collective action and the involvement shown by (Peet et al., 2016) help heighten local participation and policy change, evidencing the criticality of collective action in bridging obstacles to sustainability. Actors involved in this program highlighted community engagement and sustainable funding as key factors for success. This is to underscore the fact that local empowerment not only improves resource handling but also reinforces adherence to policy mechanisms for the protection of aquatic ecosystems. The incorporation of valid scientific information into decision-making frameworks further reinforces such measures, highlighting how empowered communities can effectively mobilize to solve their water resource issues. In looking at successful community-based projects, the spirit of collective learning arises as necessary to develop scalable solutions. Organizations that practice dialogue and collaborative learning create an innovative culture that can be translated into concrete gains in terms of water management practices. The synergy between scientific research and empowerment of the community, explained by (Peet et al., 2016), highlights the requirement to align strategies with local conditions. Resolving problems collectively tends to reduce the likelihood of free-riding, in which stakeholders leverage other's work and receive benefits without engaging themselves, an issue highlighted by (Gradl et al., 2012). Through the establishment of frameworks that foster participation and knowledge sharing, societies become stronger and better positioned to address issues of water sustainability and ultimately deliver more effective and equitable results of resource management.

KEY TERMS FROM THIS CHAPTER

Adaptive management	Agricultural communities	Capacity-building
CBWM models	Community-based projects	Community-led water projects
Data-collecting tools	Data-driven information	Economic security
Eco-tourism	Efficiency-technology synergy	Polycentric governance
Public engagement	Remote sensing	Resource distribution
localities,	Urban planner	Water governance

REFERENCES

1. Adeyolanu, D. T., Okelola, O. E. (2024), Irrigation Water Management and Food Security in Nigeria. Research Journal of Agricultural Economics and Development 3(2), 117-132. DOI: 10.52589/AJAFS-PFPU1QN7(accessed on 14 May 2025).
2. Andoni, M., Robu, V., Flynn, D., Abram, S., Geach, D., Jenkins, D., McCallum, P., et al. (2018). Blockchain technology in the energy sector: A systematic review of challenges and opportunities. *Renewable and Sustainable Energy Reviews, 100*, 143–174. https://doi.org/10.1016/j.rser.2018.10.014.
3. Ni Putu Yeni Ari Yastini, Politeknik Negeri Bali, Badung, Bali, Indonesia, I Made Agus Mahaputra Atmaja, Warmadewa, Denpasar, Bali, Indonesia, I Nengah Alit Nuriawan, Universitas Hindu Negeri I Gusti Bagus Sugriwa Denpasar(2024). The economic potential of community-based tourism management in educational tourism at Subak Teba Majelangu. *Samā Jiva Jnānam (International Journal of Social Studies).* https://doi.org/10.25078/ijoss.v2i2.4382(accessed on 14 May 2025).
4. Ash-Shiddiqie, L. (2025). Community-driven strategies for sustainable resource management, pollution control, and renewable energy transition in the Asia-Pacific. *Energy Justice.* https://doi.org/10.61511/enjust.v2i1.2025.1706(accessed on 14 May 2025).
5. Beckmann, J., & Dhawan, P. (2019). Monitor Sustainable Municipalities Report 2019: Key topic Circular Economy. Bertelsmann Stiftung Study 4 November 2019. Monitor Sustainable Municipalities Report 2019 Key topic Circular Economy. Retrieved from: https://core.ac.uk/download/287647997.pdf (accessed on 14 May 2025).
6. Bennett, G., & Carroll, N. (2014). Gaining depth: State of watershed investment 2014. Gaining Depth: State of Watershed Investment 2014 – Executive Summary. Genevieve Bennett, Nathaniel Carroll – Ecosystem Marketplace
7. . Un Viaje a las Profundidades: El Estado de las Inversiones en Protección Hídrica 2014 – Resumen Ejecutivo (accessed on 14 May 2025).
8. Font, X and Tapper, R and Schwartz, K and Kornilaki, M (2008) Sustainable supply chain management in tourism. Business Strategy and the Environment, 17 (4). 260 - 271. ISSN 0964-4733 DOI: https://doi.org/10.1002/bse.527 (accessed on 14 May 2025).
9. Calvin, K., Dasgupta, D., Krinner, G., Mukherji, A., Thorne, P., Trisos, C. H., Romero, J., et al. (2023). *IPCC, 2023: Climate Change 2023: Synthesis Report. Contribution of Working Groups I, II and III to the Sixth Assessment Report of the Intergovernmental Panel on Climate Change.* IPCC, Geneva, Switzerland. https://doi.org/10.59327/ipcc/ar6-9789291691647.
10. Cockburn, J., G. Cundill, S. Shackleton, M. Rouget, M. Zwinkels, S. Cornelius, L. Metcalfe, and D. van den Broeck. 2019. Collaborative stewardship in multifunctional landscapes: toward relational, pluralistic approaches. Ecology and Society 24(4):32. https://doi.org/10.5751/ES-11085-240432 (accessed on 14 May 2025).
11. Dewey, C. M., Hingle, S., Goelz, E., & Linzer, M. (2020). Supporting clinicians during the COVID-19 pandemic. *Annals of Internal Medicine, 172*(11), 752–753. https://doi.org/10.7326/M20-1033.
12. Gann, G. D., McDonald, T., Walder, B., Aronson, J., Nelson, C. R., Jonson, J., Hallett, J. G., et al. (2019). International principles and standards for the practice of ecological restoration.

Restoration Ecology, 27, 1–20. https://doi.org/10.1111/rec.13035.

13. Gielen, D., Boshell, F., Saygin, D., Bazilian, M., Wagner, N., & Gorini, R. (2019). The role of renewable energy in the global energy transformation. *Energy Strategy Reviews, 24*, 38–50. https://doi.org/10.1016/j.esr.2019.01.006.
14. Greiber, Thomas (Ed) (2009). Payments for Ecosystem Services. Legal and Institutional Frameworks. IUCN, Gland, Switzerland. xvi + 296 pp. (accessed on 14 May 2025).
15. Gradl, C., Knobloch, C., & Peters, A. (2012). A strategy for the commons: Business-driven networks for collective action and policy dialogue. The example of Global Compact Local Networks. *CORE*. Retrieved from: https://core.ac.uk/download/286054053.pdf (accessed on 14 May 2025).
16. Heath, T. (2010). Pragmatic but principled: Background report on integrated water resource management. https://core.ac.uk/download/140241.pdf (accessed on 14 May 2025).
17. Intergovernmental Panel on Climate Change. (2023). *Climate Change 2022–Impacts, Adaptation and Vulnerability*. https://doi.org/10.1017/9781009325844.
18. Joyce Cheruto Keter & Kenneth Mbali, 2025. "**The Impact of Community-Based Resource Management on Climate Security in Laikipia County, Kenya**," International Journal of Research and Innovation in Social Science, International Journal of Research and Innovation in Social Science (IJRISS), vol. 9(3), pages 2144-2156, March. (accessed on 14 May 2025).
19. Kruk, M. E., Gage, A., Arsenault, C., Jordan, K., Leslie, H. H., Roder-DeWan, S., Adeyi, O., et al. (2018). High-quality health systems in the Sustainable Development Goals era: Time for a revolution. *The Lancet Global Health, 6*(10), e1196–e1252. https://doi.org/10.1016/s2214-109x(18)30386-3.
20. Machuma, R. S., Odek, A., & Vundi, N. (2024). Stakeholder Participation and the Sustainability of Community-Based Water Borehole Projects in Mavoko Constituency, Machakos County, Kenya. *African Journal of Empirical Research, 5*(4), 1076–1088. https://doi.org/10.51867/ajernet.5.4.89 (accessed on 14 May 2025).
21. Madrigal-Ballestero, R., Gleeson, T., López-Ruiz, M., & Castillo-Cruz, A. B. (2025). Bright but flickering lights of sustainable, community-based groundwater supply and management: ASADAS in Costa Rica. *Environmental Research Letters*. https://www.semanticscholar.org/paper/b367275f0b9174bb7bff0d342da8b6ad62c28126 (accessed on 14 May 2025).
22. Manyi-Loh, C. E., Mamphweli, S., Meyer, E. L., & Okoh, A. I. (2018). Antibiotic use in agriculture and its consequential resistance in environmental sources: Potential public health implications. *Molecules, 23*(4), 795. https://doi.org/10.3390/molecules23040795.
23. Mgonja, R., & Massawe, P. (2024). The role of community-based initiatives in enhancing water quality and livelihoods in rural Tanzania: A case study of Mvomero District. *NG Journal of Social Development*. Vol. 15 Issue 1 (2024). ISSN(p) 0189-5958. ISSN (e) 2814-1105. https://www.semanticscholar.org/paper/f14d5a29290b9b8c9ed8b1ecc34deb4aeff0bf40 (accessed on 14 May 2025).
24. Mumararungu, I. & ya-Bititi, Gisarom, M. & Bisetsa, E. & Burny, P., 2024. "**Agricultural Cooperative and Members' Resilience in Kita and Yanfolila Cercles of Mali**," African Journal of Food, Agriculture, Nutrition and Development (AJFAND), African Journal of Food, Agriculture, Nutrition and Development (AJFAND), vol. 24(4), April.(accessed on 14 May 2025).

25. United Nations Global Compact. (2015). Private sector investment and sustainable development: The current and potential role of institutional investors, companies, banks and foundations in sustainable development. https://core.ac.uk/download/75781326.pdf (accessed on 14 May 2025).

26. Pamesa, D., Ferolin, M.C., Sison, M.P., Suson, P., Porras, M.D. (2025). Harnessing community-based aquaculture for the sustainable development of small scale fishery. *Journal of Interdisciplinary Perspectives, 3*(4), 75-88. https://doi.org/10.69569/jip.2024.0663(accessed on 14 May 2025).

27. Peet, C., Park, J., Arneson, M., & Draper, S. (2016). Collaboration for small-scale fisheries reform: Lessons in collective impact for systemic change. *CORE*. Retrieved from: https://core.ac.uk/download/80510799.pdf (accessed on 14 May 2025).

28. Purevjav, B., Klein, B., Dierkes, J. *et al.* Enhancing water sustainability in the Gobi Desert: processes based on IWRM principles. *Discov Water* **5**, 17 (2025). https://doi.org/10.1007/s43832-025-00204-2(accessed on 14 May 2025).

29. Rasheed, A., San, O., & Kvamsdal, T. (2020). Digital twin: Values, challenges, and enablers from a modeling perspective. *IEEE Access, 8*, 21980–22012. https://doi.org/10.1109/access.2020.2970143.

30. Sahana J, Rakesh H C, Pranav H Ravi, Vijesh H D, Nivyashree R (2025). Leveraging predictive analytics and smart irrigation for sustainable agriculture: A systematic literature review. *International Journal of Scientific Research in Engineering and Management.* https://www.semanticscholar.org/paper/e8801cbeb3b5364ac109f40ea90aef60f3256a2d (accessed on 14 May 2025).

31. Santoso, Gagok Imam, Prasetyo, Arief, Hermawan, Ida Bagus, Nengkoda, Ardian, and Hadi Ismoyo. "Strategic Realignment: Empowering Non-Governmental Organizations (NGOs) for Lasting Community Impact." Paper presented at the APOGCE 2024, Perth, Australia, October 2024. doi: https://doi.org/10.2118/221228-MS(accessed on 14 May 2025).

32. Shi, C., Li, Y., Li, H., Qiu, H., & Xu, T. (2024). Towards sustainable urban water management: An ecological compensation framework for sponge cities. *Environmental Research Letters.* Environ. Res. Lett. 19 123002

33. DOI 10.1088/1748-9326/ad8edf (accessed on 14 May 2025).

34. Sikhakhane Nwokediegwu, Z. Q., Ugwuanyi, E. D., Dada, M. A., Majemite, M. T., & Obaigbena, A. (2024). Urban water management: A review of sustainable practices in the USA. *Engineering Science & Technology Journal.* https://doi.org/10.51594/estj.v5i2.829. https://www.semanticscholar.org/paper/3090d6ce6178886987094098b042a53444898205 (accessed on 14 May 2025).

35. Tanpipat, V., Rassameethes, R., Chantarojsiri, J., Danusatianpong, P., Phattharakijkulthorn, S., Chitrdon, R., & Weesakul, S. (2024). Community-based water management in Thailand toward wildland fire and smoke haze issue in the Upper ASEAN. *Journal of Tropical Silviculture.* https://www.semanticscholar.org/paper/52c2426734a0773d6911dcee1858422210390991 (accessed on 14 May 2025).

36. Vadikar, P. (2024). Community-based rainwater harvesting management: A lesson from best rural practices. *World Water Policy*, 10(2), 456–479. https://doi.org/10.1002/wwp2.12188(accessed on 14 May 2025).

37. Wang, Y., Su, Z., Zhang, N., Xing, R., Liu, D., Luan, T. H., & Shen, X. (2022). A survey on Metaverse: Fundamentals, security, and privacy. *IEEE Communications Surveys & Tutorials, 25*, 319–352. https://doi.org/10.1109/comst.2022.3202047.

38. Whitmee, S., Haines, A., Beyrer, C., Boltz, F., Capon, A., Ferreira de Souza Dias, B., Ezeh, A., et al. (2015). Safeguarding human health in the Anthropocene epoch: Report of The Rockefeller Foundation–Lancet Commission on planetary health. *The Lancet, 386*(10007), 1973–2028. https://doi.org/10.1016/s0140-6736(15)60901-1.

39. Wong, L.-T., Mui, K.-W. and Zhang, D. (2025), "International service-learning projects on water sustainable management in higher education: a case study on improving water quality in a needy community", International Journal of Sustainability in Higher Education, Vol. ahead-of-print No. ahead-of-print. https://doi.org/10.1108/IJSHE-03-2024-0186 (accessed on 14 May 2025).

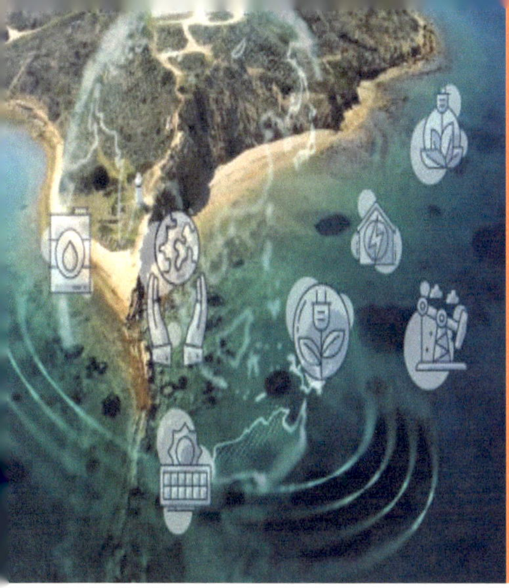

Chapter 15

FUTURE DIRECTIONS AND INNOVATIONS IN WATER AND COMMUNITY HEALTH

Contents

Introduction

Technology and nature's wellness are converging in ways that make a significant difference today. Neighborhoods are facing stresses from a changing climate, hasty urbanization, and an increasing number of neighbors, so it's not something we can do anymore, it's something we must do. New approaches don't just guarantee cleaner water but iron out the antiquated inefficiencies of how we treat and distribute it. At the heart of this transition, new technologies are disrupting every tradition. They are more refined and attached more tightly to what regular people require. In all types of situations, if we don't combine them with what they need, we embark on the path to water fixes that provide benefits now and lay the ground for healthier long-term benefits. Today, digital technologies and insights from data take center stage in improving water quality and access—no hyperbole. Consider the Internet of Things (IoT), for instance; it drives real-time information that adjusts decisions and continues to improve water systems. Such devices facilitate easier detection of problems such as contamination or deteriorating infrastructure before they get out of hand, repeating similar actions just to be on the safe side sometimes. Besides, they enable communities to see what is occurring, resulting in open discussion and other chances for people to engage, typically increasing public health choices. Naturally, the implementation of this technology requires careful and sometimes lopsided effort such that everyone is ultimately better off due to improved water services. In sustainable water management, the tale simply cannot be overlooked, particularly in a climate of unpredictable weather swings. As regulation and legislation undergo facelifts to meet pressing environmental concerns, they're beginning to adopt more intelligent regulation while accommodating a diverse array of voices. In general terms, leaning into solutions that are equipped to cope with unexpected change is an absolute necessity; policies that open the door to new tech as a contributing factor can work to unravel the complicated connection between water and health in communities. Governments, by opening the door to creative solutions and policies, could well set the path down for communities and natural areas to flourish. With concerted actions, and some strategically placed regulation adjustments, we can anticipate a time when water functions as a common good for all (Allioui et al., 2023; Yürer et al., 2023).

Importance of Water in Community Health

Clean water is at the center of community health—something most take for granted until something goes wrong. When water becomes tainted, microbes and disease can spread quickly, striking vulnerable populations particularly hard; diseases such as cholera, dysentery, and typhoid tend to plague low-income communities more than others. Effective water treatment and distribution—easy in theory, can truly make all the difference, bringing tangible improvements to a community's overall health. New technologies for water purification reduce exposure to deadly pathogens significantly, and in most instances, combining community action with technology-based treatment ultimately increases public health and the local environment. Today, advancements in water management are more critical than ever, especially with cities continuing to expand and our weather becoming a little more unpredictable. When urbanization accelerates, water shortage becomes a critical concern, pushing us to develop climate-resilient systems that deal with water resources sustainably. Methods such as rainwater collection or greywater reuse may assist local water supplies in addressing needs of quality and access, frequently in unanticipated ways. And with digital sensors watching out for water quality in real time, communities can respond quickly when something's amiss. When these new methods join forces, they provide communities with the strength they require to cope with changing water dynamics as a result of climatic variability (María et al., 2021). Digitalization is disrupting the way we perceive and utilize water by opening avenues to data-driven decisions. Sophisticated technology that captures and interprets large amounts of data enables communities to identify patterns and point their resources where they truly matter. Occasionally, technology such as geographic information systems (GIS) makes it easy to see where water quality issues are, and local stakeholders have a chance to step in with targeted solutions, such as making rash, on-the-spot modifications. This pro-active approach to problem solving not only enhances public health but also constructs some transparency and local engagement into decision making. In summary, the combination of technology with community health initiatives establishes an auspicious framework for achieving the United

Nations Sustainable Development Goals (SDGs), particularly ensuring that all people have access to clean, safe drinking water (María et al., 2021).

Overview of Current Challenges in Water Access and Quality

Access to water and water quality problems are a genuine mess of issues today. Climate change, to start with, continues to disrupt our normal weather patterns—rain arrives in odd fits and droughts linger on. This rain rollercoaster naturally stresses water supply systems and pushes existing disparities, particularly in areas already struggling. Then there's the ancient, groaning infrastructure that not only has trouble delivering water where it needs to go but sometimes manages to get water in places it shouldn't be, which, well, isn't exactly good for public health. All these elements mix together into quite a scary picture, one that cries out for new thinking and wise investments in technology and infrastructure (Almushaiti, 2024). Dealing with water quality is a pain in the head as well. From agricultural runoff, industrial effluent, and unbridled urbanization, pollution is gradually seeping into our freshwater sources. This contamination renders water dangerous and has the potential to induce unpleasant effects—consider waterborne disease and prolonged environmental degradation. To tackle this isn't a matter of throwing a switch; it requires a combination of advanced monitoring equipment and live data analysis. By engaging digital technology, communities can more easily identify where they have unwanted contaminants and how they can prevent them, which ultimately is a refinement of the general public health image (Ababii, 2024). And then there's the old problem of disparate access to clean water, a problem that's as much a matter of socio-economic divisions and governance deficits as it is a problem of water. Too many underserved communities simply lack the infrastructure to safely distribute clean water, locking them into cycles of poverty and poor health. Local solutions such as rainwater harvesting, decentralized treatment facilities, or even basic conservation education programs can make a difference. With a dash of technology added to the equation, these grassroots projects could well develop climate-resilient systems that unlock dependable water access while increasing long-term health and wellbeing (Almushaiti, 2024).

15.1. Emerging Technologies in Water Treatment

Clean water is a priority nowadays, and with increasing demand internationally, identifying new water treatment methods is paramount. Traditional methods undoubtedly have advantages, but they also often fail when urbanization, climate change, and persistent pollution are all put in the mix. Today, people are seeking methods such as advanced oxidation and membrane filtration, which—despite the surprise value of it all, can eliminate contaminants effectively. These new methods combine new materials with efficient processes and are likely to keep energy consumption minimal, while increasing cleaning effectiveness. For instance, incorporating nanomaterials into filters can enhance their effectiveness and reduce the need for chemicals, which is perfectly in line with green concepts. When these technologies converge, they even provide opportunities for real time tracking and automation that enable treatment plants to adhere to safety guidelines and, for the first time ever, serve the betterment of public health. Water management, also, is receiving a digital makeover. Intelligent systems on the Internet of Things (IoT) now collect enormous amounts of information that, in most instances, inform decisions such as when to perform predictive maintenance or how to better manage resources.

Those IoT sensors, usually quietly placed around treatment plants—continuously monitor water quality and notify officials if anything is amiss. This transition to digital practices isn't exclusively about technology; it is also a means to provide even under-resourced groups with timely interventions, in keeping with objectives established by the United Nations Sustainable Development Goals (SDGs). There is a natural, sometimes erratic, flow when technology and water services converge, creating a collaborative environment that seeks to better environmental stewardship and community wellbeing. Water treatment isn't about standing still; it's changing with a greater emphasis on climate-change resilience. In areas hardest hit by volatile weather, decentralized treatment systems and rainwater harvesting are suddenly getting a lot of attention. They assist in securing local water supplies and, as a bonus, reduce pressure on bigger, centralized plants. By embracing green infrastructure initiatives, communities become more resilient to extreme weather events and prolonged dry periods, which, in the main, increases resilience. When treatment processes begin drawing on renewable power sources, the carbon footprint is reduced overall—a point that conveniently aligns with wider sustainable principles. Overall, this better-balanced strategy doesn't only advance technology; it also connects community health and environmental stewardship, opening the door to cleaner, more accessible water and healthier communities.

15.1.1. Advanced Filtration Systems

Water treatment has evolved significantly. High-tech filtration systems now take place at the center of enhancing water quality and safeguarding communities' health (Figure 15.1). These systems—with innovative designs and new materials—draw on techniques such as nanotech and membrane filtration to remove contaminants more quickly. They are particularly crucial when drinking water is not easily accessible, as they can virtually suck up pathogens, heavy metals, and other harmful substances that compromise public health. Most studies tend to indicate that integrating these sophisticated filters into current arrangements can seriously level the playing field, industrial wastewater, for example, has a difficult mixture that requires a solid solution (Singh et al., 2023). In most instances, their distribution not only delivers improved health outcomes but also makes people feel more comfortable with their water source. Recently, digital solutions have been trending into the equation, combining with these filter designs in novel manners. Online monitoring and a dash of automation allow systems to adjust their performance in real time as water conditions fluctuate, sometimes seemingly like magic. IoT and machine learning, for instance, aren't only increasing overall productivity; they also simplify maintenance headaches by detecting problems early on and reducing system downtime. These technological advancements provide everyone an opportunity to respond to firm facts, driving water management strategies in more sustainable directions. Knowing how such digital features combine with higher-end filters is quite central, particularly where regions are struggling with climate issues, as some new research indicates (Amici et al., 2022). Going forward, the shift toward sophisticated filtration needs to go hand in hand with sustainable methods that nurture the environment and enhance community resilience. It requires a combination of engineering acumen, ecological awareness, and transparent regulations to refine water treatment possibilities. The entire concept behind circular economy thinking—waste reduction and recycling of resources—also works quite well with this agenda. When new filters are combined with an environmentally friendly attitude, industrial emissions could have a significantly smaller footprint while conserving invaluable water resources. Current research even points out that consistent collaboration between regulators, technology specialists, and native organizations is highly responsible for formulating policies for these new systems, constituting a firm move toward overall water and community health objectives (Singh et al., 2023).

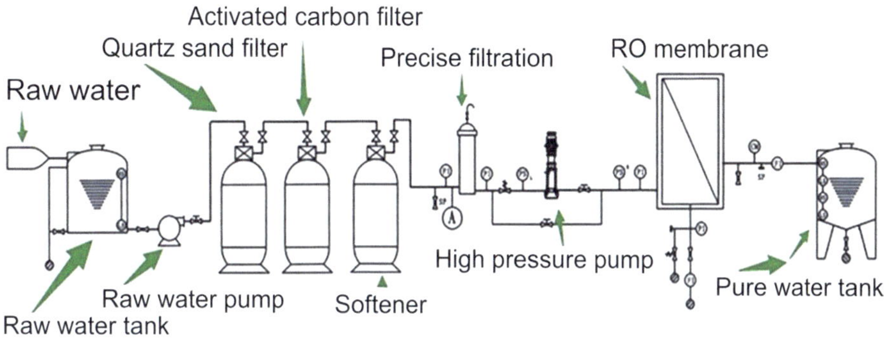

Figure 15.1. Advanced water filtration system.

Source: Numan, A. H., et al. (2022). *Advanced Water Filtration System*. In G. A. Aboud, H. Hussein, & A. H. Numan, *Effect of Temperature and Humidity Factors on Water Production Using Solar Energy with Smart Controlling*. ResearchGate.

15.1.2. Nanotechnology in Water Purification

Technological advances are transforming water purification in ways that count. Nanotechnology, for example, has captured many imaginations since it operates at the atomic scale—combining the smallest particles in unexpected ways (Figure 15.2). Scientists are now applying these nanoparticles to construct filtration systems that not only purify water more efficiently but also brush away pollutants in ways we hadn't previously witnessed. Often these filters even combine several treatments into one, which can save the day and money. As cities expand and our weather changes, these new methods could be the community health game changer and smart resource-saving solution we need. Adding nanotech to the blend of digital tools gives it still another turn of events. High-tech sensors and IoT gadgets now enable us to monitor water quality in real time, so changes are implemented nearly on the fly. This synergy of nano solutions and digital intelligence not only addresses short-term pollution but also takes care of long-term sustainability. In most instances, the information collected informs policymakers to develop water management policies prioritizing public health and environmental resilience. Notably, recent research supports this trend, demonstrating that data-driven approaches are progressively central to increasing water access and quality within communities (Ijiga et al., 2024). The advantages of nanotechnology extend beyond the instant fix, they even extend to larger concerns such as climate resilience and long-term sustainability. New technologies aren't solely focused on sanitizing today's water issues; they must also deal with climate pressures and increasing population. Nanomaterials, for instance, change based on different conditions, so treatment procedures can scale to a variety of environmental obstacles. Attempts at incorporating these new concepts into older infrastructure could potentially infuse life into our systems, allowing communities to flourish. Overall, the joint progress in nano and sustainable water management suggests a rare opportunity to transform public health and ensure that the future is secure in terms of water remaining accessible and clean (Kevin et al., 2024).

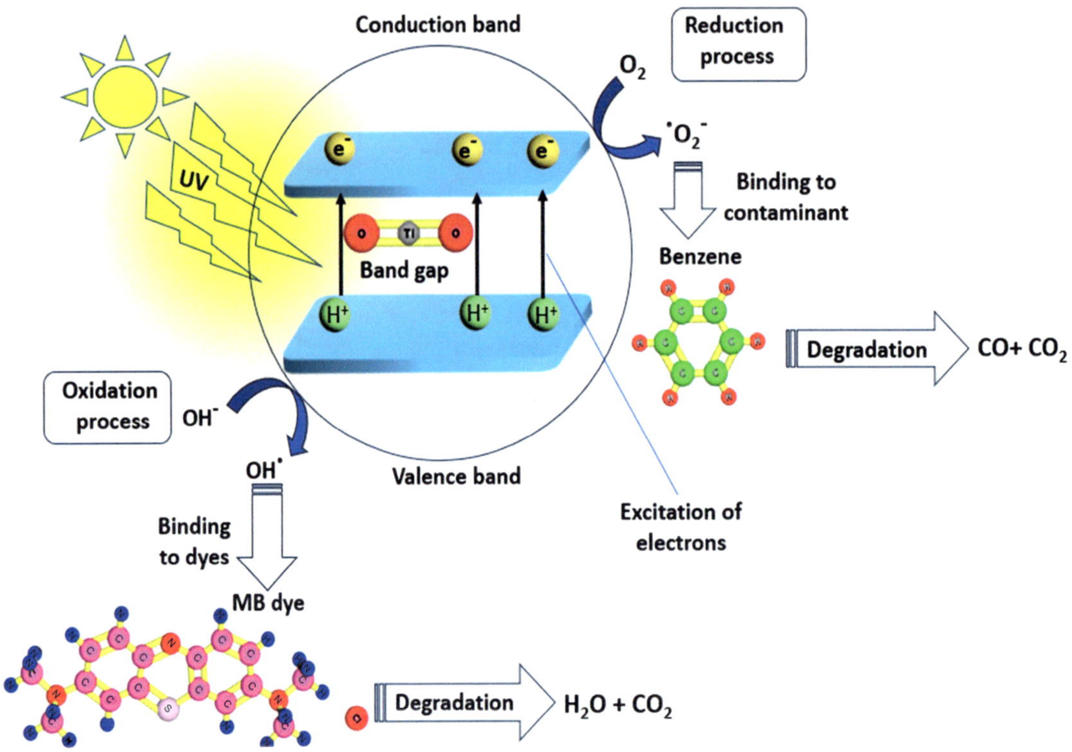

Figure 15.2. Mechanism of nanotechnology for water purification.

Source: Elhenawy S, Khraisheh M, AlMomani F, Al-Ghouti M, Selvaraj R, Al-Muhtaseb A. Emerging Nanomaterials for Drinking Water Purification: A New Era of Water Treatment Technology. *Nanomaterials*. 2024; 14(21):1707. https://doi.org/10.3390/nano14211707

15.1.3. Bioremediation Techniques

Confronting environmental toxins has driven many to experiment with nature-based clean-ups. Individuals are now using minuscule organisms or even some plants to break down or transform dangerous chemicals – a deceptively simple plan that's gaining increasing importance in repairing our environment. Consider PFAS (per- and polyfluoroalkyl chemicals), for instance; these persistent chemicals, owing to their long-lasting nature and extensive industry usage, have pushed regulators to incorporate natural approaches into their clean-up plans. In most instances, recent research is manipulating populations of microbes so that they can target these toxins, connecting environmental science with community health—clean water provides the foundation for improved public well-being and a healthy ecosystem (Panieri et al., 2022). There is also a visible change in the way that we deal with water that identifies itself with this movement. Scientists are harvesting biomass from land and sea alike, which not only combats pollution but also assists in shifting us toward a circular economy. Marine biomass is sort of unused despite having ample organic material available to clean up pollutants (Figure 15.3). By utilizing side streams such as beach wrack, the process assists in innovation in industries such as pharmaceuticals and agriculture as well. Effectively, this two-pronged strategy demonstrates how wise water management can drive economic development without damaging nature. Communities, in pursuit of more earthy means of addressing water problems, are discovering that such innovations provide avenues for blended, interdisciplinary solutions (Rudovi et al., 2021). Digital technologies and data acumen have also begun to be an integral component of these initiatives. Scientists now employ data-driven models to determine how pollutants behave and to choose the most effective natural clean-up process for a given scenario – sometimes even allowing them to monitor treatments in real time. This combination of digital methods with nature-based solutions not only increases the likelihood of successful clean-ups but also ensures that water is safe for all. Overall, combining technology, science, and an honest interest in public health appears to be charting a hopeful, sustainable course to address some of our most stubborn environmental issues (Panieri et al., 2022; Rudovi et al., 2021).

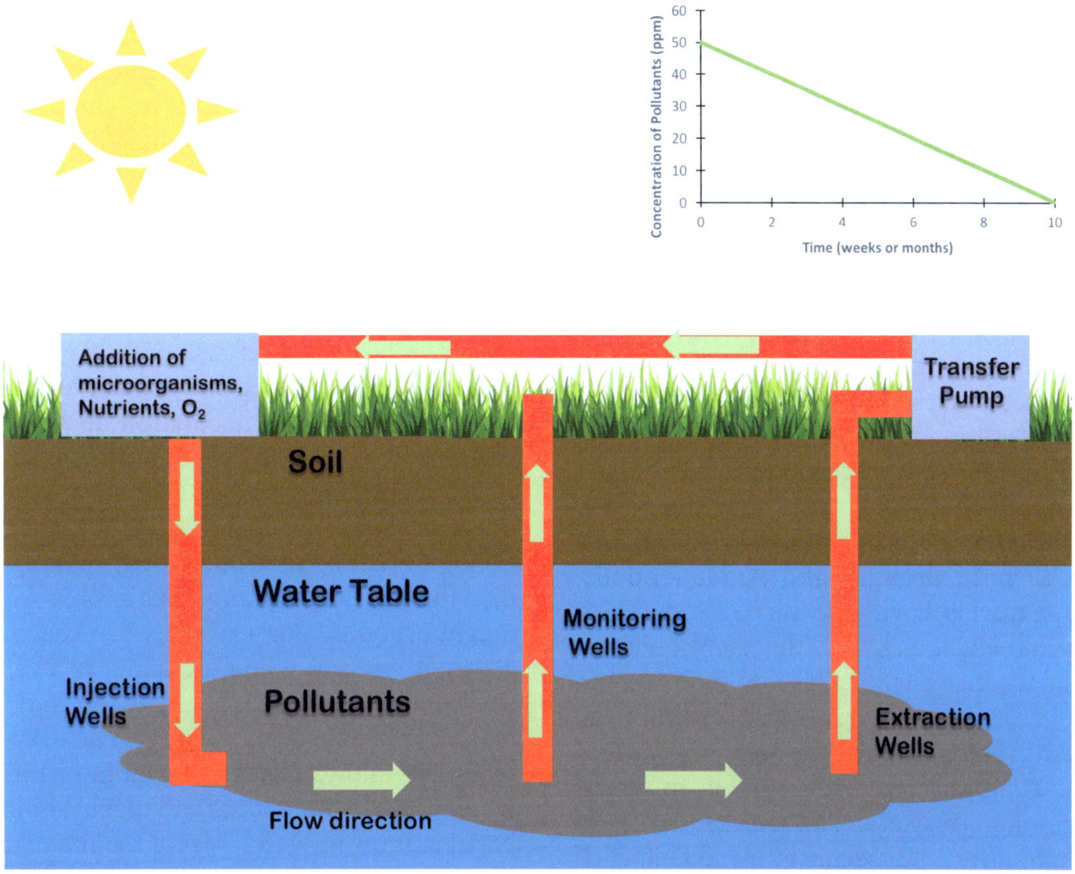

Figure 15.3. Bioremediation.

Source: By Hoodlind - Own work, CC BY-SA 4.0, https://commons.wikimedia.org/w/index.php?curid=64647624

15.2. Innovations in Water Delivery Systems

Water delivery is becoming a significant factor in local health improvement. Intelligent water meters with real-time information are appearing—monitoring pipes for leaks, maintaining water in balanced distribution and even ensuring everything is operating correctly. Towns are combining AI and data processing to maintain water consumption within limits and reduce waste. Most times, these developments not only enhance day-to-day operations but also pass on important information to people around them, which establishes a sort of trust between water utilities and the public. By and large, these developments fuel the greater concept of making water sustainable and capable of adapting to the curves of climate change and increasing urban demands. And then there is the fabulous transition to renewable energy. Fossil fuels? They're on their way out, so solar and wind are now married into water pumping and treatment systems—sometimes in surprising locations. In off-grid areas, these systems operate independently, ensuring even far-flung communities have access to safe drinking water. Picture a solar-powered well with sensors that provide real-time feedback about water quality, chiming in when there's a problem; it's a tidy solution that addresses short-term issues while also suggesting longer-term environmental stewardship. For the most part, such a shift isn't merely about short-term gains, but also about future-proofing water, particularly in regions subject to both drought and sudden floods. Digital platforms have also turned the tables on how individuals engage with water networks. Today, interactive dashboards and mobile apps provide citizens with real-time options for reporting problems on the fly, receiving notices of water quality irregularities, and even voting on local water matters. This relaxed attitude with community input seems to blend tech with daily life, repeating a point or two along the way, but as a whole making residents feel engaged. City officials receive snippets of input that can inform tweaks to services, and releasing water data openly winds up advocating for greater fairness and transparency in handling water. Overall, all of these technology-driven initiatives are paving the way for a future in which clean, safe, and secure water is accessible to all.

15.2.1. Smart Water Distribution Networks

Smart water distribution networks are fast emerging as a hot topic of buzz in urban planning conversations (Figure 15.4). Cities today rely on digital devices that allow them to see water in real time—a trick that smooths out daily operations a heck of a lot more. Sensors paired with data crunching detect leaks, test water quality, and optimize delivery systems. This interactive installation reduces lost water and ensures people have safe drinking water when they need it. With climate change continually bringing new challenges our way, this technology is a necessity to modify aged systems to respond to the changing demands of expanding urban life and green needs. Nobody can pay attention to the way digital tools and mountains of data have transformed water access and quality. Increasingly, city government officials are leveraging these smart technologies to collect reams of information about the way water is used, the way pipes perform, and what types of environmental conditions are involved. That muddle of information then informs policy decisions and budgeting, making water distribution slightly more equitable between neighborhoods. For example, forecast models at times predict water demand so even less-served neighborhoods don't get left in the dust. Making available this information on easy-to-use platforms allows residents to monitor their own water consumption, thus enhancing community participation in water resources management. When ordinary citizens and advanced technology meet, it ignites an actual transformation toward stronger—if not always smooth-as-silk—water systems. Added to that, the entire concept of smart water networks comfortably aligns with worldwide eco-objectives. By optimizing water flow and reducing inefficiencies, such systems become part of the battle to preserve vital resources and mitigate climate stress. This type of innovation all but covers the United Nations SDGs, with a special mention of clean water and sustainable cities. As new technology continues to emerge, it not only improves water quality but also converges tech, environmental, and community health initiatives in surprising ways. Studies on digitalization (María et al., 2021) even suggest that these intelligent configurations support the well-being of society as a whole while addressing grand challenges such as climate change and shortages of resources—opening up the way for a healthier future for all societies.

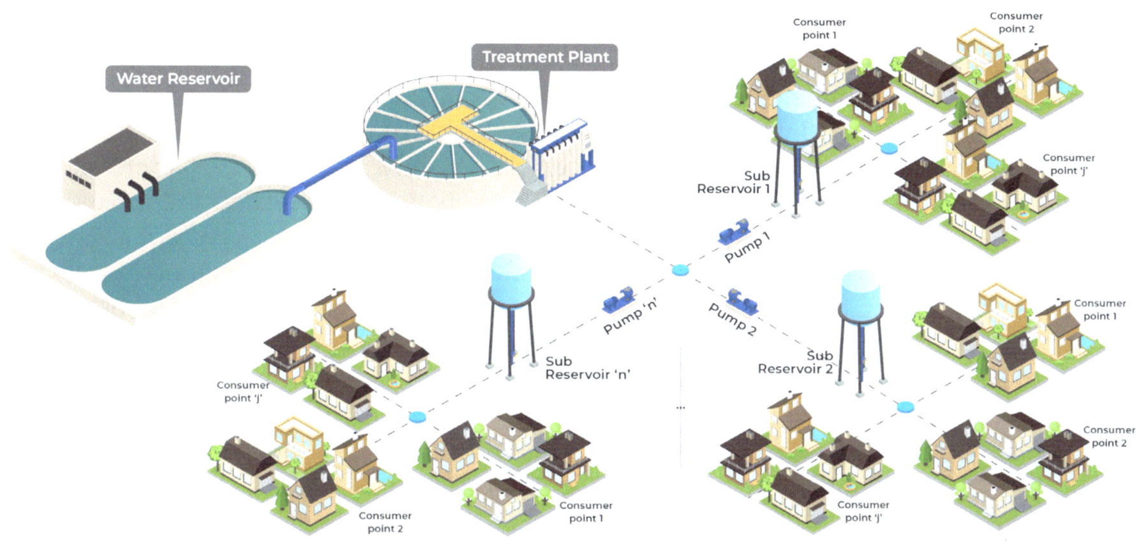

Figure 15.4. Smart water distribution.

Source: Velayudhan NK, S A, Devidas AR, Ramesh MV. Delay and Energy Efficient Offloading Strategies for an IoT Integrated Water Distribution System in Smart Cities. *Smart Cities*. 2024; 7(1):179-207. https://doi.org/10.3390/smartcities7010008

15.2.2. Use of Drones for Water Delivery

Advances in technology today have broken open new solutions for coping with water deficits in remote or underserved areas. Drones, for example, have begun appearing as a very groovy tool in the water supply arena—depending on smart navigation and timely deliveries to bring water closer to hand. With clever navigation and delivery equipment, these flying vehicles can navigate bumpy, unstable ground, reducing the time and effort that otherwise accompanies the movement of water. This feat not only streamlines the conventional procedures but also allows communities to receive a prompt response in case of emergencies—broadly improving local health levels. In most instances, climate-resilient systems are banking on such innovations to construct sustainable water systems; quick declines in disaster-struck regions translate to vulnerable individuals accessing the water they require, when they require it. Changing subjects slightly, it is difficult not to consider how data processing fits with these drone drops. Utilizing live feeds, drones are able to swap out their flight paths in real time and closely monitor water quality, which consequently optimizes resource management. This blend isn't only logistics, it's the entire IoT experience, where sensor-studded drones collect actionable nuggets on every outing. It allows the community to identify water sources, monitor usage patterns, and continuously measure quality. So when drone technology and digital intelligence meet, it opens the door for individuals to become more hands-on with their water resources, emphasizing that these tools aren't just about pumping water but also about powering a wider, data-based strategy for conservation and wellness. Considering community health projects, the application of drone technology emphasizes a tidy combination of creative solutions and simple practical solutions to the challenges of water delivery. In most instances, drone delivery for water transport tightly aligns with today's effort to go greener—either in congested cities or vast farmlands—where good water is an increasingly important priority. Lessons from other industries indicate that merging aerial shipping with earthbound water methods can create a path toward more resilient, stronger community systems. It's also worth monitoring for societal effects, such as who receives access and whether or not the system seems equitable to all. Overall, new technology such as drones appears to not only deliver water directly, but also assist in informing larger initiatives in increasing public health and environmental stewardship, with a more sustainable future ahead for all.

15.2.3. Mobile Applications for Water Access Tracking

Water shortage and delivering safe water to communities are enormous problems for public health. Recently, new smartphone apps have emerged that significantly alter how one monitors and controls water. The nifty apps enable individuals to capture data on water quality and the amount of water in a matter of seconds. The simple interfaces enable individuals to report deficits or any indications of contamination immediately. Whether in a metropolitan setting or in a rural location where the standard systems don't exist, these apps illustrate how agile mobile technology can be in dealing with water issues. Combining data analysis into water management through such telephone apps provides us with a more intimate, in-your-face view of our water systems. When you combine things such as geographic mapping (that GIS thing) with mobile technology, communities are able to readily identify trends in water access and determine where places need attention ASAP. For the most part, monitoring trends in water consumption and availability aids decision-makers in preparing for more equitable and sustainable distribution. Additionally, the exposed nature of such systems can persuade service providers to be transparent and just, to press community needs to the fore. In most instances, tools such as these online support climate-smart action and enhance local well-being. It doesn't end at merely monitoring water supply; such applications also give communities the power to manage their environment in general. They provide an entry to the sharing of data and unite local people, government, and NGOs into a single shared endeavor.

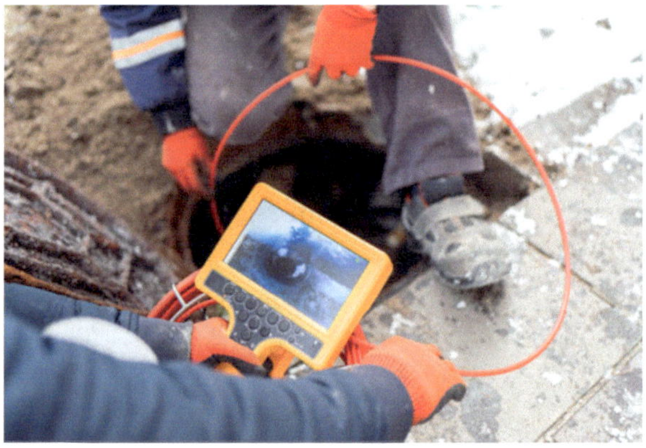

Source: https://d1v1e13ebw3o15.cloudfront.net/data/82855/pool_and_spa_master/.jpg.

That sort of collective understanding creates a more complete image of water issues and inspires directed solutions. There's also a tidy opportunity for education—people can become more comfortable with sustainable practices and why it's important to keep water clean. In the majority of instances, once communities begin to implement these technologies, they not only resolve current water concerns, but also assist in developing larger, climate-resilient frameworks that align with international sustainability targets (Conservation X Labs, 2015; Tsan et al., 2019).

15.3. The Role of Digital Tools in Water Quality Monitoring

Technology these days has revolutionized the way we monitor water quality. Electronic devices such as remote sensors and data analyzers now leap in, reversing the traditional approaches in different kinds of ecosystems. Live data arrives quickly, which translates to fast response when something goes wrong, and it even begins to identify trends that the traditional ways may have overlooked. Big data, in general, can catch on to repeat patterns, and as a whole these technological advancements complement broader aspirations of safeguarding our planet as well as public health, and are central to protecting community water sources from new threats (Dwivedi et al., 2022). The increasing use of digital tools is also revolutionizing the process of decision-making in water resource management. Intelligent systems communicating with the IoT enable communities to monitor such things as pH, turbidity, and even pathogen populations—often through remote, continuous monitoring.

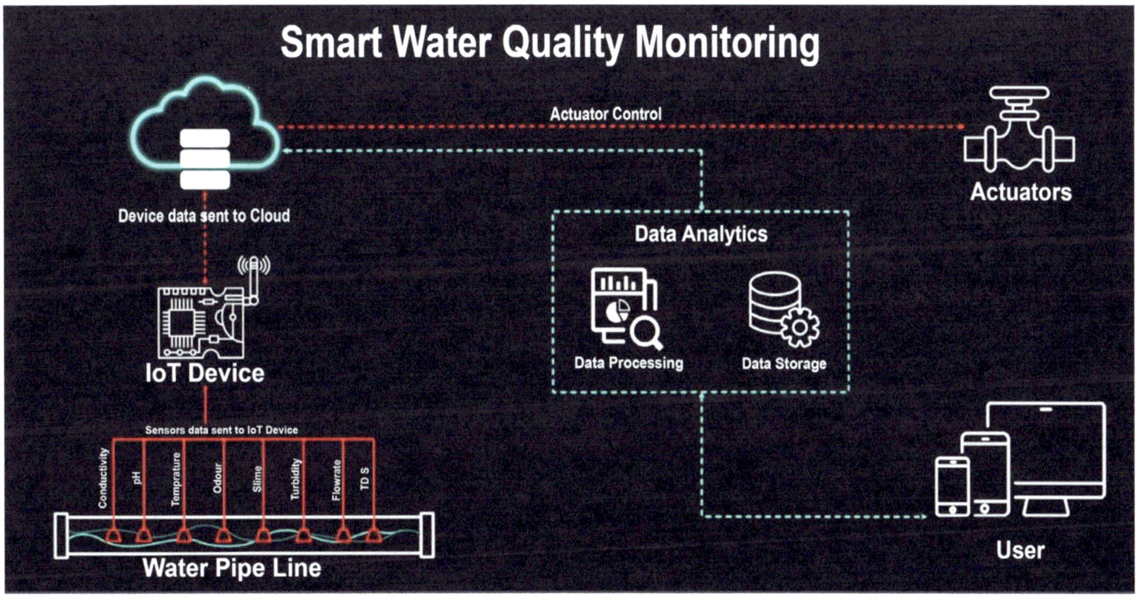

Figure 15.5. Water quality monitoring system.

Source: PsiBorg Technologies Pvt. Ltd. (2024). *Water Quality Monitoring System*.

This data-driven approach not only increases the efficiency of monitoring but also delivers the information directly to people, which generates more local interest. Occasionally, however, these technology changes initiate wider conversations about sustainability; for example, connecting such tools with initiatives like the United Nations SDGs demonstrates that water can be monitored alongside addressing food and energy security concerns in a more holistic approach to sustainability (María et al., 2021). There's plenty of potential for these new technologies to increase water quality monitoring, but obstacles still arise with implementation and equitable access for all. Closing gaps, particularly in under-resourced communities, is key if we're going to want the advantages to reach further afield. By extending digital tools to more individuals, local communities have a greater opportunity to be actively involved in caring for their water. This shift, all the while keeping public health in mind, also supports wider care for nature, corresponding to the way that water, well-being, and sustainable practices tend to overlap. As we consider what is to come in water monitoring, remaining inclusive and accessible isn't something we can do, something we must do (Figure 15.5) (María et al., 2021).

15.3.1. IoT Sensors for Real-Time Data Collection

New technology is disrupting traditional water management practices. Old methods now appear quaint when new solutions increase the speed and intelligence of water treatment systems. IoT sensors, for instance, are a true game-changer, they draw in real-time information from all sorts of sources, making it simpler to make decisions on the fly. By having these adaptable sensors on board, monitoring water quality and flow becomes much easier, and that constant flood of information is crucial to being able to detect pollutants or anomalies in time to prevent them from building up into full-blown community health crises. In the majority of instances, the application of IoT sensors addresses everyday problems with the added preparation for lasting water management sustainability since emerging data insights gradually inform policy and catalyze system enhancements (Allioui et al., 2023). Merging IoT sensors with sophisticated analytics propels real-time data collecting to unprecedented levels. These new frameworks capture and handle massive quantities of data, providing deeper insight into water use, waste tendencies, and quality checks. More often than not, the knowledge gleaned from such data aids in the creation of systems that are more capable of responding to changing environmental circumstances; for example, sensor-based monitoring can guide water distribution strategies along with disaster response planning, all leading toward healthier communities.

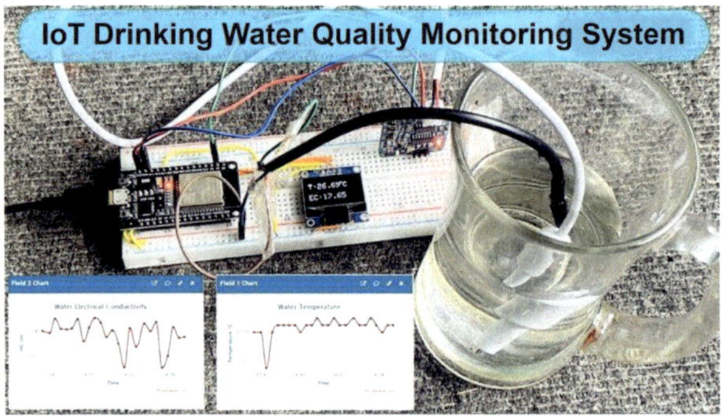

Source: How2electronics. (2022). *Water Quality Monitoring System Using ESP32*.

As more and more individuals rely on digital instruments for decision-making, it is nearly imperative to integrate these sensor networks into comprehensive environmental policy in order to secure innovative, sustainable water management strategies (Luo et al., 2023). Despite all the potential, IoT sensors also have some significant challenges to overcome in terms of widespread adoption. Integration into established water systems, managing running costs, and untangling a knot of regulation requirements can quite literally take the wind out of their rollout. And add in flexible sensors, and there's then the additional labor of ironing out performance glitches and ensuring everything remains connected. Overall, people in the water industry must come together and create systems that advance not only the technology aspects of things but also deal with ethical and business-related issues surrounding data usage. By igniting constant discussions between policymakers, engineers, and community leaders, the way can be paved for a strong IoT sensor ecosystem—finally funneling these inventions into improved public health and environmental sustainability (Allioui et al., 2023).

15.3.2. Data Analytics for Predictive Maintenance

Data analysis combined with predictive maintenance opens new avenues for enhanced water treatment and increased community well-being (Figure 15.6). Companies draw on an array of sensors and IoT devices so that they're able, in most instances, to identify potential problems before they have a chance to fully manifest—avoiding downtime and keeping services running. This proactive measure saves money while making water systems much more dependable, an aspect that is very important to public health. Recently, with IoT performing new tricks, it has become evident that water companies have to construct robust IT infrastructure just to keep up with the enormous volume of data (Allioui et al., 2023). Advanced analytics is not merely about rudimentary monitoring; it plunges into vintage and real-time data to catch up on patterns that guide decision-making. The outcome is customized maintenance schedules that respond to the unique idiosyncrasies of various water infrastructure components. For instance, wear and tear data can be filtered to determine which repairs are most critical, so resources are directed where they matter. This approach, in most instances, not only safeguards these systems but also enables environmentally friendly practices essential for climate resilience (Luo et al., 2023). Ultimately, getting predictive maintenance to mesh with data analytics relies on ironing out some real-world issues, particularly around sensor uptake and harmonizing all that streaming data. There's still a push to clean up sensor tech so it integrates neatly with current systems and communicates data smoothly. When these bugs are sorted out, overall maintenance performance is given a significant boost. Through shared overcoming of these challenges, stakeholders can unleash the game-changing promise of digital solutions, creating the way toward a more resilient water delivery system that genuinely lifts community health and environmental sustainability (Allioui et al., 2023; Luo et al., 2023).

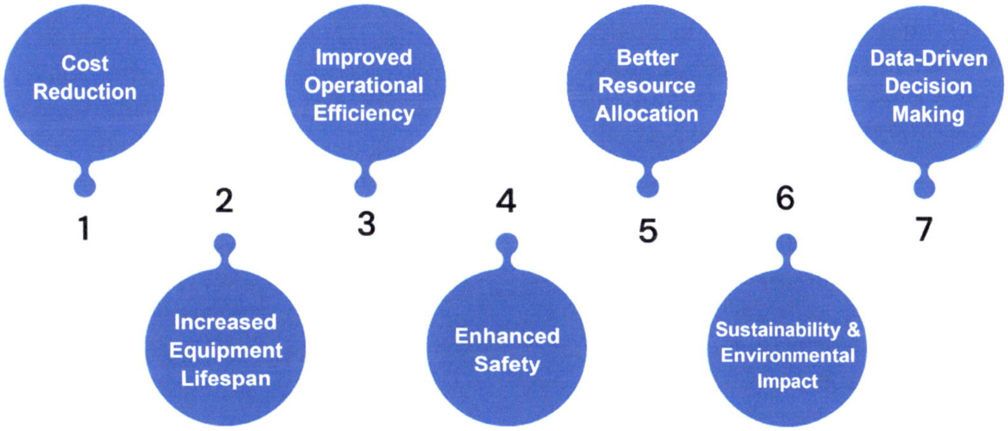

Figure 15.6. Benefits of predictive maintenance.

Source: Webflow. (2024). *Benefits of Predictive Maintenance*. https://assets-global.website-files.com/654c766f236ca78b2e2f6806/65cb6f1a24da4295db4a2f11_Benefits-of-Predictive-Maintenance.png.

15.3.3. Community Engagement Through Digital Platforms

Today, our world is more interconnected than ever before, and online platforms have moved into roles beyond mere online banter—acting as vibrant centers for community feedback, particularly when water care intersects with public health. A combination of smartphone apps and websites has emerged, allowing citizens to report concerns such as dubious water quality or obstacles to convenient access. Most often, this type of engagement makes individuals feel as if they have control as well as creates a cycle in which the local government rapidly listens to the concerns of the public and responds accordingly. As these platforms continue to be developed, you may even find some analytics added in to monitor who's being engaged and identify trouble points, enhancing community know-how and the effectiveness of water management in real-time. In addition to simply documenting issues, digital platforms explore far deeper into communal action. Research into telemedicine, for instance, indicates that remote consults have the power to assemble health, technology, and neighborhood expertise, which tends to have positive effects on communal health. It's not all about alarm systems—engagement with online forums tends to establish trust and openness, both of which are absolutely key for public health work. As hospitals and local governments collaborate increasingly, combining water quality inspections with web-based health education assists in painting a more holistic picture of well-being. Basically, making community work converge with digital technologies addresses current problems but also fosters forward-looking actions that make water and healthcare infrastructure strong. And then there's sustainability, a component oftentimes given a boost by digital citizen engagement strategies. Websites are now go-to places for collecting and exchanging key information on water usage, infrastructure health, and environmental consequences. You might refer to these centers as meeting grounds where policymakers, health professionals, and ordinary community members exchange knowledge and determine how to overcome challenges collectively. New health efforts, in the majority of instances, emphasize that integrating care of the environment into community health truly gains from multifaceted views. By harnessing technology for people's participation, the various stakeholders can initiate innovative solutions that construct systems prepared for climate crises, complementing broader green objectives, sort of reverberating what SDGs define.

15.4. Sustainable Water Management Practices

Water management for the future is not all about setting up a handful of smart sensors or running high-end data analytics, it's a blend of concepts addressing both water scarcity and quality issues that we have today and tomorrow. A combination of new technology, changes in policy, and engaging everyday people appears to be the secret. Intelligent sensors combined with data analytics assist in water systems identifying where resources are best utilized and reducing wastage. And then there are these virtual configurations—consider spaces like the metaverse—where decision-makers can simulate water scenarios to determine the outcome without any real environmental expense (Dwivedi et al., 2022). In the majority of instances, such thinking not only refines our decisions but also subtly guides communities toward adopting collective care for water resources. Industry 4.0 has entered the world of water as well, and that illustrates the potential for substantial green gains. Mobile technology, nanotechnology, and simulation software emerge as important actors in ensuring water delivery becomes both faster and more hygienic, in addition to maintaining ecological concerns in check. For instance, mobile phones have been quite useful in filling gaps in checking water quality in remote areas (Bai et al., 2020). Through combining a multi-situation decision-making strategy, one that relies on concepts borrowed from the United Nations SDGs, organizations can, in a broad sense, get the best tech mix to achieve their sustainability goals. Not only does this method enable them to comply with the law, but it also establishes a stronger protect against climate change-induced water problems. On top of everything else, public health is in the balance with how we treat and distribute water, it's as if clean water is a public well-being backbone. New methods of treating and distributing water need to keep equity in mind so that even poor areas aren't left out. Data tools, when properly applied, can highlight the areas that need the most attention, making targeted repairs more possible. Investment in bracing systems against unpredictable weather patterns is a necessity if we are to preserve our water supplies. And, of course, when governments, private enterprises, and community groups collaborate, they create an environment for an integrated approach that promotes environmentally friendly practices, which in turn raises overall community health. In most cases, this kind of multi-layered cooperation lays down the resilient groundwork we'll need to tackle water challenges in the times ahead.

15.4.1. Rainwater Harvesting Systems

Urbanization and climate change are turning the tables in terms of water management. Rainwater harvesting—literally, catching rain off roofs and other surfaces to use later, is gaining acceptance as a clever, sustainable solution (Figure 15.7). It reduces our reliance on conventional water sources and even chills the stormwater runoff problem. In many instances, it adds additional water storage with a bonus of energizing communities, which intelligent city master plans are increasingly relying on to gain efficiency in resources and reduce environmental footprints (Bouramdane, 2023).

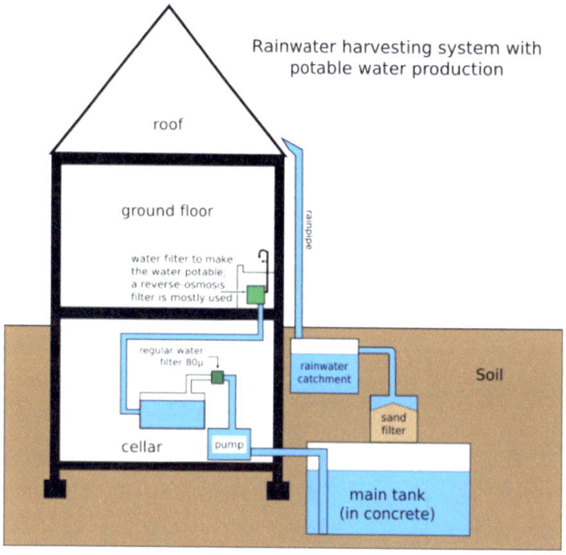

Figure 15.7. Rainwater-harvesting-system.

Source: https://commons.wikimedia.org/wiki/File:Rainwater_harvesting_system.svg

Digital solutions truly come into play to fine-tune the entire setup. Smart metering and analytics now monitor water levels, rain patterns, and system performance in real-time, providing timely glimpses of what is transpiring to both residents and urban planners. As a general rule, having all of these in-depth insights ensures the decisions are that much more informed and public engagement gets a boost, as well. With all this tech involved, common-or-garden difficulties become less hard to solve, even when now and again the tech does trail behind. If you fold everything together, though, adding rainwater systems into larger, climate-resilient configurations provides an excellent argument for sustainability. They lighten the burden on traditional supplies and even add a touch of green tech to urban landscapes. Most often, combining rainwater harvesting with other concepts, such as recycling graywater or reimagining urban gardens, produces a complete water strategy that addresses urgent needs and long-term sustainability. Urban planners are gradually recognizing that water management is not a stand-alone function; it is linked to comprehensive regional planning, bringing rainwater networks into the limelight as a primary adaptive strategy toward climate change and scarcity of resources (Bouramdane, 2023).

15.4.2. Greywater Recycling Initiatives

Water management has been an urgent issue lately, with local communities having less water to work with while giving more importance to the environment. Greywater recycling surfaces as a convenient means to recycle water from daily activities such as laundry washing, dishwashing, and showering (Figure 15.8).

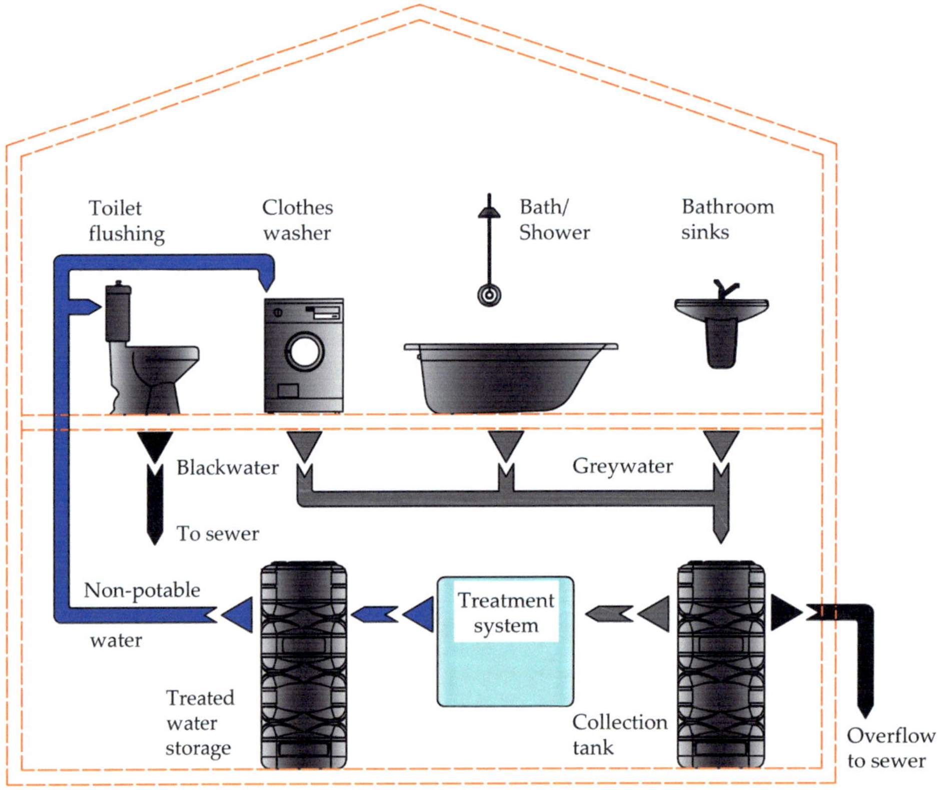

Figure 15.8. Greywater reuse.

Source: Rajski K, Englart S, Sohani A. Analysis of Greywater Recovery Systems in European Single-Family Buildings: Economic and Environmental Impacts. *Sustainability*. 2024; 16(12):4912. https://doi.org/10.3390/su16124912

Many times, employing this treated water provides much-needed relief from the continuous need for fresh water, particularly in urban locations where water may be scarce. The simple treatment process enables homes to recycle greywater for garden watering, toilet flushing, and other applications not involving potable water. This technique not only saves waste but also leads people toward a more conservationist lifestyle, which is quite significant in light of climate change and urbanization pressures. Obviously, implementing these methods requires pragmatic policies and education programs to ensure public health is protected. Technology remains key to driving greywater recycling ahead. Advanced devices such as purer filters and compact treatment systems ensure that reusing greywater does not sacrifice our health. Smart sensors and data-driven smart devices monitor water quality and usage, providing instant feedback, which frequently detects issues before they become ungovernable. Individuals discussing on local networks or via the internet sometimes state important safety points, once again strengthening community engagement within these systems. For the most part, combining ordinary technology with community attention makes greywater recycling a feasible solution that alleviates water scarcity and creates some resilience to climate ills. It's fascinating how technology and local expertise interact to make these systems functional. Meanwhile, policies must ensure they keep pace with all these thrilling advances if greywater recycling is to succeed. Strong regulations that address everything from its collection and treatment to its final application serve to establish residents' trust—collectively, sometimes a little bit of collegial cooperation really works. In general, aligning such fresh concepts with the current water infrastructure can iron out cost and installation humps; most professionals would attest that such integration is vital. Research, with continuous adjustments and trials, also influences standards that determine how pure the treated water must be. In a synthesis of viewpoints by policymakers, engineers, and even ordinary people, there is hope for having an open space where recycling greywater can take off. Overall, it's about ensuring that technology is not only saving water but is also married to initiatives that improve public health in a constantly evolving world.

15.4.3. Integrated Water Resource Management

Water resource planning isn't easy, it's a balancing act of supply, quality, demand, and the like. You just have to blend other ideas together if you want to stay in sync with development. Integrated water resource management (IWRM) attempts to satisfy everyone, balancing environmental concerns, financial concerns, and equity simultaneously. New advancements in water treatment benefit hugely by allowing it to be easier to monitor water systems. For instance, employing AI-based tools can adjust the way water is distributed and treated, and that consequently enhances access to clean water and even reduces health issues due to contamination. All this, viewed holistically, falls into larger objectives of community health and maintaining our environment well. New computer gadgets are disrupting the way water is managed today. Real-time data snapshots and analysis-fueled by IoT devices and smart sensors, all means people have a better grip on water quality and consumption almost in real-time, which in most instances makes rapid decision-making simpler. When a contamination problem arises, such devices can detect it quickly, and with a dash of clever geospatial mapping added to the mix, urban planning and policymaking become a little more agile. Climate change keeps throwing things at us—drought, flooding, and these electronic tools come in as a kind of early warning system. As communities begin to lean into these innovations, the combination of digital technology and water management becomes a primary means of increasing resource efficiency and making sure all people have access to safe water. It's starting to become apparent that water and energy are two pieces of the same sustainable development puzzle. The entire Water-Energy Nexus concept illustrates that these resources are relying on one another more than ever before, compelling us toward holistic plans for utilizing the two intelligently. Consider Smart Water Systems fueled by renewable energy—these assist in reducing the energy drain to treat and distribute water, something which reduces costs manifold but also provides our planet a much-needed relief. Obviously, getting these systems to work involves untangling a lot of regulatory and policy tangles that remain. In general, when government institutions, local organizations, and private firms get together, the system functions much more smoothly. Overall, investigating such convergent approaches is an important step toward enhancing water and energy security—a reality supported by research into urban water systems in countries such as Malawi (Munthali et al., 2025).

15.5. Climate-Resilient Water Systems

Water systems today encounter a battery of challenges, much of which is due to climate change constantly disrupting things. Communities, in most instances, are experimenting with new tech and clever solutions to enhance their resilience to unforeseen environmental changes (Figure 15.9). Novel tools and unorthodox practices blend with rule-of-thumb concepts, and tend to come together, that is, when a risk-based and nimble plan is implemented, systems become more responsive. Certain debates regarding government measures and proper monitoring even suggest that integrating innovative technology can result in better results, and harmonized regulations can enhance management efficacy as well as public health (Yürer et al., 2023).

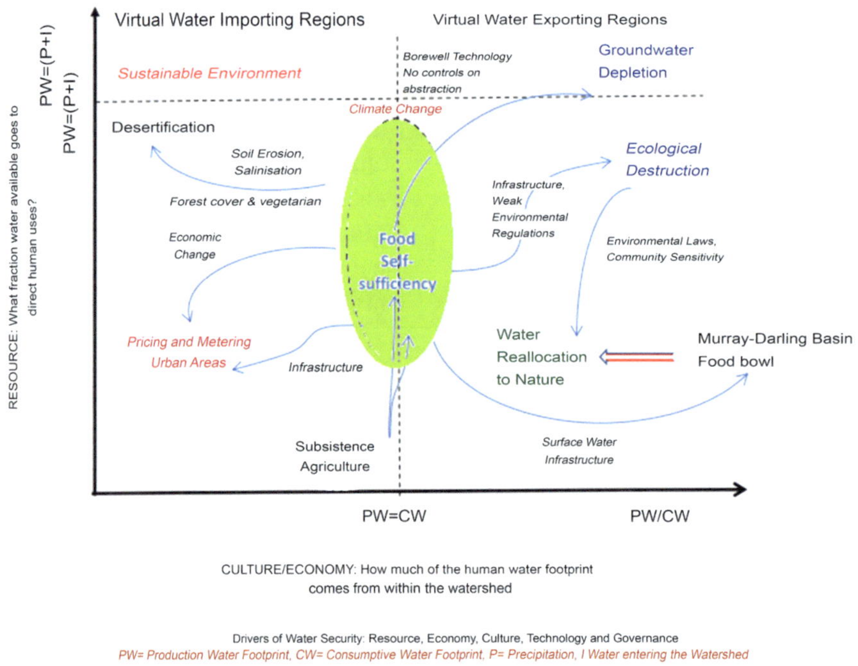

Figure 15.9. Climate-resilient water management.

Source: Abu Shoaib S, Rahman MM, Shalabi FI, Alshayeb AF, Shatnawi ZN. Climate Resilience and Environmental Sustainability: How to Integrate Dynamic Dimensions of Water Security Modeling. *Agriculture*. 2022; 12(2):303. https://doi.org/10.3390/agriculture12020303

Wastewater management also becomes relatively important in the pursuit of sustainable water networks. Recent research, for instance, has highlighted that revolutionary solutions in industrial wastewater management are desperately required. Technical and regulatory approaches would appear to need to come together at times, however, although difficulties such as outdated infrastructure and finite resources continue to stand in the way (Singh et al., 2023). As industries start embracing newer technologies—nanotechnology here, bioremediation there—the concept of a circular economy begins to take shape as the foundation of the long-term sustainability of water systems, although development can sometimes be rather patchy. Digital technology, and data analytics, are starting to enter the scene as yet another essential factor for water system reliability. When stakeholders leverage data-driven information, they are able to detect water-quality problems and act quickly, occasionally anticipating problems before they snowball. Emerging platforms and apps, in a quite cooperative manner, are engaging communities in the decision-making process; the efforts ultimately weave together an array of stakeholders that aid water systems change as climate issues change. Overall, the combination of cutting-edge technology with engaged community activism appears to hold out the prospect of a future of water delivery systems that can weather the storm of environmental transformation.

15.5.1. Adaptation Strategies for Extreme Weather

Climate change is driving communities into rougher weather than ever before. Sudden floods and heavy rains make old ways just not work any longer. Folks are now combining new technology with tried techniques to manage water problems—simple solutions such as rain gardens and permeable pavements ease flooding and increase underground water, kind of like a safety net. Technology like GIS enables municipalities to monitor water movement in real time, indicating where issues are likely to arise and triggering fast, targeted repairs. This do-it-yourself method not only takes care of our water, it also reduces local conversations about climate change. Developing more resilient infrastructure and engaging everyone, even if it gets a little complex at times, becomes crucial for weathering extreme weather, at least according to many contemporary plans for sustainability. When extreme weather hits, having adaptable water management plans is critical. Adaptive systems are typically viewed as an essential component of hardening water systems. Policymakers and water managers more and more rely on strategies that combine marketplace concepts with input from communities, even if the blend isn't necessarily ideal. Employing sophisticated data analysis, policymakers review historical climate patterns and attempt to forecast changes ahead, which in most instances enables them to better plan. Much debate regarding energy sustainability highlights that functioning systems must balance environmental, economic, social, and technical considerations simultaneously. Hearing from local communities regarding their own weaknesses makes such strategies even more specialized and efficient. A people-focused perspective, combined with the findings of academic study, typically is the prelude to regulations empowering locals and making water safe even when weather becomes erratic. New technologies, despite all their foibles, are realistically poised to support community resilience in the face of catastrophic events. Technological innovations in water treatment, supply, and stormwater management play a central role in addressing the short-term shock and long-term stress of climate change. The concept of 'smart' water systems—those that combine sensors with data analysis—sounds quite hip, as they can maximize distribution, detect leaks, monitor water quality, and even forecast changes in demand. Discussions of sustainability typically emphasize relying on renewable energy and incorporating storage systems as essential steps toward ensuring water continues to flow when the weather becomes unpredictable. Eventually, some collaboration between developers of technology, policymakers, and residents is necessary to implement these advancements well, setting solid ground for sustainable water management and enhancing climate resilience going forward.

15.5.2. Infrastructure Improvements for Flood Resilience

Floods today are affecting communities more severely and with greater frequency than in the past, so we absolutely need to redesign how buildings and infrastructure are constructed. Outdated techniques simply won't cut it, and most of the time it is found that combining new technology with real community knowledge works best. You can even discover that the installation of sensors and other IoT equipment on common buildings provides cities with an avenue to inspect water levels instantaneously. This type of instantaneous information not only assists in handling immediate threats but also defines long-term solutions and investment in important projects. In a way, these more intelligent systems can reduce economic losses and even assist in keeping water clean during floods, fitting very well into the general drive for sustainable water management and climate resilience experienced in today's debates (Allioui et al., 2023).

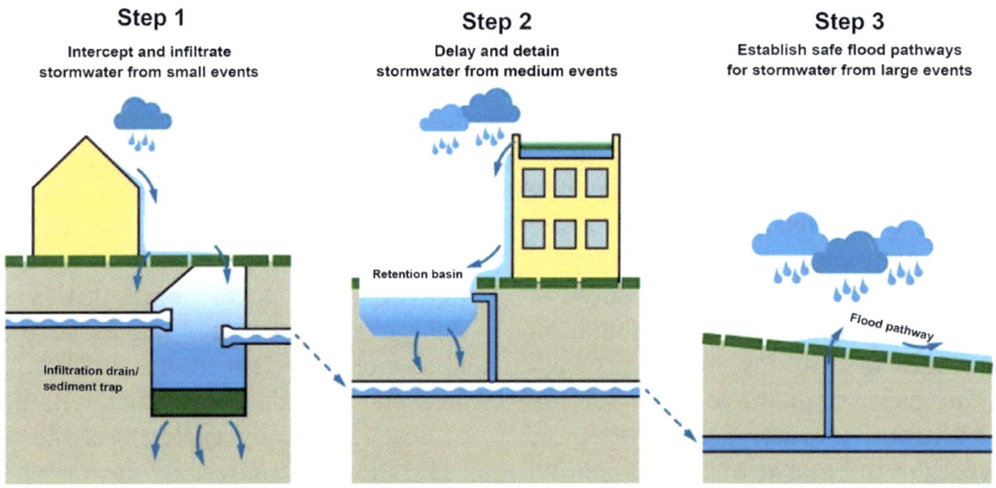

Figure 15.10. Innovative drainage solutions for flood-resilient communities.

Source: https://media.licdn.com/dms/image/v2/D5612AQEBq9l3l4EQ4w/article-cover_image-shrink_720_1280/article-cover_image-shrink_720_1280/0/1708325506768?e=2147483647&v=beta&t=0Qc728NjsXo46b7g8W7mjR9Kjp_dqR11xB-MkMWKCPg.

Meanwhile, relying on nature itself is also emerging as equally crucial. Consider green solutions such as restoring wetlands, establishing city parks, or even having surfaces that allow water to percolate through—each provides its own contribution toward lessening the burden of heavy runoff. These natural solutions are not only reducing flood risks; they're making life a little bit sweeter by forming places to sit and even fresher air to breathe. In general, when cities spend money on infrastructure that collaborates with nature, they balance urban expansion and environmental maintenance. With economic and healthcare crises piling up these days, investing in green initiatives is now almost necessary to have consistent, people-centered progress. In the future, flood-proofing's fate literally relies on engaging everyone. It is slowly becoming apparent that allowing local people to contribute to the planning process can reveal latent weaknesses that may be overlooked using command-control approaches. Occasionally, including tools such as community apps, which allow people to report flooding incidents as they occur, provides a new view and quicker communication. More often than not, combining digital tools with ground-level input constructs not only more effective technical solutions but also greater community ties (Figure 15.10). That mix of technology and community engagement is proving essential to designing systems that not only perform today against floods but are also prepared for tomorrow's emergencies (Allioui et al., 2023).

15.5.3. Policy Frameworks for Climate Adaptation

Climate change is driving individuals to find difficult policies that assist vulnerable regions to adapt ahead of time before disaster strikes. Certain communities, particularly those confronting water challenges, are threatened and require immediate interventions as well as sustained assistance. You may remember that climate catastrophes in 2018 alone cost approximately $131.7 billion, this massive number makes sense of the fact that water, health, and food are all complexed together (Fawzy et al., 2020). An intelligent strategy, therefore, needs to examine every community's specific vulnerabilities and adapt daily actions that both ward off short-term issues and enhance overall community health. New technology is disrupting the entire concept of climate adaptation, especially with regard to water management. Modern digital technology now provides us with instant feedback about water resources, so decisions can be made at the moment and a little more intelligently. Digital twins, essentially virtual representations of actual systems, allow experts to conduct rapid tests and simulate whether an idea could possibly work (Rasheed et al., 2020). These ingenious innovations not only iron out water delivery systems but also drive communities toward thinking ahead in ways that are both practical and, well, sort of inventive. Data wrangling and simulation wizardry combine strategies that address today's challenges while keeping an eye on what may be around the corner. States are racing against time to achieve the deadlines of the Paris Agreement, which amplifies the call for policies that include everyone in the picture. In most cases, a combination of all types of voices from government, residents, and private entities aid in formulating plans that make water management more adaptive and equitable. In most instances, policies that sort out who receives what resource can erode the gaps that hinder the most vulnerable people. By synergizing ideas from across the board, policymakers are usually able to ignite unexpectedly creative solutions that harden up water systems. In the end, combining a dash of tech know-how with proposals that hear what the locals want appears to be the best course of action, even if it occasionally involves tolerating a few rough edges in the process (Alumushaiti, 2024).

CLOSER LOOK

Advanced Technologies To End The Clean Water Crisis

Over the past few years, new technologies have provided for better clean water access and sanitation services for individuals all around the world. Of course, there is still much work that must be done to make sure everyone has access to clean water for a number of different reasons, but these water sanitation systems are a step in the right direction. Check out some of the technology delivering people clean water effectively.

1. **Solar-Powered Water Filtration:** Researchers at Princeton University created a Solar Absorber Gel that individuals can use on polluted water. The solar gel sucks up water at room temperature, but when it is heated, it shifts form and discharges the water. It has a second layer that is made of polydopamine, which is capable of converting the energy of the sun into heat. The third layer is alginate. When water runs through the gel, it gets purified by blocking pathogens, metals, and other molecules from passing through the water. It employs a passive gravity-driven filtering process. That is why, as a side effect, the device needs merely power from sunlight to function in the correct way. Furthermore, the device has the capability of providing clean water much faster compared to some other cutting-edge technologies for water purification.
2. **Desalination Systems:** The desalination technology is much in demand, particularly in nations in the Middle East region. During the process of desalination, salt from saltwater is removed to produce freshwater, which can be utilized for various purposes. Present methods of desalination are energy intensive, but developments in recent times have accounted for tremendous energy savings. One of the ways researchers and engineers have worked to reduce energy consumption is by enlarging the membranes used to desalinate water.4 Rather than utilizing 8-inch membranes, desalination facilities use 16-inch membranes with finer pores and four times the active surface area. This reduces the cost of operating and servicing the treatment plant and boosts the volume of water treated.
3. **Nanotechnology:** Nations may employ different nanotechnology-based water purification systems as efficient, affordable means of supplying water for those in need. Nanotechnology has the potential to remove waterborne contaminants effectively to make water more readily available. Simply put, it controls the water's atoms at a molecular level. Nanotechnology can aid in numerous water purification methods such as:

Desalination

- Filtration
- Remediation
- Water treatment

One of the most ubiquitous water purification methods in the nanotechnology field is the carbon nanotube (CNT). Filtration using CNT-based systems takes out organic, inorganic, and biological constituents from water in order to render it potable.

1. **Bioaugmentation to Treat Wastewater:** It is no secret that wastewater is a major contributor to water pollution. Not only can treating wastewater lead to synthetic fertilizer

for the farming sector but it can be converted into potable water to be consumed. Bioaugmentation is one of the most sought-after ways to treat wastewater. Scientists introduce a mixture of microbes to the liquid through this technology, which disintegrates and eliminates any impurities. Microorganisms usually include enzymes and some forms of harmless bacteria that break down contaminants such as oils or carbon substrates. Nevertheless, the researchers need to apply a step-by-step process when performing bioaugmentation — they need to remove the microorganisms safely after treating wastewater.

2. **Acoustic Nanotube Tech:** NASA originally came up with acoustic nanotube technology, which was an answer to treating and recycling wastewater in the International Space Station. The technology, though, has many uses here on Earth. In place of pressure pushing out impurities from water, the technology uses acoustics to force water through carbon nanotubes. Carbon nanotubes are embedded in a filter matrix, where water molecules go through and impurities remain behind. The acoustic system utilizes an oscillator circuit to produce an acoustic vibration, which stimulates the water molecules to de-bond and travel through the filter for cleansing.
3. **Photocatalytic Water Purification:** Another form of tech that assists in giving people water is photocatalytic water purification. The tech applies photocatalyst and ultraviolet to eliminate toxic chemicals and contaminants from water at high rates. Photocatalysis under mild conditions is an easy process and ranks as a green technology, which means it is both affordable and environmentally friendly.9 The process can take water and filter out things like pesticides, microbes, viruses, dyes, crude oil, and others.
4. **Automatic Variable Filtration:** Automatic variable filtration (AVF) is a water treatment technology that is simple yet efficient , it functions when a rising flow of influent is purified by a falling flow of filter media. The most notable advantage is the water doesn't need further filtration or washing. There are no moving parts or the need for electricity in the AVF process, making it an affordable and energy-efficient system. The technology applies to wastewater treatment and reclamation, drinking water in municipalities, and pre-treatment and desalination applications.

SUMMARY

New water treatment technologies and delivery methods hold real promise to meet our urgent requirement for a sustainable solution to water. Innovative innovations improve water quality and simplify access as well as address the issues of climate directly. Newer materials and certain alternative technologies enable various stakeholders to develop systems that are likely to care for both community health as well as for the environment. Governments, in large numbers, are now deploying supportive regulations—often accompanied by adaptive practices and global collaborations—to make sure that a combination of methods drives strong environmental goals. Flexible, inclusive regulatory systems (Yürer et al., 2023) cause efforts to hit the target by including what communities on the ground require while keeping nature's health in balance. Digital technology and big data sets have been a gigantic contributor to the change in access to water; their impact simply cannot be dismissed. People are increasingly looking to tech for on-the-spot monitoring and speedier decision-making, and this has proven to be a game-changer as far as public health is concerned. Sensor networks and big data align to detect water quality issues early, adding to our ability to efficiently manage resources. Yes, there are still some hiccups involved, such as ensuring devices communicate smoothly with each other and users remain interested all along. And, of course, ethical concerns understandably require a little extra thoughtfulness, keeping access equitable and the interests of the community in mind. For the most part, laying out a transparent map navigating through these intricacies and fostering interdisciplinary collaboration are important to increase water quality and access (Luo et al., 2023). Overall, the combination of innovation, regulation, and digital advancement provides a promising look toward the future of water management and public health. With climate challenges ongoing, developing climate-resilient systems and adaptive management plans becomes imperative flat-out. Interdisciplinary cooperation—where science and the art of well-designed policy converge, is the basis for emerging paradigms in water management that have the capacity to address the environmental challenges of today and tomorrow. Shared objectives and the exploitation of new technologies unlock the capacity to develop solutions that strengthen public health while caring for environmental integrity. This hybrid, hands-on model not only enhances water quality and supply but also charts a course for sustainable models that could influence other industries, thereby assisting society in growing slightly more resilient (Luo et al., 2023; Yürer et al., 2023).

Emerging technology is driving water purification in new and unexpected directions, particularly for those communities that so often fall through the cracks. Techniques such as membrane filtration and AOPs are emerging as credible alternatives that may treat water more effectively and reduce costs. They are doing more than just making water pure; they're also increasing access to the most marginalized people. Digital technology leaps in with real-time updates and simple data management—a huge plus when things must go more smoothly. In most instances, this translates into communities having cleaner drinking water and a little more protection against environmental change, all aligning with broader public health objectives. Digital technology makes a huge difference in delivering cleaner water to more individuals, even when the situation becomes somewhat complicated. Interconnected sensors and keen data analysis provide decision-makers opportunities to identify problems quickly and react on the fly. It's sort of neat how these technologies support green practices that largely align with the United Nations SDGs. Clever systems out on the IoT assist in constructing networks that address challenges such as water shortages and environmental pressure. With big data in their favor, communities can identify targeted areas in need of assistance, and it results in healthier lives and better community outcomes (María et al., 2021). If you consider the future of water, then climate resilience takes the prime spot. Climate change is serving up some pretty big curveballs in terms of water quantity and quality, so sustainable management is more crucial than ever. Concepts such as rainwater collection, greywater reuse, and modern drought tracking are environmentally friendly and cost-effective in your wallet. These adaptive strategies have an added advantage from modern digital solutions that facilitate planning and tracking water in a variety of environments. As societies begin to adopt these changes, they become more adept at managing climate fluctuations as well as boosting public health. Ultimately, combining new technology with wise, sustainable practices doesn't merely keep water around, it ensures it's used optimally, paving the way for a harder, more resilient world (Dwivedi et al., 2022).

KEY TERMS FROM THIS CHAPTER

Potable water	Rainwater harvesting	Compact treatment systems
Data analysis	Data processing	Drone technology
Environmental science	Environmental toxins	Fossil fuels
IoT equipment	Live data analysis	Minuscule organisms,
Mobile technology	Real-time feedback	Rudimentary monitoring
Smart water systems	Sophisticated filtration	Urbanization
Water levels	Water monitoring	

REFERENCES

1. Ababii, V. (2024). Banking supervision through SupTech. *Innovative Economics and Management.* DOI: https://doi.org/10.46361/2449-2604.11.2.2024.74-85. Retrieved from: https://www.semanticscholar.org/paper/01aca459c971ddbbcd1caf1b0d17977f18f24b86 (accessed on 14 May 2025).
2. Allioui, H., & Mourdi, Y. (2023). Exploring the full potentials of IoT for better financial growth and stability: A comprehensive survey. Sensors, 23, 8015. https://doi.org/10.3390/s23198015.
3. Amici, J., Asinari, P., Ayerbe, E., Barboux, P., Bayle-Guillemaud, P., Behm, R. J., Berecibar, M., et al. (2022). A roadmap for transforming research to invent the batteries of the future designed withi*n the European large scale research initiative* BATTERY 2030+. Advanced Energy Materials, 12. https://doi.org/10.1002/aenm.202102785.
4. Bai, C., Dallasega, P., Orzes, G., & Sarkis, J. (2020). Industry 4.0 technologies assessment: A sustainability perspective. International Journal of Production Economics, 229, 107776. https://doi.org/10.1016/j.ijpe.2020.107776.
5. Bouramdane, A. (2023). Optimal water management strategies: Paving the way for sustainability in smart cities. Smart Cities, *6, 2849–288*2. https://doi.org/10.3390/smartcities6050128.
6. Brambilla, A., Mangili, S., Dolcini, M., & Capolongo, S. (2024). Sustainability in the next generation hospital: Needs and requirements collection fr*om healthcare infrastructures supply chain stakeholders wi*th a One Health approach. The European Journal of Public Health, 34. https://www.semanticscholar.org/paper/984cb55340a3d8bc01a5d0cc1b21896859920e20 (accessed on 14 May 2025).
7. Conservation X Labs. (2015). Launching the grand challenges for ocean conservation. Working paper. https://core.ac.uk/download/84911929.pdf (accessed on 14 May 2025).
8. Dwivedi, *S. L., Lammerts Van Bueren,* E., Ceccarelli, S., Grando, S., Upadhyaya, H. D., & Ortíz, R. (2017). Diversifying food systems in the pursuit of sustainable food production and healthy diets. Tren*ds in Plant Science, 22, 842–856. https://doi.org/*10.1016/j.tplants.2017.06.011.
9. Dwivedi, Y. K., Hughes, L., Baabdullah, A. M., Ribeiro-Navarrete, S., Giannakis, M., Al-Debei, M. M., Dennehy, D., et al. (2022). Meta*verse beyond th*e hype: Multidisciplinary perspectives on emerging challenges, opportunities, and agenda for research, practice, and policy. International Journal of Information Management, 66, 102542. https://doi.org/10.1016/j.ijinfomgt.2022.102542.
10. Fawzy, S., Osman, A. I., Doran, J., & Rooney, D. W. (20*20). Strategies for mitigation of climate* change: A review. Environmental Chemistry Letters, 18, 2069–2094. https://doi.org/10.1007/s10311-020-01059-w.
11. Gielen, D., Boshell, F., Saygin, D., Bazilian, M., Wagner, N., & Gorini, R. (2019). The role of renewable energy in the global energy transformation. Energy Strategy Reviews, 24, 38–50. https:/*/doi.org/10.1016/j.esr.2019.0*1.006.
12. Hyde, K. D., Baldrián, P., Chen, Y., Chethana, K. W. T., de Hoog, S., Doilom, M., Gomes de Farias, A. R., et al. (2024). Current trends, limitations, and future research in fungi. Fungal Diversity, 125, 1–71. https://doi.org/10.1007/s13225-023-00532-5.
13. Ijiga, A. C., Peace, A. E., Idoko, P. I., Ezebuka, C. C., Harry, K. D., *Ukatu, I. E., & Agbo, D. O. (2024). Technological in*novations in mitigating winter health challenges in New York City,

USA. International Journal of Science and Research Archive, 11, 535–551. https://doi.org/10.30574/ijsra.2024.11.1.0078.

14. Kabeyi, M. J. B., & Olanrewaju, O. A. (2022). Sustainable energy transition for renewable and low carbon grid electricity generation and supply. Frontiers in Energy Research, 9. https://doi.org/10.3389/fenrg.2021.743114.

15. Kerna, N. A., Ngwu, D. C., Kadivi, K., Carsrud, N. V., Pruitt, K. D., Flores, J. V., Holets, H. M., Jomsky, B. M., Chawla, S., Azi, C. I., McKee, D., Nwokorie, U., Anderson II, J., Dugeri, J. L., Hammam, H. S. H., Chiedozie, O. B., Nnake, I., David, C. O., & Adadzi, J. (2024). Transformative Advancements in Diagnostic Imaging: Reducing Risks, Enhancing Accuracy, and Promoting Sustainability. European Journal of Medical and Health Research, 2(5), 153-172. https://doi.org/10.59324/ejmhr.2024.2(5).16 (accessed on 14 May 2025).

16. Luo, Y., Abidian, M. R., Ahn, J. H., Akinwande, D., Andrews, A. M., Antonietti, M., Bao, Z., et al. (2023). Technology roadmap for flexible sensors. ACS Nano, 17, 5211–5295. https://doi.org/10.1021/acsnano.2c12606.

17. Millar, R., Zgambo, C., & Pachalo, M. (2025). Water-energy nexus: A review of technological innovations for resource efficiency in urban water systems in Malawi. 10.59324/ejtas.2025.3(1).22 https://core.ac.uk/download/636358734.pdf (accessed on 14 May 2025).

18. Mohammad Ali Alumushaiti. (2024). Modernizing Saudi Arabia's Dates Export Market via Leveraging Technology for Sustainable Growth in the Global Economy. International Journal of Integrated Science and Technology, 2(2), 105–120. https://doi.org/10.59890/ijist.v2i2.1428 (accessed on 14 May 2025).

19. Mondéjar, M. E., Avtar, R., Baños Díaz, H. L., Dubey, R. K., Esteban, J., Gómez-Morales, A., Hallam, B., et al. (2021). Digitalization to achieve sustainable development goals: Steps toward a smart green planet. The Science of The Total Environment, 794, 148539. https://doi.org/10.1016/j.scitotenv.2021.148539.

20. Muthumanickam, D., Poongodi, C., Kumaraperumal, R., Pazhanivelan, S., & Ragunath, K. P. (2022). Smart farming: Internet of Things (IoT)-based sustainable agriculture. Agriculture, 12, 1745. https://doi.org/10.3390/agriculture12101745.

21. Noguchi, M. (2023). Prefabricated construction for sustainability and mass customization. Civil Engineering. https://doi.org/10.5772/intechopen.111181.

22. Oluseyi, S. O. (2025). Leveraging telemedicine to improve accessibility, affordability, and quality of care in rural communities. International Journal of Research Publication and Reviews. https://www.semanticscholar.org/paper/6b91e0a422da16c7934c8c9336901dbfcc0b4ae3 (accessed on 14 May 2025).

23. Panieri, E., Baralić, K., Đukić-Ćosić, D., Buha Djordjević, A., & Saso, L. (2022). PFAS molecules: A major concern for human health and the environment. Toxics, 10, 44. https://doi.org/10.3390/toxics10020044.

24. Rasheed, A., San, O., & Kvamsdal, T. (2020). Digital twin: Values, challenges, and enablers from a modeling perspective. IEEE Access, 8, 21980–22012. https://doi.org/10.1109/access.2020.2970143.

25. Rudoviča, V., Rotter, A., Gaudêncio, S. P., Novoveská, L., Akgül, F., Akslen-Hoel, L. K., Alexandrino, D. A. M., et al. (2021). Valorization of marine waste: Use of industrial by-products and beach

wrack towards the production of high added-value products. Frontiers in Marine Science, 8, 723333. https://doi.org/10.3389/fmars.2021.723333.

26. Sankari, M., Kamatchi, K. S., KarpuraDheepan, G. M., Sridevi, N., & Hemalatha, C. (2024). Innovations in irrigation: Water conser*vation in agriculture. https:*//doi.org/10.47716/978-93-92090-50-9.

27. Singh, B. J., Chakraborty, A., & Sehgal, R. (2023). A systematic review of industrial wastewater management: Evaluating challenges and enablers. Journal of Environmental Management, 348, 119230. https://doi.org/10.1016/j.jenvman.2023.119230.

28. Thürer, Y., Blanc, F., Ottimofiore, G., Castillo Morales, A., Amaral, M., Hernández, G., Karttunen, M. B., et al. *(2023). Better regulation for the green* transition. Public Governance Policy Papers. https://doi.org/10.1787/c91a04bc-en.

29. Tsan, Michael; Totapally, Swetha; Hailu, Michael; Addom, Benjamin K. 2019. The Digitalisation of African Agriculture Report 2018–2019. Wageni*ngen, The Netherlands: CTA/Dalbe*rg Advisers (accessed on 14 May 2025).

INDEX